FOOD BIOTECHNOLOGY

FOOD SCIENCE AND TECHNOLOGY

A Series of Monographs and Textbooks

Editors

STEVEN R. TANNENBAUM
Department of Nutrition and Food Science
Massachusetts Institute of Technology
Cambridge, Massachusetts

PIETER WALSTRA
Department of Food Science
Wageningen Agricultural University
Wageningen, The Netherlands

1. Flavor Research: Principles and Techniques, *R. Teranishi, I. Hornstein, P. Issenberg, and E. L. Wick (out of print)*
2. Principles of Enzymology for the Food Sciences, *John R. Whitaker*
3. Low-Temperature Preservation of Foods and Living Matter, *Owen R. Fennema, William D. Powrie, and Elmer H. Marth*
4. Principles of Food Science
   Part I: Food Chemistry, *edited by Owen R. Fennema*
   Part II: Physical Methods of Food Preservation, *Marcus Karel, Owen R. Fennema, and Daryl B. Lund*
5. Food Emulsions, *edited by Stig Friberg*
6. Nutritional and Safety Aspects of Food Processing, *edited by Steven R. Tannenbaum*
7. Flavor Research: Recent Advances, *edited by R. Teranishi, Robert A. Flath, and Hiroshi Sugisawa*
8. Computer-Aided Techniques in Food Technology, *edited by Israel Saguy*
9. Handbook of Tropical Foods, *edited by Harvey T. Chan*
10. Antimicrobials in Foods, *edited by Alfred Larry Branen and P. Michael Davidson*
11. Food Constituents and Food Residues: Their Chromatographic Determination, *edited by James F. Lawrence*
12. Aspartame: Physiology and Biochemistry, *edited by Lewis D. Stegink and L. J. Filer, Jr.*
13. Handbook of Vitamins: Nutritional, Biochemical, and Clinical Aspects, *edited by Lawrence J. Machlin*
14. Starch Conversion Technology, *edited by G. M. A. van Beynum and J. A. Roels*

15. Food Chemistry: Second Edition, Revised and Expanded, *edited by Owen R. Fennema*
16. Sensory Evaluation of Food: Statistical Methods and Procedures, *Michael O'Mahony*
17. Alternative Sweeteners, *edited by Lyn O'Brien Nabors and Robert C. Gelardi*
18. Citrus Fruits and Their Products: Analysis and Technology, *S. V. Ting and Russell L. Rouseff*
19. Engineering Properties of Foods, *edited by M. A. Rao and S. S. H. Rizvi*
20. Umami: A Basic Taste, *edited by Yojiro Kawamura and Morley R. Kare*
21. Food Biotechnology, *edited by Dietrich Knorr*

Other Volumes in Preparation

FOOD BIOTECHNOLOGY

edited by

Dietrich Knorr ed.

Biotechnology Group
Department of Food Science
University of Delaware
Newark, Delaware

MARCEL DEKKER, INC. NEW YORK AND BASEL

Library of Congress Cataloging-in-Publication Data

Food biotechnology.

(Food science and technology ; 21)
Includes bibliography and index.
1. Food industry and trade. 2. Biotechnology.
I. Knorr, Dietrich W. II. Series: Food science and technology (Marcel Dekker, Inc.) ; 21
TP370.5.F656 1987 664 86-24027
ISBN 0-8247-7578-3

MARCEL DEKKER, INC.
270 Madison Avenue, New York, New York 10016

Current printing (last digit):
10 9 8 7 6 5 4 3 2 1

PRINTED IN THE UNITED STATES OF AMERICA

To Fanny, Agnes, and Anna

Preface

The food-processing industry is the oldest and largest user of biotechnological processes (Knorr and Sinskey, 1985). Despite this fact, information on biotechnology as it relates to food production and processing is scattered throughout the publications of various scientific or technology-based disciplines. It is therefore difficult for the food scientist to obtain essential information in the field of "food biotechnology." It is the aim of this book to provide a more concentrated source of information on biotechnology as it relates to food production and processing.

Food biotechnology continues to grow in importance, and rapid developments are expected within the next few years. For example, the working committee on biotechnology of the German Gesellschaft für Chemisches Apparatewesen estimated that only 20% of the food products that will be available in 1990 were known in 1982 and that a major portion of them will be produced via biotechnology ("Biotechnologie 82", 1982). Furthermore, the production of secondary metabolites via plant tissue culture, until recently considered worthless if the product value was below $1000/kg, is now considered possible within a range of $20–25/kg (Sahai and Knuth, 1985).

Key areas of food biotechnology still in need of research have been identified by the United States food science and technology community (Liska and Marion, 1985). They include fundamental studies on the structure/function relationship of food materials and the cell physiology and biochemistry of agricultural raw materials; the improvement of enzymatic processing and food-grade microorganisms; and work on food safety and development of methods.

Future work in these research areas, along with recognition by sponsoring agencies and the food-processing industry that substantial efforts and long-range commitments are needed, will have a major impact on our food supply.

The idea for this book on food biotechnology was generated by a symposium, "Genetic Engineering in Food Production," presented at the 43rd Annual Meeting of the Institute of Food Technologists ("Genetic Engineering," 1984). It is organized in five main sections. Part One deals with the relationship between biotechnology, food production, food processing, and the nutritional quality of foods. Part Two consists of reviews on methods and processes in biotechnology, including analytical methods, fermentation processes and process control, cell culture processes, and immobilization methods. Part Three presents bioprocesses for the modification and conversion of raw material, and Part Four contains chapters on the production of food ingredients and processing aids via biotechnology. Part Five is devoted to regulatory and social aspects of food biotechnology.

As made apparent in Chapters 1, 2, 4, 7, and 8, there is still no generally accepted definition of biotechnology. However, the definition given by the European Federation on Biotechnology seems to be the most agreeable and most widely recognized. It defines biotechnology as the integrated use of biochemistry, microbiology, and engineering science to achieve the technological application of the capacities of microbes, cultured tissue cells, and parts thereof.

I am thankful to all the contributors and their commitment to this book, to Gerry Zuka for technical assistance, and to Marcel Dekker, Inc., especially to Diane Lange and Vickie Kearn, for the conversion of the raw material to a real book.

Dietrich Knorr

REFERENCES

Biotechnologie 82 (1982). Dechema Frankfurt, p. 96.

Genetic Engineering in Food Production (1984). *Food Technology* *38*(2):68-127.

Knorr D., and Sinskey, A. J. (1985). Biotechnology in Food Production and Processing. *Science* *229*:1224-1229.

Sahai O., and Knuth, M. (1985). Commercializing plant tissue culture processes: Economics, problems and prospects. *Biotechnology Progress* *1*:1-9.

Special Report (1985). America's Food Research: An Agenda for Action. *Food Technology* *39*(6):1R-44R.

Contributors

Carl A. Batt* Laboratory of Applied Microbiology, Department of Applied Biological Sciences, Massachusetts Institute of Technology, Cambridge, Massachusetts

Karl A. Bayer Department of Applied Microbiology, University of Agriculture, Vienna, Austria

Saumya Bhaduri Eastern Regional Research Center, U.S. Department of Agriculture, Philadelphia, Pennsylvania

Edward E. Bjurstrom Process Department, Advanced Technology Division, Fluor Technologies Inc., Irvine, California

Rudolf F. Bliem Cell Technology, Cambridge Life Sciences, Cambridge, England

Jeffrey Burkhardt† Department of Philosophy, University of Kentucky, Lexington, Kentucky

Lawrence Busch Department of Sociology, University of Kentucky, Lexington, Kentucky

Shing Chang Microbial Genetics, Cetus Corporation, Emeryville, California

---

Current affiliations:

*Institute of Food Science, Cornell University, Ithaca, New York
† Philosophical Studies in Agriculture and Natural Resources and Department of Philosophy, University of Florida, Gainesville, Florida

Lowell E. Coker The Hubinger Company, Subsidiary of H. J. Heinz Company, Keokuk, Iowa

David A. Evans DNA Plant Technology Corporation, Cinnaminson, New Jersey

David H. Gelfand Microbial Genetics, Cetus Corporation, Emeryville, California

Robert J. Griesbach Florist and Nursery Crops Laboratory, U.S. Department of Agriculture, Beltsville, Maryland

Norman F. Haard* Department of Biochemistry, Memorial University of Newfoundland, St. John's, Newfoundland, Canada

Frank E. Hammer Fermco Development Inc., Subsidiary of Finnsugar LTD, Elk Grove Village, Illinois

Michael Hansen† Department of Sociology, University of Kentucky, Lexington, Kentucky

Dallas G. Hoover Department of Food Science, University of Delaware, Newark, Delaware

Michael A. Innis Microbial Genetics, Cetus Corporation, Emeryville, California

Hermann W. D. Katinger Department of Applied Microbiology, University of Agriculture, Vienna, Austria

George G. Khachatourians Department of Applied Microbiology and Food Science, College of Agriculture, University of Saskatchewan, Saskatoon, Saskatchewan, Canada

John E. Kinsella Institute of Food Science, Cornell University, Ithaca, New York

Dietrich Knorr Biotechnology Group, Department of Food Science, University of Delaware, Newark, Delaware

Edward L. Korwek Law Firm of Keller and Heckman, Washington, D.C.

William B. Lacy Department of Sociology, University of Kentucky, Lexington, Kentucky

Alan R. McCurdy Department of Applied Microbiology and Food Science, College of Agriculture, University of Saskatchewan, Saskatoon, Saskatchewan, Canada

---

Current affiliations:
*Department of Food Science and Technology, Institute of Marine Resources, University of California - Davis, Davis, California
†Institute of Consumer Policy Research, Mt. Vernon, New York

James H. Meade Microbial Genetics, Cetus Corporation, Emeryville, California

Joop A. Roels Industrial Pharmaceutical Products Division, Gist-brocades nv, Delft, The Netherlands

Heinz Ruttloff Central Institute of Nutrition, Academy of Sciences of the GDR, Bergholz-Rehbrücke, German Democratic Republic

Don Scott Fermco Development Inc., Subsidiary of Finnsugar LTD, Elk Grove Village, Illinois

Sharon P. Shoemaker* Fermentation–Research and Development, Cetus Corporation, Emeryville, California

Benjamin K. Simpson Department of Biochemistry, Memorial University of Newfoundland, St. John's, Newfoundland, Canada

Anthony J. Sinskey Department of Applied Biological Sciences, Massachusetts Institute of Technology, Cambridge, Massachusetts

Thomas J. Szalkucki† Fermco Development Inc., Subsidiary of Finnsugar LTD, Elk Grove Village, Illinois

Rita A. Teutonico Department of Biology, University of Pennsylvania, Philadelphia, Pennsylvania

Henricus A. C. Thijssen‡ Research and Development, Gist-brocades nv, Delft, The Netherlands

K. Venkatasubramanian Business and Technical Development, H. J. Heinz Company, Pittsburgh, Pennsylvania, and Department of Chemical and Biochemical Engineering, Rutgers University, New Brunswick, New Jersey

Patricia M. Walsh Department of Food Science, University of Delaware, Newark, Delaware

Ming C. Wen Institute of Food Science, Cornell University, Ithaca, New York

Robert J. Whitaker Plant Secondary Products and Organelle Genetics, DNA Plant Technology Corporation, Cinnaminson, New Jersey

---

Current affiliations:
*Genencor, Inc., South San Francisco, California
†Finnsugar Biochemicals Inc., Subsidiary of Finnsugar LTD, Elk Grove Village, Illinois
‡Thijssen Process Engineering BV, Son, The Netherlands

Thomas J. White Research Department, Cetus Corporation, Emeryville, California

Ludger Witte Physikalische Messtechnik/Instrumentelle Analytik, Gesellschaft für Biotechnologische Forschung, Braunschweig, Federal Republic of Germany

Contents

Preface v
Contributors vii

Part One Biotechnology in Food Production and Processing

1 Biotechnology: Applications of Genetics to Food Production
George G. Khachatourians and Alan R. McCurdy 3
2 Impact of Biotechnology on the Food Industries
Joop A. Roels and Henricus A. C. Thijssen 21
3 Impact of Biotechnology on Food and Nutrition
Heinz Ruttloff 37
4 Impact of Biotechnology on the Nutritional Quality of Foods
Rita A. Teutonico 95

Part Two Methods and Processes in Biotechnology

5 Methods and Applications of Molecular Cloning
Saumya Bhaduri 139
6 Analytical Methods in the Structure Elucidation of Fermentation Products: Low Molecular Weight Compounds
Ludger Witte 163
7 Fermentation Systems and Processes
Edward E. Bjurstrom 193

8 Bioprocess Control
Karl A. Bayer 223
9 Animal Cell Culture Methods
Hermann W. D. Katinger and Rudolf F. Bliem 253
10 Methods in Plant Tissue Culture
Robert J. Griesbach 271
11 Immobilization of Microbial and Cultured Plant Cells
Dietrich Knorr 287

Part Three Modification and Bioconversion of Raw Materials

12 Technology for the Development of New Breeding Lines and Plant Varieties for the Food Industry
David A. Evans and Robert J. Whitaker 323
13 Single-Cell Protein: Production Modification and Utilization
Carl A. Batt and Anthony J. Sinskey 347
14 Functional Proteins from Yeast Nucleoprotein for Food Uses: Methods for Isolation
John E. Kinsella 363
15 Molecular Cloning of Carbohydrases for the Food Industry
James H. Meade, Thomas J. White, Sharon P. Shoemaker, David H. Gelfand, Shing Chang, and Michael A. Innis 393
16 Bioconversions: Enzyme Technology
Don Scott, Frank E. Hammer, and Thomas J. Szalkucki 413

Part Four Food Ingredients and Processing Aids from Biotechnological Processes

17 Corn Sweeteners
Lowell E. Coker and K. Venkatasubramanian 443
18 Plant Tissue Culture for Lipid Production
Ming C. Wen and John E. Kinsella 461
19 Cold-Adapted Enzymes from Fish
Benjamin K. Simpson and Norman F. Haard 495
20 Bacterial Starter Cultures
Patricia M. Walsh and Dallas G. Hoover 529

Part Five Regulatory and Social Aspects of Biotechnology

21 Regulatory Aspects of the Use of Modern Biotechnological Methods in the Food Industry
Edward L. Korwek 559

22 Biotechnology and Food: A Social Appraisal
Jeffrey Burkhardt, Lawrence Busch, William B. Lacy, and Michael Hansen 575

Index 601

ONE

Biotechnology in Food Production and Processing

1

Biotechnology: Applications of Genetics to Food Production

GEORGE G. KHACHATOURIANS and ALAN R. McCURDY / University of Saskatchewan, Saskatoon, Saskatchewan, Canada

INTRODUCTION

Between 1980 and 1984, biotechnology has generated an explosive evolution of technical literature and scientific results. In the area of agriculture and more specifically that portion which deals with food and beverage production, this is clearly evident. Although many of the highlights of biotechnology occurred in the area of genetic engineering related to human health care products, a cursory examination of the literature in the last 6 years has yielded more than 350 publications, a great proportion of which dealt with food production. This reflects how biotechnology is generating new questions and answers to some of the fundamental problems of food production. The reasons are primarily due to improvements in the production and transformation of materials used in the food and beverage industry which cannot be done through conventional technologies. To exemplify an area which is common to many food and beverage transformations and production, that is, the use of yeasts, it has been shown that there are current biotechnological capabilities in dealing with yeasts which were impossible just 10 years ago.

PATHWAYS OF BIOTECHNOLOGICAL DEVELOPMENT

The biotechnological research needs for production in the food and beverage industries of the future have been the subject of numerous recent articles (see *Science*, 1983; *Developments in Industrial*

Microbiology, 1983; *Food Technology*, 1984). To place these needs in proper perspective the major aspects of the subject are discussed below.

The discipline called biotechnology has been defined in several ways (Bull et al., 1982). We prefer the definition used by the Canadian Government Task Force on Biotechnology, which defines biotechnology as the utilization of the biological process, be it microbial, plant, or animal cells or their constituents, to provide goods and services (Biotechnology; A Development Plant for Canada, 1981). In order for biotechnology to develop there is a need for the contribution from various interdisciplinary sciences, such as biology, chemistry, engineering, mathematics, and physics. From the outgrowth of these bases, we see additional disciplines such as biochemistry, microbiology, and genetics as major players. The components which lead to the development of biotechnolgy as an industry can be defined by a pathway containing (1) techniques, (2) process applications, and (3) the products. The general techniques employed in current biotechnology include genetic engineering, the development of enzyme and enzyme systems, cell fusion, the culture and cultivation of plant cells, and process and system engineering, including the scale-up and computerization of these processes. There are a number of applications of these techniques, for example, dinitrogen fixation, which are entirely process oriented. Through symbiotic organisms this process relates to the applications of genetic engineering, enzymes, and cell-manipulative technologies to enhance the utilization and fixation of dinitrogen into plant cell proteins. Other areas of biotechnological process application include the utilization of cellulose, waste treatment, and the production of various food and beverages. In addition, the substances or products that are generated by the plants or animals with high product yields could include materials that are of high nutritional value or those which are unique in that they can be synthesized at will and in any geographical location. Indeed, we can see that the pathways of biotechnological development are scientifically complex and technologically interrelated. We need to accelerate the development in this area to encompass the contribution of biotechnology to food production. We need to recognize the pivotal role of the basic sciences and specifically that of genetics (Morris, 1981, 1983; Khachatourians and Haffie, 1985).

PRINCIPLES OF GENETICS

The scientific and commerical aspects of food production and development ultimately depend on the biotechnological principles that govern the experimental manipulation of genetics. The discipline of genetics has contributed significantly to modern biology as well as to the genesis of biotechnology. Thus many of the biotechnological realities that are presently commercialized have been in part made possible by the advances made in molecular genetics and gene manipulation. Ultimately the driving force for biotechnology to experimentally manipulate genetics will depend on the market opportunities in the area of food production. It is therefore pertinent to review the basic concept of genetics, the importance of gene expression and regulation, and finally the processes that are required in gene transaction.

Analysis of Heredity

The inheritance of genetic characters in most organisms resides in the DNA molecule or chromosome. It is organized into a genophore in bacteria and into a nucleus in eukaryotic cells. In the organelles found within cells there might be additional forms of DNA, such as those found in mitochondria. Here the organelle DNA contains the information necessary for additional functions required for the cell. The fundamental difference between the genetic organization of bacteria and that of higher organisms is that the eukaryotic cell is comprised of a number of chromosomes, each of which contains histones and specialized arrangements of the transcriptional units, termed introns and exons (Bainbridge, 1980; Stewart and Hunt, 1982). The unique configuration of the DNA which leads to its stability and chemical structure resides in the two complementary strands of DNA chains, which form the basis for the acquisition and inheritance of the genetics of each cell in nature. On the DNA, genes are found in prokaryotic and eukaryotic cells, which are organized from a simple to a fairly complex form, respectively. The nuclear material in the eukaryotic cells contains repeating units of DNA structurally organized in the form of chromatin. A high-resolution study of this material shows that the right-handed DNA superhelix contains several additional structural features. For example, there are sharp bends to allow for the interactions between the DNA and histones (Richmond et al., 1984).

The purpose of the genes is to encode for fundamental biological structures which give an organism a self-identity or expression. Genetic analysis examines these traits, permits the synthesis of gene products, and allows for the manipulation of such genes and hence their product. The ultimate goal, therefore, is to gather all the necessary information so as to understand and then be able to alter such organizations within the chromosome of an organism. In this context we know the genetic maps of several bacterial viruses, animal viruses, bacteria, yeasts, fungi, various invertebrates, and finally some vertebrate species, including some of the genes in primates and humans. The compilation of genetic maps prepared at the

National Institutes of Health (O'Brien, 1982) is an impressive collection showing the genetic linkage and DNA restriction enzyme mapping of several organisms. Such studies are important, as they provide the fundamental basis for the utilization of such knowledge in the biotechnology research industry.

Gene Expression and Regulation

From the experiments that were conducted in the early 1960s to those done today, we have a fairly clear understanding of the principles governing gene expression. The development of methods that were used to identify the steps involved in transcribing DNA into an RNA and translation into polypeptides is a milestone in the history of molecular biology. Orthodox genetic analysis revealed that genes were on DNA (see Davern, 1982) and the RNA made from one of the two strands, the "sense" strand, of the DNA. Current research indicates that the anti-"sense" RNA is capable of inhibiting gene expression in both eukaryotic and prokaryotic organisms.

To understand gene expression and regulation, it is important to detail some of the above points. DNA can be dissected into sequences involved in regulation and those involved in structural products, that is, proteins. The structural portions of genes could be dissected and fused to regulatory regions of other genes, giving rise to composite DNA structures where such cloned material can result in maximum expression. There are several examples of such experimental manipulations of genes from bacteria, yeast, plant cells, and animal cells (for a general reference, see Inouye, 1983, and references therein). (Knowledge in this area has reached the point where various genes coding for food production-related products such as hormones, seed storage proteins, regulatory proteins, and enzymes can be inserted, expressed, and amplified in any biological system) (Barton and Brill, 1983; Nagley et al., 1983, and references therein). The "central dogma" of one-gene, one-enzyme and one-gene, one-polypeptide, which was the foundation of the early concepts of molecular biology (Davern, 1982), is much better understood now. The control of inducible enzyme synthesis is governed by negative regulation, that is, the presence or absence of repressor molecules. The key aspect of a repressor molecule is to function by binding to the operator site on the DNA and prevent the RNA polymerase from synthesis of the corresponding message. The bacterial genes which relate to functions that are shared are found in an organization called operons. Operons are preceded by two sequences called operators and promoters. These are the signals to indicate the initiation of messenger RNA synthesis. In the 1960s repressors were isolated and identified (Gilbert and Müller-Hill, 1966; Ptashne, 1967) and currently the DNA sequences for many repressors are known. In addition to repressor control, some genes are regulated by a positive regulation of gene transcription. In these cases the regulation occurs through the presence of an intracellular regulator molecule, for example, cyclic adenosine monophosphate (cAMP) and a protein known as CAP, or cAMP-binding protein (Epstein et al., 1975; Simpson, 1980; McKay et al., 1982). The cAMP and CAP complexes bind to promoters to help activation of the operons which are under their control. The expression of some other bacterial operons involved in the synthesis of amino acids is also controlled by another process known as the attenuator. The attenuator was discovered by Yanofsky (1981) for the tryptophan biosynthetic operon in *Escherichia coli*. He found that the lead region of the tryptophan operon contained a number of sequences rich in a codon which relates to tryptophan. Thus, in addition to tryptophan repressor, the attenuation is responsible for a several-fold increase in the biosynthesis of the tryptophan by biosynthetic enzymes. Tryptophan starvation, for example, increases the biosynthesis of tryptophan by first removing the tryptophan-activated repressor, which results in a 70-fold increase in the transcription of this operon. By relieving the normal attenuation there is an additional 10-fold increase in the transcription of the operon. In total, one can see an expression increase 600- to 700-fold when the two systems are operating. In addition to the above, gene expression in bacteria is also under translational control by the presence of specific nucleotides responsible for ribosome binding. These sequences, which are named Shine–Dalgarno sequences, determine the efficiency of translation (Shine and Dalgarno, 1974; Gold et al., 1981).

In the eukaryotic organism the DNA is organized into a nucleosome which represents a complex of DNA molecules with chromatin or nucleoproteins. They appear to have a beaded structure when viewed with the electron microscope. The histone proteins fall into several categories or classes termed H1, H2a, H2b, H3 and H4. They come together to form the nucleosome complex. The current structure of the nucleosome core particle has been visualized at the 7Å resolution level to show that the right-handed B-DNA on the outside has several sharp bends and numerous interactions with octomeric units of histones (Richmond et al., 1984). These interactions often contain symmetries which allow for the regulation of gene expression. In contrast to the single RNA polymerase of the prokaryotic cells, in eukaryotic cells gene expression occurs by the successful employment of three RNA polymerases. These different RNA polymerases interact with different promoters to synthesize an RNA corresponding to each of these structures. Finally the eukaryotic RNA transcribed from the nucleus traverses the nuclear membrane, reaching the cytoplasm, where the translation and processing of such messengers take place (for details see Watson et al., 1983).

Genetic Manipulation: Mutants and Recombinant DNA

Organisms used in the production of food, feed, and fermentation are categorized under either the prokaryotes, such as bacteria, or eukaryotic organisms such as yeast, plant, and animal cells. The bulk of fermentation, metabolite synthesis, and production of enzymes, cofactors, vitamins, and other food ingredients used by industry is carried out by microorganisms. Selection and construction of mutants for the purpose of genetic and biochemical analysis has been a fundamental tool of genetic research. Classic examples of this are improvements in the production of antibiotics and amino acids through the selection of higher-yield mutants. In such cases simple blockage of the regulatory aspects of metabolite production has achieved overproduction of the end-products in the biosynthetic pathway. In terms of current potential, there are additional techniques which allow for a much more rapid attainment of the same end result. Thus the enhancement of specific genetic mutations, the isolation of mutants in ill-defined strains of yeast, and the specific insertion of sequences which would affect the regulation of biosynthesis in any gene sequence are some of the possibiliites (see Conde and Fink, 1976; Jimenez and Davis, 1980). While we know that such improvements are possible, the large-scale industrial utilization of some of these technologies has lagged. For example, the application of genetic mutations in agriculturally important plants for separation technology, improvement in flavor, and reduction of toxic or undesirable materials in the oil seed production is not too far from becoming a commercial reality (Chaleff, 1983), but the techniques are not yet in full commercial practice.

In addition to the selection and use of mutants, there are methods for creating recombinant DNA molecules and effecting recombination in vitro which could potentially affect the future of the food production industry.

In the early 1960s research revealed the sequence of various DNA molecules. At that time a group of enzymes known as restriction endonucleases was discovered. These restriction endonucleases have the ability to make specific breaks in unique regions of DNA molecules. The mapping of DNA by such enzymes led to a powerful new method for sequencing and delineating the structural and nonstructural regions of "genes" within a DNA molecule. Between then and now about 300 such restriction enzymes have been identified and the exact sequence of segments of DNA cut by such nucleases have also been deciphered. In addition, a series of specific techniques were developed which allowed for the creation and sequencing of such DNAs (Watson et al., 1983). The development of these methodologies allowed the synthesis of DNA pieces containing elements of DNA from diverse organisms. In fact, this was where the species barrier was traversed. In the early 1970s experiments carried out at the University of California and Stanford University produced a new species of DNA molecule. The end result of this genetic engineering, using recombinant DNA molecules, was the possibility of recombining the DNA of higher organisms into that of bacteria. However, the limits of the bacterial expression of such DNA and the concerns about the possible hazards of such research hindered progress in this area.

Isolation and Transfer of Cloned Genes

In most cases of genetic engineering, isolation of new cloned genes occurred through the insertion of foreign DNA into transposons, phages, and cosmids (Watson et al., 1983). These phages and transponsons contain an easily assayable marker whose expression indicates the presence of a cloned gene. As such, cloned DNAs could be found within any number of transformed microbial colonies using appropriate molecular manipulation. The procedures led to cloning genes that contained material from various gene libraries and vectors that were used for the isolation of specific eukaryotic cloned DNA. This was followed by more sophisticated radioisotopic and immunological screening of such genes and their expression in microbial organisms. The history of the transposon is interesting, as this phenomenon was first observed in the early 1950s by Barbara McKlintock. She observed that the control of the dormant genes in corn were often unstable. The instability could not be explained in terms of mutation, but in terms of controlling elements that could get in and out of genes and generate new phenotypes. Transposons, through their insertion and excision across the DNA, can create new features and mutations in many organisms. Such movable genetic elements have been found in fruit flies, yeasts, bacteria, and several plants. In bacteria an additional aspect of the transposable element is that it is often found in conjunction with conjugal plasmids responsible for the transfer of such genetic elements to appropriate recipient bacteria. Thus, through a process of conjugation or mating, transformation, and transduction, we find that some genetic information can be transmitted to another cell to generate a new character(s). In eukaryotic cells such as in yeasts and plants, not only these processes but also those of protoplasm fusion and hybridization are observed. In these cases, aside from genetic exchange, mixing of the cytoplasmic material of the two cells can occur.

Protoplast formation is generally simple in that it requires digestion of the cell wall and liberation of membranous structures called protoplasts. It can be carried out in species of potato, tomato, petunia, tobacco, various fungi, and yeasts. These protoplasts are brought into direct contact in the presence of polyethylene glycol and calcium ions. The product is a somatic cell hybrid protoplast containing genetic and cytoplasmic elements of the two parental protoplasts. They are subsequently grown to regenerate their cell walls and stable hybrids are formed. Many examples of intraspecific, interspecific, and intergeneric crosses using protoplasts can be found (Carlson et al., 1972; Constable, 1972; Wilson et al., 1982; Shepard et al., 1983). In the case of yeast cells, the resultant recombinants have shown improved characters, including that of fermentation or sporulation. Similar advances in the case of plants have been fairly slow and no commercially valuable hybrids have yet been produced asexually by the above process. Other achievements in this area are probably forthcoming, for example, the inclusion of DNA into liposomes and their uptake by higher eukaryotic cells, which is currently in the research stage. The successful outcome of these processes would be most valuable for the production of exotic food products.

Hybridization and fusion of yeasts is industrially important because in most cases there is a lack of mating-proficient strains and, more importantly, of those that have defined ploidy and genetic characters. As such, the cryophilic killer character in wine yeasts were successfully bred by Hara et al. in 1981. Hybridization is particularly valuable in the transfer of genetic traits that are controlled by a number of linked genes. This technique has been successfully employed by Steward et al. (1980) to construct an isogenic series of triploid yeasts in order to examine the gene dosage effect on maltose–maltotriose metabolism. Additionally, rare mating techniques have been developed by Spencer and Spencer (1977, 1983), allowing for the hybridization of commercially important yeast strains on which there was only sparse genetic information. Indeed, this protocol was used by Young (1981) to construct a killer brewing yeast.

GENETIC APPLICATIONS TO BIOTECHNOLOGY: FOOD PRODUCTION AS A SYSTEM

The wide variety of genetic principles described above can be applied to the production of food and beverages. Genetics can be used to enhance and change the quantity and quality of ingredients that are used in human and animal food and feed systems. This can be done by alterations in the material used for obtaining substances from plants and animals or the production of chemicals or pharmacological ingredients. Such items can also be changed to provide higher-value material or more readily utilizable materials for the food and chemical industry. We will give a basic overview of the possibilities and present a few biotechnological examples that illustrate this point. There are other chapters in the book which provide a more complete review and presentation of specific examples of the utilization of biotechnology relating directly to food production technologies.

Several aspects of biotechnology relating to food production were discussed above. This section emphasizes the link that exists between genetics and biotechnology and discusses how this link can be exploited for future food production developments.

Genomic Banks and Libraries

To make greater use of biotechnology, the food industry must make profitable use of current genetic activity such as recombinant DNA technology, gene transfer technology, and gene expression and regulation. These activities must eventually translate to lower cost and higher yields so that the manufacture of these substances will become dramatically cost effective when compared to conventional systems. Toward this end, the next step should be to collect genomic banks and libraries for all organisms which are important in the food production industry.

Until recently, production of food through conventional technologies has, in general, been sufficient in developed countries. However, trends indicate that the continuous expansion of both the population and world food markets will require a different strategy. For example, presently most of the world protein and food is provided by animals and plants. It is estimated that the need for fortifying animal feeds by amino acids for nutritional improvement or enhancement will continue. It is conceivable that at some future point this would be a much wider requirement for the food production system. To accomplish this we would need genomic banks for the synthesis of various amino acids, vitamins, peptide hormones, and nucleotides, which are essential to the enhancement of the nutritional value of food. Thus the marriage of recombinant DNA to the production of essential amino acids and other ingredients to generate new products requires the acquisition and maintenance of specialized genomic banks. Present genomic banks are few and primarily derived from microorganisms and, in some instances, higher eukaryotes. However, we need to have such banks from various fungi, yeasts, and animals. Various laboratories have made moves to collect and generate such genomic banks and libraries (Williams, 1981). The availability of such banks would facilitate the applications of biotechnology to the food and beverage industry.

Cloned Natural Genes

The impact of enzymes involved in the biosynthesis or biodegradation of various substrates is staggering. There are some exciting possibilities for increasing either enzyme activities, allosteric properties, or enzyme yields through mutations and genetic engineering. For example, examination of a number of natural and mutant enzymes and isoenzymes indicates that some enzymes function better than others for a specific enzymatic change of a substrate to its corresponding product. As such it is important that natural "genes" of such enzymes be identified and separated. For example, to enhance the kinetics of an enzymatic process one may wish to use an enzyme from a thermophilic or a psychrophilic organism to convert substrates to products at corresponding temperatures. Thus coupling of the natural genetic information with that obtained through biotechnology (e.g., gene machines and recombinant DNA technologies) could replace the "natural" genes of an organism to achieve new applications. It is imperative that we understand gene products in functional and molecular terms and that we secure cloned DNA for these gene products (see Davies, 1982) from a large number of species. At present, most of the species that have been analyzed have special applications in the areas of human and animal pharmaceuticals. Soon this list should extend to include items relating to the area of food production.

Enzyme Engineering

Most of our information about the biological conversion of various substrates to products or their transformation to newer products comes from the study of enzymes. The use of enzymes in terms of both traditional and immobilized states requires the isolation of natural enzymes which, under a number of physical conditions, can carry out the changes required for substrate transformation. Enzymes, which are in general proteins containing amino acids and having various physical constraints such as folding and structural features, are amenable to other additional changes. These include changes in the native structure, thermal and cryodenaturation, and inactivation. Being biological catalysts, enzymes are made of 100–1000 amino acid residues linked together to give a specific structure and function. The physical requirements of enzyme action are those of pH, temperature, and other cofactors to allow the catalytic activity to proceed. Each enzyme contains an active site and cofactor-binding sites which activate the enzymes for a specific purpose. Through the process of in vitro genetic engineering and computer modeling one can therefore synthesize enzymes containing altered recognition specificity, active center(s), and improved enzymatic action (Ulmer, 1983). Thus there are several enzyme engineering techniques that can be applied to food production (Wasserman, 1984; White et al., 1984). The successful adaptation of these technologies remains in the distant future because of the costs of manufacturing synthetic genes and their products, the examination of the stability and status of the products and the conversion efficiency of such enzymes. Nonetheless, the possibilities are real and could revolutionize the food processing industry.

The Concept of Organismic Barriers

From the above discussions, it is clear that the scientific data indicate unlimited possibilities for biotechnology and genetics to interact and to be of particular service to the food production industry. One of the greatest difficulties in genetics has been our inability to cross desired genetic characters from one species to another in nature. This impedes our ability to achieve the goal of value-added food products. In the final analysis, it would be desirable to have methodologies of cell fusion, spheroplast and protoplast formation, microencapsulation, and the transfer of such genetic information to a system(s) that provides the material required for future food production. While the remarkable process of the "green revolution" has served to quickly provide food and feed for most of the world population, it is a limiting step. The greater food production requirements in the last two decades in combination with unfavorable environmental conditions require a new examination of what can be done when environmental conditions, the soil, and its nutrient supply and utilization do not match consumer demands. In this regard the fate of such agricultural changes depends on the successful employment of biotechnology to cross the organismic barriers through specialized genetic engineering. A number of methodologies would aid crop improvement as well as fermentation products such as single-cell proteins (Litchfield, 1983; Batt and Sinskey, 1984) for food production. Recent evidence shows that Ti plasmid genes of *Agrobacterium tumefaciens* can be expressed in monocotyledonous plants (Hooykaas-Van Slogteren et al., 1984), suggesting the types of possibilities that exist in edible plants. However, the potential of emerging biotechnological methods to increase the availability of new organisms which contain genetic material from yet other species would considerably enhance the possibility of meeting the expectations of food production and demand in future years.

Biotechnological research and the application of genetics would have the greatest impact in the Third World countries and regions of the globe where tolerance to salt or cold temperatures is a disadvantage to plants. The transformation of various simple carbohydrates or substrates to alternate proteins, food, and feed has the greatest potential. Thus, when we examine the aspects of biotechnology in relation to world food supplies and Third World agriculture and food production, we see that genetic engineering will probably be the primary mechanism for achieving these goals. For further discussion the reader is referred to articles by Brady (1982) and Swaminathan (1982).

Future Trends and Perspectives in Food Production

Food production and processing have placed an emphasis on traditional processing procedures and techniques. These methods have included canning, freezing, dehydration, and the incorporation of antimicrobial agents. The major emphasis of the processing was to preserve food and thus make it available to the marketing system and consumers over longer periods. From these basic methods of preservation food processing grew into areas of new product development and the reformulation of traditional products. This growth in the food processing area has resulted in such a wide variety of available foods that the average supermarket contains some 8000 food items (Labuza and Erdman, 1984). The genetic aspects of biotechnology are having a great impact in all areas of food processing, from raw material production to new processing aids and food additives that enable the food processor to improve the shelf life, acceptability, and nutritive value of foods.

Genetic alterations of plant products to the benefit of the food industry have been the area of the most obvious impact of genetics on food processing. Every aspect of plant production, including augmentation of conventional plant breeding, new plant varieties, pesticide screening, herbicide resistance, growth regulators, and increased dinitrogen fixation, can be manipulated by biotechnology. The genetic techniques utilized to accomplish these improvements in plant production have been tissue culture, recombinant DNA and genetic transformation, protoplast fusion, as well as somaclonal and gametoclonal variation (Kidd, 1984; Sharp et al., 1984; Morris, 1983; Teutonico and Knorr, 1984). The applications of these techniques can be found in the above-named sources, along with Chapter 10 of this book.

Unlike the use of animal growth hormones, physiological aspects of animal production factors such as feed efficiency, fertility, and meat quality and quantity have not been as greatly influenced by genetic manipulation. This is probably because many traits have not yet been genetically characterized (Haas, 1984) and the public has raised objections to gene transfer experiments in animals (Beardsley, 1984). On the other hand, animal tissue culture methods (see Chap. 9) have made significant progress and should potentiate biotechnological use for future food production.

Modern food processing requires the use of several food processing aids. These include preservatives, antioxidants, sequestrants, surfactants, stabilizers, bleaching and maturing agents, colors, sweeteners, nutrient supplements, and flavoring compounds (Luckey, 1972). As an example, Glicksman (1969) lists 21 functions of plant and microbially produced gums in food systems. Many gums utilized by the food industry are seed extracts from plants native to underdeveloped countries, and, as a result, the reliability of supply has been erratic. Many new gums utilized by the food industry can be produced by microorganisms, and thus the production of these gums lends itself nicely to productivity enhancement by genetic engineering. Examples of gums produced by these newer, more reliable techniques are xanthan (Glicksman, 1982) and gellan (Hannigan, 1983).

Flavorings are added to new food products for consumer appeal. The flavoring compounds can often be produced in fermentation processes with the aid of genetic alterations. The reader is referred to reviews by Morris (1983) and Haas (1984).

Enzymes produced by either plants or microorganisms have many uses in the food industry. One of the most novel uses is the utilization of immobilized enzymes to monitor final product quality and microbiological safety (Dunnill, 1984). The production of rennin by recombinant DNA techniques (Anonymous, 1984a) and the availability of glucose isomerase (Anonymous, 1984b) are but two of the most recent examples of these new techniques at work in the food industry.

CONCLUSIONS

In this chapter we have attempted to define the pathways of biotechnological development and the role of one of the basic sciences, genetics, in the application of biotechnology to food production. We find that a number of major breakthroughs to enhance the many facets of food production industries are possible. Almost all of the problems of food production are at present amenable to biotechnological changes. For example, the isolation of mutants would permit better fermentation or the elimination of undesirable characters. On the other hand, genetic engineering applied with ingenuity would be useful in devising new organisms which would carry out additional biosynthetic or biodegradative processes integral to food production.

Food production as an industry also creates special challenges for biotechnology and genetics as a scientific endeavor. Genetic engineering and the commercial production of single-cell proteins are now commercially possible as a result of major scientific breakthroughs (see Chap. 13). Genetics in baking, brewing, wine making, and the production of microbial polysaccharides, enzymes, sweeteners, flavors, and fragrances should be a great challenge to many microbiologists, geneticists, and biotechnologists.

There is a question as to whether the scientific community is willing to accept the challenges presented by these new technologies. If they are ready, are the resources going to be made available that are needed for the research and development required to bring these new products to commercial reality?

At the time of this writing it is already clear that biotechnological applications to food production are a reality. Public support in terms of economic, legal, and social comprehension are obviously needed (Cape, 1984). Among the limiting factors are the funding and incentive necessary to undertake this key endeavor. This would, through the provision of food and healthy life-styles, continue to make this planet inhabitable, not only in geographically well-suited areas but also in areas that are currently in significant need of food and health care.

ACKNOWLEDGMENTS

We are grateful to Jean Oliver for typing this manuscript. Special thanks are due to J. V. Cross and L. Khachatourians, who contributed to the ideas and proofing of the manuscript. Biotechnological work in our laboratories was supported by The Natural Sciences and Engineering Research Council of Canada and The Saskatchewan Agricultural Research Fund.

REFERENCES

Anonymous (1984a). Gene splicing applied to cheese production. *Chem. Eng. News. 62*:6.

Anonymous (1984b). HFCS—production enzyme. *Food Eng. 56*:56.

Bainbridge, B. W. (1980). *Genetics of Microbes*, Wiley, New York, pp. 1–194.

Barton, K. A. and Brill, W. J. (1983). Prospects in plant genetic engineering. *Science 219*:671–676.

Batt, C. A. and Sinskey, A. J. (1984). Use of biotechnology in the production of single–cell protein. *Food Technol. 38*:108–111.

Beardsley, T. (1984). Rifkin strikes against gene transfer experiments. *Nature 311*:495.

Biotechnology; A Development Plant for Canada (1981): A Report of the Task Force on Biotechnology to the Minister of State for Science and Technology, Department of Supply and Services, Government of Canada, Ottawa, Ontario, p. 50.

Brady, N. C. (1982). Chemistry and world food supply. *Science 218*:847–853.

Bull, A. T., Holt, G., and Lilly, M. D. (1982). *Biotechnology: International Trends and Perspectives.* Organization for Economic Cooperation and Development (OECD), Paris, France, p. 84.

Cape, R. E. (1984). On deserving awe and envy. *Biotechnology 10*:912.

Carlson, P. S., Smith, H. H., and Deering, R. (1972). Parasexual interspecific plant hybridization. *Proc. Nat. Acad. Sci. U.S.A. 74*:5109–5112.

Chaleff, R. S. (1983). Isolation of agronomically useful mutants from plant cell cultures. *Science 219*:676–682.

Conde, J. and Fink, G. R. (1976). A mutant *Saccharomyces cerevisiae* defective for nuclear fusion. *Proc. Nat. Acad. Sci. U.S.A. 73*:3651–3655.

Constable, F. (1972). Somatic hybridization in higher plants. *In Vitro 12*:743–748.

Davern, C. J. (1982). *Genetics, Readings from Scientific American,* Freeman, San Francisco, pp. 1–331.

Davies, K. E. (1982). A comprehensive list of cloned eukaryotic genes. In *Genetic Engineering* (R. Williams ed.). Academic Press, New York, pp. 143–173.

Dunnill, P. (1984). Biotechnology and the British industry. *Chem. Ind. 2*:470–475.

Epstein, W., Rothman, G. B., and Hesse, J. (1975). Adenosine 3':5'–cyclic monophosphate as the mediator of catabolite repression in *E. coli. Proc. Nat. Acad. Sci. U.S.A. 72*:2300–2304.

Food Technology (1984). *Overview: Genetic Engineering in Food Production, Food Technol. 38*:69–127.

Gilbert, W., and Müller-Hill, B. (1966). Isolation of the *lac* repressor. *Proc. Nat. Acad. Sci. U.S.A. 56*:1891–1898.

Glicksman, M. (1969). *Gum Technology in the Food Industry,* Academic, New York.

Glicksman, M. (1982). Food applications of gums. In *Food Carbohydrates* (D. R. Linebeck and G. E. Inglett, eds.), AVI, Westport, Conn., pp. 270–295.

Gold, L., Prinbow, D., Schneider, T., Shinedling, S., Singer, B. S., and Stormo, G. (1981). Translational initiation in prokaryotics. *Ann. Rev. Microbiol. 35*:365–403.

Haas, M. T. (1984). Methods and applications of genetic engineering. *Food Technol. 38*:69–77.

Hannigan, K., (1983). Fermentation yields a new gum. *Food Eng. 55*:52–53.

Hara, S., Iimura, Y., Oyama, H., Kozeki, T., Kitano, K., and Otsuka, K. (1981). The breeding of cryophilic killer wine yeasts. *Agric. Biol. Chem. 45*:1327–1334.

Hooykaas-Van Slogteren, G. M. S., Hooykaas, P. J. J., and Schilperoort, R. A. (1984). Expression of triplasmid genes in monocotyledonos plants infected with *Agrobacterium tumefaciens. Nature 311*:763–764.

Inouye, M. (ed.) (1983). *Experimental Manipulation of Gene Expression*, Academic, New York, p. 328.

Jiminez, A. and Davis, J. (1980). Expression of a transposable antibiotic resistance element in *Saccharomyces cerevisiae. Nature 289*:33–37.

Kidd, G. N. (1984). Agricultural and food production. *Brew. Dig. 59*:14–20.

Khachatourians, G. G. and Haffie, T. L. (1985). Biotechnology: Applications to genetics. In *Biotechnology Handbook* (P. Cheremisinoff and R. P. Ouellette, eds.), Technomic, Lancaster, Mich., pp. 242–249.

Labuza, T. P. and Erdman, J. W. (1984). *Food Science and Nutritional Health*, West, Minn.

Litchfield, J. H. (1983). Single-cell proteins. *Science 219*: 740–746.

Luckey, T. D. (1972). Introduction. In *Handbook of Food Additives* (T. E. Furia, ed.), CRC Press, Cleveland, Ohio.

McKay, D. B., Weber, I. T., and Steitz, T. A. (1982). Structure of catabolite gene activator protein at 2.9Å resolution: Incorporation of amino acid sequence and interaction with cyclic-AMP. *J. Biol. Chem. 257*:9518–9524.

Morris, C. E. (1981). Genetic engineering: Its impact on the food industry. *Food Eng. 53*:57–69.

Morris, C. E. (1983). Developments in genetic engineering. *Food Eng.* 55:18–21.

Nagley, P., Linnane, A. W., Peacock, W. J., and Pateman, J. A. (1983). *Manipulation and Expression of Genes in Eukaryotes*, Academic, New York, p. 416.

O'Brien, S. J. (1982). *Genetic Maps. A Compilation of Linkage and Restriction Maps of Genetically Studied Organisms*, Vol. 2, National Institutes of Health, Frederick, Md., pp. 1–400.

Ptashne, M. (1967). Isolation of the λ-phage repressor. *Proc. Nat. Acad. Sci. U.S.A. 57*:306-313.

Richmond, T. J., Finch, J. T., Rushton, B., Rhodes, D., and Klug, A. (1984). Structure of the nucleosome core particle at the 7Å resolution. *Nature 311*:532–537.

Science (1983). *Biotechnology. Science 219*:609–746.

Sharp. W. R., Evans, D. A., and Ammirato, P. U. (1984). Plant genetic engineering: Designing crops to meet food industry specifications. *Food Technol. 38*:112–119.

Shepard, J. F., Bidney, D., Barsby, T., and Kemble, R. (1983). Genetic transfer in plants through interspecific protoplast fusion. *Science 219*:683–688.

Shine, J. and Dalgarno, L. (1974). The 3'-terminal sequence of *E. coli* 16S ribosomal RNA: Complementarity to nonsense triplets and ribosome binding sites. *Proc. Nat. Acad. Sci. U.S.A. 71*: 1342–1346.

Simpson, R. B. (1980). Interaction of the cAMP receptor protein with the *lac* promoter. *Nucl. Acid Res. 8*:759–766.

Society of Industrial Microbiology (1983). *Developments in Industrial Microbiology 24*:71–162.

Spencer, J. F. T. and Spencer, D. M. (1977). Hybridization of non-sporulating and weakly sporulating strains of brewer's and distiller's yeast. *J. Inst. Brew. 83*:287–289.

Spencer, J. F. T. and Spencer, D. M. (1983). Genetic improvement of industrial yeasts. *Annu. Rev. Microbiol. 37*:121–142.

Stewart, A. D. and Hunt, D. M. (1982). *The Genetic Basis of Development*, Wiley, New York, pp. 1–221.

Stewart, G. G., Russell, I., and Panchal, P. (1980). The genetic manipulation of industrial yeast strains. In *Current Developments in Yeast Research: Advances in Biotechnology, Proceedings of the Fifth International Yeast Symposium* (G. G. Stewart and I. Russell, eds.), Pergamon, Willowdale, Ontario, pp. 17–24.

Swaminathan, M. S. (1982). Biotechnology research and Third World agriculture. *Science 218*:967–972.

Teutonico, R. and Knorr, D. (1984). Plant tissue culture: Food applications and the potential reduction of nutritional stress factors. *Food Technol. 38*:120–127.

Ulmer, K. M. (1983). Protein engineering. *Science 219*:666–671.

Wasserman, B. C. (1984). Thermostable enzyme production. *Food Technol. 38*:78–89.

Watson, J. D., Tooze, J. and Kurtz, D. T. (1983). *Recombinant DNA: A Short Course*, Freeman, New York, p. 260.

White, T. J., Meade, J. H., Shoemaker, S. P., Koths, K. E., and Innis, M. A. (1984). Enzyme cloning for the food fermentation industry. *Food Technol. 38*:90-98.

Williams, R. (ed.) (1981). *Genetic Engineering*, Vols. 1–3, Academic, New York.

Wilson, J. J., Khachatourians, G. G., and Ingledew, W. M. (1982). Protoplast fusion in the yeast *Schwanniomyces alluvius*. *Mol. Gen. Genet. 186*:95–100.

Yanofsky, C. (1981). Attenuation in the control of expression of bacterial operons. *Nature 289*:751–758.

Young, T. W. (1981). The genetic manipulation of killer character into brewing yeast. *J. Inst. Brew. 87*:292–295.

2

Impact of Biotechnology on the Food Industries

JOOP A. ROELS and HENRICUS A. C. THIJSSEN* /
Gist-brocades nv, Delft, The Netherlands

INTRODUCTION

The food industry plays an important role in our present-day society: Without the food industry, urbanization as we know it today would not have been possible. Also, along more economic lines, the gross money value output of the food industry is two or three times that of the chemical industry. Of course, the fact that the raw material costs are much higher in the food industry has to be taken into account; however, even based on gross added value, the food industry is larger than the chemical industry.

Presently the food industry employs biobased processes which account for about 95% of the industrial applications of living systems (Bronn, 1976). This does not, however, necessarily imply that food technology accounts for roughly 95% of the applications of biotechnology, at least if we define it as "the integrated use of (bio)-chemistry, (molecular) genetics, microbiology and process engineering with the objective to arrive at commercial applications of the reactions performed by microorganisms, cell cultures or parts of microorganisms or cells."

Food technology, or, better, food process engineering, should be based on a profound understanding of the physical or (bio)chemical mechanisms, underlying the processes and conversions relevant in food processing and storage. However, food process engineering, including biobased processing, is still removed from the fully science-based approach defined in the preceding description of biotechnology. Moreover, the degree to which science has penetrated the industry strongly varies among the various branches of the industry. The reason for this is that the food industry, in contrast

*Current affiliation: Thijssen Process Engineering BV, Son, The Netherlands

to the large-scale chemical industry, is not yet really integrated from a technological point of view. The food industry contains the separate "nationalisms" of the dairy industry, bakery industry, brewing industry, and so on, each with its own types of engineers, professional organizations, and journals. The technology in the food and food-associated industries is, as opposed to the more science-based industrial sectors, strongly product oriented and relatively weakly process oriented. As a consequence, the biobased process developments in certain areas of the food industry are not readily translated to other branches.

With respect to the potential impact of biotechnology on the food industry, one has to be aware of the fact that the food industry cannot be considered as a coherent industry overall. Not only, as remarked above, is it widely differentiated with respect to its product branches, but it also shows strongly varying degrees of aptitude with regard to the implementation of more science-based approaches, such as biotechnology in the science-based interpretation given above. In the "traditional" food industry, in which the processing methods are rooted in empiricism, the basic skills for the exploitation of biotechnology in the processing routes are mainly lacking. On the other hand, a small group of large-turnover science- and technology-based companies recognizes the potential of biotechnology and is progressively taking advantage of it (Holmes and Jarvis, 1982).

The total annual turnover in biobased processes (Thijssen and Roels, 1983) can be assumed to be well over $100 billion, and about two-thirds of this figure is accounted for by alcoholic beverages. Fermented foods account for another 20–25% of the applications of biobased processes. Baker's yeast, organic acids, amino acids, enzymes, and a variety of other compounds make up the remaining approximately 10% of the industrial applications of biobased processes. Even in this latter category the food industry accounts for an important share, and overall this industrial sector accounts for around 95% of industrial applications of biobased processes.

It would, however, be incorrect to combine this figure of 95% with the overall market volume of well over $100 billion on a yearly basis to get an idea of the significance of biotechnology in relation to food and food-related processes. The market share of traditional processes in the beverages and fermented foods sector has been stated to be very large, and, although modern science-based biotechnology will certainly have an impact on the processing routes employed in these sectors, it would not be very realistic to state that modern biotechnology is responsible for the total market volume in these industries. Rather, it indicates the potential of modern biotechnology to improve food processing technology.

BIOBASED PROCESSES IN THE FOOD INDUSTRY: CLASSIFICATION ACCORDING TO OBJECTIVES

Synthesis of Consumer End-Products

A large number of the biobased processes in the food industry are directed to the synthesis of consumer products, and the biological process is mainly directed toward adding flavor and fragrances and/or toward preservation. Typical examples are the production of alcoholic beverages, fermented dairy foods, cheese, sauerkraut, and fermented fish. Many of these processes have a long history indeed and modern biotechnology has relatively minor but increasingly significant impacts in these sectors. These will be discussed in some detail later on.

Synthesis of Food Additives

Biobased processes are having an increasing impact on the synthesis of food additions. Examples are the following:

- The synthesis of food acidulants like lactic acid, gluconic acid, and citric acid
- The synthesis of sweeteners such as glucose syrups and high-fructose corn syrups
- The production of flavors and fragrances other than acidulants or sweeteners, for example, yeast extract, glutamic acid, and nucleic acid hydrolysates
- The production of thickeners and gelling agents like xanthan gum or other microbial polysaccharides

Directed Modification of Foods or Food Additives

In this category a multitude of examples can be mentioned, such as the tenderization of meat with the enzyme papain and the improvement of the functional properties of proteins using proteases. Also the in situ liquefaction of sucrose in candies, using invertase, can be considered an example of the processes under consideration.

Production of Processing Aids

The production of processing aids for the food industries is another typical example of the impact of biobased processes on the food industries. A broad subdivision of this category can be made as follows:

- The production of microbes or microbial populations to be used as "starter" cultures in the production of dairy products.

The use of yeast in bread baking can be also considered an example of this type of application. The activities of the "starter" cultures have to be tailored toward a variety of functions, the formation of flavors, preservation, acidulation, and the formation of gases. Furthermore, the mode of action can be direct or through the excretion of extracellular enzymes by the microbes.

The production of enzymes for food production. This important aspect of the impact of the more modern biotechnological approach on food processing will be discussed in more detail later on. Here we will mention only cell wall-degrading enzymes; for example, pectinase preparations are widely used in the production of fruit and vegetable juices. Furthermore, proteases are used in improving the shelf life of beers.

Analytical Applications

A number of applications do exist or are in development in a variety of procedures for the analysis of foods and food additives, for example, the use of enzymes for analytical purposes and the use of monoclonal antibodies in the detailed analysis of proteinaceous materials.

Waste Treatment

Biotechnology is a very important factor in the treatment of wastes from food production or food processing operations. In some instances food wastes can be used for the production of single-cell protein as food or feed. Furthermore, aerobic and preferably anaerobic wastewater treatment can be applied to reduce the chemical oxygen demand of industrial wastewater. Anaerobic treatment, such as the upflow anaerobic sludge blanket process, has proved to be an important asset to the beet sugar industry. Recent developments have extended the use of anaerobic treatment beyond liquid wastes to the treatment of solid and semisolid wastes.

As typical representatives of the state of the art in the food industries, most of the processes categorized above still bear signs of an artisanal nature. In the past the emphasis has been on scaling up and to a much lesser extent toward real process improvements, this latter approach often being hampered by a lack of mechanistic knowledge of the details of the processes used. Processing breakthroughs will become increasingly likely if this obstacle is overcome. Particularly for the category of existing but yet to be improved processes for existing products, the requirements of lengthy toxicity testing accompanying the introduction of new foods and food additives and the problems of social acceptance will become less hampering in the introduction of new biotechnological approaches.

THE SWEETENERS MARKET: A RECENT EXAMPLE OF THE IMPACT OF BIOTECHNOLOGY

One relatively straightforward example of the impact of biotechnology on the food industries relates to the developments in the sweeteners market (Van Tilburg, 1983), which was traditionally the realm of sucrose, derived from cane and beet crops, and glucose syrups derived from starchy crops. The competition between starch-based glucose syrups and sucrose is governed by the relative sweetness and prices of these compounds. Glucose has a relative sweetness of 72% that of sucrose. Fructose, an isomer of glucose, has a sweetness of about 160% that of glucose.

Owing to both the local differentiation in the availability of sucrose-containing and starchy crops and the relative variation of their market prices, means of influencing the competitive positions of starch-derived products and sucrose with respect to the sweeteners market have been a target of extensive research for several decades. A number of breakthroughs in the availability of enzymes and the technology of their applications have drastically influenced this competitive position during recent years: Biotechnology had its impact on the sweeteners market.

Relatively recently efficient enzymatic processes were developed for the liquefaction and subsequent saccharification of starch syrups into glucose syrups with a free glucose content of 93% or more. The conventional acid-based saccharification technology resulted in syrups with a much lower free glucose content. In addition, the acid-catalyzed process was characterized by the formation of often objectionable by-products. In all, the application of the enzymes α-amylase in starch liquefaction and glucoamylase in saccharification has made the production of glucose syrups much more cost effective.

Owing to the above-mentioned high sweetness of fructose compared to its isomer glucose, which could, aided by enzyme technology, be produced from starch, the isomerization of glucose into fructose has been a target of active research. However, despite extensive studies, the alkaline isomerization of glucose did not produce the desired results: The resulting fructose-containing syrups contained undesirable, nonmetabolizable materials such as psicose and colored materials, which are costly to remove. Developments in enzyme technology such as the discovery of a thermostable xylose isomerase, which also catalyzes the conversion of glucose into fructose, and the subsequent development of techniques allowing the fixation of enzymes into (or onto) suitable carrier particles paved the way for the advancement of high-fructose corn syrup (HFCS) technology. In fact, the dramatic increase in the world market sucrose price in 1974 led to a rapid penetration of HFCSs in the U.S.

Table 1. Per Capita Nutritive Sweetener Consumption Trends in the United States

Year	Total (kg/year)	Sucrose (%)	Corn syrups other than HFCSs	HFCSs (%)
1970	55.0	84.1	15.9	—
1972	56.3	82.8	16.3	0.9
1974	55.3	79.2	18.6	2.2
1976	56.6	75.9	18.7	5.5
1978	57.8	73.1	17.3	9.7
1980	58.2	68.0	15.6	16.4

Source: Van Tilburg (1983).

sweeteners market, as illustrated in Table 1. In 1981 the market for the immobilized enzyme used in the process was about $26 million and several million metric tons of HFCSs (on a dry substance base) were produced.

The developments in the sweeteners market are still far from completion: The processes of enzymatic liquefaction, saccharification, and isomerization are the subjects of active research, and significant developments are to be expected. Furthermore, biotechnology has opened the way to new noncalorific sweeteners such as aspartame, a dipeptide ester, and the plant protein thaumatin, which in principle can be produced using recombinant DNA-modified production organisms.

The sweeteners market is also illustrative of the importance of political factors in the penetration of a new technology into an existing market. In the United States political preferences and technological possibilities had a synergistic effect on the deployment of HFCSs and the market share of the new sweetener rapidly increased. On the other hand, in the European community the prospects of increasing beet sugar surpluses if HFCSs were to take a substantial part of the sweeteners market led to a conflict between political and technological forces which resulted in several restrictions, including a production levy on HFCSs. This effectively inhibited the penetration of both the product and the technology in the European market.

POTENTIAL IMPACT OF BIOTECHNOLOGY

It is not likely that genetic engineering by itself will provide a major thrust in the impact of biotechnology on the food industries. However, most likely it will provide additional tools in the development of better organisms for the production of consumer products and better production organisms for processing aids or food additives.

Perhaps a more significant impact of genetic engineering on the food industries will be of a nature which has little to do with biotechnology as defined here. Genetic engineering will contribute strongly to the development of cultivars with improved resistance against pests, drought, salt, increased productivity of conventional raw materials for the food industry.

In the following some selected areas in which new biotechnological or biotechnology-based developments may affect the food industries will be discussed. This list is, however, by no means exhaustive.

Developments in the Synthesis of Consumer End-Products

The production of consumer products such as alcoholic beverages, butter, cheese, and yogurt are traditionally batch processes in which several reactions take place simultaneously. The result is a variety of physical and chemical transformations which give the product its final appearance. A number of developments have been of characteristic note in the changing state of the art in these processes and can be expected to have an increasing impact in the future:

- The use of a more industrial, often continuous processing-based approach toward the process, for example, of yogurt production (Lelieveld, 1984)
- The staging of the integral complex process into a more sequential mode of operation, for example, the decoupling of the coagulation, acid formation, and flavor formation processes in butter production (Lankveld, 1981)
- The use of starter cultures, perhaps genetical engineering modified in the more removed future
- The use of immobilized cells in, for example, the production of alcoholic beverages
- The use of enzymes such as lipases in the flavor formation in cheeses
- A more extensive use of additives such as thickeners and flavorings

Base Raw Materials for the Food Industries

It is well known that proteins (Cooney et al., 1980), fats (Ratledge, 1978), and oils can be produced in fermentation processes in submerged culture, and a strong effort has been directed toward a highly integrated biotechnological approach to the development of cost-effective processes for the production of proteins, more specifically. The Imperial Chemical Industries' single-cell protein (Senior, 1980) developments in particular have exploited a highly science-based approach, including sophisticated reactor technology and the development of efficient production organisms via genetic engineering. However, it still remains questionable if fermentation routes toward proteins and oils will ever become competitive compared to agricultural production. Certainly if the genetic engineering-induced advances in the efficiency of agriculture are taken into account, the production of raw materials for the food industry has to be expected to largely stay in the "niche" of agriculture.

Food Flavors and Fragrances

As far as food flavors and fragrances are concerned, the debate over the natural versus nature-identical versus synthetic plays an important role. A presently unresolved question is whether the products of biotechnological processes, for example, using microbes or enzymes, would be considered natural or nature-identical compounds if the starting materials were natural compounds. In the realm of flavors and fragrances, there certainly remains considerable room for growth, since 90% of the total sales in this sector are currently derived from synthetic products.

For many of the natural, plant-derived flavors and fragrances the costs and availability of the raw materials and therefore the prices of the food additives are subject to concern. Therefore plant tissue cultures have been considered as a means of producing raw materials for these compounds. The economics of these endeavors seem questionable, since the costs of plant tissue culture-derived products are expected to remain high if previous cost estimates and development are extrapolated. A number of breakthroughs could alter this picture:

1. The development of highly productive genetic engineering-modified plant cell lines.
2. The expression of plant metabolites in a microbial production organism. One has to recognize, however, that the present developments in the exploitation of recombinant DNA refer mainly to the expression of so-called primary gene products, that is, proteins which are, through messenger RNA-medi-

ated synthesis at the ribosomes, more or less directly derived from a discrete genetic code. The approach to nonproteinaceous secondary metabolites, which are products of a metabolic pathway based on the processing of material by a sequence of enzymatic reactions, is still a largely unexplored area.

In addition to the above-mentioned product groups, newer routes to the synthesis of amino acids, for example, the aspartame raw materials aspartic acid and phenylalanine, are expected to affect the production technology (Poldermans and Roels, 1985). Furthermore, new enzymatic methods are expected to have an increasing impact on the synthesis of peptides from proteins or amino acids.

Production of Polysaccharides and Carbohydrate Processing

Polysaccharides of various origins, such as starches, various plant gums, and algal gums, are widely used in the food industries as thickeners, stabilizers, or, in the case of starch, as a source of raw material for the production of sweeteners and ethanol. Apart from the developments in the sweeteners market, which have already been discussed, developments can be foreseen in the production of microbial gums by fermentation with xanthan gum being a notable example.

The present world production and market prices for a number of polysaccharides used by the food industries are summarized in Table 2. The market prices range between $2000 and $20,000 per metric ton, and this does not, at least for the higher-value compounds, exclude microbial production.

Important technological problems, however, still exist. A real breakthrough in production costs could be achieved if alternatives were developed for the aqueous phase fermentation processes, which inevitably result in very viscous solutions if the polysaccharide yield in the process is high. Substantial developments would also result if enzymatic processes could be applied to the modification of starches and other carbohydrates. The approach already widely exploited in the treatment of starch is based on the action of hydrolytic enzymes, and although there is some room for development in this direction, real future breakthroughs are unlikely. A less exploited approach is the use of enzymes, like phosphorylases, which appear in the synthetic pathways in microorganisms. The applications of phosphorylated monomers as such and in the modification of carbohydrates merit further investigation and may provide room for new developments.

Table 2. Polysaccharide Sources, Properties, Applications, and Market Volume and Price

Polysaccharide	Source	Application	Market volume (tons/year)	Market price (dollars/kg)
Agar	Red seaweeds	Gelling agent, adhesive, emulsifier, stabilizer	5,000	20
Carrageenan	Red seaweeds	Gelling agent, stabilizer	5,000	6.4
Alginate	Brown seaweeds	Gelling agent, emulsifier, stabilizer, thickener, film forming	10,000	4–8
Pectin	Plants	Gelling agent, stabilizer	10,000	6.7
Xanthan	Microbial	Gelling agent, stabilizer, emulsifier, thickener, swelling agent	—	8–11
Arab gum	Acacia tree	Emulsifier, thickener, adhesive, coating, stabilizer	23,000–68,000	1.6–3.0
Locust gum	*Ceratonia* seeds	Gelling agent, stabilizer, thickener, swelling agent, film forming	15,000–18,000	4.0–4.6
Guar gum	*Cyaniopsis* seeds	Emulsifier, stabilizer, swelling agent, thickener	60,000–90,000	1.6–1.8

Source: Bus et al. (1984).

Use of Enzymes in Chemical Synthesis and as Processing Aids

The use of enzymes in the food industries has shown considerable progress in the past few decades and will no doubt continue to do so in the near future. Table 3 gives a summary of some important markets and sales volumes. In fact there are a number of important reasons for predicting progress in this area. First, there are developments by the enzyme producers. The deployment of a truly interdisciplinary biotechnology in the last decade has turned the technology for enzyme production into a highly science-based activity, and, in fact, given sufficient market volume expectations, almost any enzyme tailored to specific processing needs can presently be offered on the market at reasonable costs. In fact, in most cases the existing industrial enzymes have become relatively cheap processing aids (see Table 4).

Second, enzymes as they exist in nature are highly suited to the treatment of proteins, oils, carbohydrates, and other products of natural origin. In the food industries the potential for large-scale applications of enzymes is much brighter than in the chemical industries, where the most important treatment and conversion processes employ compounds or conditions which are less suited to an enzymatic approach.

A further impact of enzyme technology can be foreseen in the recovery of compounds from plant, animal, or microbial material, for example, in a more efficient or cost-effective degradation of cell

Table 3. Enzyme Sales in the Food Industries

Industrial sector	Sales (U.S. dollars × 10^6)
Starch	55
Dairy	10
Ethanol, industrial	10
Brewing	5
Juices and wines	15
Bakery	10
Other	10
Total	180

Source: Grampp (1981).

Table 4. Direct Enzyme Costs in Enzyme Processes

Process	Units	Enzyme costs (U.S.¢)
Starch liquefaction	1 kg of starch	0.25
Starch saccharification	1 kg of starch	0.42
Starch isomerization	1 kg of starch	0.9
Cheese manufacture	1 liter of milk	0.05
Alcohol production	1 liter of alcohol	1.0
Brewing	1 liter of beer	0.09
Baking	1 kg of flour	0.01
Juice production	1 liter of juice	0.05–0.1
Wine production	1 liter of wine	0.05–0.1

tissue. Also the modification of carbohydrates, lipids, and proteins shows much room for the growth of enzyme use. For example, applications can be foreseen in cheese manufacture (the production of a microbial calf rennet by means of genetic engineering-modified microorganisms), the inter-esterification of fats and lipids, and the production of sugar esters. The full deployment of enzyme technology in the food industries calls for a number of specific developments, which will be briefly summarized.

First, there exists room for the introduction of enzymes which, as far as their mode of action, pH optimum, and temperature optimum are concerned, are optimally suited to the desired application. Second, only a limited number of the enzymes potentially available in nature are actually used. The majority of these are hydrolytic enzymes, one isomerase, and a few redox enzymes (glucose oxidase). The wide variety of other redox enzymes, ligases, lyases, and other enzymes with synthetic rather than degradative properties is hardly exploited. In the exploitation of new enzymes, for example, the redox enzymes, or the use of enzymes under unusual conditions, that is, in heterogeneous or multiphase systems such as in fat inter-esterification, there is substantial room for growth. The technological problems, however, are in many instances still great and in some cases, for example, in the use of redox enzymes, which depend on complex and expensive cofactors like NADH, the feasibility of developing a cost-effective technology may still be questioned.

New Antimicrobial Systems

In view of the trend toward products that contain no chemical preservatives or which have not been extensively sterilized, it would seem rewarding to take a closer look at the antimicrobial systems that appear in nature. Certain hydrolytic enzymes, like lysozymes, keratinases, and D-aminopeptidases, may be promising in this respect.

Waste Treatment

Most of the solid wastes of the food industries are sold as animal feed or as an energy source (boiler feed). Biotechnology could contribute to the development of higher added value applications for these materials, either by microbe- or enzyme-aided partial digestion or combinations thereof.

The liquid wastes are generally too dilute to be used as feedstocks for fermentation, and the costs of the disposal of these wastes are significant and increasing. In this respect a strong impact in the future is to be expected from rather recent developments which allow the very efficient conversion of dilute wastes to methane. At present in most cases the costs of this treatment are almost balanced by the gain of useful energy. A very interesting development in this respect is the high-technology fluid bed-immobilized cell reactor for efficient methane generation from a wide variety of liquid, sediment-containing wastes (Heijnen, 1984).

LIMITING FACTORS IN THE BIOTECHNOLOGY OF FOOD PROCESSING

The main factors which will impede the further applications of biotechnological processing methods in the food industry, although probably to a gradually decreasing extent, are the following:

The very complex nature of many foods and the fact that the relationship between the functional properties of the product, on the one hand, and the properties of the raw materials and processes, on the other hand, is difficult to establish.

The often rather weak relationship between market value and the real intrinsic quality of many foodstuffs. Food is a consumer product and its functional properties, such as taste, fragrance, and texture, are judged subjectively by the consumer. An attractive package and a catchy promotion often appear to have more effect on consumer acceptance than the products themselves. On the other hand, this provides an opportunity for biotechnology in view of the tendency to a larger scale of operation and rational production methods, which is typical for today's food industry. Processing aids like enzymes and tailored microorganisms may be necessary to retain consumer acceptance in the newer approaches to food processing. An example is found in the industrial baking process.

Consumer conservatism. If a product has already been on the market for some time, the manufacturer is often rightly wary of introducing drastic changes in the product characteristics. Consequently changes have to be brought about in rather small and careful steps. It is important that consumer organizations be kept well informed of the changes introduced so that they can critically evaluate and appreciate them and are capable of providing a rational judgment as to the appropriateness of the new technologies in the production of foodstuffs of the future. In this respect the recombinant DNA debate, which has accompanied the new appraisal of biotechnology, and the identification of biotechnology with recombinant DNA may still have adverse effects on the rate of the further penetration of biotechnology in the food industries.

Official regulations, more specifically the requirements for the toxicological testing of new products or of existing products produced along different bioprocess lines. The authorities may also intervene on the relative economic positions of various raw materials and finished products via quota systems and levies at a level that is prohibitive to the introduction of a new technology. This point was already discussed with respect to HFCS developments.

The shortage of properly trained food engineers with sufficient knowledge in bioprocess technology to be able to fully implement the fruits of biotechnological developments. The relatively low emphasis on food engineering and technology in academic circles may be an important factor in this respect.

REFERENCES

Bronn, W. K. (1979). *Branntweinw. 116*:211–217.

Bus, W. C. et al. (1984). *Chemisch Weekblad Magazine*, July, p. 427 (in Dutch).

Cooney, C. L., Rha, C., and Tannenbaum, S. R. (1980). *Adv. Food. Res. 26*:45.

Grampp, E. (1981). "Enzymtechnologien in der Lebensmittelindustrie," *Voedingsmiddelentechnologie 14*:22, 29 Oktober, p. 32 (in German).

Heijnen, J. J. (1984). "Biological industrial waste-water treatment minimizing biomass production and maximizing biomass concentration," Ph.D. Thesis, Delft University Press, Delft.

Holmes, A. W., Jarvis, B. (1982). *J. Chem. Technol. Biotechnol. 32*:224.

Lankveld, J. M. G. (1981). *Voedingsmiddelentechnologie 14*, 22, October, 15 (in Dutch).

Lelieveld, H. L. M. (1984). *Proc. Biochem. 19* (3), 112.

Poldermans, B., Roels, J. A. (in press). "Enzymes," in *Encyclopedia of Polymer Science and Engineering*.

Ratledge, C. (1978). In *Economic Microbiology*, Vol. 2, p. 263.

Senior, P. J. (1980). In A. Verbraek (ed.), *Biotechnology: A hidden past a shining future*, p. 97.

Thijssen, H. A. C., Roels, J. A. (1983). Paper presented at the Third International Food Engineering Conference, Dublin.

van Tilburg, R. (1983). "Engineering Aspects of the Application of Enzymes in Starch Conversion Technology," Ph.D. Thesis, Delft University of Technology, Delft.

3

Impact of Biotechnology on Food and Nutrition

HEINZ RUTTLOFF / Central Institute of Nutrition, Academy of Sciences of the GDR, Bergholz-Rehbrücke, German Democratic Republic

INTRODUCTION

For a long time microbial processes have been used to produce beer, wine, other alcoholic beverages, bread, curdled milk beverages, cheese, sauerkraut, vinegar, and other foods. The predecessors of up-to-date food biotechnologists were brewers, distillers, and cheese makers, who first achieved a combination of bacteriology, engineering, and chemistry. At that time personal engagement and empirical work · were the basis of any progress. The uses of all these fermentation processes in housekeeping and trade did not change in principle until about 100 years ago. Often the procedures had a touch of the supernatural. On the basis of the development of modern natural sciences, empirical fermentation techniques became a technology and many of the procedures originally performed for small trades were developed into industrial processes.

The worldwide increase in the prices of raw materials and the precarious energy situation in the 1970s required a constant increase in primary production as well as increased efficiency of food technologies and the development of substitutes for existing products. There is still much loss during production, distribution, and consumption of food. Every year agriculture, forestry, and food processing create enormous amounts of waste and by-products. At the same time, the consumption of energy-rich food in developed countries is so high that more and more diseases can be attributed to malnutrition. Unfortunately most people have too little awareness of nutritional requirements and the relationship of food preference judgements to these needs.

Table 1. Selected Foods, Food Additives, and Feed Produced by Fermentation Processes

Microbial biomass (single-cell protein)	Yeast (baker's yeast, fodder yeast), bacteria, fungi, mushrooms, algae
Soluble enzymes	Amylases, pectinolytic enzymes, cellulases, proteases, lipases, and other enzymes
Immobilized enzymes	Glucose isomerase, β-galactosidase, aminoacylase
Microbial polysaccharides	Xanthan, dextran, pullulan, alginate, curdlan, scleroglucan
Organic edible acids	Citric acid, vinegar, lactic acid, gluconic acid, malic acid, tartaric acid
Amino acids	Glutamic acid, lysine, methionine, phenylalanine, tryptophan, threonine, cysteine
Aroma compositions	Protein hydrolysates, fat hydrolysates, fruity flavors, flavor enhancers, sour milk products, cheese aroma, butter aroma, sausage ripeners, mushroomlike aroma, bread aroma, fermented foods

These problems are important to the national economy and public health and have incited an international interest in the efficiency of agriculture, the processing of its products into foodstuffs, and the optimal use of all conventional and nonconventional resources available. To satisfy these requirements we must make use of all our present knowledge. Biotechnology is a science of increasing importance in this regard (Rehm, 1981; Ruttloff, 1981a; Kirsop, 1981; Hulse, 1984).

Food and food additives of actual biotechnological relevance are cited in Table 1 and will be discussed in the following sections. Some interesting products concerning animal breeding will also be mentioned.

SUBSTRATES FOR FERMENTATION PROCESSES

Besides classic feedstocks, in the 1960s and 1970s fossil resources, methane from wastewater-clearing basins, and methanol were increasingly offered as carbon sources (Table 2). Since the energy crisis of

Table 2. Substrates for Fermentation Processes on the Industrial Scale

Conventional substrates	Nonconventional substrates	Waste and by-products of agriculture, forestry, the food industry, and industrial centers
Starch, starch-containing products	Petroleum, petroleum fractions and distillates (gas oil, kerosene, diesel oil, n-paraffins)	Wood, wood pulp, sawdust
Sucrose	Natural gas	Bagasses (sugar cane, citrus)
Molasses	Methane	Straw
Scraps of cereals	Ethane	Plant residues
Extraction scraps of oil seeds	Methanol	Peels, seeds, husks, cones, stones of fruit and vegetable
Processed grains	Ethanol	Rejected whole fruits
Soybean		Liquor stillage
Hydrol		Animal wastes
Distiller's wash		Wastewater
Corn-steep liquor		Starch water
Yeast extract		Spent water
Sulfite liquor		Spent sludges
Whey		Paper, paper residues
Fish meal		Pasteboard residues
Bran		Slaughter residues

the 1970s, however, interest in using mineral oil and its crude or purified fractions has strongly decreased. Instead, more and more low-value agricultural residues have been used in the bioconversion processes.

MICROBIAL BIOMASS: SINGLE-CELL PROTEIN

Currently the world population is rapidly increasing. Whereas in 1950 nearly 2.5 billion and in 1980 about 4.4 billion people inhabited the earth, this number is calculated to reach 6.1 billion by 2000 (United Nations Organization, 1981). In this connection single-cell protein (SCP)—in the form of biomass from yeasts, bacteria, fungi, and algae (unfortunately this term is used for microbial protein and biomass alike)—is employed more and more frequently as an ingredient of feed in animal breeding (Fritsche, 1978; Drews, 1979; Faust, 1984; Tusé, 1984). In the production of animal protein into foodstuff, a transformation loss of 80% must be calculated. In the future, therefore, single-cell protein may be directly applied to human nutrition, but only in an isolated, purified form. It should be taken into consideration that the productivity of protein synthesis in microorganisms is much greater than in higher plants or animals (Table 3).

Yeasts consist of 40–60% protein, fungi 30%, bacteria up to about 70%, and phototropic microorganisms 60–70% protein in dry matter. In addition, single-cell protein has a high content of B vitamins (e.g., the biomass of *Methylomonas* contains 1 mg of vitamin B_1, 8 mg of B_2, 2 mg of B_6, and 35 µg of B_{12} per 100 g of dry matter). The high amount of nucleic acids (yeasts, 5–8%; fungi, 10%; bacteria, 10–15%; algae, 6%) must be mentioned as disadvantageous. Moreover, numerous microorganisms store fat that is not

Table 3. Comparison of Protein Production by 1000 kg of Living Substance

Origin	Protein produced per day (Hkg)
Steer	1
Soybean	10^2
Yeast	10^5
Bacteria	10^{14}

Source: Yousri (1982).

utilized by humans (e.g., with poly-β-hydroxybutyric acid as the fatty acid component and lipopolysaccharides). The presence of traces of heavy metals has been reported. Branched-chained fatty acids as well as some with odd numbers of carbon atoms have been found in microorganisms cultivated on paraffin; however, these compounds are said to be metabolized by the organism of mammals.

With regard to amino acid composition, the microbial proteins generally have lower contents of methionine and cysteine than the Food and Agriculture Organization (FAO) reference protein (Table 4); on the other hand, they often exceed soy protein with regard to biological value. Scientists are trying to culture yeast strains with a more favorable protein composition and a lower content of nonprotein substances (glycogen, fat, steroids), as well as produce appropriately purified protein isolates.

Bacterial protein is often more valid for animal feeding and human nutrition than the protein of other microorganisms, especially that of yeasts. Above all, the high content of nucleic acids connected with the high growth rate of bacteria is disadvantageous.

Single-cell protein from yeasts using carbohydrates as a carbon source (Oura, 1983) is already applied worldwide on a large scale in animal nutrition, whereas microorganism production using mineral oil as well as n-paraffins as a carbon source (Bauch et al., 1978; Einsele, 1983; Ringpfeil, 1983) has not always been successful. Actually, already started large-scale projects have not been completed. One main reason for this is the fact that other protein-containing food, such as soybean and fish meal, are very strong competitors on the world market.

At present some companies consider methanol to be a very promising carbon substrate for single-cell protein; in this case methylotrophic bacteria—sometimes yeasts too—are used (Faust and Präve, 1983). At the same time possibilities of cell disintegration, isolation, and purification and chemical or enzymatic modification of the proteins are being tested to make the microbial protein directly available to human nutrition (Table 5, Fig. 1).

At the moment the role of single-cell protein in human nutrition is not yet clear. This is due to the costs of purification steps, and is therefore an economic problem. It is possible that microbial protein, even after the required processing and cleaning, may be used in the future.

The known production of single-cell protein, preferably for supplementing feed, is summarized in Table 6.

Other protein sources for future animal and human nutrition are being studied, such as phototropic microorganisms (Richmond, 1983). Their protein productivity exceeds that of higher plants and animals (Table 7). On this point it may be pointed out that people in different parts of the world supplement their food with algae (e.g., *Spirulina maxima* biomass is dried in the sun along Lake Chad in Africa and in Mexico).

Table 4. Essential Amino Acids in Several Proteins (g/16 gN)

Amino acid	Single-cell proteins: Alkane yeast	*Methylomonas* bacterium	*Scenedesmus* alga	Leaf protein concentrate	Fish meal	Soybean	Wheat	FAO reference protein
Lysine	7.8	6.9	5.7	6.5–7.5	7.9	6.2	2.8	5.4
Methionine + cysteine	2.5	3.1	2.3	2.7–3.7	3.9	2.9	3.8	3.5
Isoleucine	5.3	4.3	4.1	4.6–5.4	4.8	4.9	3.7	4.0
Leucine	7.8	7.9	8.0	7.2–8.5	7.6	7.6	6.6	7.0
Phenylalanine + tyrosine	8.8	6.8	7.6	8.3–10.1	7.9	8.1	7.3	6.1
Threonine	5.4	4.3	5.2	5.3–5.8	4.5	4.0	2.8	4.0
Tryptophan	1.3	1.1	1.3	1.3–1.5	1.1	1.3	1.1	1.0
Valine	5.8	5.9	6.4	5.5–7.0	5.6	4.8	4.5	5.0

Source: Kübler and Schulz (1978).

Table 5. Composition of Proteins from *Methylomonas clara*

Component	Spray-dried crude protein (%)	Isolated and purified "bioprotein type S" (%)
Crude protein (N × 6.25)	80	
Purified protein (ΣAS)	72	88–95
Crude fat	9	1–2
Nucleic acids	12	1–2
Ash	6	6
Crude fiber	3	3
Resting water	5	5

Source: Scharf and Schlingmann (1983).

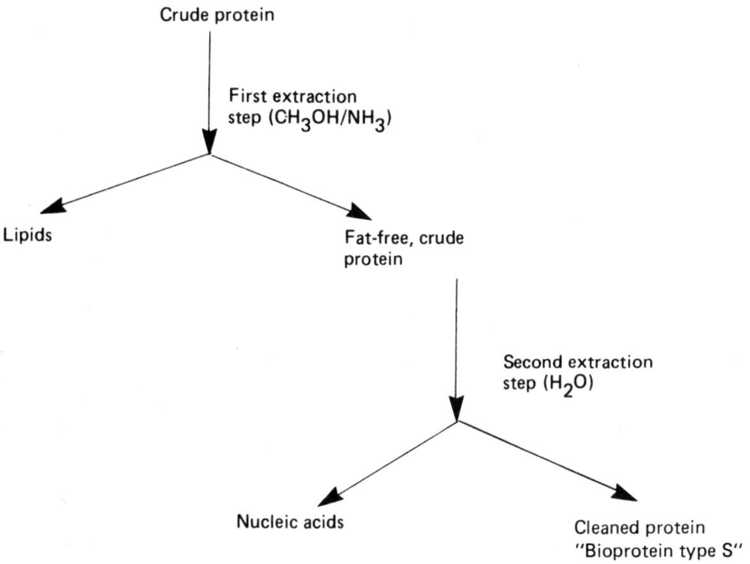

Fig. 1. Hoechst/Uhde flow sheet of the isolation and purification procedure of bioprotein (Scharf and Schlingmann, 1983).

Table 6. SCP-Producing Companies (Industrial and Pilot Scale): 1982

State	Company	Organism	Substrate	Trademark	Capacity (tons/year)	Status
England	Imperial Chemical Industries, Ltd.	*Methylophilus methylotrophus*	Methanol	Pruteen	50–70,000	Production
	Ranka Hovis McDougall Ltd.	*Fusarium graminearum*	Glucose syrup		100	Pilot plant
					25,000	In realization phase
Finland	Serlachius Oy Mänttä	*Paecilomyces varioti*	Sulfite liquor	Pekilo	8,000	Production
United States	Pure Culture Products Corp., Hercules Chemical Co.	*Candida utilis*	Ethanol	Zyest	7,000	Production
	Amber Laboratories, Universal Foods Corp.	*Kluyveromyces fragilis*	Whey		5,000	Production

Mexico	Pemex	*Methylophilus methylotrophus*	Methanol	Amberex	50,000	In planning
German Democratic Republic	VEB Petrochemisches Kombinat Schwedt	*Candida* sp.	Petroleum distillate	Fermosin	60,000	In realization phase
Romania	Romiport, Dainnippon	Yeast	n-Paraffins		60,000	Production
					60,000	In planning
USSR	Government companies	Yeast	Petroleum distillate, n-paraffins, sulfite liquor		1,000,000	Production
					1,200,000	In planning
Federal Republic of Germany	Hoechst/Uhde	*Methylomonas clara*	Methanol	Probion	1,000	Pilot plant

Source: Scharf and Schlingmann (1983).

Table 7. Protein Productivity Data for Algae Compared with Other Sources

Protein source	Protein yield (kg dry weight/ha per year)
Spirulina platensis	24,300
Chlorella pyrenoidosa (Emerson)	15,700
Clover meal	1,680
Grass	670
Peanuts	470
Peas	395
Wheat	300
Milk from cattle on grassland	100
Meat from cattle on grassland	60

Source: Yousri (1982).

SOLUBLE ENZYMES

Of the six main classes of enzymes, emphasis is on the large-scale production of hydrolases. The ones to be mentioned first are amylases (α-amylase, glucoamylase), cellulases, proteases (microbial rennin included), glucanases (e.g., brewery enzyme), lipases, pectin-splitting enzymes, and some others belonging to other main classes. The important enzymes for food technology purposes are sufficiently known and are described in detail in the literature (Johnson, 1977; Ruttloff, 1978; 1981b; Taylor and Richardson, 1979; Ruttloff et al., 1979; Halpern, 1981; Schwimmer, 1981; Aunstrup, 1983; Kula, 1984). These water-soluble—that is, not immobilized—enzyme preparations are said to belong to the first enzyme generation. They are used as solvated preparations and cannot be regenerated and are produced by submerged or emerged fermentation. Their degree of purity is generally low, which is actually desirable in many cases. They do not need coenzymes to be active and their production costs are relatively low. Crude preparations of hydrolytic enzymes are relatively stable and can be well stored without excessive expenditure in comparison to other enzymes, such as the intracellular ones.

Some of them are of special actual importance in nutrition and/or food technology. They will be discussed below.

Pectin-Splitting Enzymes

Fruits and vegetables are highly valued foodstuffs because of their high content of crude fiber, minerals, and vitamins, good taste and aroma, vivid color, and low energy content. The industrial processing of fruits and vegetables is carried out worldwide. The conventional process is juice making, but liquefaction is becoming more common.

Pectinolytic enzymes (Fogarty and Kelly, 1983), such as pectinesterase, polygalacturonase, pectin and pectate lyases, as well as cellulases, hemicellulases, and amylases, are effective in decomposing the plant cell wall (Table 8). In fruit and vegetable cell walls, especially in young tissues, the incrustation of cellulose with lignin has not advanced very far. This makes the application of cellulolytic enzymes easier, although not entirely without problems.

When *macerating* enzymes are used under suitable conditions of reaction, only the middle laminae of the plant tissue are decomposed. The cellular wall rich in fibers remains intact, for example, as in the formation of monocellular suspensions. This means that the crude fiber-rich material—cellulose, hemicellulose, lignin, pectin—forming the cellular wall, and which is very important in nutrition physiology, gets into the intestinal tract. It is not attacked by the enzymes of the proximal small intestine, but only later by the microflora in the distal sphere. However, the main portion is excreted from the body unchanged. Such products are also suited for elderly people, who often neglect to eat meals rich in crude fiber. The plant cell walls may be separated from the serum; the serum can be concentrated and mixed. On the whole, there are many possibilities for additional appreciation of low-energy products (Table 9).

In the *total liquefaction* of fruits and vegetables, the middle lamina of plant tissue containing pectin and also the cellular wall (composed of cellulose, hemicellulose, lignin, and pectin) must be degraded. This can easily be accomplished via the synergistic action of pectinolytic and cellulolytic enzymes.

The following example with carrot juice illustrates the nutritional importance of enzyme application (Table 10). Not only is it of great importance to public health (food for babies and children), but also in general it will be a valuable raw material of the future for the production of mixed fruit drinks (Dongowski and Bock, 1984). In the conventional production of pressed carrot juice (i.e., by expression without enzyme application) the yield of juice is about 65%. The maximal carotene content of the juice is 2 mg/100 g, which is about 7% of the total carotene content. By the application of

Table 8. Degradation of Plant Tissue by Pectinolytic and Cellulolytic Enzymes

Enzymes and effects	Biochemical reaction	Desirable process
Pectinolytic enzymes: tissue softening	Partial decomposition of unsoluble protopectins	Natural ripening of fruits and vegetables
Pectinolytic enzymes: tissue loosening	Partial destruction of cell tissue	Juice production; production of carrot juice
Pectinolytic enzymes: tissue maceration	Destruction of the middle lamina; crude fiber fraction as well as cell substances remain intact	Production of drinkable monocellular suspensions or macerates
Pectinolytic and cellulolytic enzymes: total liquefaction	Destruction of the cell wall; liberation and partial destruction of cell substances	Total liquefaction of the plant tissue; production of drinkable hydrolysates

Source: Adapted from Bock (1978).

Table 9. Production of Fruit and Vegetable Products by Application of Macerates

Fruit nectar
Fruit and vegetable juices
Concentrates of fruit and vegetable pulp
Foods for children, dietary foods
Fruit and vegetable powder
Products containing cream and mayonnaise
Instant products
Products of dried potatoes
Structured products

Source: Bock (1978).

Table 10. Yields of Juice, Macerate, and Hydrolysate and β-Carotene upon Liquefaction of Carrots

Technology	Product	Yield of product (%)	Yield of β-carotene (%)
Pressing in traditional manner	Carrot juice	65	7
Pressing after enzyme treatment with pectinase–macerase (i.e., 1% Rohament P; decanter)	Carrot juice	75	60
Passing after enzyme treatment with pectinase–macerase (e.g., 4% Rohament P; passing sieve)	Carrot macerate	95–100	85
Passing after enzyme treatment with pectinase–macerase + cellulase (passing sieve)	Carrot total hydrolysate	95–100	85

Source: Adapted from Bock, personal communication (1982).

pectinase–macerase preparations the juice yield can be increased to 75% (or even 80%) and the carotene content of the juice is about 60% of the total carotene content. However, in the enzymatic production of carrot juice about 20–25% of the carrot pulp remains as residue. If macerates (monocellular suspensions) are produced, then 95–100% of the total carrot substance may be used for nutrition. The application of pectinase–macerase *and* cellulase preparations results in total hydrolysis of the plant tissue. In this case the cell structures are destroyed and no residues remain (hydrolysates).

Cellulases

Cellulose is the world's most abundant organic substance. If it were possible to convert cellulose and cellulose-containing material from forestry, agriculture, and industrial centers (i.e., wood, wood wastes, sawdust, straw, bagasses, plant residues, paper, wastes of paper plants) biotechnologically to single-cell protein, glucose, ethanol, and other substances, this would represent an inexhaustible source for the feed, food, and chemical industries. Therefore the enzymatic degradation of cellulose is internationally being studied with great intensity (Vanbelle et al., 1982; Enari, 1983; Holm and Sahm, 1983).

Unfortunately the insolubility, crystallinity, and small surface of cellulose give rise to difficult problems in its enzymatic degradation. The fibrous micelles complicate enzymatic hydrolysis because the large cellulase molecules cannot penetrate the intercrystalline spaces. The incrustation by lignin likewise strongly reduces the enzymatic attack on cellulose. Nevertheless, enzymes are interesting for cellulose degradation because of their specificity and high efficiency. For example, 1 mol of cellulase has the same catalytic effect as 10^6 mol of hydrochloric acid.

There has been a long-lasting dispute concerning the enzymes participating in cellulose degradation. As we know, the cellulose complex consists of amorphous and crystalline regions. According to our present knowledge, the enzymatic attack on the system takes place as shown in Figure 2. The C_x and C_1 cellulases demonstrate a synergistic effect. The lignin content of cellulose acts as a great barrier to splitting. In principle, certain saprophytic microorganisms (i.e., white rot fungi and some brown rot fungi) are able to decompose lignin; however, up to now no economically satisfactory cellulase and ligninase activities have been obtained to split the cellulose within the lignocellulose complex. Therefore pretreatments with chemical agents (e.g., mineral acids) or physical processes (e.g., grinding and heating) are necessary.

Figure 3 demonstrates the possible variants of biotechnological cellulose utilization. For the production of ethanol and/or biomass, appropriate microorganisms are required. These are cultivated on the cellulose-containing material that has been prehydrolyzed with cellulase preparations or they produce the cellulase complex themselves in order to decompose the available lignocellulose. Probably intact cellulase-producing microorganisms are given preference as compared to decomposition of cellulose substrates by purified enzymes.

Because of the relatively low lignin content involved, in fruits and vegetables the enzymatic degradation of cellulose is associated with fewer problems. Commercial cellulase preparations (for this particular application mainly in combination with pectinolytic enzymes) are able to carry out total hydrolysis of the vegetable substrates.

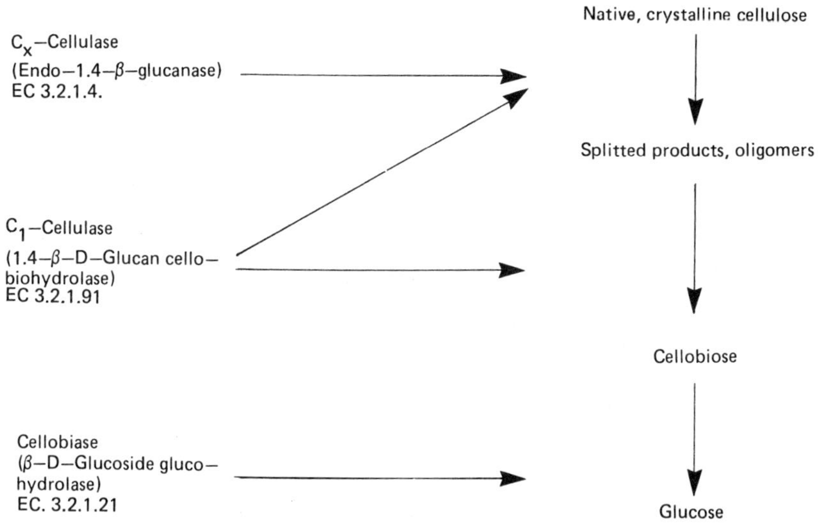

Fig. 2. Mechanisms of the degradation of crystalline cellulose by cellulolytic enzymes (adapted from Hirte and Philipp, 1983).

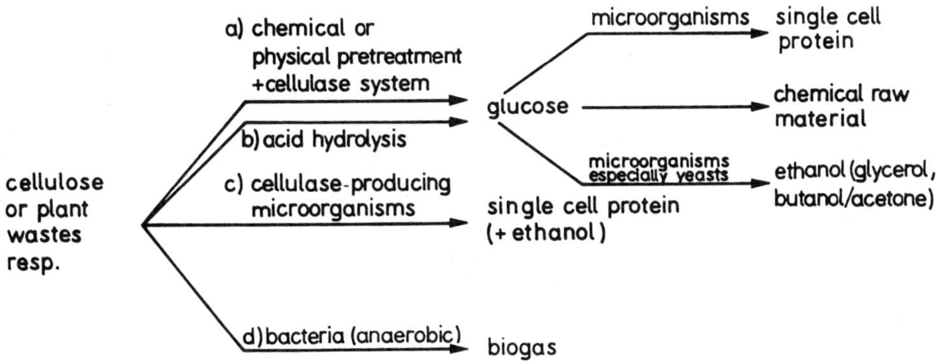

Fig. 3. Enzymatic, acid, and/or microbial degradation of cellulose or cellulolytic material.

Proteinases

Within the last years many experiments have been carried out to produce, characterize, and apply proteinases (Ward, 1983). Proteinases can change the functional properties of different protein substrates in order to obtain a rationalization of food technologies or an improvement of the quality of final products.

When dough is prepared, the proteins of wheat flour form a gluten network that is responsible for the mechanical properties of the dough, such as kneadability, elasticity, and gas-preserving capacity (Gabor et al., 1982a). When special cereal-based foodstuffs are produced, certain rheological demands are made on the dough. Thin liquid flour suspensions are required to have a low water content in order to limit energy consumption in the baking process; flours low in gluten are needed for these doughs. In the past there was wheat available for this purpose, but now, following the international trend, more and more wheat types are rich in gluten. This fact can result in problems of processing and quality. Here the additional use of technical proteinase preparations is desired. The advantage is a reduction of kneading time and improvements in crumb pores, mellowness, browning, taste, and aroma. The gluten can be decomposed to such an extent that its typical properties of plasticity and elasticity disappear. In this way conventional procedures for the production of instant semolina, instant flours, bread crumbs, wafer sheets, biscuits, and other products could be improved (Drechsel and Ruttloff, 1975; Ter Haseborg, 1981). In some cases more effective technologies have been developed (Fig. 4).

Despite a comparatively *low gluten decomposition* (splitting of only 1–2% of the peptide bonds), the rheological properties of products treated by the above-mentioned processes are considerably changed. Figure 5 shows the fractionation of gluten washed out from flour before and after treatment with Thermitase, a serine-proteinase obtained from *Thermoactinomyces vulgaris* (Ruttloff et al., 1983). The splitting of enzyme-treated gluten samples on a Sepharose 4B column shows a decrease of the highly molecular glutenin fraction in favor of compounds with molecular masses below 5×10^5. Components that have the same molecular mass as the gliadines will be increased.

With another group of enzymatically modified proteins the aim is to reach a *higher degree of hydrolysis* (10–25% of the peptide bonds). This includes the splitting of conventional and nonconventional proteins to change their functional properties, as in blood plasma, thick blood, waste poultry meal, wheat or corn gluten, ground bonds from slaughterhouses, egg albumin, whey protein, and *vicia faba* protein (Behnke et al., 1984).

An important possible application of partially hydrolized proteins is their use for dietary or clinical purposes, as they are needed by

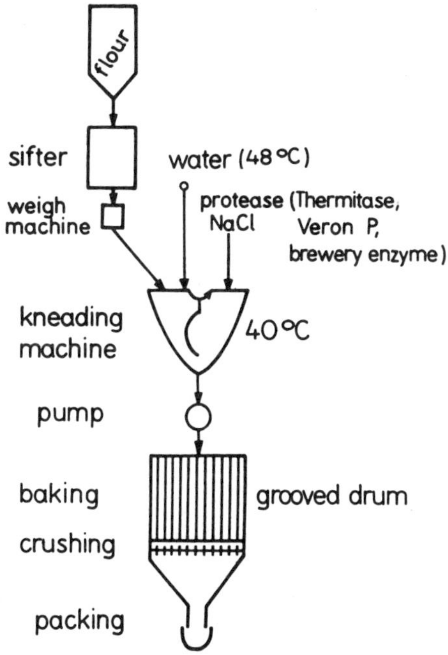

Fig. 4. Flow chart for the production of bread crumbs (Täufel et al., 1982).

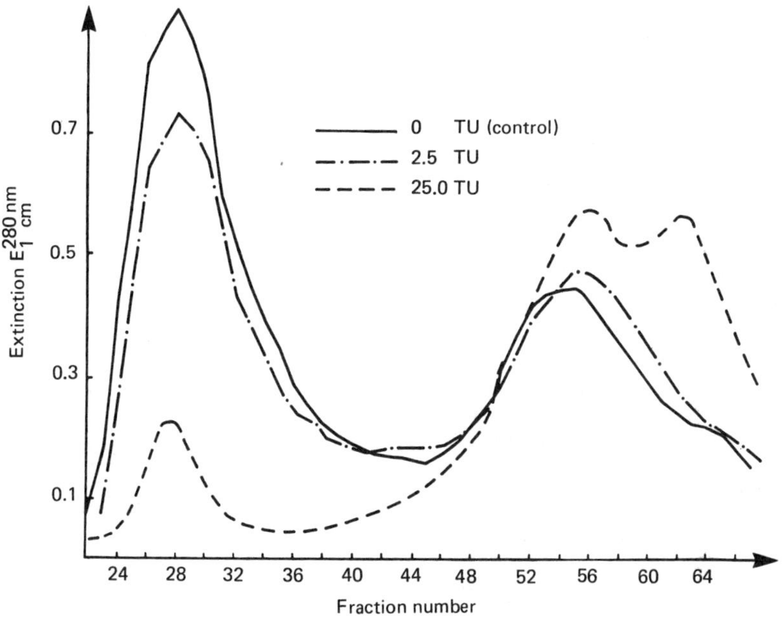

Fig. 5. Fractionation of isolated gluten treated with the protease Thermitase on a Sepharose 4B column (Gabor et al., 1982b).

Table 11. Production and Application of Enzymatically Hydrolyzed Proteins

Applied enzymes	
	Thermitase
	Brewery enzyme
	Pancreatine
Applied substrates	
	Casein
	Whey protein
	Egg albumin
	Muscle protein
Fields of application	
	Babies
	Premature babies
	Patients with pre- or postoperative conditions
	Patients with gastrointestinal diseases
	Convalescents
	Patients in intensive care

Source: Ruttloff (1983).

special groups of people and patients. For this proteins with a high biological value are necessary as substrates (Table 11). They must be converted to low molecular weight peptides to facilitate digestion. The conditions for enzymatic action must be chosen in such a way that a high degree of hydrolysis is achieved—if possible, above 30% (up to 40%)—as well as a low trichloroacetic acid-precipitable sediment (less than 2%). Substrates can be whey protein, muscle protein, egg albumin, and casein.

A disadvantage of the use of enzymatic protein hydrolysates is the bitterness of peptide mixtures (Fig. 6). This depends mainly on the hydrophobicity of the side chains of peptide-forming amino acids, the degree of decomposition, and, of course, the protein used (Behnke, 1985).

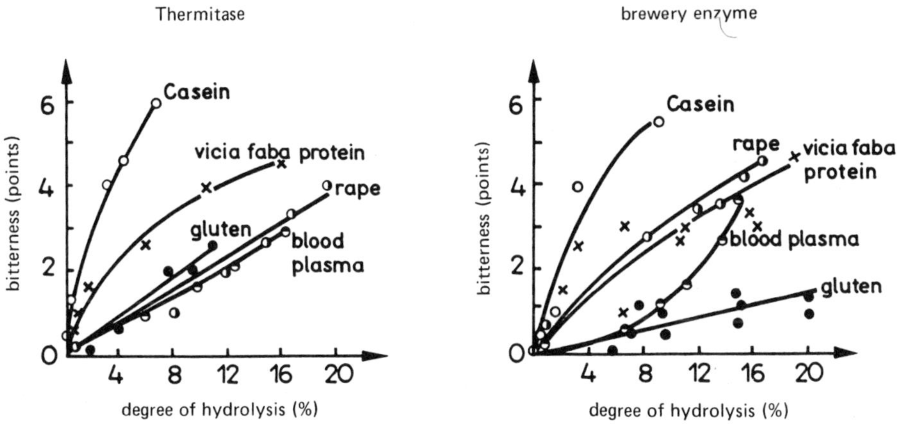

Fig. 6. Influence of protein hydrolysis on protein bitterness (Behnke and Ruttloff, personal communication).

Table 12. Advantages of Enzymatic Protein Partial Hydrolysates Compared with Acid Protein Total Hydrolysates

Chemical advantages
No destruction of amino acids
No supplement required
No formation of by-products (humine substances, discoloration)
Reduced osmolarity of the hydrolysates
Technical and economic advantages
Shorter incubation times
Reduced indubation temperatures
No time-consuming cleaning operations

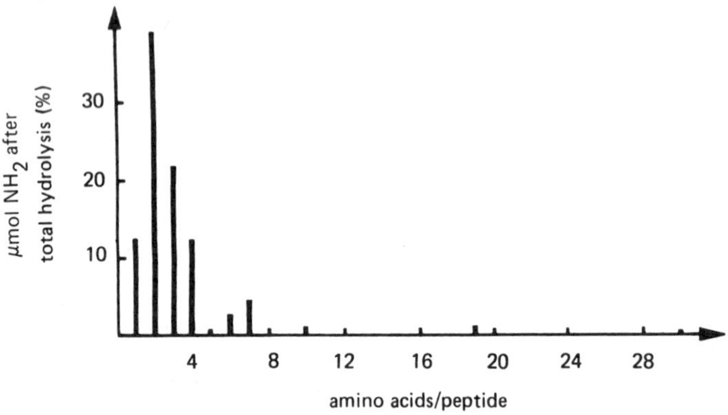

Fig. 7. Size distribution of the peptides of muscle protein partially hydrolyzed by enzymatic action (Behnke and Ruttloff, personal communication).

Enzymatic protein hydrolysates have several advantages compared to total acid hydrolysates (Table 12). Recent investigations in perfused rat intestine showed that the amino acids in the peptide molecule are absorbed at least as quickly as the corresponding free amino acids of equimolecular mixtures (Friedrich et al., 1985). According to preliminary tests, this result can also be achieved in the intestinal tract of the infant. Figure 7 shows the peptide distribution of enzymatically hydrolyzed muscle protein.

IMMOBILIZED ENZYMES

A second generation of enzymes was introduced by their immobilization (Konecny, 1975; List and Knechtel, 1980; Hultin, 1983; Klibanov, 1983). These immobilized enzymes are acting without coenzyme (in the first-line hydrolases) which are fixed to a carrier or entrapped in certain structures. The advantages and disadvantages of their production and application are shown in Table 13. Furthermore, the pH profiles as well as specific kinetic properties of certain enzymes can be changed by variation of the functional groups present on the surface of the carrier. Several carriers with high loading capacities were developed. However, immobilized enzymes cannot replace soluble preparations in every case.

According to literature of the 1970s, several application fields in the food sector are possible and a great future had been predicted for immobilized enzymes (Table 14). However, in food production so far, only three of the enzymes discussed in the literature

Table 13. Advantages and Disadvantages of Enzyme Immobilization

Advantages	Disadvantages
Continuous process possible	Losses of enzyme with immobilizing process
Improved product quality	Leaching effects
Reuse of enzyme	Expenses for carrier substances and immobilizing
Product free of enzyme	Raised expenditure for equipment and techniques
Inactivation of enzyme (e.g., heat) not necessary	Danger of microbial contamination
Immobilizing of multistep enzyme process possible	

Source: Adapted from Uhlig (1984).

Table 14. Possibilities for the Application of Immobilized Enzymes Within the Food Industry

Enzyme	Application
Glucoamylase	Starch conversion
Glucose isomerase[a]	Production of isomerate sugar
Invertase	Production of invert sugar
Lactase[a]	Hydrolysis of lactose (milk, whey)
β-Amylase	Production of maltose
β-Glucanase	Viscosity reduction of wort and beer
Pectinase (polygalacturonase–pectine esterase)	Clarification of fruit juices
Protease	Chill proving of beer; production of protein partial hydrolysates
Rennin	Cheese production
Glucose oxidase + catalase	Oxygen elimination in beverages
Glucose isomerase + glucose oxidase	Production of gluconic acid and fructose from glucose
Catalase	Elimination of H_2O_2 after chemical sterilization
Aminoacylase[a]	Production of L-amino acids from racemic mixtures

[a]Immobilized enzymes in large-scale production.
Source: Hartmeier (1977).

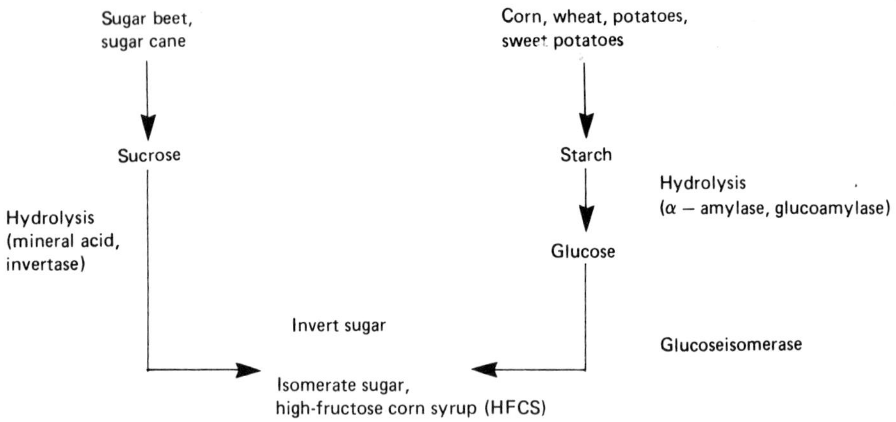

Fig. 8. Starting material and intermediate steps for the production of invert sugar and isomerate sugar, high-fructose corn syrup, HFCS).

have been produced and applied on a large scale: glucose isomerase, aminoacylase, and β-galactosidase. Maybe one day soluble glucoamylase will be changed to its immobilized form, but for such a replacement to be undertaken in industry, the immobilized enzyme must deomonstrate economic and technical advantages. Up to now its large-scale application in dextrose preparation could not be enforced. This may be due to the fact that the soluble enzyme is very cheap and economically superior to the immobilized preparation.

Glucose Isomerase

The enzymatic isomerization of glucose (Venkatasubramanian, 1980; Bucke 1983a) leads to an equilibrium mixture of 42% fructose, 52% glucose, and 6% other sugars in dry matter—isomerate sugar, high-fructose corn syrup, HFCS (Fig. 8). The application of immobilized preparations shows considerable economic advantages compared with the expensive soluble enzyme. The production of HFCS from corn starch as raw material is more cost efficient than the production of cane or beet sugar. Isomerate sugar is used for sweetening soft drinks, alcoholic beverages, ice cream, sauces, fruits, and sweets, and it is already often preferred over sucrose. It does not crystallize easily, which is a special advantage in the production of syrups and liqueurs.

Lactase

The increasing interest in lactase may be explained by the fact that whey contains 70% lactose in dry matter. This sugar has only 33% of the solubility of glucose and galactose and scarcely half the sweetening effect of sucrose. The glucose–galactose mixture is sweeter, more soluble, and more fermentable than lactose.

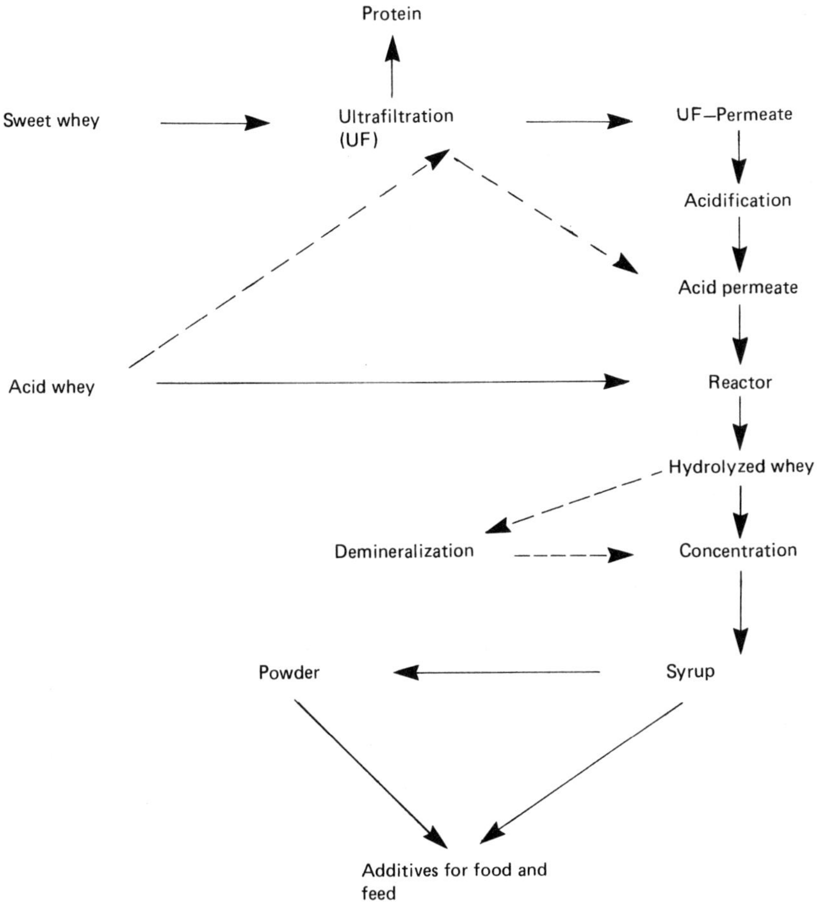

Fig. 9. Flow sheet of the hydrolysis of sweet and acid whey into lactose-hydrolyzed whey and further processing (adapted from Sprössler and Plainer, 1983).

At present whey is used mainly in animal nutrition while another part remains as wastewater, thus considerably affecting the environment in some countries. But chances for an economic hydrolysis of lactose are increasing because of raising costs for the treatment of wastewater, the continuously growing demand for sweetening agents, and a growing interest in whey protein. Moreover, the incompatibility of milk observed in adults due to an intestinal lactase deficiency (lactose intolerance) is much more widespread than formerly thought. This fact may result in an increasing demand for lactase-pretreated milk.

Lactase application in its immobilized form seems to have chances, but it is presently still very expensive. Current developments are aimed toward the desalting of whey after protein separation (ultrafiltration) and lactose hydrolysis (Fig. 9). The resulting product can be used as a sweetening agent or a substitute for starch syrup or converted via fermentation to biomass and/or ethanol. The first commercial low lactose milk was produced by "Centrale del Latte" of Milan, Italy utilizing the Snamprogetti technology. This plant is working with cellulose acetate fiber immobilized lactase (Pastore and Morisi, 1976).

IMMOBILIZED CELLS

Immobilization of whole cells has been carried out since about 1975 (Bucke, 1983b; Mosbach, 1983). According to Chibata (1983), the preparation techniques in the cases of immobilized cells and enzymes are the same: "Immobilized enzymes and immobilized cells are physically confined or localized in a certain defined region of space with retention of their catalytic activities, and which can be used repeatedly and continuously" (Table 15).

For microorganisms the entrapment method has proved to be the best one. Among the numerous gels principally applicable are the following:

- Polyacrylamide
- Polysaccharides
  - κ-Carrageenan
  - Ca-alginate
- Proteins
  - Collagen

Immobilized cells represent a multicomponent enzyme system. Depending upon the pretreatment and utilization purpose, however, only one single enzyme, one enzyme sequence, or the total enzyme system of the cell must be intact. In the latter case the cell is still vital and the population is able to grow in the gel with high

Table 15. Methods for Cell Immobilization

Carrier binding method	
	Covalent binding
	Ionic binding
	Adsorptive binding
Crosslinking method	
	Application of bifunctional agents
	Application of multifunctional agents
Entrapping method	
	Involvement in a gel matrix
	Encapsulation in a semipermeable polymer membrane
Heating of the biomass	

growth rates. Also, many activities are underway to immobilize plant and animal cells.

For the production of some food and dietary products, various interesting compounds can be synthesized without problem by means of biotransformation with immobilized cells (Chibata, 1983). With the use of polyacrylamide and later on carrageenan as the gel matrix, L-aspartic acid (since 1973) and L(−)-malic acid (since 1974) have been in large-scale production with *Escherichia coli* (aspartase) and *Brevibacterium ammoniagenes* (fumarase) from fumaric acid, respectively (with the addition of NH_3 and H_2O, respectively). The industrial production of L-alanine from fumaric acid via L-aspartic acid by means of *two different* kinds of immobilized microorganisms (*E. coli* and *Pseudomonas dacunhae*) is possible. Here we may mention the dipeptide methyl ester aspartame (L-aspartyl-β-L-phenylalanine methyl ester), which is approved in several countries as a sweetening agent. Phenylalanine can also be produced from the ammonium salt of cinnamic acid by means of immobilized *Rhodotorula gracilis* (phenylalanine ammonialyase). Malic acid is a valuable organic acid that is used as a flavoring substance in lemonades and fruit products.

Additional enzymes of interest for food technology and nutrition and immobilized within dead cells are given in Table 16. Corresponding procedures are already used on a large scale (e.g., glucose isomerase).

Table 16. Immobilized Cells with Enzymes of Importance in Food Technology or Nutrition

Enzyme	Substrate	Product
Glucose isomerase (xylose isomerase) EC 5.3.1.5	Glucose	Isomerate sugar (high-fructose corn syrup)
α-D-Galactosidase, EC 3.2.1.22	Raffinose	Galactose + sucrose (beet sugar production)
β-D-Fructofuranosidase (invertase), EC 3.2.1.26	Sucrose	Invert sugar
Tryptophanase, EC 4.1.99.1	Indole, pyruvic acid, NH_3	L-Tryptophan
Tyrosine phenolyase (β-tyrosinase), EC 4.1.99.2	Phenol, pyruvic acid, NH_3	L-Tyrosine

The use of *vital* immobilized cells is an area of recent interest. Alcohol-producing yeasts (e.g., *Saccharomyces carlsbergensis*)—included in a carrageenan matrix—continuously transfer sugar into ethanol (14% alcohol in eluate) for up to 90 days. In the near future this procedure will also be applied on a large scale.

Further reactions are being studied worldwide. The coimmobilization of microorganisms and enzymes (Hartmeier, 1983) is a part of such programs. A comparison of the immobilization of yeasts and the coimmobilization of enzymes and microorganisms is provided below.

Immobilization of yeasts.

D-Xylose ⟶ ethanol
Inulin ⟶ ethanol } special yeasts
Whey ⟶ ethanol

(lactose ⟶ ethanol and lactose ⟶ glucose + galactose ⟶ ethanol, respectively)

Coimmobilization of enzymes and microorganisms.

$$\text{D-Xylose} \xrightarrow{\text{glucose isomerase}} \text{xylulose} \xrightarrow{\text{yeast}} \text{ethanol}$$

$$\text{Cellobiose} \xrightarrow{\text{cellobiase}} \text{glucose} \xrightarrow{\text{yeast}} \text{ethanol}$$

$$\text{Starch} \xrightarrow{\text{glucoamylase}} \text{glucose} \xrightarrow{\text{yeast}} \text{ethanol}$$

It is thought that intact immobilized microorganisms can be used for the production of organic acids, amino acids, enzymes, and vitamins, among other things.

MICROBIAL POLYSACCHARIDES

The commercial polysaccharide-based hydrocolloids are derived from gums, mucilages, exudates, and extracts of plant origin (Pilnik and Voragen, 1984). The known compounds of this class of substances are listed in Table 17. They have different functional properties owing to their structural diversity. In aqueous systems they are of major importance to food technology and—more indirectly—to nutrition (Table 18). Numerous areas of application result from these properties; the following are a few examples:

Quality improvement of foodstuffs
Development of substitutes
Improvement of certain products
Economy in using valuable raw materials

With regard to nutritional and physiological aspects, such hydrocolloids are mainly important as thickening agents, filling materials, and gel forming, "body-giving," and "mouth-feeling" substances, especially in the production of low energy foods. In addition, during passage through the gastrointestinal tract, they cannot be degraded by pancreatic and mucosal enzymes. Thus they represent nutritionally valuable ballast material. Their application in the production of foodstuffs and dietary products can only be recommended, as the low amount of fiber in the diet of highly developed industrial countries is a serious problem (Ruttloff, 1980).

Table 17. Natural Polysaccharides of Plant Origin

Type of polysaccharide	Example
Seaweed extracts	Agar-agar, carrageenan, Irish moss, alginate, laminarin, furcellaran
Lichen extracts	Icelandic moss
Plant extracts	Pectin, arabinogalactan (larch gum)
Plant exudates	Gum arabic, karaya gum, tragacanth gum, gum ghatti (Indian gum)
Seed mucilages and gums	Locust bean gum, guar gum, tamarind mucilage
Plant starches	Cereals, potatoes, artichokes
Other natural hydrocolloids	Salep mannan

Source: Adapted from Sanderson and Clark (1983).

Within the last years the natural hydrocolloids available were subjected to continuously rising prices. This is due to the increasing demand for such products and the climatic fluctuations, harvest problems, and other events in producing countries.

These and other reasons have prompted the development of a large number of microbial polysaccharides (Jeans, 1974; Lawson and Sutherland, 1978; Catley, 1983; Fyfe and Govan, 1983; Kenne and Lindberg, 1983; Sutherland, 1983; Voelskow, 1983; Alsop, 1983; Phillips and Lawford, 1983). At first they were provided for medical or biochemical and analytical purposes (e.g., dextran), as bore media (e.g., xanthan), additives for paints, latex emulsions, rust-preventing agents, for the production of ceramics, the textile industry, and so on. In the meantime their application within the food industry has proved to be successful. Part of the compounds mentioned below (e.g., xanthan) are already permitted by the FAO and the health administrations of many countries. More compounds are currently being introduced or are undergoing toxicological and food hygiene testing.

With the microbial polysaccharides one must distinguish between neutral and acid (anionic) products, as well as between homopolysaccharides (consisting of only one monomer sugar) and heteropolysaccharides (composed of various monomers).

Table 18. Desired Functional Properties of Polysaccharides in the Production and Kitchen-Technical Preparation of Foods

Foam formation	Precipitation prevention
Foam stability	Protective colloid effectivity
Emulsifiability	Prevention of crystal formation
Emulsion stability	Turbidity stability
Water solubility for ingredients	Suspension stability
Water-binding capacity	Structure formation
Effectiveness as a swelling agent	Texture formation
Effectiveness as a filling agent	Film and foil formation
Effectiveness as an adhesive agent	Mouth-feel characteristic
Effectiveness as a binding agent	Body-giving capacity
Gelling activity	Protein stabilization
Gel strength	Freeze—thaw stability
Gel brittleness	Resistance to microbial and enzymatic degradation
Gel softness	Syneresis prevention
Gel hardness	Consistency variation
Gel clarity	Plasticity promotion
Thickening capacity	Glaze-forming capacity
Stabilizing capacity	

Table 19 characterizes important microbial polysaccharides. Xanthan is already used in the food industry. Bacterial alginates are other interesting products. They are very similar to the alginates derived from brown algae and are used as stabilizers and thickening agents for ice creams and a number of other foods. Their physical properties are also similar. Compared with the plant-derived products, they have the advantage of better consistency and greater purity concerning color and optical purity.

Table 19. Microbial Polysaccharides

Polysaccharide	Microorganism	Carbon source	Monomer components of the polysaccharide	Application in food production or preparation
Xanthan (Keltrol, Kelzan, Rhodogel, xanthan gum)	*Xanthomonas campestris*, *Xanthomonas juglandis*, *Pseudomonas aeruginosa*, *Azotobacter vinelandii*	D-Glucose, sucrose, starch syrup, whey	D-Glucose, D-glucuronic acid, D-mannose, acetate, pyruvate	Puddings, soft drinks, alcoholic beverages and drinks, fruit beverages, fruit juices, jellies, confectionaries, jams, canned goods, mayonnaises, seasonings, dressings, instant foods, toppings, foams, sauces, gravies, frozen foods, aroma stabilization, calorie-reduced foods, cake fillings, pie fillings, gelling agents
Dextran	*Leuconostoc mesenteroides* ("*dextranicum*"), *Streptobacterium dextranicum*, *Streptococcus mutans*, *Streptococcus viridans*, *Betacoccus arabinosaceus*	Sucrose	D-Glucose	Baked goods, beverages, sweets, ice creams, fruit syrups

Pullulan	*Pullularia pullulans* (syn. *Aureobasidium pullulans*, *Dematium pullulans*	D-Glucose, sucrose, maltose	D-Glucose	Airtight and edible films or foils, food coatings, sausage skins, calorie-reduced foods
Alginate	*Azotobacter vinelandii*, (*Pseudomonas aeruginosa;* toxicological problems)	Sucrose, D-glucose, (mannitol)	β-D-Mannuronic acid, α-L-guluronic acid, acetate	Ice creams, beer, jellies, dairy products, fruit juices, dressings, puddings, jams, calorie-reduced foods, food coatings, edible sausage skins
Curdlan	*Alcaligenes faecalis* var. *myxogenes*, *Agrobacterium* sp.	D-glucose	D-Glucose	Heat-resistant gels, jellies, mayonnaises, boiling-resistant egg dough foods

Pullulan consists of maltotriose and maltotetraose units combined by 1,6-linkages. It is an odorless, tasteless, fine white water-soluble powder. It increases the stability of foods, gives mouth feeling, and is not metabolized. At high concentrations it is a fungistatic and reduces spoilage in high-moisture products. It seems especially useful for the packing and wrapping of foods. Since pullulan films are of low oxygen permeability, foods with a high fat content can be better protected by pullulan films than by cellophane or polyethylene foil. Pullulan can be made water insoluble by etherification or esterification. Two microbial polysaccharides of future importance in food and nutrition are dextran and curdlan, among others.

EDIBLE ORGANIC ACIDS

Edible acids are indispensable for the production of various foods. They are mainly applied in the confectionary industry, the production of soft drinks, alcoholic beverages, and liqueurs and special diets for certain consumer groups, as buffer substances and acid carriers in baking powder, in the production of jams, jellies, ice creams, processed cheese, and so on.

The most important edible acids are citric acid, malic acid, tartaric acid, acetic acid, lactic acid, and gluconic acid (Miall, 1978; Buchta, 1984).

Citric acid

Originally citric acid was isolated from citrus fruit. In 1893 Wehmer discovered citric acid to be a by-product of the metabolism of the mold *Penicillium glaucum*. *Aspergillus niger* eventually became the most important strain for citric acid production (Röhr et al., 1983; Hossain et al., 1984; Panda et al., 1984). For a very long time citric acid was produced by emerged cultivation or solid-state fermentation (Koji process). Submerged fermentation is being introduced worldwide; however, emerged and solid-state production cannot be totally replaced by the stirred-tank reactor process as of yet.

The biochemical reaction involves the conversion of sugars (normally from molasses) into citric acid. In recent years unconventional media have been increasingly used as carbon sources, n-paraffins (Arima, 1977) being an example. In the latter case special strains of *Corynebacterium*, *Arthrobacter*, and *Brevibacterium* were used. In the meantime *Candida lipolytica* has become the main strain for this substrate. With n-paraffins a large quantity of isocitric acid is produced, which is a disadvantage for the crystallization step; however, from a nutritional and physiological point of view, it is a normal intermediate product of the citric acid cycle, is found in many fruits (citrus fruits and blackberries), and is therefore harmless. Recently citric acid was biosynthesized by immobilized cells of *Saccharomycopsis lipolytica* (Maddox and Kingston, 1983). Now some 100,000 tons of citric acid are produced annually worldwide.

Malic Acid

In nature only the L(−) form of malic acid occurs. The racemate is produced synthetically by the addition of water to fumaric or maleic acid. The L form is derived from the fruits of mountain ash and barberry via the calcium salt. It is used to a limited extent in fruit products and lemonades.

One of the most successful procedures for its biotechnological production was developed by applying immobilized cells (Chibata, 1983) as outlined below:

Brevibacterium flavum in carrageenan (fumarase)

Fumaric acid ⟶ L(−)-malic acid

In Japan it was industrially introduced in 1974 with *B. ammoniagenes* and in 1977 with *B. flavum*. The half-life of the enzymatically active cells is 160 days at 37°C.

Tartaric Acid

Traditionally the acid K^+ salt of D(+)-tartaric acid (tartar) precipitated during the production of wine is used for the production of the free acid. Because of their pleasantly sour taste, tartaric acid and tartar are used in the food industry as acid carriers in baking powder, sweeteners, ice creams, lemonades, various fruit products, baked goods, and complex components for the exclusion of prooxidative metal ions in order to prevent fat autoxidation (lard, tallow). Chemical synthesis always leads to the racemate.

It is also possible to prepare tartaric acid by fermentation using the following reaction and immobilized cells (Kamatani et al., 1976):

Maleic acid ⟶ (chemical oxidation (H_2O_2))

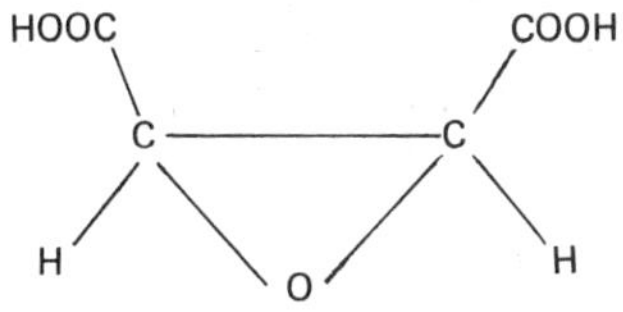

cis-epoxy succinic acid (Na salt)

↓ asymmetrical hydrolysis of the epoxide by immobilized cells (or enzyme solution) of *Alcaligenes levotartaricus* or *Achromobacter tartarogenes* (PAA-gel)

D(+)-tartaric acid (Na salt)

Gluconic Acid

D-Gluconic acid is used as an acid component in the production of various foodstuffs (e.g., fruit juices and lemonades). Its δ-lactone (1,5-lactone ring) serves as a rapid ripening agent for raw sausages. With the addition of gluconic acid (as well as starter cultures), within a few days the required ripening is achieved, as well as reddening and firmness. δ-Gluconolactone is also used for the production of baking powder. In Japan 3000 tons of gluconolactone are required annually for the precipitation of soybean protein in the production of tofu. A further application is in the pharmaceutical sector in the form of Ca-gluconate (oral and intravenous calcium therapy).

Gluconic acid is easily obtained by *A. niger*, as well as other strains of microorganisms—for example *Gluconobacter*, *Pseudomonas*, and *Penicillium* (Röhr et al., 1983b).

Lactic Acid

Lactic acid has a mild, pleasant, characteristic odor and taste. It is not simply "sour" and is often used instead of tartaric or citric acid. It has various food applications: lemonades, essences, fruit juices, jams, syrups, canned fruits, less acidic fruit wines, sweets and baked goods, and in the meat and fish industry. Sodium and calcium lactates are applied in mixtures of baking powders because the liberated lactic acid protects the dough against butyric and acetic acid fermentation; otherwise it supports the growth of sourdough yeasts. Lactic acid is used extensively for preservation (e.g., sour vegetables and sour milk products).

The physiologically useful form of lactic acid is L(+)-lactic acid (Buchta, 1983). Since the turn of the century, already, it has been industrially produced by homofermentative bacteria of lactic acid (chiefly *Lactobacillus delbrückii*, *Lactobacillus leichmannii*, and *Lactobacillus bulgaricus*). Since 1982 immobilized *Lactobacillus delbrückii* cells (entrapped in Ca-alginate) have been used on a laboratory scale with a yield of 90% L(+)-lactic acid. The half-life of the pellets arranged in the reactor (43°C) is 100 days. It is expected that these continuous technologies will soon be brought to the industrial scale.

AMINO ACIDS

Out of the 20 amino acids contained in food proteins, 8 are essential to humans and therefore of special nutritional importance (Table 20). Certain amino acids are necessary for patients in clinical nutrition. For this purpose mainly essential amino acids are needed, as well as glycine as the basic material.

Table 20. Essential Amino Acid Requirements for Adults

	Daily requirement (g)	
Amino acid	Minimal	Recommended
L-Valine	0.8	1.6
L-Leucine	1.1	2.2
L-Isoleucine	0.7	1.4
L-Phenylalanine	1.1	2.2
L-Tryptophan	0.25	0.5
L-Methionine	1.1	2.2
L-Threonine	0.5	1.0
L-Lysine	0.8	1.6
L-Arginine[a]		
L-Histidine[a]		

[a] Essential for infants only.

Within the medical sector arginine (hyperammonemia, liver damage), aspartic acid (heart insufficiency, liver disease, diabetes), cysteine (protects thiol enzymes of the liver, acts as an antioxidant, mercury detoxicant), phenylalanine (DOPA synthesis with Parkinson syndrome) find special application.

In the food industry, furthermore, glutamic acid (in the form of its Na-salt) is important as a flavor enhancer (often synergistically effective together with certain nucleotides).

Large amounts of amino acids are required to supplement feed in animal nutrition (especially with pigs and poultry). This is especially the case for methionine (soybean), lysine (cereals), tryptophan (corn), and threonine (rice, wheat, rye). At present methionine and lysine are still partially produced via chemosynthetic processes and consequently occur as racemates. With the progress of biotechnological procedures, production seems to aim increasingly toward the natural L forms.

In 1982 approximately 450,000 tons of amino acids were produced worldwide, of which nearly 300,000 tons were Na-glutamate and 150,000 tons were for animal breeding. Only 1–2% was reserved for the medical and cosmetic sectors; however, these branches claimed 18% of the total amino acid market, with $1.15 billion.

At present there are several ways of producing L-amino acids (Arima, 1977; Kinoshita and Nakayama, 1978; Chibata, 1983; Soda et al., 1983; Buchta, 1984; Leuenberger and Kieslich, 1984). One can differentiate between three groups:

The chemical synthesis of racemates with subsequent isolation of the L form by the use of aminoacylase

Preparation by the cultivation of microorganisms in stirred tank reactors:

- Wild strains after screening
- Auxotrophic and regulatory mutants

Biotransformation from precursors by means of the following:

- Microorganism culture
- Soluble enzymes
- Immobilized enzymes
- Immobilized microorganisms

These investigations started around the end of the 1950s and reached a climax in the 1970s; they are, however, still not completed.

Chemical Synthesis of Racemates with Subsequent Isolation of the L Forms by the Use of Aminoacylase

The racemic mixture of the desired amino acid is produced by chemical synthesis. The racemates are firstly acetylated (N-Acetyl-D/L-amino acid) and then applied to a reactor with immobilized aminoacylase (e.g., DEAE-Sephadex) or cells. The acylase can split only the N-acyl-L-amino acid. The N-acyl-D-amino acid can be reracemized and transferred to the process again (Fig. 10). The relatively expensive derivatization of amino acids is a disadvantage. The L forms of methionine, phenylalanine, tryptophan, valine, and alanine are produced in this way by a continuous and automatic procedure.

Preparation by Cultivation of Microorganisms in Stirred Tank Reactors

The strains applied to amino acid production must have a defect in their amino acid intermediate metabolism. This makes it possible for the steady state to be interrupted and for unphysiologically high concentrations of a single intermediate product to be secreted into the culture medium. Generally, there are two possibilities:

1. By appropriate screening, a wild strain is selected that has a natural defect and produces a high yield at appropriated phenotypical optimization.
2. By the use of chemical or physical mutagens, the gene expression is blocked for special enzymes so that only special routes of metabolism can be utilized while others are blocked.

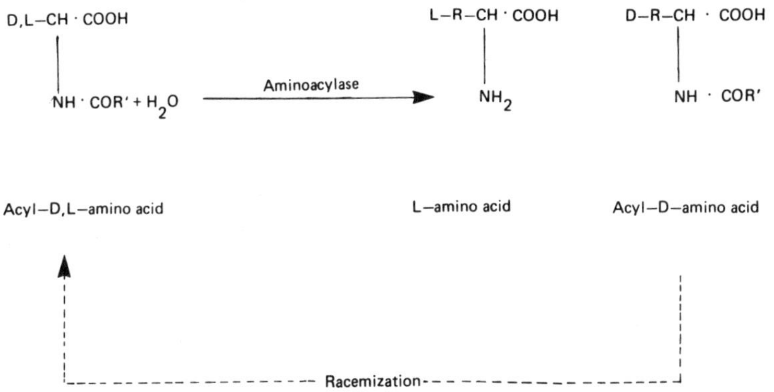

Fig. 10. Isolation of L-amino acids from racemates with immobilized aminoacylase (Tosa et al., 1967).

The principle of direct fermentation on cheap carbon sources (glucose, saccharose, starch hydrolysates, and n-paraffins) is favorable with regard to costs because the expensive chemo- or biosynthesis of precursors is not necessary. This is without doubt the method to be recommended.

By these procedures, numerous amino acids, such as glutamic acid, lysine, threonine, methionine, and isoleucine, are produced on a large scale.

Preparation by Biotransformation from Precursors

Here a precursor of the amino acid to be produced is required which is synthesized with chemosynthetic or biochemical procedures. In principle, four variants exist for the biotransformation:

1. The compound serving as a precursor is inserted into a microorganism culture which carries out the biotransformation. In general, there must be enough cheap culture substrate in the fermenter so that the required energy is not supplied by the precursor metabolism.
2. The reaction of the precursor is completed in an aqueous system by the addition of a purified, soluble enzyme.
3. An immobilized enzyme reactor is used.
4. An immobilized microorganism reactor is used.

The last two methods mentioned here are the most effective. The production of aspartic acid and alanine involves methods applied at an industrial scale.

AROMA PRODUCTION

Natural food flavors are produced by biochemical or chemical processes in plant or animal tissues or they are formed by microorganisms during the ripening, processing, refining, or storage of foods or their raw materials (Table 21). In many cases aroma precursors are formed in a first step and then transferred enzymatically or chemically (by physical influences) into the actual aroma substances. The complexity of the reaction processes linked together results in the formation of a multitude of single components the sum total of which creates the aroma impression (Rothe, 1978; Heath and Allen, 1982–1983).

In the past the aroma-producing industry dealt mainly with the production of natural extracts and the composition of suitable synthesized compounds. The latter procedure is only promising if it succeeds in finding some substances from multicomponent mixtures that have a key character and which decisively represent the total flavor. Numerous natural flavors, however, are only insufficiently produced by this method. Here one might consider the more intensive use of biological aroma-forming systems (Table 22).

Use and Effect of Enzymes

Protein Hydrolysates and Plastein Reaction

Meat aroma concentrates can be produced by heating enzymatic animal and plant protein hydrolysates with reducing sugars in a Maillard reaction. They are used as additives to soups, sauces, gravies, broths, and other specialities. Bitter substances developed by protease reactions (formation of bitter peptides) should be avoided.

In the plastein reaction (Yamashita et al., 1976) proteins with an off-flavor (e.g., beanlike aroma with leguminous proteins) are enzymatically hydrolyzed and then—also by protease reaction—repolymerized or condensed. The off-flavor is then lost. Furthermore, it is possible to introduce essential amino acids into the macromolecule and to increase the biological value of the product. The use of the plastein reaction has not yet reached an industrial scale.

Fat Splitting

Animal lipases are used for improving the flavor of special kinds of cheese (e.g., provolone, Romano). They act as pacemaker enzymes for the microorganisms of the cheese flora which further metabolize the fatty acids. Lipases are also recommended to produce "lipolyzed butter fat" for the intensification of the butter aroma of different foods (Table 23) or commercial butter aroma products.

Table 21. Aroma Formation During Ripening, Processing, and Refining in the Production of Food

Type of reaction	Food
Biochemical (animal or plant enzymes)	Fruits, vegetables, spices, ripened fish or ripened meat
Biochemical (microbial enzymes, partially with enzymes inherent in the substrates)	Butter, cheese, curdled milk products, beer, wine, fermented foods
Biochemical (plant or animal enzymes + microbial enzymes)	Tea, tobacco, ripened dry sausage
Biochemical and chemical (enzymes and physical influences, e.g., heat and distillation processes)	Bread, cocoa, coffee, malt, alcoholic drinks
Chemical (partially with enzymes)	Cooked meat, cooked fish

Source: Ruttloff (1982).

Aroma-Producing Enzymes in Fruit

The investigation of aroma-forming enzymes of fruits and vegetables revealed an interesting effect. Several plant flavors are produced at a higher rate after the destruction of the cell tissue. Obviously the enzymes are thus coming into closer contact with the precursors. Examples are the formation of 2-hexenal in apples, 2,6-nonadienal in cucumbers, and 2- or 3-hexenal in tomatoes. According to Guadagni et al. (1971a,b), an intensive apple aroma is formed within 1 or 2 days if apple peels are stored in a closed vessel at room temperature (Fig. 11). Vamós et al. (1984) used apple peels—as it results as a waste product—for their experiments in aroma production. The juice obtained in the laboratory was two to seven times more aroma intensive than that from untreated peels.

Application of Microorganisms

Flavor Enhancers

The flavor enhancers monosodium glutamate and 5'-ribonucleotides are produced microbiologically. The commercial importance of 5'-ribonucleotides is limited to 5'-inosine monophosphate and

Table 22. Enhancing, Producing, or Keeping Aroma by the Application of Biotechnological Knowledge

Application and action of enzymes
Protein hydrolysates and plasteins
Fat splitting
Aroma-forming enzymes in fruits and vegetables
Use of microorganisms
Flavor enhancers
Glutamate
5'-Ribonucleotides
Milk products
Curdled milk products
Cheese aroma
Butter aroma
Dry sausage ripening
Fruit aroma
Mushroom aroma
Alcoholic beverages
Bread aroma
Fermented foods

Source: Ruttloff (1982).

5'-guanosine monophosphate. They intensify the aroma impression of meat and are used mainly for soups, sauces, canned meat, fish products, tinned greens, and tomato juice. Possible ways of producing them are given in Figure 12.

Milk Products

Curdled milk products of different specialities are being increasingly consumed worldwide. Besides numerous cheese varieties, yogurt, curdled milk, kefir, buttermilk, as well as whey-based beverages (with sugar, fruit pulp, citric acid, citrus, pineapple, orange, mango, and other additives) are to be mentioned. Beverages made of fermented whey (application of lactose yeasts) are also gaining importance.

To rationalize cheese production, one might think of the natural ripening acceleration due to microorganisms or lipolytic and proteolytic enzymes. For example, proteolytic enzyme cultures as well as autolysates of microorganisms have been developed that cause an acceleration in the ripening of different cheeses. It is also possible to cultivate microorganisms of the ripening flora in an aerated fermenter (Ruttloff et al., 1984). Under favorable conditions these

Table 23. Products Conveniently Flavored by the Addition of Lipolyzed Products

Bakery and cereal products
Cake and cookie mixes
Chemically leavened bakery formulations
Sweet doughs
Cheesecake mixes
Pancake mixes
Cereals
Candy and confectionary products
Milk chocolate
Creams and cream centers
Toffee and caramel fudges
Dairy products
Cheese dips
Coffee whiteners
Miscellaneous products
Margarines, imitation dairy products
Popcorn oils
Salad dressings
Sauces, soups, snack foods

Source: Shanani et al. (1976).

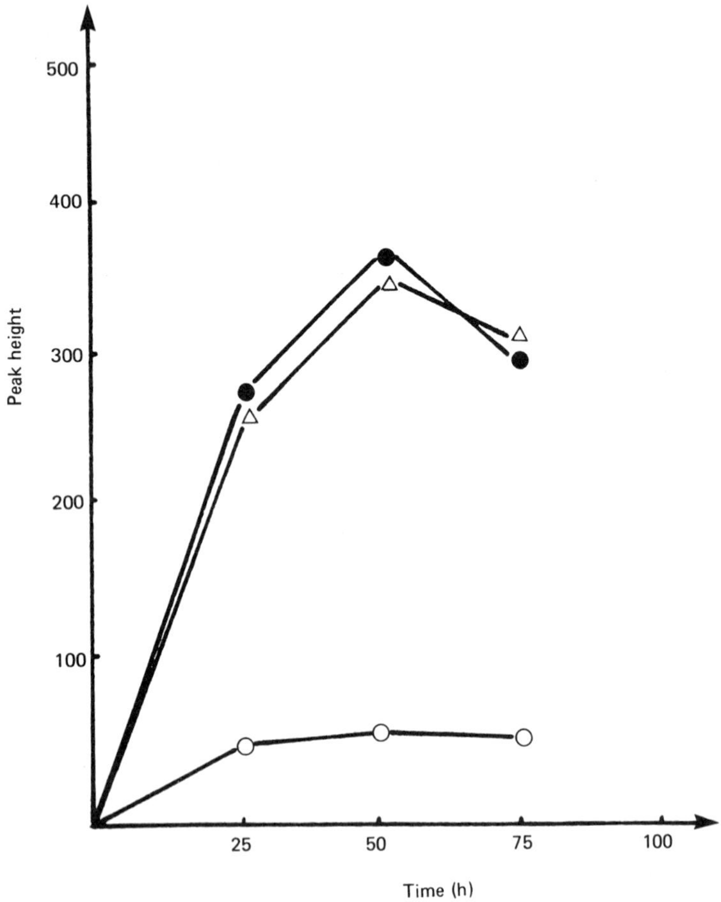

Fig. 11. Development of peak 10 (ethylbutyrate, hexenal, butylacetate) in the flesh and peel of Gravenstein apples at 22°C (Guadagni et al., 1971a,b). ○ flesh; ● unwashed peels; △ washed peels.

microorganisms release the aroma into the fermentation medium. One such system that has been experimentally investigated is lipase—*Penicillium roqueforti*. The fatty acids released by the activity of the enzyme are decarboxylated during the growth of *P. roqueforti* and transformed into methyl ketones which serve as key substances for the Roquefort aroma (Fig. 13). The aroma concentrate (Fig. 14) can be applied to processed cheese, cream cheese preparations, cheese pastes, curd—fat mixtures, and Roquefort butter.

1. RNA —microorganisms→ 5′-nucleotides (1961-)

2. medium —microorganisms→ nucleosides
↓ chemically
5′-nucleotides (1964-)

3. medium —microorganisms→ 5′-nucleotides (1966-)

4. RNA —chemically→ nucleosides
↓ chemically
5′-nucleotides (1967-)

Fig. 12. Industrial production of nucleotides (Arima, 1977).

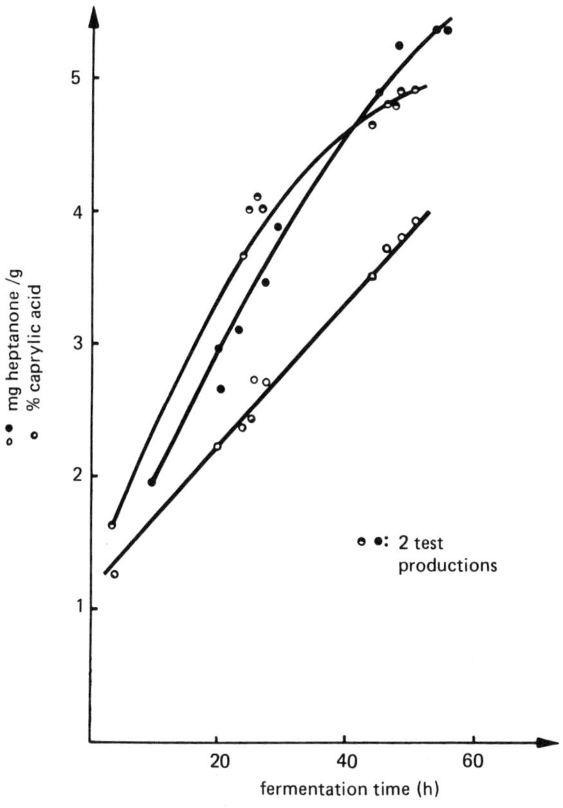

Fig. 13. Biotechnological production of fatty acids and methyl ketones by *P. roqueforti* during fermentation (Rothe and Ruttloff, 1983).

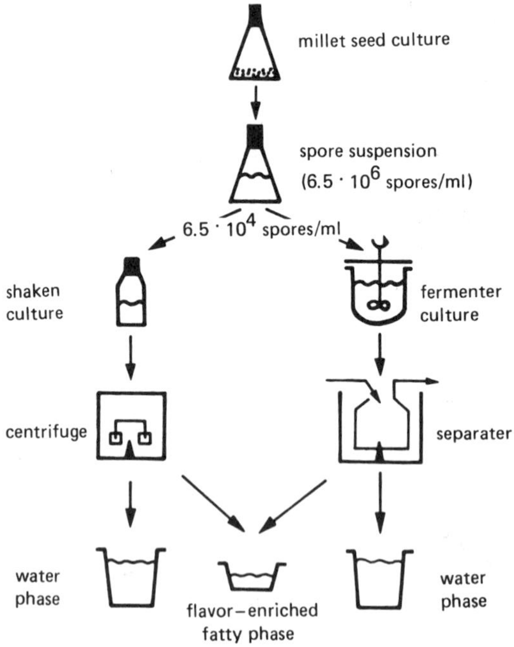

Fig. 14. Biotechnological production of blue cheese flavor concentrate (Ruttloff et al., 1981).

Commercial butter aroma concentrates are frequently needed for the aromatization of food (Table 24). At present they are based mainly on a complex mixture of chemosynthetic compounds, but these mixtures do not always meet the consumer's full acceptance, since a "background aroma" is missing. The microbial production of butter aroma is carried out in principle by inoculating a culture medium containing milk or skimmed milk powder, whey, or other milklike components with microorganisms used in the dairy industry—often together with lipase—and by cultivating it at optimum conditions.

Ripening of Raw Smoked Sausages

As is well known, the ripening of raw smoked sausage takes place during ripening and refining processes that are microbially started or controlled. Mainly strains of *Micrococcus*, *Lactobacillus*, and *Streptomyces* are responsible for this. The considerable variations in the microflora of the raw material have led to the use of starter cultures about 10 years ago. These consist of lyophilized mixed populations of the above-mentioned strains. This makes the ripening more reliable and reproducible and accelerates the process (Table 25).

Fruit Aroma

The 1960s concept of the formation of fruit aroma by so-called aroma-forming enzymes or plant extracts has not yet been successful, so the question for economically suitable sources of enzymes has become the center of interest. According to Hattori et al. (1974), microorganisms might be suited for this, since they are in principle able to synthesize fruit esters. The authors isolated the *Candida* yeast *Oospora suaveolens* from overripe strawberries. This

Table 24. Possible Applications of Butter Aroma

Improvement of the quality of fresh cream butter
Aromatization of products of the oil and margarine industry
Margarine
Frying and baking fats
Grained fat powder
Aromatization of bakery and confectionary goods
Enhancement of the butter taste with calorie-reduced products
Pound cake masses
Snack food products, crackers
Aromatization of products of the cereal products industry
Dried soups
Instant flours
Alimentary pastes
Other products
Ice creams
New foods

Table 25. Advantages of the Application of Starter Cultures at Dry Sausage Ripening

Desired ripening process (prevention of misripening)
Reduced ripening time; dry sausages on sale earlier
Quicker and secured reddening
Decreased water loss
Improved color stability

strain, cultivated on different kinds of heated mashed fruit, synthesizes aroma compositions that, according to gas chromatography results—coincide well or nearly so with those of fresh, that is, nonheated, fruit. Fruit aroma has also been formed upon cultivation of that strain on a synthetic medium. It remains to be seen whether these results can be used for practical purposes in the future.

Mushroomlike Flavor

Mushroomlike flavors are very desirable in the production of soups, sauces, instant products, and vegetable dressings. The commercial preparations are preferably based on chemosynthetic compounds. Mushrooms are cultivated on agricultural and forestry wastes. Obviously basidiomycetes can also be cultivated in a liquid medium (i.e., in aerated fermenters), even though in nature they normally grow only on solid media. At suitable conditions the submerged mycelium synthesizes flavors that are similar to the fruit bodies of *basidiomycetes*. However, up till now it was not possible to obtain economically reasonable quantities of mushroom flavor by the submerged cultivation of the mycelia of mushrooms (Torev, 1968; Dijkstra, 1976; Ghosh and Sengupta, 1978; Hanssen, 1982).

Bread Aroma

The application of modern processing technologies in bread production is often associated with the loss of aroma (Rothe and Ruttloff, 1983). This might also be a reason for the steady drop in bread consumption in the industrialized countries in favor of food rich in energy, especially in fat.

In bread production diverse factors can influence aroma quality (Rothe, 1974). These biochemical, chemical, and physical reactions

Table 26. Factors Influencing Aroma in the Production of Bread and Baked Goods

Influencing factors	Reaction processes
Ingredients	
Flour, yeast, microorganisms, water, sodium chloride, milk, sugar, fat, improvers	
Dough making	
Mixing	Formation of sugars, peptides, amino acids, alcohols
Fermentation	Lactic acid, aldehydes, ketones, keto acids, other reactive organic compounds
Temperature, time, sugar concentration, salt content, enzyme activites, strange germs	
Dividing	Different intensities of the baking process in various parts of the baked goods
Size of dough pieces	
Baking	Crust browning, distillation of ethanol, water, low-boiling-point acids, aldehydes, etc.
Temperature, time, sugar concentration, amino acids, reactive NH_2 groups	

take place simultaneously and successively (Table 26). Great efforts have been made to obtain an aroma of high quality and intensity despite the reduced dough-processing and baking times that are necessary for economic reasons. Biotechnologists should also be involved in solving these problems. One should consider the application of microbial systems promoting aroma formation, as well as optimized or modified fermentation. Up to now such systems have only been optimized from an economic point of view.

Screening and Optimization in Microbial Aroma Production

The methods of screening and process optimization that are routinely used in industrial microbiology are based on certain exactly defined and easily determined quantities (e.g., biomass, amount of an antibiotic, enzyme activity). With the biotechnological production of aromas things are more difficult, for it involves mixtures of many

Table 27. Evaluation of Aroma Production by *P. roqueforti* in Shaken Culture and Submerged Culture

Goal parameters
Aroma quality
Aroma intensity
Tested parameters
Sensory indices
Total flavor quality
Roquefort note
Sharp
Bitter
Soapy
Fruity
Rancid
Instrumental indices
Methyl ketones
Free fatty acids
Volatile fatty acids
Volatile carbonyls
Headspace components
Water and steam volatile components

different components that determine the total quality or create the desired sensory impression only by their complexity.

Sensory evaluations in general are associated with greater costs, which complicates the establishment of screening and optimization programs. It is therefore necessary to complement sensory methods with the increasing use of instrumental methods of qualitative and quantitative evaluation (Table 27). These and related problems require that microbiologists, biochemists, and aroma experts speak the "same language" in the development of processes for the biotechnological production of aroma, that they agree on their goals, and that the qualitative and quantitative evaluation criteria be considered as a unity.

Fermented Foods

An interesting development is taking place in the field of fermented foods (Table 28), which have been used especially in East Asia but also in other regions of the world for centuries (Hesseltine, 1981, 1983; Chang et al., 1983; Chu et al., 1983; Steinkraus, 1983). These products are increasingly consumed in the Western Hemisphere (Kretschmer, 1982). The products in question are produced from raw materials rich in protein and/or carbohydrates that are fermented by fungi and bacteria.

Table 28. Fermented Foods

Foods and products	Raw ingredients	Area where commonly used
Bongkrek	Coconut press cake	Indonesia
Soy sauce (shoyu)	Soybean	Japan
Sufu	Soybean	China
Tao-si	Soybean	Philippines
Tempeh	Soybean	Indonesia, New Guinea, Surinam
Acidophilus milk	Milk	Many countries
Kefir	Milk	Southwestern Asia
Koumiss	Raw mare's milk	Soviet Union (western region)
Yogurt	Milk	Worldwide
Taette	Milk	Scandinavia
Fish sauces	Small fish	Southeast Asia
Katsuobushi	Skipjack tuna	Japan
Kaffir beer	Kaffir corn	Malawi
Magon	Corn	South Africa

Source: Vandamme (1982).

Plant Cell Cultures

An increasingly important field of biotechnological research and development is the cultivation of plant cells. The results of the past 15 years have revealed that plant cell cultivation can already be carried out in fermenters of up to 1000 liters. The production of pharmacologically important preparations is now in the foreground of interest. It is obvious that this method can also be used for the production of aroma compounds; however, its practical use here cannot be expected in the near future (Rehm, 1981): The growth of the cell population is still too slow; the cells suffer from dedifferentiation as the cultivation progresses, and the analytical control of the complex system with several secondary plant stuffs is difficult.

CONCLUSION

All biosynthetic compounds can be decomposed by microorganisms and naturally recycled. Wastes and by-products of the chemical industry do not follow this principle. In many cases they differ in structure from natural substances or microorganisms do not have the necessary enzyme systems to decompose such products. Biotechnology, however, always produces nonpolluting substances or wastes and by-products; their further processing can be far better reconciled with the demands for a nonpolluting product than in the case of synthetic compounds and wastes, which are an increasing burden on our environment. A modern food technology must consider the preservation of the good health, joy of life, and efficiency of the consumer by means of the right nutrition and must also meet the requirements of the environment. In these respects biotechnology may make a valuable contribution.

REFERENCES

Alsop, R. M. (1983). Industrial production of dextrans. In *Progress in Industrial Microbiology*, Vol. 18 (M. E. Bushell, ed.), Elsevier, Amsterdam, pp. 1–44.

Arima, K. (1977). Recent developments and future direction of fermentations in Japan. *Rev. Ind. Microbiol.* *18*:78–116.

Aunstrup, K. (1983). Enzymes of industrial interest in traditional products. *Am. Rep. Ferment. Proc.* *6*:175–201.

Bauch, J., Koslowa, L. I., Sobek, K., Triems, K., Meschtschankin, G. I., and Roschkowa, M. I. (1978). Verfahren zur Gewinnung von "Fermosin"-Futterhefe aus Erdöldestillaten. *Chem. Techn.* *30*:284–287.

Behnke, U. (1985). Bedeutung von Peptiden enzymatisch abgebauter Proteine als Bestandteile von Nahrungsmitteln. *Nahrung* *29*:979–992.

Behnke, U., Ackermann, E., and Ruttloff, H. (1984). Untersuchungen zur enzymatischen Hydrolyse von Rinderknochenschrot. *Nahrung* *28*:397–407.

Bock, W. (1978). Anwendung von pektinolytischen und zellulolytischen Enzymen in der Lebensmittelproduktion. *Lebensm. Ind.* *25*:27–30.

Buchta, K. (1983). Lactic acid. In *Biotechnology*, Vol. 3 (H. Dellweg, ed.), Verlag Chemie, Weinheim, pp. 409–417.

Buchta, K. (1984). Primärmetabolite. In *Handbuch der Biotechnologie*, Vol. 2 (P. Präve, U. Faust, W. Sittig, and D. A. Sukatsch, eds.), R. Oldenbourg Verlag, Munich, pp. 349–376.

Bucke, C. (1983a). Glucose transforming enzymes. In *Microbial Enzymes and Biotechnology* (W. M. Fogarty, ed.), Applied Science, London, pp. 93–129.

Bucke, C. (1983b). Immobilized cells. *Philos. Trans. R. Soc. London B* *300*:369–389.

Catley, B. J. (1983). Regulation of yeast and fungal polysaccharides excluding chitin and cellulose. In *Progress in Industrial Microbiology*, Vol. 18 (M. E. Bushell, ed.), Elsevier, Amsterdam, pp. 129–200.

Chang, S. T., Khor, G. L., NG, C. L., Ong, K. C., Quimio, T. H., Stanton, W. R., and Wang, W. C.-W. (1983). Mushrooms: Producing single cell (microbial) protein on lignocellulosic or other food and agricultural wastes. In *Handbook of Indigenous Fermented Foods* (K. H. Steinkraus, ed.), Marcel Dekker, New York, pp. 573–604.

Chibata, I. (1983). Industrial production of optically active compounds using immobilized biocatalysts. *Basis Life Sci.* *25*: 465–496.

Chu, F. S., Hesseltine, C. W., Lim, G., Nga Been Hen, Stanton, W. R., Tang, T. C., and Wang, H. L. (1983). General papers related to indigenous fermented foods. In *Handbook of Indigenous Fermented Foods* (K. H. Steinkraus, ed.), Marcel Dekker, New York, pp. 605–636.

Dijkstra, F. I. (1976). Submerged cultures of mushroom mycelium as sources of protein and flavour compounds. *Dissertation, Technical Highschool,* Delft, Netherlands.

Dongowski, G., and Bock, W. (1984). Untersuchungen zum Abbau der Pektinstoffe durch Polygalakturonase während der Gewinnung von Möhrensaft. *Lebensm. Ind.* *31*:161–165.

Drechsel, W. and Ruttloff, H. (1975). Zum Einsatz von Proteasen bei der Waffelherstellung. *Baecker Konditor.* *23*:212–213.

Drews, G. (1979). Mikroorganismen-Eiweiss für die Ernährung. *Naturwiss. Rundsch.* *32*:11–17.

Einsele, A. (1983). Biomass from higher n-alkanes. In *Biotechnology,* Vol. 3 (H. Dellweg, ed.), Verlag Chemie, Weinheim, pp. 43–81.

Enari, T.-M. (1983). Microbial cellulases. In *Microbial Enzymes and Biotechnology* (W. M. Fogarty, ed.), Applied Science, London, pp. 183–223.

Faust, U. (1984). Mikrobielle Biomassegewinnung. In *Handbuch der Biotechnologie,* Vol. 2 (P. Präve, U. Faust, W. Sittig, and D. A. Sukatsch, eds.), R. Oldenbourg Verlag, Munich, pp. 485–501.

Faust, U. and Präve, P. (1983). Biomass from methane and methanol. In *Biotechnology,* Vol. 3 (H. Dellweg, ed.), Verlag Chemie, Weinheim, pp. 83–108.

Fogarty, W. M. and Kelly, C. T. (1983). Pectic enzymes. In *Microbial Enzymes and Biotechnology* (W. M. Fogarty, ed.), Applied Science, London, pp. 131–182.

Friedrich, M., Noack, J., Proll, J., and Noack, R. (1985). Vergleichende Untersuchungen zur Absorption enzymatischer Proteinhydrolysate am Dünndarm der Ratte. 2. Mitt. Die Absorption von tryptischen, thermitatischen und tryptisch-thermitatischen Caseinhydrolysaten im Vergleich zum äquimolaren Gemisch freier Aminosäuren. *Nahrung* *29*:167–178.

Fritsche, W. (1978). *Biochemische Grundlagen der Industriellen Mikrobiologie,* VEB Gustav Fischer Verlag, Jena.

Fyfe, J. A. M. and Govan, J. R. W. (1983). Synthesis, regulation and biological function of bacterial alginate. In *Progress in Industrial Microbiology,* Vol. 18 (M. E. Bushell, ed.), Elsevier, Amsterdam, pp. 45–83.

Gabor, R., Täufel, A., and Ruttloff, H. (1982a). Zur Wirkungsweise varschiedener mikrobieller Proteasepräparate auf Weizengluten und -mehl. *Nahrung* *26*:37–46.

Gabor, R., Täufel, A., and Ruttloff, H. (1982b). Veränderungen der Molmassen von Weizenkleberproteinen nach schwacher Proteolyse. *Z. Lebensm. Unters. Forsch.* *175*:399–402.

Ghosh, A. K., and Sengupta, S. (1978). Studies on biochemistry of higher fungi. II. Submerged growth of a few mushrooms in synthetic media. *J. Food Sci. Technol.* *15*:237–242.

Guadagni, D. G., Bomben, J. L., and Hudson, J. S. (1971a). Factors influencing the development of aroma in apple peels. *J. Sci. Food Agric.* *22*:110–114.

Guadagni, D. G., Bomben, J. L., and Harris, J. G. (1971b). Recovery and evaluation of aroma development in apple peels. *J. Sci. Food Agric.* *22*:115–119.
Halpern, M. G. (1981). *Industrial Enzymes from Microbial Sources. Recent Advances*, Noyes Data Corp., Park Ridge, N. J.
Hanssen, H.-P. (1982). Pilzaromen—Aromen aus Pilzen? *Dtsch. Lebensm. Rundsch.* *78*:435–440.
Hartmeier, W. (1977). Immobilisierte Enzyme für die Lebensmittelindustrie. *Gordian* *77*:202–210, 232–236.
Hartmeier, W. (1983). Preparation, properties and possible application of coimmobilized biocatalysts. In *Enzyme Technology. III. Rotenburg Fermentation Symposium 1982* (R. M. Lafferty and E. Maier, eds.), Springer-Verlag, Berlin, pp. 207–217.
Hattori, S., Yamaguchi, Y., and Kanisawa, T. (1974). Preliminary study on the microbiological formation of fruit flavors. Paper presented at IV. International Congress on Food Science and Technology, Madrid.
Heath, H. B. and Allen, B. B. (1982–1983). The application of flavor in food processing. *Perfum. Flavorist* *7*:27–38.
Hesseltine, C. W. (1981). Future of fermented foods. *Proc. Biochem.* *16*:2–13.
Hesseltine, C. W. (1983). The future of fermented foods. *Nutr. Rev.* *41*:293–301.
Hirte, W. and Philipp, B. (1983). Möglichkeiten und Probleme des Einsatzes von Zellulasen in der Landwirtschaft und Lebensmittelindustrie. *Wiss. Z. Humboldt Univ. Berlin Math. Naturwiss. Reihe* *32*:235–245.
Holm, H. P. and Sahm, H. (1983). Induction of cellulases in Trichoderma reesei. In *Enzyme Technology. III. Rotenburg Fermentation Symposium 1982* (R. M. Lafferty and E. Maier, eds.), Springer-Verlag, Berlin, pp. 55–68.
Hossain, M., Brooks, J. D., and Maddox, I. S. (1984). The effect of the sugar source on citric acid production by *Aspergillus niger*. *Appl. Microbiol. Biotechnol.* *19*:393–397.
Hulse, J. H. (1984). Biotechnology: New horns for an old dilemma. *Food Technol. Aust.* *36*:271–277.
Hultin, H. O. (1983). Current and potential uses of immobilized enzymes. *Food Technol.* *37*:66–82.
Jeans, A. (1974). Extracellular microbial polysaccharides. *Food Technol.* *28*:34–40.
Johnson, J. C. (1977). *Industrial Enzymes. Recent Advances*, Noyes Data Corp., Park Ridge, N.J.
Kamatani, Y., Okazaki, H., Imai, K., Fujita, N., Yamazani, Y., and Ogino, K. (1976). Verfahren zur Herstellung von Weinsäure. *German Patent* No. 26 00 589.

Kenne, L. and Lindberg, B. (1983). Bacterial polysaccharides. In *The Polysaccharides*, Vol. 2 (G. O. Aspinall, ed.), Academic, New York, pp. 287–363.
Kinoshita, S. and Nakayama, K. (1978). Amino acids. In *Economic Microbiology*, Vol. 2 (A. H. Rose, ed.), Academic, London, pp. 209–261.
Kirsop, B. H. (1981). Biotechnology in the food processing industry. *Chem. Ind. 7*:218–222.
Klibanov, A. M. (1983). Immobilized enzymes and cells as practical catalysts. *Science 219*:722–727.
Konecny, J. (1975). Enzymes as industrial catalysts. *Chimia 29*:95–102.
Kretschmer, K. F. (1982). Zukünftige Ernährungsmöglichkeiten durch Fermentation aus US-amerikanischer Sicht. *Monatsschr. Brau. 35*:366–368.
Kübler, W. and Schulz, E. (1978). Ernährungsphysiologische und toxikologische Bewertung neuartiger Lebens- und Futtermittel. In *Biotechnologie Forschung Aktuell* (Bundesminister Forschung und Technologie, ed.), Umschau Verlag Breidenstein KG, Frankfurt-am-Main, pp. 36–50.
Kula, M.-R. (1984). Enzyme. In *Handbuch der Biotechnologie*, Vol. 2 (P. Präve, U. Faust, W. Sittig, and D. A. Sukatsch, eds.), R. Oldenbourg Verlag, Munich, pp. 379–411.
Lawson, C. J. and Sutherland, I. W. (1978). Polysaccharides. In *Economic Microbiology*, Vol. 2 (A. H. Rose, ed), Academic, London, pp. 327–392.
Leuenberger, H. G. W. and Kieslich, K. (1984). Biotransformationen. In *Handbuch der Biotechnologie*, Vol. 2 (P. Präve, U. Faust, W. Sittig, and D. A. Sukatsch, eds.), R. Oldenbourg Verlag, Munich, pp. 453–482.
List, D. and Knechtel, W. (1980). Immobilisierte Enzyme in der Lebensmitteltechnologie. *Ind. Obst Gemueseverwert. 65*:415–419.
Maddox, I. S. and Kingston, P. J. (1983). Use of immobilized cells of the yeast *Saccharomycopsis lipolytica* for the production of citric acid. *Biotechnol. Lett. 5*:795–798.
Miall, L. M. (1978). Organic acids. In *Economic Microbiology*, Vol. 2 (A. H. Rose, ed.), Academic, London, pp. 47–119.
Mosbach, K. (1983). The potential in biotechnology of immobilized cells and of immobilized multistep enzyme-coenzyme systems. *Philos. Trans. R. Soc. London B 300*:355–367.
Navarro, A. and Callieri, D. (1984). Horizontal reactor for the continuous production of ethanol by yeasts immobilized in pectin. *Biotechnol. Lett. 6*:465–470.
Oura, E. (1983). Biomass from carbohydrates. In *Biotechnology*, Vol. 3 (H. Dellweg, ed.), Verlag Chemie, Weinheim, pp. 3–41.

Panda, T., Kundu, S., and Majumdor, S. K. (1984). Studies on citric acid production by *Aspergillus niger* using treated Indian cane molasses. *Proc. Biochem. 19*:183–187.

Pastore, M. and Morisi, F. (1976). Lactose reduction of milk by fiber-entrapped β-galactosidase. Pilot plant experiments. *Methods Enzymol. 44*:822–830.

Phillips, K. R. and Lawford, H. G. (1983). Curdlan: Its properties and production in batch and continuous fermentation. In *Progress in Industrial Microbiology*, Vol. 18 (M. E. Bushell, ed.), Elsevier, Amsterdam, pp. 201–229.

Pilnik, W. and Voragen, A. G. J. (1984). Polysaccharides and food. *Gordian 7 and 8*:144–148, 166–171, 195–199.

Rehm, H.-J. (1981). Biotechnologie: Möglichkeiten und Grenzen. *Naturwiss. Rundsch. 34*:494–502.

Richmond, A. (1983). Phototrophic microalgae. In *Biotechnology*, Vol. 3 (H. Dellweg, ed.), Verlag Chemie, Weinheim, pp. 109–143.

Ringpfeil, M. (1983). SCP-Produktion auf der Basis von Kohlenwasserstoffen. *Acta Biotechnol. 3*:227–240.

Röhr, M., Kubicek, C. P., and Kominek, J. (1983a). Citric acid. In *Biotechnology*, Vol. 3 (H. Dellweg, ed.), Verlag Chemie, Weinheim, pp. 419–454.

Röhr, M., Kubicek, C. P., and Kominek, J. (1983b). Gluconic acid. In *Biotechnology*, Vol. 3 (H. Dellweg, ed.), Verlag Chemie, Weinheim, pp. 455–465.

Rothe, M. (1974). Aroma von Brot. In *Handbuch der Aromaforschung* (M. Rothe, ed.), Akademie-Verlag, Berlin, pp. 44–107.

Rothe, M. (1978). Einführung in die Aromaforschung. In *Handbuch der Aromaforschung* (M. Rothe, ed.), Akademie-Verlag, Berlin, pp. 26–32.

Rothe, M. and Ruttloff, H. (1983). Aroma retention in modern bread production. *Nahrung 27*:505–512.

Rothe, M., Ruttloff, H., Herrmann, H., and Engst, W. (1984). Problems of technical production and characterization of blue cheese aroma concentrate. Paper presented at third International Aroma Symposium of Socialistic Countries, Kecskemet, Hungary.

Ruttloff, H. (1978). Entwicklungstrends der Anwendung von Enzymen bei der Lebensmittelproduktion. *Nahrung 22*:883–906.

Ruttloff, H. (1980). Kohlenhydrate. In *Ernährungslehre und Diätetik*, Vol. 1 (H.-D. Cremer, D. Hötzel, and J. Kühnau, eds.), Georg Thieme Verlag, Stuttgart, pp. 60–75.

Ruttloff, H. (1981a). Bedeutung biotechnologischer Verfahren für Nahrung und Ernährung. *Ernaehrung Nutr.* 5:411–420.

Ruttloff, H. (1981b). Stand und Entwicklungstendenzen der mikrobiellen Enzymproduktion. In *Mikrobielle Enzymproduktion* (H. Ruttloff, ed.), Akademie-Verlag, Berlin, pp. 11–21.

Ruttloff, H. (1982). Biotechnology and aroma production. *Nahrung 26*:575–589.

Ruttloff, H. (1983). Biotechnology and its importance for food and nutrition. Paper presented at third Symposium of Socialistic Countries on Biotechnology, Bratislava, Czechoslovakia.

Ruttloff, H., Huber, J., Zickler, F., and Mangold, K.-H. (1979). *Industrielle Enzyme*, Dr. Dietrich Steinkopff Verlag, Darmstadt, pp. 246–358.

Ruttloff, H., Quehl, A., Leuchtenberger, A., Rothe, M., and Engst, W. (1981). Biotechnological production of blue cheese flavour concentrate. Poster on the Second International Aroma Symposium of Socialistic Countries, Rydzyna, Poland.

Ruttloff, H., Körner, D., and Jacob, H. E. (1983). Importance of carbon dioxide for the cultivation of *Thermoactinomyces vulgaris* from spores. *Enzyme Microb. Technol.* 5:129–132.

Ruttloff, H., Quehl, A., and Leuchtenberger, A. (1984). Fermentationstechnische Gewinnung von Käsearoma unter besonderer Berücksichtigung der Richtung Roquefort. 1. Mitt. Literaturüberblick. *Nahrung 28*:873–881.

Sanderson, G. R. and Clark, R. C. (1983). Laboratory-produced microbial polysaccharide has many potential food applications as a gelling, stabilizing, and texturizing agent. *Food Technol. 37*:63–70.

Scharf, U. and Schlingmann, M. (1983). Lebensmitteltechnologie im Aufbruch: Nichtkonventionelle funktionelle Lebensmittelproteine. *Int. Z. Lebensm. Technol. Verfahrenstech. 4*:302–306.

Schwimmer, S. (1981). *Source Book of Food Enzymology.* AVI, Westport, Conn.

Shanani, K. M., Arnold, R. G., Kitara, A., and Dwivedi, B. K. (1976). Die Rolle mikrobieller Enzyme für die Aromabildung in Lebensmitteln. *Biotechnol. Bioeng. 18*:891–907.

Shiotani, T. and Yamane, T. (1981). A horizontal packed bioreactor to reduce CO_2 gas holdup in the continuous production of ethanol by immobilized yeast cells. *Europ. J. Appl. Microbiol. Biotechnol. 13*:96–101.

Soda, K., Tanaka, H., and Esaki, N. (1983). Amino acids. In *Biotechnology*, Vol. 3 (H. Dellweg, ed.), Verlag Chemie, Weinheim, pp. 479–530.

Sprössler, B. and Plainer, H. (1983). Immobilized lactase for processing whey. *Food Technol. 37*:93–95.

Steinkraus, K. H. (1983). *Handbook of Indigenous Fermented Foods.* Marcel Dekker, New York.

Sutherland, I. W. (1983). Extracellular polysaccharides. In *Biotechnology*, Vol. 3 (H. Dellweg, ed.), Verlag Chemie, Weinheim, pp. 531–574.

Täufel, A., Ruttloff, H., and Schlobach, C. R. (1982). Eine neue Technologie für die Herstellung von Semmelmehl. *Lebensm. Ind. 29*:317–320.

Taylor, M. J. and Richardson, T. (1979). Application of microbial enzymes in food systems and in biotechnology. *Adv. Appl. Microbiol. 25*:7–35.

Ter Haseborg, E. (1981). Enzymes in flour and baking applications, especially waffle batters. *J. Proc. Biochem. 16*:16–19.

Torev, A. (1968). Submerged culture of higher fungi mycelium on an industrial scale. *Mushroom Sci. 7*:585–589.

Tosa, T., Mori, T., Fuse, N., and Chibata, I. (1967). Studies on continuous enzyme reactions. IV. Preparation of a DEAE-Sephadex aminoacylase column and continuous optical resolution of acyl-D,L-amino acids. *Biotechnol. Bioeng. 9*:603–615.

Tusé, D. (1984). Single cell protein: Current status and future prospects. *CRC Crit. Rev. Food Sci. Nutr. 19*:273–325.

Uhlig, H. (1984). Einsatz von Enzymen in der Lebensmitteltechnik. *Swiss Food 7–8*:25–36.

United Nations Organization (1981). World population prospects as assessed in 1980. *United Nations*, New York.

Vamós, L., Hersiczky, A., and Kiss-Kutz, N. (1984). Third International Aroma Symposium of Socialistic Countries, Kecskemet, Hungary.

Vanbelle, M., Meurens, M., and Crichton, R. R. (1982). Enzymes in foods and feeds. *Rev. Ferment. Ind. Aliment. 37*:124–135.

Vandamme, E. (1982). Fermented foods and fermentation: Mystique, art and science. *Rev. Ferment. Ind. Aliment. 37*:115–123.

Venkatasubramanian, K. (1980). High fructose corn syrup: Plant design and process economics. In *Enzymes, the Interface Between Technology and Economics* (J. P. Danelny and B. Wolnak, eds.), Marcel Dekker, New York, pp. 53–73.

Voelskow, H. (1983). Extrazelluläre mikrobielle Polysaccharide: Biopolymere mit interessanten Anwendungsmöglichkeiten. *Forum Mikrobiol. 6*:273–282.

Wada, M., Kato, J., and Chibata, I. (1980). Continuous production of ethanol using immobilized growing yeast cells. *Europ. J. Appl. Microbiol. Biotechnol. 10*:275–287.

Ward, O. P. (1983). Proteinases. In *Microbial Enzymes and Biotechnology* (W. M. Fogarty, ed.), Applied Science, London, pp. 251–317.

Yamashita, M., Arai, S., and Fujimaki, M. (1976). Plastein reaction for food protein improvement. *J. Agric. Food Chem.* *24*: 1100–1104.
Yousri, R. M. (1982). Single cell protein: Its potential use for animal and human nutrition. *World Rev. Anim. Prod.* *18*:49–67.

4

Impact of Biotechnology on the Nutritional Quality of Foods

RITA A. TEUTONICO / University of Pennsylvania, Philadelphia, Pennsylvania

NUTRITIONAL QUALITY OF FOODS AND NUTRITIONAL STRESS FACTORS

The nutritional quality of foods depends on the total amount of nutrients present in the food consumed, as well as the levels of antinutritive factors. Nutritional stress factors are defined as elements which increase human nutritional requirements by destroying essential nutrients, making essential nutrients unavailable, interfering with the utilization of essential nutrients, interfering with the digestion of food, and/or decreasing food intake (Table 1). Several stress factors occur as components of plant or animal tissue, while others originate in processing, spoilage of foods, or from the environment, that is, the soil, water, and air (Knorr, 1981).

Some nutritional stress factors present in foods are given in Table 2. For example, phytic acid, the essential storage form of phosphorus in plants (Sutardi and Buckle, 1985), chelates ions such as calcium, magnesium, iron, and especially zinc to form compounds of low solubility (Oberleas, 1973), while oxalates affect absorption by forming insoluble salts with calcium (Hodgkinson, 1977), iron (Gillooly et al., 1983), and to some extent zinc (Kelsay, 1982). Cottonseed meal contains the polyphenol gossypol, which chelates metals and has been reported to cause anemia, as well as poisoning, in nonruminants (Singleton and Kratzer, 1973). Tannins—polyphenolic compounds present in legumes, cereals, and leafy vegetables—inactivate enzymes and make proteins indigestible (Reddy et al., 1985). They also have been shown to reduce the bioavailability of iron and vitamin B_{12} in rats (Liener, 1980). Epidemiological observations have correlated the intake of tannins with esophageal cancer in humans (Morton, 1978).

Table 1. Stress Factors Associated with Food

Deficiencies of essential nutrients in the diet
Imbalance among the essential nutrients
Presence of deleterious compounds which
Destroy essential nutrients
Make essential nutrients unavailable
Interfere with the utilization of essential nutrients
Interfere with the digestion of food
Decrease the intake of food

Source: Lepkovsky (1953).

Raw egg white contains the protein avidin, which forms a stable complex with biotin in the intestinal tract and makes it biologically unavailable (Somogyi, 1973). Avidin also inactivated biotin-containing enzymes such as pyruvate carboxylase in vitro (Cazzulo and Stoppani, 1967).

Other stress factors interfering with the enzymatic digestion of foods are trypsin inhibitors, which were found in significant amounts in legumes (Liener and Kakade, 1980), as well as in cereal grains, leafy vegetables, and sweet corn (Chen and Mitchell, 1973). The trypsin inhibitors present in raw soybean meal accounted for 30–50% of the growth-inhibiting effect and for nearly all of the pancreatic hypertrophic response of rats (Rackis, 1965). In addition, the polyphenol chlorogenic acid present in sunflower seed meal inhibited the activity of digestive enzymes (Delic et al., 1972), while the alkaloid solanine in potatoes inhibited cholinesterase activity (Whitaker and Feeney, 1973).

Goitrogenic stress factors, such as thioglycerides, were present in high levels in rapeseed (Liener, 1977). Since livestock forage on the leaves of *Brassica* species, which are known to yield thiocyanate ion (Tookey et al., 1980), many researchers have investigated the goitrogenic potential of milk, but it does not seem that enough thiocyanate ion would be transferred to milk to make it goitrogenic (Piironen and Virtanen, 1963).

Lima beans, sorghum, and cassava contain cyanogenetic glucosides which release cyanide when the plant cells are disrupted and can result in chronic toxicity (Conn, 1973).

Naturally occurring antivitamins of thiamine, the thiaminases, are structure-modifying antagonists present predominantly in the

Table 2. Nutritional Stress Factors in Food

Stress factor	Chemical nature	Occurrence	Action	Dietary effect
Phytates	Organic acid	Cereals, legumes	Chelate metals	Reduce mineral availability
Oxalates	Organic acid	Spinach, amaranth	Chelate cations	Calcium and iron unavailable
Gossypol	Polyphenol	Cottonseed	Chelate metals	Anemia
			Reactive	Potential poisoning
Tannins	Polyphenol	Beans	Bind proteins	Proteins insoluble, inactivate enzymes
		Sorghum		Reduce iron and B_{12} availability
Avidin	Protein	Egg white	Binds biotin	Biotin unavailable
Trypsin inhibitors	Protein	Legumes, cereals	Inhibit proteolysis	Reduce protein digestibility
Solanine	Alkaloid	Potato	Inhibits cholinesterase	Gastrointestinal or neurological disorders, potential poisoning
Goitrin	Glucosinolate	Rapeseed	Goiterogenic	Reduces iodine uptake
Limarin	Cyanogenetic glucoside	Cassava	Releases cyanide	Potential poisoning
Thiaminases	Protein	Fish	Destroy thiamine	Possible thiamine deficiency

Source: Berardi and Goldblatt (1980), Hodgkinson (1977), Lepkovsky (1953), Liener (1980), Liener and Kakade (1980), Montgomery (1980), Oberleas (1973), Reddy et al. (1985), Singleton and Kratzer (1973), and Tookey et al. (1980).

viscera of carp, as well as in other freshwater and marine fishes and shellfish (Somogyi, 1973). Thiaminases have also been isolated from the tissues of warm-blooded animals (Sure and Ford, 1943).

EFFECTS OF PROCESSING ON NUTRITIONAL QUALITY

Traditional processing methods can improve nutritional quality by increasing food palatability and digestibility or increasing nutrient availability by destroying toxic factors or minimizing their effects (Hudson, 1980). Processing also may create stress factors by destroying or removing essential nutrients, making them unavailable, or decreasing digestibility (Lepkovsky, 1953).

Processing methods can be categorized as separation, preservation, and assembly–formulation–preparation methods, involving mechanical, physical, chemical, and biological modes of operation (Knorr, 1985; see Table 3). Some examples of their application are given below.

Dehulling (*mechanical separation*) significantly decreased the tannin level in some dry beans and increased iron absorption but also produced substantial losses of protein (Reddy et al., 1985). Milling of flour resulted in the removal of phytate (Kirk, 1979) but also caused a reduction of more than 70% in total ash, copper, iron, zinc, vitamins E and B_6, thiamine (B_1), riboflavin (B_2), and niacin (Nesheim, 1974).

Physical separation methods such as extraction methods are very effective for the removal of some nutritional stress factors, including separation of gossypol from cottonseed in a cyclone or by solvent treatments (Damaty and Hudson, 1975; Hudson, 1980) and thioglycosides from rapeseed by extraction with hot water, acetone, or alkali (Liener, 1977). Alkali treatment also substantially reduced the amount of tannin in sorghum (Price et al., 1979), but it decreases protein quality by forming artifact amino acids, such as lysinoalanine (Hudson, 1980), and converting polyphenols to quinones which oxidize amino acid side chains (Finot, 1983).

The principal effect of heat treatment, a *physical preservation* method, is protein denaturation (Karmas, 1975), thus destroying undesirable microorganisms, inactivating enzymes (Nesheim, 1974), and improving digestibility (Synge, 1976). Beneficial effects of moist heat treatment on plant products include the liberation of bound niacin in cereals (Bender, 1978), the destruction of antidigestive factors in legumes and cereals (Anantharaman and Carpenter, 1969; Lee, 1977), the removal of hydrogen cyanide from cassava

Table 3. Simplified Organization of Unit Operations Used in Food Processing

Method	Mode of operation	Examples
Separation	Mechanical	Cleaning, grinding, filtration, centrifugation
	Physical	Crystallization, extraction, membrane separation
	Chemical	Hydrolysis
	Biological	Fermentative separation, enzymatic treatment
Preservation	Mechanical	Washing, soaking
	Physical	Dewatering, temperature modification, protective packaging
	Chemical	Smoking, curing, pH modifications, salting
	Biological	Fermentation
Assembly–formulation–preparation	Mechanical	Mixing, extruding
	Physical	Cooking, baking
	Chemical	Aging
	Biological	Sprouting, malting

Source: Knorr (1985); reprinted from *Food Technol. 39* (1985).

(Hudson, 1980), the conversion of much free gossypol to the bound, nontoxic form (Singleton and Kratzer, 1973), and the reduction of the chlorogenic acid level of sunflower meal (Sastry and Subramanian, 1985). Phytic acid, though, was only heat labile at high temperatures—as in autoclaving soy isolates for 4 hr at 115°C, for example (Sutardi and Buckle, 1985; Rackis, 1974)—and excess heat adversely affected the nutritive value of soy products and sunflower meal by destroying cystine and lysine (Liener, 1978; Sastry and Subramanian, 1985), reducing protein availability due to Maillard browning (Lee, 1977), forming new linkages between and within proteins (Ford, 1973), and destroying vitamins A, B_1, B_2, C, and E (Lee, 1977).

While freezing and dehydration did not cause major losses in vitamins (Nesheim, 1974), water-soluble vitamins and minerals were lost during the preparative steps of washing, trimming, and blanching vegetables (Carlsson and Hallqvist, 1981).

Heat treatment also has both positive and negative effects on animal products. For example, there was no significant decrease in the biological value or digestibility of milk due to pasteurization (Smith, 1970), but pasteurization resulted in almost complete destruction of vitamin C, a 10% loss of vitamin B_{12} (Bender, 1978), thiamine losses of 3–20%, and only slight losses in niacin (Wanner, 1971). Vitamins A and D, and biotin were stable during the heating of milk (Bender, 1978), while riboflavin was destroyed by exposure to light (Wanner, 1971).

Spray-drying milk did not affect lysine availability, but roller drying reduced both total and available lysine levels (Mauron et al., 1955). Instantization of dried skim milk had no effect on B vitamins and only a slight effect on the vitamin C present (Bender, 1978).

There was no loss of essential amino acids when bacon, pork, beef, chicken, and shrimp were freeze-dried, cooked, canned, or irradiated (Thomas and Calloway, 1961), but the frying of bacon at 170°C for 6 min destroyed 20–30% of the vitamin C (Newmark et al., 1974).

Effects of irradiation on nutrients vary with the food and dose applied, with thiamine being the most sensitive vitamin (Bender, 1978). Irradiation had little or no effect on the vitamin C and carotene content of fruits and vegetables, such as the mango, tomato, and potato, while irradiation of orange juice and carrot pulp produced a 23–48% loss of vitamin C and a 30% loss of beta-carotene, respectively. Maize which had been disinfected and then stored for 4 years showed no changes in protein content and quality or vitamin contents. Beef and poultry irradiated at −40°C had only minor changes in protein and did not contain free radicals or antithiamine properties (Murray, 1983). Up to 50% of the thiamine was lost when fish was treated with 0.6 Mrad, while niacin was unaffected (Kennedy and Ley, 1971). Irradiation of milk with 440 Krad destroyed 40% of its carotenoids, 70% of its retinol, and 60% of its tocopherol content (Kung et al., 1953), while a 1-Mrad dose can destroy 90% of the vitamin C, 80% of vitamin B6, 75% of the riboflavin, and some of the niacin (Kon, 1961).

Chemical preservation through salting usually has a small but variable effect on nutrients (Karmas, 1975), though removal of brine in the preparation of fresh cucumber pickles resulted in a loss of water-soluble constituents.

The salting and smoking of herring destroyed 30–40% of the iodine (Bender, 1978). Curing is an advanced form of salting in which not only salt but also nitrate and/or nitrite, sugar, and other ingredients are added (Daun, 1975). Liquids exude from the meat during curing, resulting in a 0.35–1.2% loss of protein in the curing of ham (Hoagland et al., 1947). Losses of thiamine were 20% in the curing and smoking of pork hams, but mostly due to smoking, and there was no loss of riboflavin or niacin (Dunker et al., 1953). Ascorbic acid is added to increase the rate of curing and block formation of nitrosamines (Bender, 1978). In general, losses of nutrients due to curing are small, and the vitamin, mineral, and macronutrient content of processed meat products is similar per unit protein to that of unprocessed meats (Watt and Merrill, 1963).

Chemical additives can alter nutrient losses, such as sulfur dioxide, which preserved vitamin C in dehydrated potatoes but caused an increased loss of thiamine (Nesheim, 1974), or additives can affect nutrient availability, such as caffeine or polyvinylpyrrolidone, which interacted with tannins in beans and cereals to liberate proteins and increase digestibility (Reddy et al., 1985). Sulfite added to comminuted meats destroyed thiamine (Bender, 1978), while hydrogen peroxide addition to milk destroyed vitamin C completely and reduced protein quality by 6% (Kon, 1961).

Physical assembly—formulation—preparation methods include the baking of bread and the cooking of meats. Bread baking increased the availability of amino acids, especially methionine, tryptophan, and threonine, relative to unground wheat (Hepburn et al., 1966), but there was a 10% decrease in protein quality due to loss of available lysine, especially in the crumb (Rosenberg and Rohdenburg, 1951). There was no loss in riboflavin or niacin on bread baking, but 15–30% of the thiamine was lost (Zaehringer and Personius, 1949), while in breads baked for a long time, such as pumpernickel, almost all of the thiamine was destroyed (Spicher, 1983).

Proteins suffer little or no damage when meats are cooked, even at the high temperatures of roasting, except for a decrease in amino acid availability through Maillard browning (Bender, 1978). Thiamine was the most heat-labile vitamin, with 40—50% lost in braised beef and 20—30% from pork (Farrer, 1955). In contrast, cooking increased the available thiamine in fish by destroying the thiaminases present in raw fish (Wittlife and Airth, 1970).

Thus physical, chemical, and mechanical processes can increase nutrient availability and reduce the level of some nutritional stress factors in foods.

EFFECTS OF BIOLOGICAL UNIT OPERATIONS ON NUTRITIONAL QUALITY

According to the European Federation of Biotechnology, biotechnology is the integrated use of biochemistry, microbiology, and engineering sciences in order to achieve the technological application of the capabilities of microorganisms, cultured tissue cells, and parts thereof (Kuenzi et al., 1985). Many classic food processes, such as the production of vinegar and alcoholic beverages, cheese making, the ripening of cured meats, and enzymatic meat tenderizing, are based on biotechnological principles (Jarvis and Holmes, 1982; Knorr and Sinskey, 1985). Biological processes traditionally, though, have not been included as unit operations in food processing and there is limited information on the effects of these processes on nutritional quality (Teutonico and Knorr, 1985a).

Enzymatic Treatment (Separation)

Enzymes are used for fruit and vegetable juice production. For example, the combined use of pectinases and cellulases for carrot juice production increased juice yield from 65 to 95% and carotene content from 7 to 60% (Ruttloff, 1985).

Enzymatic treatment also can reduce the level of nutritional stress factors. For example, raffinose and stachyose present in soybeans cause flatulence in humans and animals because there is no α-galactosidase activity in the mammalian intestine (Rackis, 1977), thus decreasing the intake of soy products. Treatment of soybean meal with invertase and α-galactosidase resulted in conversion of these oligosaccharides to monosaccharides (Delente and Ladenburg, 1972). α-Galactosidase, produced by culturing *Aspergillus awamori* on wheat bran, was used in a hollow fiber reactor to convert the oligosaccharides of soy milk to their constituent hexoses (Smiley et al., 1976).

Lactase (β-galactosidase) catalyzes the breakdown of lactose in milk or whey to glucose and galactose, thus making these products digestible for lactose-intolerant people (Hultin, 1983; Ruttloff, 1985) and immobilized lactase has already been used commercially to produce lactose-free milk (Cooney, 1983).

Addition of phytase (on a 2% flour basis) and phosphatase (0.11%) reduced the initial phytate phosphorus concentration of whole wheat flour dough to 12.5 and 8.3% of its initial values, respectively, with a further reduction in phytate content occurring during the baking and storage of the whole wheat breads (Knorr et al., 1981). Similarly, treating raw white beans with wheat germ phytase decreased their phytate level (Kon et al., 1972). In addition, Liener (1977) suggested adding microbial enzymes to such foods as rapeseed and cassava to selectively detoxify them.

Industrial production of amino acids for food or feed suplementation has utilized immobilized aminoacylase since 1969 to isolate the natural L isomer amino acids from chemically synthesized racemic mixtures (Hultin, 1983; Ruttloff, 1985).

Fermentation (Preservation)

Besides its preservative effect, fermentation also affects the texture, flavor, and nutritive quality of the raw substrate. Nutrient losses may occur due to leaching, destruction by light, heat, or oxygen, or by microbial utilization (Jones, 1975), though the loss of nutrients during fermentation is commonly small and there may even be an increase in the nutrient level through microbial synthesis (Karmas, 1975).

Effects of Fermentation on Macronutrients

Fermentation did not change the protein content of fermented *grains and oilseeds* (Table 4), but protease production by *Rhizopus oligosporus* in tempeh (fermented, partially cooked soybeans) and oncom (fermented peanut press cake) increased the free amino acid levels by as much as 85-fold (Murata et al., 1967) and digestibility increased over unfermented beans (Zamora and Veum, 1979; van Veen and Steinkraus, 1970). The protein efficiency ratio (PER) of most fermented oilseed products was the same as that of the properly heated, unfermented substrate (Wang and Hesseltine, 1981; Quinn et al., 1975), while an increase in PER was reported for miso (steamed soybeans mixed with *Aspergillus oryzae*-fermented rice and inoculated with *Saccharomyces rouxii* or *Streptococcus faecalis*) and wheat–soybean tempeh (Beuchat, 1983; Wang et al., 1968). The total fat content of fermented rice, wheat, soy, and peanut was unchanged by fermentaiton, but lipid hydrolysis resulted in an increase in the free fatty acid levels (Beuchat, 1983; van Buren et al., 1972).

Fermentation of grains led to a highly significant increase in available lysine in wheat, oats, rice, millet, and maize (Hamad and Fields, 1979) and in isoleucine and leucine levels in fermented rice meal (Tongnual and Fields, 1979). The protein quality of the final products was found to vary, depending on the particular organisms used for fermentation (Beuchat, 1983).

In addition to mold fermentations, the nutritive value of grain proteins was improved by fermentation with sourdough bacteria and yeast. Lactic acid fermentation is used to preserve many foods through the production of acids which inhibit undesirable microbial growth (Pederson, 1960), but relatively little information is available on the effect of such fermentation on the nutritive value of plant foods (Fleming and McFeeters, 1981). The proteinases and peptidases of the lactic acid bacteria increased the levels of free amino acids, especially leucine, phenylalanine, methionine, tyrosine, isoleucine, and lysine (Spicher, 1983). The total protein content of acid-leavened idli (rice and black gram fermented by lactic acid bacteria) was unchanged, though the amino-nitrogen level increased (Akolkar, 1977). Though the fat, crude fiber, crude protein, and ash content of maize meal are not affected significantly by fermentation (Akinrele and Bassir, 1967), traditional preparation of ogi (*Lactobacillus plantarum*, yeast, and mold fermentation of maize)

Table 4. Effects of Fermentation on Macronutrients in Grains and Oilseeds

Nutrient or product	Quality factor[a]				Reference
	Protein efficiency ratio	Digestibility	Free amino acids	Free fatty acids	
Protein					
Grains					
Wheat tempeh	+				Wang et al. (1968)
Wheat			++ lysine		Hamad and Fields (1979)
Maize, oats, rice, millet			+ lysine		Hamad and Fields (1979)
Rice meal			+ isoleucine, + leucine		Tongnual and Fields (1979)
Oilseeds					
Miso	+	+			Beuchat (1983)
Wheat–soybean	+				Wang et al. (1968)
Soybean	N.D.	N.D.			Wang et al. (1968)

		+	++		Murata et al. (1967)
	N.D.	+			Zamora and Veum (1979)
	N.D.	+			van Veen and Steinkraus (1970)
			+		Jones (1975)
	+				Liener (1978)
Natto	+				Liener (1978)
Oncom	N.D.	N.D.			Wang and Hesseltine (1981)
		+			Beuchat (1983)
	N.D.	+			van Veen and Steinkraus (1970)
Sunflower meal			+ lysine		Canella et al. (1984)
Lipid					
Oilseeds					
Miso				+	Beuchat (1983)
Soybean tempeh				+	Murata et al. (1967)
Oncom				+	Beuchat (1983)

[a] +, increase; ++, ⩾ fivefold increase; −, decrease; N.D., not different from unfermented product.
Source: Reprinted from *Food Technol.* 39 (1985).

resulted in substantial losses in lysine (Banigo and Muller, 1972) and tryptophan (Makinde and La Chance, 1976), as well as a reduction in PER (Akinrele and Bassir, 1967).

Lactic acid bacteria metabolized stachyose and raffinose during soy milk fermentation, which increased its digestibility and acceptability (Mital and Steinkraus, 1979). Likewise, fermented soy idli batter contained elevated free sugar levels and the total sugar content was reduced (Akolkar, 1977).

Fermentation of doughs by yeast decreased the caloric content by 20% owing to conversion of sugars to ethanol and carbon dioxide (Reed, 1981). In addition, use of 5–7% yeast (based on the weight of flour) increased the level of the limiting amino acid lysine in bread, since yeast contains 1.3% lysine (Spicher, 1983).

The primary *cultured dairy products* include sour cream, cultured buttermilk, *acidophilus* milk, and yogurt, which result from inoculation with selected lactic acid bacteria; kefir and koumiss, which are acidic–alcoholic products of fermentation by lactic acid bacteria and yeast (Jones, 1975); as well as cottage cheese, which is creamed milk coagulated by lactic bacteria and a small amount of rennet (Bottazzi, 1983).

Most fermented milk products have nutrient contents comparable to the milks from which they are prepared (Table 5), though the lactose content is reduced (Jones, 1975). Lactic acid accumulated to a maximum of 1.5% in cultured milk, which inhibited undesirable microbial growth, and reduced the lactose content by 30% (Vedamuthu, 1982). Lactose-intolerant persons can thus consume cultured milk products without illness (Gallagher et al., 1974).

In addition to lactose metabolism, starter cultures also hydrolyze proteins to obtain nitrogen for growth (Speck, 1981). This protein breakdown produced the desired curd characteristics of the products, as well as improved digestibility by humans (Davis and Latto, 1957; Breslaw and Kleyn, 1973). In the preparation of dahi, an Indian food, from lactic fermentation of cow or buffalo milk, the total nitrogen content was unchanged, the protein nitrogen decreased slightly, and the nonprotein and ammonia–nitrogen levels increased (Khambatta and Dastur, 1951). Fermentation increased the amount of free amino acids in yogurt, while bacterial cell proteins contributed to the overall protein content and amino acid composition (Bottazzi, 1983).

The nutrient levels in cheese depend upon the method of curd coagulation, the extent and method of whey removal, and the ripening process (Jones, 1975). The greatest losses of nutrients occurred at the whey separation stages (Kon, 1959), in which water-soluble nutrients were partitioned into the whey while protein and fat formed the curd. Soluble proteins, such as globulins and albumins, though, remained in the whey and resulted in a 25% loss in total protein content. The processes which affected nutrients during ripening, including proteolysis, lipolysis, and lactose fermentation (Jones, 1975), not only produced the flavor and texture characteristics of the different cheese varieties but also released free fatty acids and amino acids (Law, 1982).

Fermentation of *meat* products prolongs their shelf life and substitutes for alternative means of preservation, such as high heat and chemical treatments, that may reduce nutritive value (Bacus and Brown, 1981). The major changes produced in sausages by fermentation included conversion of sugars to lactic acid and nitrate to nitrite (Palumbo and Smith, 1977). In addition, dry sausage ripening involves lipolysis, which decreased triglyceride levels with corresponding increases in free fatty acids and diglycerides (Demeyer et al., 1974), as well as proteolysis, which resulted in increased free ammonia and free amino-nitrogen levels (Dierick et al., 1974).

Effects of Fermentation on Vitamins (Micronutrients)

Microorganisms differ in their ability to synthesize vitamins, thus affecting the final composition of fermented *grains and oilseeds*. The tempeh mold, *R. oligosporus*, has a great capacity to synthesize both niacin and riboflavin but requires thiamine for maximum growth (Wang and Hesseltine, 1981), and researchers (Table 6) have reported three- to fivefold increases in niacin and riboflavin levels in tempeh relative to raw soybeans (Beuchat, 1983; Roelofsen and Talens, 1964). While products fermented by *R. oligosporus* had decreased thiamine levels, natto (partially cooked soybeans fermented by *Bacillus subtilis*) contained threefold higher thiamine levels than raw soybeans, as well as increased riboflavin and B_{12} (Sano, 1961). Therefore the nutrient composition of the final fermented product can be affected by the choice of fermenting microorganisms.

Lactic acid fermentation of idli produced increased levels of thiamine and riboflavin (Rajalakshmi and Vanaja, 1967), as well as free and total niacin (Rajalakshmi et al., 1964). Preparation of Nigerian gari (lactic acid and yeast fermentation of cassava), though, resulted in losses of 95% of the ascorbic acid originally present in the cassava pulp (Ogunsua, 1977), while riboflavin, thiamine, and niacin were lost from fermented maize meal (ogi), mostly owing to washing and steeping of the meal (Akinrele, 1970).

While fermentation of *vegetables* has little effect on their nutrient content, water-soluble constituents were lost when the brine was discarded during the desalting of cucumbers (Jones, 1975; Fellers, 1971). Since sauerkraut is fermented with only 2.25% salt, there was no desalting and thus no major leaching losses of nutrients (Jones, 1975), so sauerkraut had the same vitamin C content as raw cabbage (Pederson et al., 1939). In addition, the amount of ascorbic acid in sauerkraut canned immediately after fermentation remained relatively constant, owing to the protective effect of the

Table 5. Effects of Fermentation on the Composition of Animal Products

Products	Components[a]	Reference
Cultured dairy products	Macronutrients	
	− lactose	Vedamuthu (1982)
	+ protein digestibility	Speck (1981), Davis and Latto (1957), Breslaw and Kleyn (1973)
Yogurt	+ free amino acids	Bottazzi (1983)
	Micronutrients	
	+ riboflavin	Kon (1972)
Cottage cheese	+ niacin, B_6, B_{12}, folic acid	Reif et al. (1976)
Dahi	− vitamin A	Narayanan et al. (1954)
Dahi[b]	− thiamine (B_1), B_2, nicotinic acid	Rao and Basu (1952)
Dahi[c]	+ B_1	Rao and Basu (1952)
Yogurt	− vitamin C	Watt and Merrill (1963)
	Nutritional stress factors	
	− nitrosamines	Rowland and Grasso (1975)
Lactobacillus acidophilus	− procarcinogen activation	Goldin and Gorbach (1977), Goldin et al. (1980)
Yogurt	− serum cholesterol	Mann (1977), Mann and Spoerry (1974)

Cheese		
	Macronutrients	
Ripened cheeses	+ free amino acids	Law (1982)
Ripened cheeses	+ free fatty acids	Law (1982)
	Micronutrients	
Ripened cheeses	− vitamin C, N.D. vitamin A	Kon (1972)
Cheddar cheese	− calcium, − phosphorus	Mattick (1951)
Cottage cheese	− calcium, − phosphorus	Lampert (1970)
	Nutritional stress factors	
	+ tyramine	Liener (1980)
Meat		
	Macronutrients	
Dry fermented sausage	+ free fatty acids	Demeyer et al. (1974)
Dry fermented sausage	− histidine, − tyrosine	Dierick et al. (1974)
Dry fermented sausage	+ free amino nitrogen	Dierick et al. (1974)
	Micronutrients	
Cured ham	(−) B_1, B_2, niacin	Rice et al. (1947)
	Nutritional stress factors	
Dry fermented sausage	++ histamine, ++ tyramine, ++ putrescine, + cadaverine	Dierick et al. (1974)
Dry fermented sausage	++ histamine	Taylor et al. (1978)

[a] +, increase; ++, ⩾ 10−fold increase; −, decrease; (−), slight decrease; N.D., not different from unfermented product.
[b] *Lactobacillus bulgaricus* + *Lactobacillus cremoris* fermentation.
[c] *Streptococcus lactis* + *Streptococcus cremoris* fermentation.

Table 6. Effects of Fermentation on Vitamins in Plant Foods

Product	Vitamin[a]								Reference
	B_1	B_2	Niacin	B_6	B_{12}	C	A	E	
Grains									
Wheat tempeh[b]	–	+	++						Wang and Hesseltine (1966)
Oilseeds									
Soy tempeh[b]	–	+	++						Steinkraus et al. (1961)
	–	+	+	++	+				Murata et al. (1967)
	–	++	+						Roelofsen and Talens (1964)
								(+)	Chen et al. (1972)
		+	++		+				Beuchat (1983)
	–		++		++				van Veen and Steinkraus (1970)

Miso[c]						+	Beuchat (1983)
Natto[d]	+	+	++				Sano (1961)
Vegetables							
Pickles[e,f]				–	–		Jones (1975)
Pickles, salt stock[e,f]	–			–	–		Fellers (1971)
Pickles, dill[e,f]				–	N.D.		Fellers (1971)
Beets, peas, turnips[e,f]				–	–		Fellers (1971)
Sauerkraut[e]				N.D.			Pederson (1960)

[a]+, increase; (+), antioxidant, not definitively identified as α–tocopherol; ++, ⩾ fivefold increase; –, decrease; N.D., not different from unfermented substrate.
[b]*Rhizopus oligosporus.*
[c]*Aspergillus oryzae* and *Saccharomyces rouxii* or *Streptococcus faecalis.*
[d]*Bacillus subtilis.*
[e]Lactic acid bacteria.
[f]Leaching losses during desalting.
Source: Reprinted from *Food Technol.* 39 (1985).

carbon dioxide formed during fermentation (Pederson, 1960). In contrast, nonfermented vegetables lost 20–90% of their ascorbic acid, riboflavin and thiamine during canning (Kirk, 1979). Thus fermentation of vegetables can result in shelf-stable products which do not require further heat processing (Fleming and McFeeters, 1981), as well as protect the nutrient content of subsequently heated products.

Since yeasts are good sources of B vitamins, they can replace some of the vitamins lost during the milling and baking of bread (Reed, 1981), particularly thiamine, which is present at 15–30μg per gram of yeast (Spicher, 1983). In addition, yeast fermentation of ciders resulted in a small increase in riboflavin content, with considerable increases in thiamine, nicotinic acid, and pantothenic acid levels (Goverd, 1975).

Microbial utilization and synthesis during fermentation affect the micronutrient content of *cultured dairy products*. Lactic acid fermentation increased the niacin, B_6, B_{12}, and folic acid contents of cottage cheese (Reif et al., 1976), increased the riboflavin content of some products (Kon, 1972), reduced the vitamin A content in dahi (Narayanan et al., 1954), and destroyed almost all of the vitamin C in yogurt (Watt and Merrill, 1963). The temperature and length of incubation influence synthesis (Reif et al., 1976), as does the particular microorganism used. For example, *Lactobacillus bulgaricus* and *Lactobacillus cremoris* reduced the thiamine, riboflavin, and nicotinic acid content of dahi, while *Streptococcus lactis* and *Streptococcus cremoris* increased the thiamine content over that of the original milk (Rao and Basu, 1952).

While most of the vitamin A and calcium remained in the *cheese* curd during whey separation, there was little retention of riboflavin, thiamine, and vitamin C (Kon, 1959). The small amount of vitamin C present in the curd was lost during ripening (Kon, 1972), while vitamin A and the other vitamins were fairly stable. Additionally, certain molds and bacteria can synthesize the B vitamins and so increased the levels of these nutrients in ripened cheeses, though only the crust of cheese contained the additional vitamins (Jones, 1975).

The direct contribution of microbial vitamin synthesis to the nutritive value of fermented *meat* products has not been studied extensively (Bacus and Brown, 1981).

Effects of Fermentation on Nutritional Stress Factors

Fermentation also can affect the nutritive value of *grains and oilseeds* by altering the levels of nutritional stress factors (Table 7). Fermentation reduced the phytate content of wheat flour (Kirk, 1979; Reinhold, 1975), tempeh (Sutardi and Buckle, 1985; Sudarmadji and Markakis, 1977), and oncom owing to the phytase activity of the

Table 7. Effects of Fermentation on Nutritional Stress Factors in Plant Foods

Product	Stress factor[a]	Reference
Grains		
Wheat flour	– phytate	Kirk (1979)
Whole wheat bread	+ zinc solubility (– phytate)	Reinhold (1975)
Oilseeds		
Soybean tempeh[b]	– phytate	Sudarmadji and Markakis (1977)
	– phytate	Sutardi and Buckle (1985)
	– trypsin inhibitor[c]	Van Veen and Schaeffer (1950)
	– trypsin inhibitor[c]	Smith et al. (1964)
Oncom[b]	– phytate	Fardiaz and Markakis (1981)
Sunflower meal[d]	– chlorogenic acid	Canella et al. (1984)
Cottonseed meal[e]	– free gossypol	Baugher and Campbell (1969)
Vegetables		
Sauerkraut[d]	– goitrogens	Pederson (1960)
Gari[d,f]	– cyanogenetic glucosides	Collard and Levi (1959)

[a]+, significant increase; –, significant decrease.
[b]*Rhizopus oligosporus.*
[c]Probably destroyed by heat treatment prior to fermentation (Liener and Kakade, 1980).
[d]Lactic acid bacteria.
[e]*Diploida.*
[f]Yeast.
Source: Reprinted from *Food Technol.* *39* (1985).

microorganisms, with the amount of reduction depending on the specific organism used for fermentation (Fardiaz and Markakis, 1981). Idli fermentation decreased the phytate phosphorus level by 45%, with only a slight decrease in total phosphorus, and resulted in elevated phytase activity compared to the raw batter (Akolkar, 1977).

The actual effect of fermentation on protease inhibitors is not known, but tempeh did not cause pancreatic enlargement when fed to rats (Smith et al., 1964), indicating that the trypsin inhibitors in raw soybeans had been destroyed, most likely by the heat treatment before fermentation (Liener and Kakade, 1980). Roozen and de Groot (1985) also found that only 5% of the original trypsin inhibitor activity was present in fermented tempeh and they attributed this decrease to the leaching of low molecular weight inhibitors during the soaking and washing of beans (Gatfield, 1980) and the inactivation of proteinaceous inhibitors during steaming prior to fermentation (Rackis, 1972).

Fermentation also caused partial detoxification of sunflower meal (natural lactic acid fermentation) by reducing chlorogenic acid (Canella et al., 1984), cottonseed meal (with *Diploida* fungus) by decreasing the free gossypol and increasing the bound, nontoxic form (Baugher and Campbell, 1969), cabbage by hydrolyzing goitrogenic sulfur glucosides (Pederson, 1960), and cassava (with *Corynebacterium*) by causing hydrolysis of cyanogenetic glucosides (Collard and Levi, 1959), especially linamarin, and significantly reducing the cyanide content (Olarewaju and Boszormenji, 1975).

The possible production of toxic substances, such as aflatoxin, during fermentation was investigated, but the industrial koji mold was found to be nonaflatoxigenic (Beuchat, 1983). No aflatoxin was found in peanuts fermented by *A. oryzae* (Quinn et al., 1975), and *Rhizopus* spp. even were able to degrade aflatoxin to a nontoxic form (Cole et al., 1972; van Veen and Steinkraus, 1970). In addition, an antibacterial agent was produced by *R. oligosporus* and found to have a growth-promoting effect on animals (Wang and Hesseltine, 1970).

Another beneficial effect of fermentation was the synthesis of compounds by tempeh molds which make the final product very stable to lipid oxidation (Gyorgy et al., 1974). Murakami et al. (1984) confirmed that this antioxidative activity of tempeh is generated by the liberation of lipophilic isoflavones from glucosides by β-glucosidase.

Recently the anticarcinogenicity or antimutagenicity of fermented foods has been reported, with soy sauce decreasing the incidence of tumors in rats and the daily ingestion of miso soup significantly reducing the risk of gastric cancer in the Japanese population (Fukushima, 1985). This antimutagenic activity of miso was attributed to fatty acid ethyl esters formed in miso during fermentation, with linoleic acid ethyl ester having the strongest activity (Okazaki et al., 1984).

Fermentation of *dairy products* not only preserves the nutrients present in perishable fluid milk and provides a variety of food products (Vedamuthu, 1982) but also provides milks with some probiotic actions (see Table 5). For example, lactic acid had beneficial effects on digestion, stimulated normal intestinal functions, and inhibited harmful microorganisms (Bottazzi, 1983).

Feeding studies with Masai males revealed that large intakes of fermented milk (8 liters/day) led to a decrease in cholesteremia despite weight gain and a high intake of cholesterol (960–1200 mg/day), with the greatest milk intakes causing the largest reduction in serum cholesterol (Mann and Spoerry, 1974). A subsequent study reported that both whole- and skim-milk yogurt produced a significant reduction of cholesteremia in U.S. adult subjects while intake of the same quantity of fresh milk (2 liters/day) had no effect (Mann, 1977). These results led Mann (1979) to propose that certain bacteria produce a hypocholesteremic milk factor which inhibits cholesterol synthesis, though Jaspers et al. (1984) found the hypocholesteremic effect of yogurt to be transient.

In addition to the production of milk factor, certain species of lactic acid bacteria can adapt and grow in the intestine, thus producing their enzymes which intervene in intestinal processes and affect the growth of other bacteria (Bottazzi, 1983). For example, lactobacilli in the intestine have been reported to degrade nitrosamines (Rowland and Grasso, 1975). In addition, feeding of viable *Lactobacillus acidophilus* to omnivorous rats decreased the activities of β-glucuronidase, nitroreductase, and azoreductase, which are bacterial enzymes believed to be involved in the conversion of procarcinogens to proximal carcinogens (Goldin and Gorbach, 1977), with the same results achieved with humans on meat diets (Goldin et al., 1980). Thus *Lactobacillus* supplements could be used to alter the metabolic activity of the human microflora.

Certain types of *cheeses* are rich in tyramine, a pressor amine which acts as a vasoconstrictor and elevates blood pressure (Liener, 1980).

Histamine is formed from bacterial decarboxylation of histidine and thus is a normal constituent of fermented *meats*, such as sausages, as well as cheese, wine, and sauerkraut. High histamine levels detected in some samples of Italian dry salami and pepperoni indicated that the potential exists for producing toxic levels, but proper control of the natural fermentations was found to prevent histamine accumulation (Taylor et al., 1978). Other amino acids can be decarboxylated during dry sausage ripening to produce significant amounts of tyramine, putrescine, and even cadaverine (Dierick et al., 1974).

Germination (Assembly—Formulation—Preparation)

Germination can be used to prepare foods with improved nutritional quality, with examples presented in Table 8. Germination affected protein quality by increasing the PER of soybeans (Liener, 1978) and increasing available lysine levels in wheat, barley, oats, and rice (Hamad and Fields, 1979). In addition, germination produced a 10-fold increase in the vitamin C content of peas and beans (Fordham et al., 1975) and resulted in higher levels of vitamins B_1, B_2, B_6, and C, niacin, folic acid, and biotin in soybeans (Liener, 1978).

Germination also can reduce or eliminate antinutritional factors, such as the tannins in pigeon peas, chick pea, and gram (Reddy et al., 1985), which were reduced by 50%, and the phytate in soybeans (Sutardi and Buckle, 1985). The effects of germination on trypsin inhibitor varied, with the activity found to increase in kidney beans (Palmer et al., 1973), decrease in field peas (Hobday et al., 1973), and remain unchanged in soybeans (Desikachar and De, 1942). Germination resulted in an increase in the nutritive value (PER) of kidney beans (Palmer et al., 1973) and soybeans (Desikachar and De, 1942), though this increase was not correlated with the effects of germination on protease inhibitor activity.

ROLE OF TISSUE CULTURE METHODS IN QUALITY IMPROVEMENT OF PLANT FOODS

While the traditional and biological processing methods discussed affect the nutritive value of the final food product, plant tissue culture can be used to improve the quality of the raw material. In addition, tissue culture can supplement both traditional and biological processes to achieve optimum food quality.

Conventional breeding has been used to improve crop plants, specifically utilizing induced mutants to improve disease resistance (Bliss, 1984) and to alter the amino acid composition of maize (Mertz et al., 1964), barley (Munck et al., 1970), and wheat (Corpuz et al., 1983). Traditional breeding, though, requires recurrent cycles of hybridization and selection which are time- and resource-consuming (Scowcroft, 1977). In addition, selective breeding requires the existence of biological variability for the desired trait within the particular species (Downton, 1984). Intensive breeding for desirable features in commercial cultivars unintentionally has reduced the variability for other traits such as salt and cold tolerance, and interspecific hybrids are difficult to achieve (Scowcroft, 1977), so the genetic variability generated in tissue culture can provide a solution (Nabors et al., 1980).

Table 8. Effects of Germination on Nutritional Quality of Food Plants

Component	Food plant	Effect on quality factors[a]	Reference
Protein	Soybeans	+ PER	Liener (1978)
	Wheat, barley, oats, rice	+ lysine	Hamad and Fields (1979)
Vitamins	Soybeans	+ B_1, + B_2, + niacin, + B_6, + C, + folic acid, + biotin	Liener (1978)
	Beans, peas	− B_1, N.D. B_2, + C	Fordham et al. (1975)
Stress factors	Soybeans	+ PER, N.D. trypsin inhibitor	Desikachar and De (1942)
	Soybeans	− phytate	Sutardi and Buckle (1985)
	Field peas	− trypsin inhibitor	Hobday et al. (1973)
	Field peas	N.D. trypsin inhibitor	Liener and Kakade (1980)
	Kidney beans	+ PER, + trypsin inhibitor	Palmer et al. (1973)

[a] +, increase; −, decrease; N.D., not different from nongerminated product.
Source: Reprinted from *Food Technol. 39* (1985).

Plant tissue culture, a blanket term for the culture of cells, tissues, organs, and protoplasts under aseptic conditions (Bhojwani and Razdan, 1983), offers advantages for plant breeding and improvement. These include the capacity to screen large numbers of individuals in one suspension culture, the ability to select for natural and induced mutations, and the ability to produce many copies (or clones) of an individual cell selected for a desired trait (Welsh, 1981). The major advantage of cell culture, though, is the possibility of direct selection in vitro. Novel phenotypes are selected from large populations of physiologically and developmentally uniform cells grown under defined conditions (Chaleff, 1983). The cell culture is exposed to selective conditions, usually based on a chemical difference in the medium, that only allow variant cells to grow (Tomes and Swanson, 1982). The high frequency of variation induced in tissue culture, combined with the selection pressure applied, results in cells with enhanced tolerance to the selective agent (Downton, 1984). Plants are then regenerated from resistant cells to determine whether the selected trait is heritable.

Improvement of Stress Tolerance

In the area of crop improvement through in vitro selection, most research has focused on increasing the stress tolerance of plants, with disease resistance being the first trait for which selection at the cellular level led to expression by plants (Chaleff, 1983). Gengenbach et al. (1977), for example, selected for variant maize cell cultures which were resistant to the T toxin of *Drechslera maydis* and exhibited heritable resistance.

Alfalfa (*Medicago sativa*) cells were selected for freezing tolerance, but plants were not regenerated to see whether the induced tolerance was maintained (Orr et al., 1985). Alfalfa cells also were selected for salt tolerance, but regenerated plants lost the tolerance (Croughan et al., 1978), indicating that the changes seen in culture were not due to mutations but, rather, to changes in gene expression (Downton, 1984). Aluminum tolerance has been achieved with the tomato (*Lycopersicon esculentum*) (Meredith, 1978). Additional examples of in vitro selection for stress tolerance(s) are discussed by Tomes and Swanson (1982).

Improvement of Nutritional Quality

Nutritional quality improvement through tissue culture is possible and can involve increasing levels of certain nutrients and/or decreasing the amount of nutritional stress factors. An example of the former is increasing amino acids which are deficient in plant foods, such as lysine in all cereal grains, threonine in wheat and rice, and tryptophan in corn (Widholm, 1977). While supplementation of foods with purified amino acids or proteins is a possible solution to these deficiencies, the costs are too high and acceptability (Widholm, 1977) and stability (Shemer and Perkins, 1975) are potential problems.

Alternatively, plant amino acid biosynthesis can be manipulated by exposing cultured cells to amino acid analogs which inhibit the growth of normal cells and then selecting for variant cells that acquire analog resistance by overproducing the corresponding amino acid (Widholm, 1977). In vitro selection for amino acid overproduction has been attempted in a number of species, with successes reported for the carrot (*Daucus carota*) (Widholm, 1972a,b), alfalfa (*M. sativa*) (Reisch et al., 1981), the soybean (*Glycine max*) (Das and Widholm, 1983), rice (*Oryzae sativa*) (Chaleff and Carlson, 1975; Schaeffer and Sharpe, 1981, Schaeffer et al., 1984), and maize (*Zea mays*) (Hibberd et al. 1980; Hibberd and Green, 1982).

Chaleff and Carlson (1975) selected for resistant rice cell cultures which had elevated lysine both in the free amino acid pool and in total amino acids, but plants were not regenerated to determine whether the grain protein had elevated lysine levels (Scowcroft, 1977). Schaeffer and Sharpe (1981) regenerated rice plants which had increased levels of protein and increased lysine within the protein, while Schaeffer et al. (1984) found that anther-derived cell lines had increased seed protein but also reduced seed yields.

Maize plants are inhibited by lysine and threonine addition because the presence of these two amino acids blocks methionine synthesis. Therefore addition of both of these amino acids to cell culture medium selects for resistant variant cells whose enzymes lack feedback inhibition and accumulate either methionine, lysine, and/or threonine (Widholm, 1977). Hibberd et al. (1980) selected maize cell culture variants which grew vigorously in the presence of lysine plus threonine and accumulated threonine (ninefold increase), methionine, lysine, and isoleucine, with no reduction in the levels of other amino acids. Regenerated plants were fertile and had increased free amino acid levels in the kernel, especially threonine, suggesting that the observed increases were due to a stable, heritable mutation. This is encouraging, because in order for such traits of amino acid overproduction selected in tissue culture to be useful for crop improvement, the traits must be heritable, expressed in the regenerated plant, and expressed in the plant part consumed, that is, the mature grain of cereals.

Little work has been done on the use of tissue culture techniques to improve the nutritional quality of plants by reducing the levels of nutritional stress factors. Our results with cultured cells of vegetable amaranth (*Amaranthus tricolor*) indicated that tissue culture can be used to decrease the level of specific stress factors while maintaining the concentrations of other, desirable nutrients (R. A. Teutonico and D. Knorr, unpublished results, 1985). Specifically, amaranth seedlings and cultured cells were grown on nine medium variations which differed only in the relative amounts of nitrogen sources. After the same growth period cultured amaranth cells had significantly lower concentrations of oxalate and nitrate than seedlings, while the concentration of ascorbic acid, an indicator of food plant quality, was the same or slightly lower in the cells and seedlings for each medium variation (Table 9). In addition, the variations in the medium composition also had a significant effect on the nutrient content of the cells. Therefore tissue culture can be used as a source of "sterile," "detoxified" biomass with a defined composition.

In addition, the significantly lower levels of oxalate and nitrate found in suspended *A. tricolor* cells compared to those in seedlings and the fact that spontaneous mutants are known to occur in tissue culture (Gamborg and Shyluk, 1981) indicated that it should be possible to isolate low-oxalate and/or low-nitrate variants from populations of suspended amaranth cells without selection. Therefore a nondestructive screening method was developed (Teutonico and Knorr, 1985b) to provide the means for the isolation of low-oxalate variants which can be regenerated into plants and examined for inheritance of the low-oxalate trait.

Food Applications of Plant Tissue Culture

In summary, the food applications (Table 10) of plant tissue culture include crop improvement, as well as the area of food production, both of biomass in general and of specialty foods. In the area of crop improvement many nutritional stress factors have potential for reduction through in vitro selection. For example, reduction in the tannin content of plants would be desirable, especially in sorghum, which may contain up to 3% dry weight as tannins (Oberthur et al., 1983). Polyphenols, such as tannins, are not removed by physical and chemical treatments and are only partially removed by fermentation or germination. On the other hand, selection for decreased phytate levels does not seem desirable, because, although phytate inhibits mineral availability, it is the major storage form of phosphorus in plants (Sutardi and Buckle, 1985).

Elimination of trypsin inhibitors from some plant species also would be desirable, especially in maize, barley, rye, and buckwheat, where the trypsin inhibitor is not heat labile (Bender, 1978). However, research is needed on the effects of a reduction in nutritional stress factors on the plant's metabolism. For instance, protease inhibitors may be involved in the defense mechanism of plants against invading microbes and insects (Ryan, 1974) and so their removal may have adverse effects on resistance.

Table 9. Effects of Medium Variations on the Oxalate, Nitrate, and Ascorbic Acid Concentrations[a] of *Amaranthus tricolor* Seedlings and Cultured Cells

			Oxalate		Nitrate		Ascorbic acid	
Medium variation	Molar ratio $NO_3^-:NH_4^+$	Total nitrogen (mM)	Seedlings (N=8)	Suspended cells (N=8)	Seedlings (N=4)	Suspended cells (N=4)	Seedlings (N=4)	Suspended cells (N=4)
1	12.5:1	27.0	48.97±13.09[b]	8.09±4.29[c]	57.25±6.56[d]	10.77±3.39[e]	2.62±0.66[f]	3.07±0.80[g]
2	1:1	27.0	15.56±2.50[b]	2.67±1.29[c]	66.16±4.27[d]	4.11±4.67[e]	5.54±0.52[f]	3.06±0.57[g]
3	1:12.5	27.0	29.66±14.23[b]	5.36±4.45[c]	34.63±2.67[d]	1.20±1.32[e]	6.8±1.20[f]	3.25±0.53[g]

[a]Mean ± SD (mg/g dry matter).
[b,c]Different letters within one row indicate significant differences ($p<.01$) between the means of oxalate content.
[d,e]Different letters within one row indicate significant differences ($p<.01$) between the means of nitrate content.
[f,g]Different letters within one row indicate significant differences ($p<.01$) between the means of ascorbic acid content.
Source: R. A. Teutonico and D. Knorr, unpublished results (1985).

Table 10. Food Applications of Plant Tissue Culture

Crop improvement		
	Stress tolerance	
		Disease and pest resistance
		Salt and cold tolerance
		Aluminum tolerance
		Pesticide resistance
	Nutritional quality	
		Increase nutrient content (e.g., amino acids)
		Reduce nutritional stress factors (e.g., oxalate)
Food production		
	Biomass	
	Specialty foods	

In the area of food production, it has been demonstrated that large amounts of biomass can be produced in culture, with Tulecke and Nickell (1960) obtaining 3.1 g of plant matter per liter of media per day and Byrne and Koch (1962) yielding 4.6 g of *D. carota* plant material per liter of media per day. The biomass produced in tissue culture has the advantage of being sterile, of defined composition, and free of environmental pollutants. Specialty items from culture, such as baby foods, geriatric diets, specific nutrient supplements, and specialty ingredients with desired characteristics, could be produced with minimal further processing.

CONCLUSIONS

The information presented in this chapter has shown that there are a number of possible approaches to improving the nutritional quality of foods. Traditional processing methods have long been used to reduce many naturally occurring stress factors in foods and to increase nutritive value. Biological processes also have positive effects on nutritional quality and need to be recognized as unit operations in food processing and better utilized for food quality improvement. Recently plant tissue culture has been identified as an additional method for improving nutritional quality and it provides an alternative or a supplement to processing in situations where traditional and biological processes cannot remove a particular nutritional stress factor. Future research must be directed toward utilizing interactions of these methods to design strategies which maximize the nutritional value of foods during production and attempt to minimize nutrient losses during processing.

REFERENCES

Akinrele, I. A. (1970). Fermentation studies on maize during the preparation of a traditional African starch-cake food. *J. Sci. Food Agric. 21*:619–625.

Akinrele, I. A. and Bassir, O. (1967). The nutritive value of ogi, a Nigerian infant food. *J. Trop. Med. Hyg. 70*:279–280.

Akolkar, P. N. (1977). Cited by Steinkraus, K. H., ed. (1983), *Handbook of Indigenous Fermented Foods*, Marcel Dekker, Inc., New York.

Anantharaman, K. and Carpenter, K. J. (1969). Effect of heat processing on the nutritional value of groundnut products 1. Protein quality of groundnut cotyledons for rats. *J. Sci. Food Agric. 20*:703–708.

Bacus, J. N. and Brown, W. L. (1981). Use of microbial cultures: Meat products. *Food Technol. 35*:74–78.

Banigo, E. O. I. and Muller, H. G. (1972). Manufacture of ogi (a Nigerian fermented cereal porridge): Comparative evaluation of corn, sorghum, and millet. *Can. Inst. Food. Sci. Technol. J. 5*:217–221.

Baugher, W. L. and Campbell, T. C. (1969). Gossypol detoxication by fungi. *Science 164*:1526–1527.

Bender, A. E. (1978). *Food Processing and Nutrition*, Academic, London.

Berardi, L. G. and Goldblatt, L. A. (1980). Gossypol. In *Toxic Constituents of Plant Foodstuffs* (I. E. Liener, ed.), Academic Press, New York, pp. 183–237.

Beuchat, L. R. (1983). Indigenous fermented foods. In *Biotechnology*, Vol. 5 (G. Reed, ed.), Verlag Chemie, Weinheim, pp. 477–528.

Bhojwani, S. S. and Razdan, M. K. (1983). *Plant Tissue Culture: Theory and Practice*, Elsevier, Amsterdam.

Bliss, F. A. (1984). The application of new plant biotechnology to crop improvement. *Hort. Sci. 19*:43–48.

Bottazzi, V. (1983). Other fermented dairy products. In *Biotechnology,* Vol. 5 (G. Reed, ed.), Verlag Chemie, Weinheim, pp. 315–363.

Breslaw, E. S. and Kleyn, D. H. (1973). *In vitro* digestibility of protein in yogurt at various stages of processing. *J. Food Sci. 38*:1016–1021.

Byrne, A. F. and Koch, R. B. (1962). Food production by submerged culture. *Science 135*:215–218.

Canella, A., Bernardi, A., and Marghinotti, D. (1984). Improvement of germinated sunflower meal by fermentation. *Food Sci. Technol. 17*:314–318.

Carlsson, R. and Halqvist, C. W. (1981). *Atriplex hortensis* L. Revival of a spinach plant. *Acta Agric. Scand. 31*:229–234.

Cazzulo, J. J. and Stoppani, A. O. M. (1967). Purification and properties of pyruvate carboxylase from baker's yeast. *Arch. Biochem. Biophys. 121*:596–608.

Chaleff, R. S. (1983). Isolation of agronomically useful mutants from plant cell cultures. *Science 219*:676–682.

Chaleff, R. S. and Carlson, P. S. (1975). Higher plant cells as experimental organisms. In *Modifications of the Information Content of Plant Cells* (R. Markham, D. R. Davies, D. A. Hopwood, and R. W. Horne, eds.), North Holland, Amsterdam. pp. 127–137.

Chen, I. and Mitchell, H. L. (1973). Trypsin inhibitors in plants. *Phytochemistry 12*:327–330.

Chen, L. H., Packett, L. V., and Yun, I. (1972). Tissue antioxidant effect of ocean hake fish and fermented soybean (tempeh) as protein sources in rats. *J. Nutr. 102*:181–186.

Cole, R. J., Kirksey, J. W., and Blankenship, B. R. (1972). Conversion of aflatoxin B1 to isomeric compounds by *Rhizopus* spp. *J. Agric. Food Chem. 20*:1100–1102.

Collard, P. and Levi, S. (1959). A two–stage fermentation of cassava. *Nature 183*:620–621.

Conn, E. E. (1973). Cyanogenetic glycosides. In *Toxicants Occurring Naturally in Foods,* 2nd ed., National Research Council, National Academy of Sciences, Washington, D. C., pp. 229–308.

Cooney, L. L. (1983). Bioreactors: Design and operation. *Science 219*:728–730.

Corpuz, L. M., Heyne, E. G., and Paulsen, G. M. (1983). Increasing grain protein content of hard red winter wheat (*Triticum aestivum* L.) by mutation breeding. *Theor. Appl. Genet. 65*:41–46.

Damaty, S. M. and Hudson, B. J. F. (1975). Preparation of low–gossypol cottonseed flour. *J. Sci. Food Agric. 26*:109–115.

Das, P. K. and Widholm, J. M. (1983). Amino acid analog resistance in the species of soybean and tobacco. In *Plant Cell Culture in Crop Improvement* (S. K. Sen and K. L. Giles, eds.), Plenum Press, New York, pp. 411–417.

Daun, H. (1975). Effects of salting, curing, and smoking on nutrients of flesh foods. In *Nutritional Evaluation of Food Processing* (R. S. Harris and E. Karmas, eds.), AVI, Westport, Conn., pp. 355–381.

Davis, J. G. and Latto, D. (1957). Yogurt in gastro–enteritis of infancy. *Lancet 272*(1):274–275.

Delente, J. and Ladenburg, K. (1972). Quantitative determination of the oligosaccharides in defatted soybean meal by gas–liquid chromatography. *J. Food Sci. 37*:372–374.

Delic, I., Vucurevic, N., and Stajanovic, S. (1972). Cited by Liener (1980). Miscellaneous toxic factors. In *Toxic Constituents of Plant Foodstuffs*, 2nd. ed. (I. E. Liener, ed. Academic Press, New York, pp. 429–467.

Demeyer, D., Hoozee, J., and Mesdom, H. (1974). Specificity of lipolysis during dry sausage ripening. *J. Food Sci. 39*:293–296.

Desikachar, H. S. R. and De, S. S. (1942). Role of inhibitors in soybean. *Science 106*:421–422.

Dierick, N., Vandekerchove, P., and Demeyer, D. (1974). Changes in nonprotein nitrogen compounds during dry sausage ripening. *J. Food Sci. 39*:301–304.

Downton, W. J. S. (1984). Salt tolerance of food crops: Prospectives for improvements. *CRC Crit. Rev. Plant Sci. 1*:183–201.

Dunker, C. F., Berman, M., Snider, G. G., and Tubiash, H. S. (1953). Quality and nutritive properties of different types of commercially cured hams. III. Vitamin content, biological value of the protein and bacteriology. *Food Technol. 7*:288–291.

Fardiaz, D. and Markakis, P. (1981). Degradation of phytic acid in oncom (fermented peanut press cake). *J. Food Sci. 46*:523–525.

Farrer, K. T. H. (1955). The thermal destruction of vitamin B1 in foods. *Adv. Food Res. 6*:257–311.

Fellers, C. R. (1971). Effects of fermentation on food nutrients. In *Nutritional Evaluation of Food Processing* (R. S. Harris and H. von Loesecke, eds.), AVI, Westport, Conn., pp. 161–165.

Finot, P. A. (1983). Influence of processing on the nutritional value of proteins. *Qual. Plant. Plant Foods Hum. Nutr. 32*:439–453.

Fleming, H. P. and McFeeters, R. F. (1981). Use of microbial cultures: Vegetable products. *Food Technol. 35*:84–88.

Ford, J. E. (1973). Some effects of processing on nutritive value. In *Proteins in Human Nutrition* (J. W. G. Porter and B. A. Rolls, eds.), Academic, New York, pp. 515–530.

Fordham, J. R., Wells, C. E., and Chen, L. M. (1975). Sprouting of seeds and nutritional composition of seeds and sprouts. *J. Food Sci. 40*:552–556.

Fukushima, D. (1985). Fermented vegetable protein and related foods of Japan and China. *Food Rev. Int. 1*:149–209.

Gallagher, C. R., Moleson, A. L., and Caldwell, J. H. (1974). Lactose tolerance and fermented dairy products. *J. Am. Diet. Assoc. 65*:418–421.

Gamborg, O. L. and Shyluk, J. P. (1981). Nutrition, media, and characteristics of plant cell and tissue cultures. In *Plant Tissue Culture: Methods and Applications in Agriculture* (T. A. Thorpe, ed.), Academic, New York, pp. 21–44.

Gatfield, I. L. (1980). Loss of dry matter during the industrial preparation of legumes: Leaching of trypsin inhibitors during the soaking step. *Food Sci. Technol. 13*:46–48.

Gengenbach, B. G., Green, C. E., and Donovan, C. M. (1977). Inheritance of selected pathotoxin resistance in maize plants regenerated from cell cultures. *Proc. Nat. Acad. Sci. U.S.A. 74*:5113–5117.

Gillooly, M., Bothwell, T. H., Torrance, J. D., MacPhail, A. P., Derman, D. P., Bezwoda, W. R., Mills, W., and Charlton, R. W. (1983). The effects of organic acids, phytates, and polyphenols on the absorption of iron from vegetables. *Br. J. Nutrit. 49*:331–335.

Goldin, B. R. and Gorbach, S. L. (1977). Alterations in fecal microflora enzymes related to diet, age, *Lactobacillus* supplements, and dimethylhydrazine. *Cancer 40*:2421–2426.

Goldin, B. R., Swenson, L., Dwyer, J., Sexton, M., and Gorbach, S. L. (1980). Effect of diet and *Lactobacillus acidophilus* supplements on human fecal bacterial enzymes. *J. Nat. Cancer Inst. 64*:255–261.

Goverd, K. A. (1975). Changes in some B group vitamin levels in fermenting ciders. *J. Inst. Brew. 81*:450–453.

Gyorgy, P., Murata, K., and Sugimoto, Y. (1974). Studies on antioxidant activity of tempeh oil. *J. Am. Oil Chemist's Society 51*:377–380.

Hackler, L. R., Van Buren, J. P., Steinkraus, K. H., El Rawi, I., and Hand, D. B. (1964). Effect of heat treatment on nutritive value of soy milk fed to weanling rats. *J. Food Sci. 30*:723–728.

Hafez, Y. S., Singh, G., McLellan, M. E., and Monroe-Lord, L. (1983). Effects of microwave heating on nutritional quality of soybeans. *Nutr. Rep. Int. 28*:413–421.

Hamad, A. M. and Fields, M. L. (1979). Evaluation of the protein quality and available lysine of germinated and fermented cereals. *J. Food Sci.* *44*:456–459.

Hepburn, F. N., Calhoun, W. K., and Bradley, W. B. (1966). The biological availability of essential amino acids in wheat, flour, bread and gluten. *Cereal Chem.* *43*:271–283.

Hibberd, K. A. and Green, C. E. (1982). Inheritance and expression of lysine plus threonine resistance selected in maize tissue culture. *Proc. Nat. Acad. Sci. U.S.A.* *79*:559–563.

Hibberd, K. A., Walter, T., Green, C. E., and Gengenbach, B. G. (1980). Selection and characterization of a feedback–insensitive tissue culture of maize. *Planta* *148*:183–187.

Hoagland, R., Hankins, O. G., Ellis, N. R., Hiner, R. L., and Snider, G. G. (1947). Composition and nutritive value of hams as affected by method of curing. *Food Technol.* *1*:540–552.

Hobday, S. M., Thurman, D. A., and Barber, D. J. (1973). Proteolytic and trypsin inhibitory activities in extracts of germinating *Pisum sativum* seeds. *Phytochemistry* *12*:1041–1046.

Hodgkinson, A. (1977). *Oxalic Acid in Biology and Medicine*, Academic, London.

Hudson, B. J. F. (1980). Detoxification of foods in food processing. In *Food and Health: Science and Technology* (G. G. Birch and K. J. Parker, eds.), Applied Science, London, pp. 305–317.

Hultin, H. O. (1983). Current and potential uses of immobilized enzymes. *Food Technol.* *37(10)*:66–82, 176.

Jarvis, B. and Holmes, A. W. (1982). Biotechnology in relation to the food industry. *J. Chem. Tech. Biotechnol.* *32*:224–232.

Jaspers, D. A., Massey, L. K., and Luedecke, L. O. (1984). Effect of consuming yogurts prepared with three culture strains on human serum lipoproteins. *J. Food Sci.* *49*:1178–1181.

Jones, I. D. (1975). Effects of processing by fermentation on nutrients. In *Nutritional Evaluation of Food Processing* (R. S. Harris and E. Karmas, eds.), AVI, Westport, Conn., pp. 324–354.

Karmas, E. (1975). Nutritional aspects of food processing methods. In *Nutritional Evaluation of Food Processing* (R. S. Harris and E. Karmas, eds.), AVI, Westport, Conn., pp. 11–15.

Kelsay, J. (1982). Effect of fiber and oxalic acid on zinc balance of adult human subjects. U.S. Department of Agriculture, Beltsville, MD.

Kennedy, T. S. and Ley, F. T. (1971). Studies on the combined effects of gamma radiation and cooking on the nutritive value of fish. *J. Sci. Food Agric.* *22*:146–148.

Khambatta, J. S. and Dastur, N. N. (1951). Changes in chemical composition of milk during souring. II. Changes in nitrogen constituents. *J. Dairy Sci. 4*:73–80.

Kirk, J. R. (1979). Nutritional changes upon processing. In *Food Science and Nutrition: Current Issues and Answers* (F. Clydesdale, ed.), Prentice–Hall, Englewood Cliffs, N. J., pp. 62–91.

Knorr, D. (1981). The influence of food processing on the nutritional quality of food. In *Soil, Food, and Health in a Changing World* (K. Barlow and P. Bunyard, eds.), Academic, London, pp. 34–46.

Knorr, D. (1985). Unit operations and processing equipment in small scale food processing. In *Small Scale Food Processing* (R. J. Gray and D. Knorr, eds.), Marcel Dekker, New York, (in press).

Knorr, D. and Sinskey, A. J. (1985). Biotechnology in food production and processing. *Science 239*:1224–1229.

Knorr, D., Watkins, T. R., and Carlson, B. L. (1981). Enzymatic reduction of phytate in whole wheat breads. *J. Food Sci. 46*: 1866–1869.

Kon, S. K. (1959). *Milk and Milk Products in Human Nutrition*, FAO Nutritional Series #17, Food Agric. Org., United Nations, Rome.

Kon, S. K. (1961). Nutritional effects on milk of chemical additives and processing. *Fed. Proc. Suppl. 7*:209–216.

Kon, S. K. (1972). *Milk and Milk Products in Human Nutrition*, FAO Nutritional Series #27, Food Agric. Org., United Nations, Rome.

Kuenzi, M., Assi, F., Chmiel, A. K., Collins, C. H., Donikan, M., Dominguez, J. B., Financsek, L., Fogarty, L. M., Frommer, W., Hasko, F., Hovland, J., Houwink, E. H., Mahler, J. L., Sandkvist, A., Sargent, K., Sloover, C., and Tuijnenburg Mujis, G. (1985). Safe biotechnology: General considerations. *Appl. Microbiol. Biotechnol. 21*:1–6.

Kung, H., Gaden, E. L., and King, C. G. (1953). Vitamins and enzymes in milk. Effect of gamma radiation on activity. *J. Agric. Food Chem. 1*:142–144.

Laakso, I., Hiltunen, R., Hovinen, S., von Schants, M., and Huhtikangas, A. (1982). Selection of high linoleic acid content in summer turnip rape (*Brassica campestris* L.). *Acta Agric. Scand. 32*:397–404.

Lampert, L. M. (1970). *Modern Dairy Products*, Chemical Publishing Co., New York.

Law, B. A. (1982). Cheeses. *Econ. Microbiol. 7*:147–198.

Lee, C. Y. (1977). Influence of processing on nutritive values of foods. In *Nutrition Council Seminar* (D. L. Downing and C. A. Bisogni, eds.), New York State Experiment Station, Geneva, New York, pp. 17–20.

Lepkovsky, S. (1953). Nutritional stress factors and food processing. *Adv. Food Res.* *4*:105–131.

Liener, I. E. (1977). Removal of naturally occurring toxicants through enzymatic processing. In *Food Proteins: Improvement through Chemical and Enzymatic Processing* (R. E. Feeney and J. R. Whitaker, eds.), American Chemical Society, Washington, D. C., pp. 283–300.

Liener, I. E. (1980). Miscellaneous toxic factors. In *Toxic Constituents in Plant Foodstuffs*, 2nd ed. (I. E. Liener, ed.), Academic, New York, pp. 283–300.

Liener, I. E. and Kakade, M. L. (1980). Protease inhibitors. In *Toxic Constituents of Plant Foodstuffs*, 2nd ed. (I. E. Liener, ed.), Academic, New York, pp. 7–71.

Makinde, M. A. and La Chance, P. A. (1976). Tryptophan: First limiting amino acid in ogi. *Nutr. Rep. Int.* *14*:671–679.

Mann, G. V. (1977). A factor in yogurt which lowers cholesteremia in man. *Atherosclerosis* *26*:335–340.

Mann, G. V. (1979). Milk factor—A regulator of cholesteremia. *Clin. Res.* *27*:554A.

Mann, G. V. and Spoerry, A. (1974). Studies of a surfactant and cholesteremia in the Massai. *Am. J. Clin. Nutr.* *27*:464–469.

Mattick, E. C. V. (1951). The calcium and phosphorous of Cheddar and Stilton cheese. *J. Dairy Res.* *18*:305–316.

Mauron, J., Mottu, F., Bujard, E., and Egli, R. H. (1955). The availability of lysine, methionine, and tryptophan in condensed milk and milk powder in *in vitro* digestion studies. *Arch. Biochem. Biophys.* *59*:433–451.

Meredith, C. P. (1978). Selection and characterization of aluminum-resistant variants from tomato cell cultures. *Plant Sci. Lett.* *12*:25–34.

Mertz, W. T., Bates, L. S., and Nelson, O. E. (1964). Mutant gene that changes protein composition and increases lysine content of maize endosperm. *Science* *145*:279–280.

Miflin, B. J., Bright, S. W. J., Rognes, S. E., and Kueh, J. S. H. (1983). Amino acids, nutrition and stress: The role of biochemical mutants in solving problems of crop quality. In *Genetic Engineering of Plants* (T. Kosuge, C. P. Meredith, and A. Hollander, eds.), Plenum Press, New York, pp. 391–414.

Mital, B. K., and Steinkraus, K. H. (1979). Fermentation of soy milk by lactic acid bacteria. A review. *J. Food Protect.* *42*: 895–899.

Montgomery, R. D. (1980). Cyanogens. In *Toxic Constituents of Plant Foodstuffs*, 2nd ed. (I. E. Liener, ed.), Academic, New York, pp. 143–160.

Morton, J. F. (1978). Economic botany in epidemiology. *Econ. Bot. 32*:111–116.

Munck, L., Karlsson, A., Hagber, A., and Eggum, B. O. (1970). Gene for improved nutritional value in barley seed protein. *Science 168*:985–987.

Murakami, H., Asakawa, T., Terao, J., and Matsushita, S. (1984). Antioxidative stability of tempeh and liberation of isoflavones by fermentation. *Agric. Biol. Chem. 48*:2971–2975.

Murata, K., Ikehata, H., and Miyamoto, T. (1967). Studies on the nutritional value of tempeh. *J. Food Sci. 32*:580–586.

Murray, T. K. (1983). Nutritional aspects of food irradiation. In *Recent Advances in Food Irradiation* (P. S. Elias and A. J. Cohen, eds.), Elsevier, New York, pp. 203–216.

Nabors, M. W., Gibbs, S. E., Berstein, C. S., and Meis, M. E. (1980). NaCl–tolerant plants from cultured cells. *Z. Pflanzenphysiol. 97*:13–17.

Narayanan, K. M., Shroff, N. B., Anankrishman, C. P., and Sen, K. C. (1954). Vitamin A in dairy products. Part 2. Vitamin A in curd and ghee from fortified milk. *Indian J. Dairy Sci. 7*: 76–82.

Nesheim, R. O. (1974). Nutrient changes in food processing: A current review. *Fed. Proc. 33*:2267–2269.

Newmark, H. L., Osadca, M., Araujo, M., Gerenz, N., and DeRitter, E. (1974). Stability of ascorbate in bacon. *Food Technol. 28*:28–31, 60.

Oberleas, D. (1973). Phytates. In *Toxicants Occurring Naturally in Foods*, National Research Council, National Academy of Sciences, Washington, D. C., pp. 363–371.

Oberthur, E. E., Nicholson, R. L., and Butler, L. G. (1983). Presence of polyphenolic materials, including condensed tannins, in sorghum. *J. Agric. Food Chem. 31*:660–662.

Ogunsua, A. O. (1977). Cited by Steinkraus, K. H., ed. (1983). *Handbook of Indigenous Fermented Foods*, Marcel Dekker, New York.

Olarewaju, O. C. and Boszormeji. (1975). The process of detoxification and residual cyanide content of commercial gari samples. *West African J. Biol. Appl. Chem. 18*:7–14.

Ozakaki, S., Akiba, M., and Kimura, S. (1984). Cited by Fukushima, D. (1985).

Orr, W., Singh, J., and Brown, D. C. W. (1985). Induction of freezing tolerance in alfalfa cell suspension cultures. *Plant Cell Rep. 4*:15–18.

Palmer, R., McIntosh, A., and Pusztai, A. J. (1973). The nutritional value of kidney beans (*Phaseolus vulgaris*): The effect on nutritional value of seed germination and changes in trypsin inhibitor content. *J. Sci. Food Agric.* *24*:937–940.

Palumbo, S. A. and Smith, J. L. (1977). Chemical and microbiological changes during sausage fermentation and ripening. In *Enzymes in Food and Beverage Processing* (R. L. Ory and A. J. St. Angelo, eds.), American Chemical Society, Washington, D. C., pp. 279–294.

Pederson, C. S. (1960). Sauerkraut. *Adv. Food Res.* *4*:31–85.

Pederson, C. S., Mack, G. L., and Athawes, W. L. (1939). Vitamin C content of sauerkraut. *Food Res.* *10*:233–291.

Piironen, E. and Virtanen, A. I. (1963). Cited by Tookey et al. (1980).

Price, M. L., Butler, L. G., Rugler, J. C., and Featherston, W. R. (1979). Overcoming the nutritionally harmful effect of tannin in sorghum grain by treatment with inexpensive chemicals. *J. Agric. Food Chem.* *27*:441–445.

Quinn, M. R., Beuchat, L. R., Miller, J., and Worthington, R. E. (1975). Fungal fermentation of peanut flour: Effects on chemical composition and nutritive value. *J. Food Sci.* *40*:470–474.

Rackis, J. J. (1965). Physiological properties of soybean trypsin inhibitors and their relationship to pancreatic hypertrophy and growth inhibition of rats. *Fed. Proc.* *24*:1488–1493.

Rackis, J. J. (1972). Biologically active components. In *Soybeans: Chemistry and Technology I* (A. K. Smith and S. J. Circle, eds.), AVI, Westport, Conn., pp. 158–202.

Rackis, J. J. (1974). Biological and physiological factors in soybeans. *J. Am. Oil Chem. Soc.* *51*:161A–174A.

Rackis, J. J. (1977). Enzymes in soybean processing and quality control. In *Enzymes in Food and Beverage Processing* (R. L. Ory and A. J. St. Angelo, eds.), American Chemical Society, Washington, D. C., pp. 244–265.

Rajalakshmi, R., and Vanaja, K. (1967). Chemical and biological evaluation of the effects of fermentation on the nutritive value of foods prepared from rice and gram. *Br. J. Nutr.* *21*: 467–473.

Rajalakshmi, R., Nanvaty, K., and Gumazha, A. (1964). Effect of cooking procedures on the free and total niacin content of certain foodstuffs. *Indian J. Nutr. Diet.* *1*:276–280.

Rao, R. V. and Basu, K. P. (1952). Effect of dahi formation (souring) on the thiamine, riboflavin, and nicotinic acid contents of milk. *Indian J. Dairy Sci.* *5*:1–8.

Reddy, N. R., Pierson, M. D., Sathe, S. K., and Salunkhe, D. K. (1985). Dry bean tannins: A review of nutritional implications. *J. Am. Oil Chem. Soc.* *62*:541–549.

Reif, G. D., Shahani, K. M., Vakil, J. R., and Crowe, L. K. (1976). Factors affecting B–complex vitamin content of cottage cheese. *J. Dairy Sci.* *59*:410–415.

Reinhold, J. G. (1975). Phytate destruction by yeast fermentation in whole wheat meals. *J. Am. Diet. Assoc.* *66*:38–41.

Reisch, B., Duke, H., and Bingham, E. T. (1981). Selection and characterization of ethionine–resistant alfalfa (*Medicago sativa* L.) cell lines. *Theor. Appl. Genet.* *59*:89–93.

Rice, E. E., Beuk, J. F., and Fried, J. F. (1947). Effect of commercial curing, smoking, storage, and cooking operations upon vitamin content of pork hams. *Food Res.* *12*:239–246.

Roelofsen, P. A. and Talens, A. (1964). Changes in some B vitamins during moulding of soybeans by *Rhizopus oryzae* in the production of tempeh kedelee. *J. Food Sci.* *29*:224–226.

Roozen, J. P. and de Groot, J. (1985). Electrophoresis and assay of trypsin inhibitors in different stages of tempeh production. *J. Food Biochem.* *9*:37–48.

Rosenberg, H. R. and Rohdenburg, E. L. (1951). The fortification of bread with lysine. 1. The loss of lysine during baking. *J. Nutr.* *45*:593–598.

Rowland, I. R. and Grasso, P. (1975). Degradation of N–nitrosamines by intestinal bacteria. *Appl. Microbiol.* *29*:7–12.

Ruttloff, H. (1985). Impact of biotechnology on food and nutrition. In *Food Biotechnology*, D. Knorr, ed., Marcel Dekker, New York.

Ryan, C. A. (1974). Assay and biochemical properties of the proteinase inhibitor–inducing factor, a wound hormone. *Plant Physiol.* *54*:328–332.

Sano, T. (1961). Feeding studies with fermented soy products (natto and miso). In *Meeting Protein Needs of Infants and Children*, Publ. No. 843, National Research Council, Washington, D. C., pp. 257–268.

Sastry, M. C. S. and Subramanian, N. (1985). Effect of heat processing on phenolic constituents and nutritional quality of sunflower flours. *J. Am. Oil Chem. Soc.* *62*:1131–1134.

Schaeffer, G. W. and Sharpe, F. T., Jr. (1981). Lysine in seed protein from S–aminoethyl–cysteine resistant anther–derived tissue cultures of rice. *In Vitro* *17*:345–352.

Schaeffer, G. W., Sharpe, F. T., Jr., and Cregan, P. B. (1984). Variation for improved protein and yield from rice anther culture. *Theor. Appl. Genet.* *67*:383–389.

Scowcroft, W. R. (1977). Somatic cell genetics and plant improvement. *Adv. Agron.* *29*:39–81.

Shemer, M. and Perkins, E. G. (1975). Degradation of methionine in heated soybean protein and the formation of β–methylmercaptopropionaldehyde. *J. Agric. Food Chem.* *23*:201–204.

Singleton, V. L. and Kratzer, F. H. (1973). Plant phenolics. In *Toxicants Occurring Naturally in Foods*, 2nd ed., National Research Council, National Academy of Sciences, Washington, D. C., pp. 309–345.

Smiley, K. L., Hensley, D. E., and Gasdorf, H. J. (1976). Alpha-galactosidase production and use in a hollow–fiber reactor. *Appl. Environ. Microbiol.* *31*(*4*):615–617.

Smith, A. K., Rackis, J. J., Hesseltine, C. W., Smith, M., Robbins, D. J., and Booth, A. N. (1964). Tempeh: Nutritive value in relation to processing. *Cereal Chem.* *41*:173–181.

Smith, J. A. B. (1970). Milk and Milk products. In *Proteins as Human Food* (R. A. Lawrie, ed.), AVI, Westport, Conn., pp. 213–224.

Somogyi, J. C. (1973). Antivitamins. In *Toxicants Occurring Naturally in Foods*, 2nd Ed. National Research Council, National Academy of Sciences, Washington, D. C., pp. 254–275.

Speck, M. L. (1981). Use of microbial cultures: Dairy products. *Food Technol.* *35*:71–73.

Spicher, G. (1983). Baked goods. In *Biotechnology*, Vol. 5 (G. Reed, ed.), Verlag Chemie, Weinheim, pp. 1–80.

Steinkraus, K. H., Hand, D. B., van Buren, J. P., and Hackler, L. R. (1961). Pilot plant studies on tempeh. In *Proceedings of the Conference on Soybean Products for Protein in Human Foods*, U. S. Res. Service, Washington, D. C.

Sudarmadji, S. and Markakis, P. (1977). The phytate and phytase of soybean tempeh. *J. Sci. Food Agric.* *28*:381–383.

Sure, B. and Ford, Z. W. (1943). Influence of incubation at 37°C on the stability of thiamine and riboflavine in cow's milk: *Proc. Soc. Exp. Biol.* *54*:83–85.

Sutardi and Buckle, K. A. (1985). Reduction in phytic acid levels in soybeans during tempeh production, storage and frying. *J. Food Sci.* *50*:260–263.

Synge, R. L. M. (1976). Damage to nutritional value of plant proteins by chemical reactions during storage and processing. *Qual. Plant. Plant Foods Human Nutr.* *26*(*1*/*3*):9–27.

Taylor, S. L., Leatherwood, M., and Lieber, E. R. (1978). A survey of histamine levels in sausages. *J. Food Protect.* *41*(*8*): 634–637.

Teutonico, R. A. and Knorr, D. (1985a). Impact of biotechnology on the nutritional quality of food plants. *Food Technol.* *39*: 127–134.

Teutonico, R. A. and Knorr, D. (1985b). A simple, non–destructive method for the determination of soluble oxalate in cultured *Amaranthus tricolor* cells. *J. Agric. Food Chem.* *33*(*1*):60–62.

Thomas, M. H. and Calloway, D. H. (1961). Nutritional value of dehydrated foods. *J. Am. Diet. Assoc.* *39*:105–116.

Tomes, D. T. and Swanson, E. B. (1982). Application of *in vitro* selection to plant improvement. In *Application of Plant Cell and Tissue Culture to Agriculture & Industry* (D. T. Tomes, B. E. Ellis, P. M. Harney, K. J. Kasha, and R. L. Peterson, eds.), University of Guelph, Guelph, Ontario, pp. 25–43.

Tongnual, P. and Fields, M. L. (1979). Fermentation and relative nutritive value of rice meal and chips. *J. Food Sci. 44*:1784–1785.

Tookey, H. L., Vanetten, C. H., and Daxenbichler, M. E. (1980). Glucosinolates. In *Toxic Constituents of Plant Foodstuffs* (I. E. Liener, ed.), Academic, New York, pp. 103–142.

Tulecke, W. and Nickell, L. G. (1960). Methods, problems, and results of growing plant cells under submerged conditions. *Trans. N. Y. Acad. Sci. 22*:196–205.

Van Buren, J. P., Hackler, L. P., and Steinkraus, K. H. (1972). Solubilization of soybean tempeh constituents during fermentation. *Cereal Chem. 49*:208–211.

Van Veen, A. G. and Schaeffer, G. (1950). The influence of the tempeh fungus on the soya bean. *Doc. Neerl. Indones. Morbis Trop. 11*:270–281.

Van Veen, A. G. and Steinkraus, K. H. (1970). Nutritive value and wholesomeness of fermented foods. *J. Agric. Food Chem. 18*:576–578.

Vedamuthu, E. R. (1982). Fermented milks. *Econ. Microbiol. 7*: 198–226.

Wang, H. L. and Hesseltine, C. W. (1966). Wheat tempeh. *Cereal Chem. 43*:563–566.

Wang, H. L. and Hesseltine, C. W. (1981). Use of microbial cultures: Legumes and cereal products. *Food Technol. 35*: 79–83.

Wanner, R. L. (1971). Effects of commercial processing of milk and milk products on their nutrient content. In *Nutritional Evaluation of Food Processing* (R. S. Harris and H. von Loesecke, eds.), AVI, Westport, Conn., pp. 173–196.

Watt, B. K. and Merrill, A. L. (1963). *Composition of Foods: Raw, Processed, Prepared.* Handbook 8, U. S. Department of Agriculture, Washington, D. C.

Welsh, J. R. *Fundamentals of Plant Genetics and Breeding.* Wiley, New York.

Whitaker, J. R. and Feeney, R. E. (1973). Enzyme inhibitors in foods. In *Toxicants Occurring Naturally in Foods,* National Research Council, National Academy of Sciences, Washington, D. C., pp. 276–298.

Widholm, J. M. (1972a). Cultured *Nicotiana tabacum* cells with an altered anthranilate synthetase which is less sensitive to feedback inhibition. *Biochim. Biophys. Acta 261*:52–58.

Widholm, J. M. (1972b). Anthranilate synthetase from 5-methyl-tryptophan-susceptible and -resistant cultured *Daucus carota* cells. *Biochim. Biophys. Acta 279*:48–57.

Widholm, J. M. (1977). Selection and characterization of amino acid analog resistant plant cell cultures. *Crop Sci. 17*:597–600.

Wittlife, J. L. and Airth, R. L. (1970). Thiaminase I, II. *Methods Enzymol. 18a*:229–269.

Zaehringer, M. V. and Personius, C. J. (1949). Thiamine retention in bread and rolls baked to different degrees of brownness. *Cereal Chem. 26*:384–392.

Zamora, R. G. and Veum, T. L. (1979). The nutritive value of dehulled soybeans fermented with *Aspergillus oryzae* or *Rhizopus oligosporus* as evaluated by rats. *J. Nutr. 109*:1333–1339.

TWO

Methods and Processes in Biotechnology

5

Methods and Applications of Molecular Cloning

SAUMYA BHADURI / U.S. Department of Agriculture, Philadelphia, Pennsylvania

INTRODUCTION

The development of molecular cloning methods (the isolation of specific DNA fragments from complex genomes and their multiplication and expression in bacterial cells) probably represents the major biological breakthrough of the decade. Not only has DNA cloning led to totally new approaches in most fields of biological research but also it promises to profoundly affect the future of mankind by its applications. Several compounds of medical and industrial importance have already been produced and are currently being marketed at competitive prices.

Among the most significant scientific achievements resulting from DNA cloning are (1) the isolation and characterization of functional genes from both prokaryotes and eukaryotes, which led to the discovery of intervening sequences that separate coding sequences of eukaryotic genes, and (2) the demonstration that the genomic organization in eukaryotic cells is not static but, rather, that genome rearrangements occur frequently. Basically, the cloning of DNA involves the in vitro joining of DNA molecules (passenger DNA to vector DNA) and the propagation of the resulting hybrid molecule into suitable host cells to obtain a clone, that is, a colony of identical cells derived from a single parental cell. The steps leading to the isolation of such clones constitute what is called molecular cloning (recombinant DNA technology). The rapid development of molecular cloning techniques resulted from progress made in several fields and has led to (1) the characterization and purification of a wide collection of enzymes that permit the modification and specific cleavage of nucleic acids, (2) the construction of cloning vehicles or vectors derived from either bacterial plasmids, bacteriophages, or animal viruses, (3) the development of techniques that allow the efficient introduction of large pieces of DNA into bacterial and eukaryotic cells, and (4) the development of techniques to rapidly screen transformants for their DNA content or expression of cloned sequences. To put all this into perspective, this chapter will present the basic experimental methods of recombinant DNA (rDNA) techniques and their limitations, possible applications to the food industry, and future trends. An understanding of the methods and applications of recombinant DNA technology requires familiarity with the structure of genes and gene products, the nature of the genetic code, the differences in how proteins are synthesized in prokaryotes and eukaryotes, and the approaches for developing new specialized organisms. The biochemical reactions in bacteria by which genetic information is stored, transferred, and converted into proteins are reviewed in Figures 1–3.

BASIC RECOMBINANT DNA TECHNOLOGIES

Progress in genetic engineering has been highly dependent upon the development of new methods, which have been used to establish new conceptual advances in biology. Recombinant DNA technology involves in vitro DNA recombination and the transfer of rDNA into a suitable foreign host. (For detailed methods in rDNA technology, the manual on molecular cloning by Maniatis et al., 1982, is recommended.) This process can be divided into five different stages: (1) gene selection, (2) DNA isolation, fragmentation, and purification to permit cloning of the gene of interest into a vector, (3) a suitable choice of vector, (4) gene insertion into the vector and introduction of rDNA into the host, and (5) the screening and selection of clones. Figure 4 depicts the fundamental steps in rDNA technology.

Gene Selection

The desired final product will determine the source of the genes. Although the genetic code is universal, the appreciable differences—such as introns and eukaryotic transcriptional controls—between prokaryotic (bacterial) and eukaryotic (animal, plant, and fungal) genes must be evaluated to ensure subsequent expression of the desired traits.

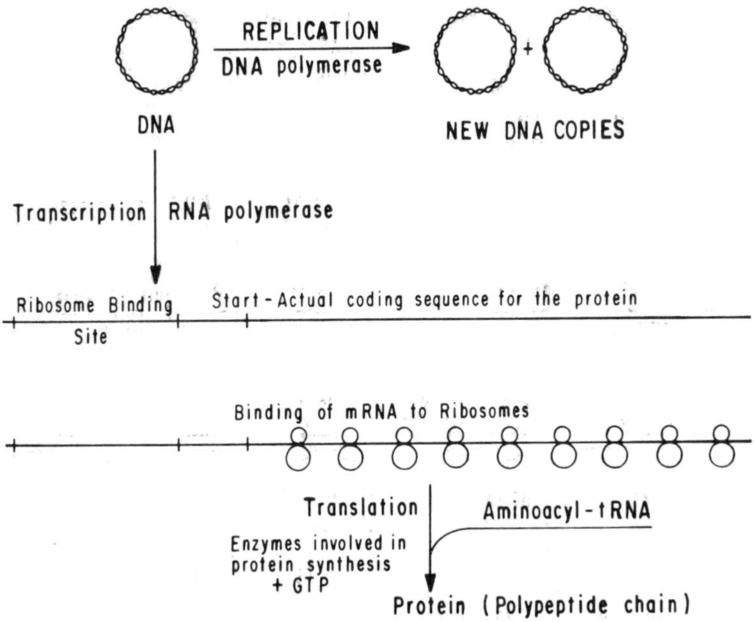

Fig. 1. The storage and conversion of genetic information is shown schematically in Figures 1 and 2. Both the *Escherichia coli* chromosome and plasmids useful in recombinant DNA methods are closed, circular, double-stranded DNA molecules. The chromosomal DNA is replicated by the enzyme DNA polymerase before cell division. Thus, genetically, both daughter cells are identically endowed (Davidson, 1969). Plasmid DNA, however, replicates independently of the chromosome (Sherratt, 1974; Helinski, 1976); one plasmid inserted into an *E. coli* may generate a hundred or more copies of itself within the cell. Expression begins with transcription of a section of DNA by the action of DNA-dependent RNA polymerase into messenger RNA (mRNA) molecules, which are single-stranded polyribonucleotides that mediate the conversion of DNA into protein (Davidson, 1969; Zillig et al., 1970; Watson, 1976). Ribosomes bind the mRNA molecules and, with these as templates, link amino acids to form proteins according to the genetic code (see Fig. 3) (Watson, 1976; Lewin, 1974; Nirenberg et al., 1966). Amino acids do not attach directly to mRNA templates. First they combine with transfer RNA (tRNA) molecules to form "activated" aminoacyl-tRNA (AA-tRNA) by a specific activating enzyme (aminoacyl synthetase) for the accurate reading of the genetic code. DNA polymerase, RNA polymerase, aminoacyl synthetase, and ribosomes owe their great fidelity of translation to the specific interactions of nucleic acids known as sequence complementarity (see Fig. 2).

```
CODING STRAND

5'—\\—C C T A G G A G G T T T G A C C T A T G C G A G C T T T T A G T T A A A G C A A C—\\—3'
                                                                                             DNA
3'—\\—G G A T C C T C C A A A C T G G A T A C G C T C G A A A A T C A A T T T C G T T G—\\—5'

TEMPLATE STRAND

                            fMET—ARG—ALA—PHE—SER          PROTEIN

5'————C C U A G G A G G U U U G A C C U A U G C G A G C U U U U A G U U A A A G C A A C—3'   mRNA
                                                                      STOP
```

Fig. 2. Transcription and translation of genetic information is stored in the structure of double-stranded DNA. A DNA is a chain of nucleotides, each consisting of a deoxyribose sugar ring, a phosphate group, and four organic bases: adenine (A), guanine (G), thymine (T), and cytosine (C). The sugars and phosphates constitute the backbone of the strand, and paired bases linked by hydrogen bonds connect two strands. The bases linked by hydrogen bonds connect two strands. The bases are complementary: A is always opposite to T and G is always opposite to C. The genetic information depends on sequence complementarity. Expression begins when mRNA is transcribed by RNA polymerase using the lower DNA strand as a template and inserts A, C, G, and uracil (U) (chemically analogous to T) monomers according to the same complementarity rules to generate a sequence identical in biological information to the upper DNA strand. At the ribosome the complementary interaction between the triplet codon in the mRNA and the anticodon of the appropriate aminoacyl-tRNA determines which amino acid is inserted next to the growing polypeptide chain. The example here shows initiation of protein synthesis at a "start" codon (methionine codon AUG) and termination of synthesis at UAA, which is one of three possible "stop codons" in the genetic code.

THE GENETIC CODE

1ST↓ 2ND →	U	C	A	G	↓3rd
U	PHE	SER	TYR	CYS	U
	PHE	SER	TYR	CYS	C
	LEU	SER	OCHRE	?	A
	LEU	SER	AMBER	TRP	G
C	LEU	PRO	HIS	ARG	U
	LEU	PRO	HIS	ARG	C
	LEU	PRO	GLUN	ARG	A
	LEU	PRO	GLUN	ARG	G
A	ILEU	THR	ASPN	SER	U
	ILEU	THR	ASPN	SER	C
	ILEU	THR	LYS	ARG	A
	MET	THR	LYS	ARG	G
G	VAL	ALA	ASP	GLY	U
	VAL	ALA	ASP	GLY	C
	VAL	ALA	GLU	GLY	A
	VAL	ALA	GLU	GLY	G

Fig. 3. The genetic code consists of a one-to-one correspondence between each of the 64 best allocations (codons) for the 4 nucleotides (A,G,C, and U) and the 20 amino acids used by ribosomes for protein synthesis. There are definite assignments of specific amino acids to 61 out of the 64 codons. Methionine codon AUG initiates the protein synthesis and synthesis terminates at any chain-terminating (formerly called "nonsense") codons.

DNA Isolation, Fragmentation, and Purification

Isolation

DNA is readily isolated from lysed cells by phenol extraction followed by precipitation with alcohol. Various methods of cell lysis for DNA isolation have been developed which are suitable and

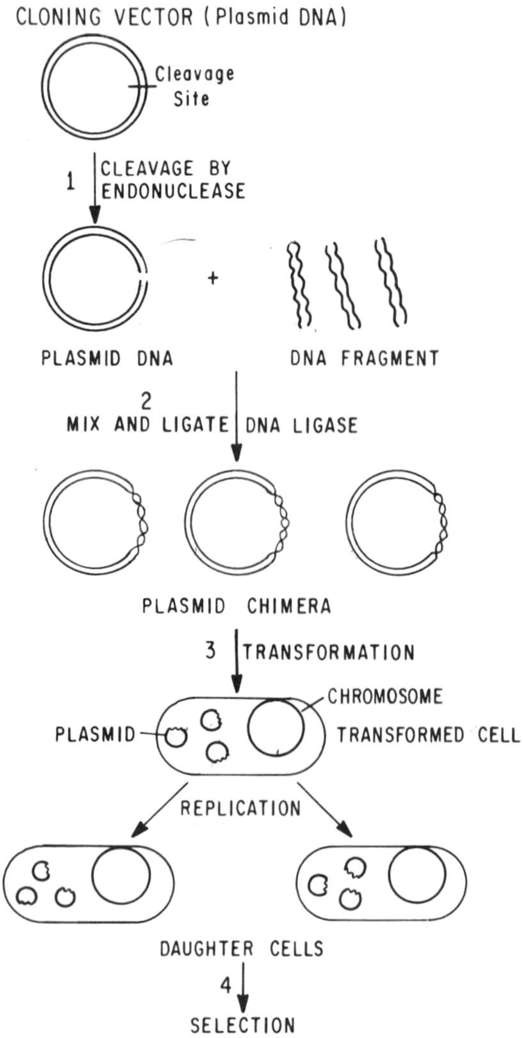

Fig. 4. Generalized scheme in gene cloning. (1) Isolation of DNA which bears the gene of interest by digestion with restriction endonuclease to generate the restriction fragment containing the gene of interest. The cloning vector is also digested with the same restriction endonuclease. (2) Fragments of the cleaved DNA containing the target gene are joined to the digested plasmid DNA by DNA ligase. (3) The ligated DNA (rDNA), each consisting of the entire plasmid, and the target gene are introduced into the host (*E. coli*) by transformation and DNA is replicated by virtue of the replication of the plasmid. (4) Selection of transformants containing the appropriate gene of interest.

Table 1. Cleavage Patterns of Restriction Endonucleases[a]

Blunt cleavage, Hae III	—GC ↓ CC—
	—CC ↑ GG—
Staggered cleavage, Eco RI	—G ↓ AATT C—
	—C TTAA ↑ G—

[a]Arrows represent recognition sequences and DNA cleavage sites by restriction endonuclease.

efficient for a variety of organisms (animals, plants, fungi, gram-positive and gram-negative bacteria, phages, and viruses) (Kolodner and Tewari, 1975; Schleif and Wensink, 1981; Crosa and Falkow, 1981; Perbal, 1984). The DNA fragments generated are usually purified further by techniques such as sucrose density gradients and dye-buoyant density gradient centrifugation (Schleif and Wensink, 1981; Crosa and Falkow, 1981; Perbal, 1984).

DNA Fragmentation and Purification

Physical shearing forces (vigorous mixing, drawing through a syringe needle or pipette, and ultrasonication) can be useful to generate short DNA fragments, some of which will contain the gene of interest. These procedures, however, produce random and irreproducible DNA fragments and are not generally suitable for the production of rDNA molecules. Instead, restriction endonucleases are usually used for the fragmentation of DNA (Nathans and Smith, 1975). More than 250 of these enzymes have been described, each having the ability to cleave double-stranded DNA at particular nucleotide sequences (Roberts, 1981). Table 1 illustrates the actual cleavage location in each strand relative to the recognition sequence for two common restriction endonucleases used in molecular cloning. Since the distribution of restriction sites within a DNA molecule is random, the average length of the fragments depends on the statistical occurrence of the particular restriction site in DNA. In most cases the fragments are about the size of a gene and therefore ideal for experiments involving gene cloning. These fragments can then be separated by agarose gel electrophoresis (Fig. 5) and the fragment containing the gene of interest is subsequently isolated and purified from the gel by electroelution (Perbal, 1984) or freezing and thawing techniques (Bhaduri et al., 1980; Goldenberg et al., 1981).

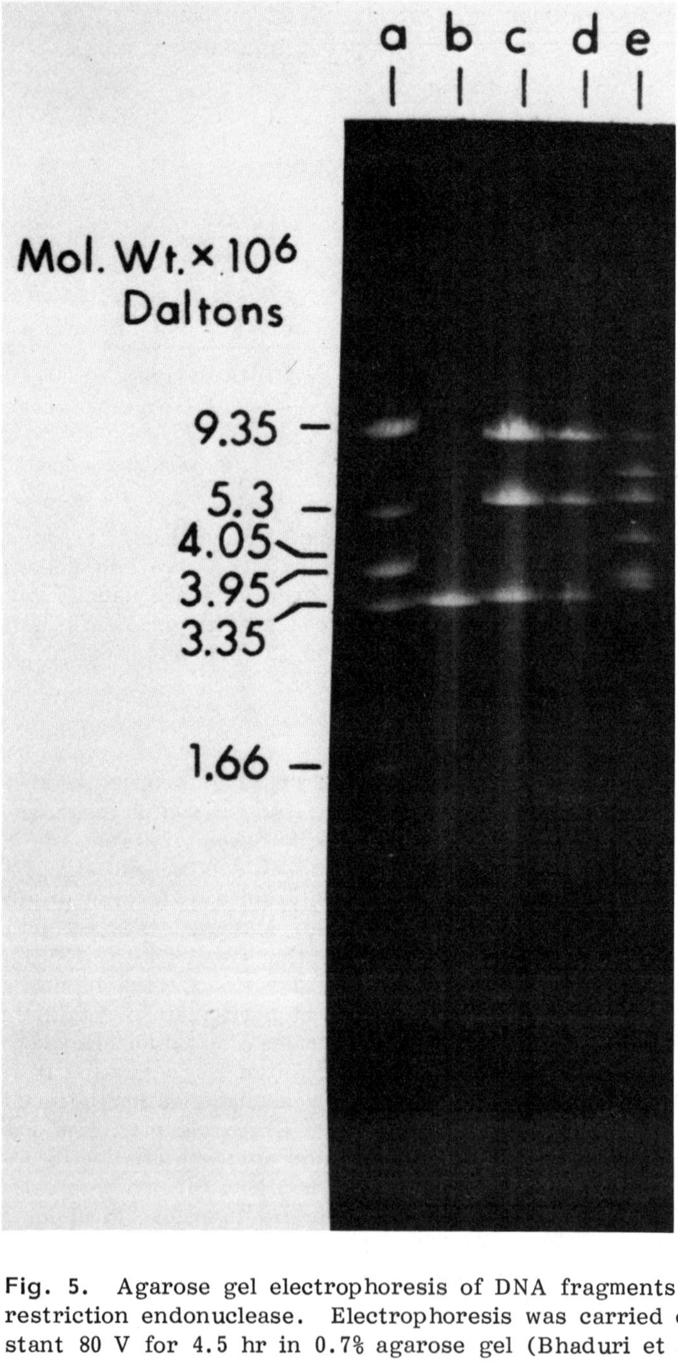

Fig. 5. Agarose gel electrophoresis of DNA fragments generated by restriction endonuclease. Electrophoresis was carried out at a constant 80 V for 4.5 hr in 0.7% agarose gel (Bhaduri et al., 1980).

Suitable Choice of Vector

Vectors are vehicles used to transfer and maintain DNA in foreign hosts. They are divided into two classes: plasmid and lambdoid phages. Since lambdoid phages can be expressed by only a few hosts, the following discussion will focus on plasmids. Plasmids are double-stranded, circular pieces of DNA found in bacteria which replicate independently of the bacterial chromosome. Genes for resistance to many antibiotics are often carried on plasmids (Fig. 6).

For ease of gene cloning, most researchers use small nonconjugative (low molecular weight) plasmids that posses readily identifiable markers (e.g., resistance to drugs or antibiotics). These plasmids must be capable of undergoing replication and amplification in an appropriate host. Additionally, plasmid DNA should posses a single restriction endonuclease cleavage site within resistance genes.

Several such vectors have been developed and specifically engineered for use in *Escherichia coli*. Two general types of plasmids should be selected for cloning: (1) those that are capable of very high copy numbers but restricted to a very small number of bacterial species, for example, pBR 322 in *E. coli* (Fig. 6) (Bolivar and Backman, 1979; Helinski, 1979), and (2) those that are derivatives of plasmids that can be maintained in a large number of bacterial species but which occur in relatively low copy numbers, for example, pRK 290 (Ditta et al., 1980). The high-copy number plasmid (1) is more useful for cloning any protein or peptide in a suitable host. The second type of plasmid (2) has potential application where modification of a "commercial microbe" is the objective; an example would be the cloning of useful genes (e.g., cellulase) into the nitrogen-fixing bacterium *Rhizobium* to obtain an organism that can convert wood (cellulose) into microbial protein. Table 2 lists some cloning vectors and their properties.

Gene Insertion into Vector and Introduction of Recombinant DNA into the Host

The gene (DNA fragment) to be cloned must be covalently joined to the cloning vector to generate an rDNA molecule. Such manipulations generally involve the specific cleavage of DNA preparation (passenger) with a restriction endonuclease. These DNA fragments are then mixed with a correspondingly cleaved vector DNA and joined end to end by DNA ligase followed by transfer (transformation or transfection) of circular rDNA molecules into a suitable host. Several strategies can be employed for ensuring that the desired DNA fragment is inserted in the correct position and orientation.

Cleavage of the DNA by a specific restriction endonuclease as indicated by arrows in Table 1 yields DNA fragments with either complementary single-stranded termini (i.e., Eco R1) causing

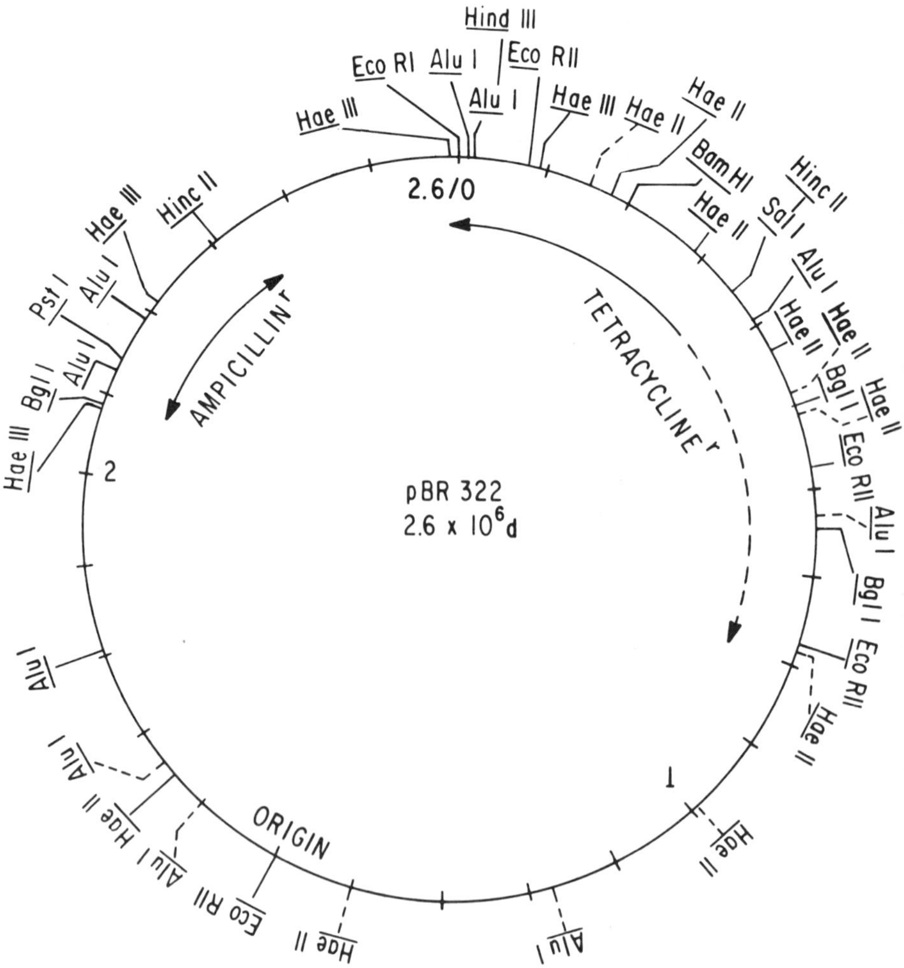

Fig. 6. Restriction map of pBR 322. Regions of the vector which confer resistance to the antibiotics ampicillin and tetracycline are indicated.

staggered or "sticky" cohesive ends. As is also shown in Table 1, cleavage can be opposite the phosphodiester bonds of the DNA duplex (i.e., Hae III), giving rise to blunt ends. The joining of passenger DNA (genes of interest) and vector DNA is easier in the case of the sticky ends. However, ligation can be achieved with T4 DNA ligase, which acts on both cohesive and blunt end DNA to yield rDNA.

Table 2. Plasmid Vectors for Gene Cloning

Vector	Host range	Comments
Gram-negative bacteria		
Col E1	*E. coli*	Can be amplified.
pBR 322	*E. coli*	The most common vector for general purpose use; can be amplified.
RSF 1010	*E. coli*	Some *Pseudomonas* spp. can be used as host.
pRK 290	*Klebsiella aerogenes*	Most gram-negative bacteria can be used as host.
RP1	*Pseudomonas aeruginosa*	Most gram-negative bacteria can be used as host.
Gram-positive bacteria		
pUB 110	*Bacillus*	Suitable for other *Bacillus* spp.
SCP–2	*Streptomyces*	Some *Streptomyces* spp. can also be used.
Fungi		
YEp; YRp	*Saccharomyces*	A broad-range vector system for yeast.
Plant cells		
Ti	*Agrobacterium tumefaciens*	At present only effective vector for cloning in plants.
Animal cells		
Defective SV40	Mammalian cell line	Control of transmittance is obtained in part by use of defective virus.

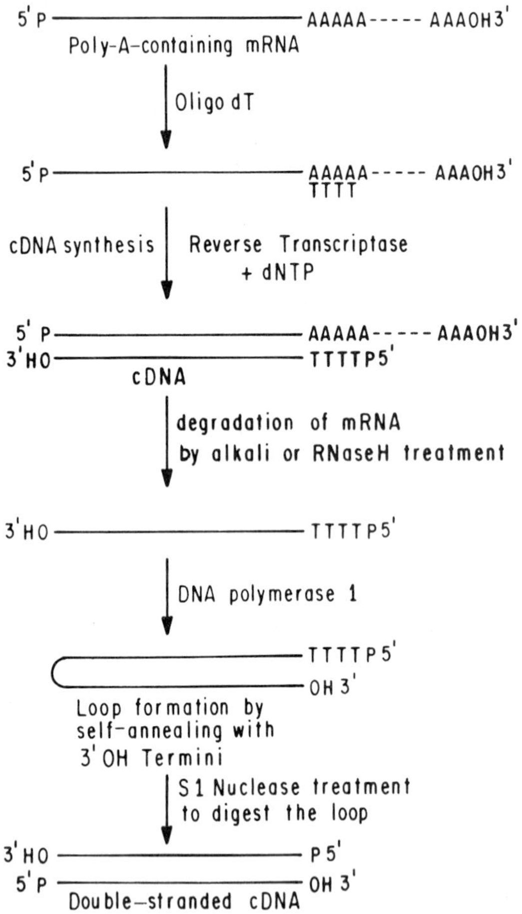

Fig. 7. Synthesis of double-stranded cDNA from poly-A containing mRNA. The schematic diagram is self-explanatory.

In certain cases problems arise. The restriction endonuclease cleavage site may be present within the structural gene of interest or the DNA fragment to be cloned may be extremely difficult to purify. In these cases different approaches have been employed (Craig and Hall, 1983; Harris, 1983). For example, a DNA fragment containing a gene (e.g., in the production of somatostatin and insulin) can be synthetically synthesized and then introduced into a plasmid. One effective approach to producing synthetic DNA is to use the messenger RNA (mRNA) for a desired cell product in conjunction with enzyme reverse transcriptase plus four deoxynucleoside triphosphates. This enzyme uses the mRNA as a template to generate the complementary DNA (called cDNA). This method is preferred in cases where mRNA can be purified easily from a particular tissue. A schematic diagram is shown in Figure 7.

A second approach to gene cloning is chemical synthesis of DNA by a combination of organic and nucleic acid chemistry. Recent developments on the methods initiated by Khorana have made it possible to synthesize gene-sized fragments of DNA in several months, as with the synthesis of the insulin gene (Itakura et al., 1977; Crea et al., 1978). In this approach a DNA sequence is designed, based on the genetic code for a particular protein. In addition, cDNA and synthetic DNA do not contain the internal nontranslated sequence (introns) found in eukaryotic chromosomal DNA and are thus more suitable for expression of the gene in prokaryotes (Goldenberg et al., 1981). Synthetic DNA can also be cloned if a DNA contains the proper restriction site in the molecule.

When end-to-end ligation is not suitable to insert passenger DNA (particularly in the case of synthetic DNA) into the vector, homopolymeric tailing techniques (Deng and Wu, 1981) or the addition of synthetic linkers (Perbal, 1984) at the site of insertion can be employed. With homopolymeric tailing procedures, 15--20 nucleotides can be added to small amounts of DNA sequences. This process can be achieved with considerable accuracy over a reasonable time course (Fig. 8). Linkers containing the recognition and cleavage sites for specific restriction enzyme are joined to the passenger DNA by ligase and then inserted into the cloning vector as shown in Figure 9. A number of these linker molecules for different restriction enzymes are commercially available.

The introduction of rDNA into suitable hosts for the purpose of gene amplification or to obtain gene expression is carried out by the process of transformation. This involves inducing cells to incorporate rDNA. The cells which are capable of incorporating exogenous DNA without degradation are known as competent cells. Competence can often be induced by treatment with magnesium chloride and calcium chloride (Bhaduri et al., 1980; Goldenberg et al., 1981). Transformation is relatively inefficient, but if transformants (bacteria which have taken up plasmids) can be readily selected directly, the desired clone can usually be isolated.

Screening and Selection of Clones

Following transformation, the clone containing the desired gene must be identified. Clones constructed using the method described above contain plasmids with a range of inserts. The efficiency of the screening or selection method determines the success of a cloning

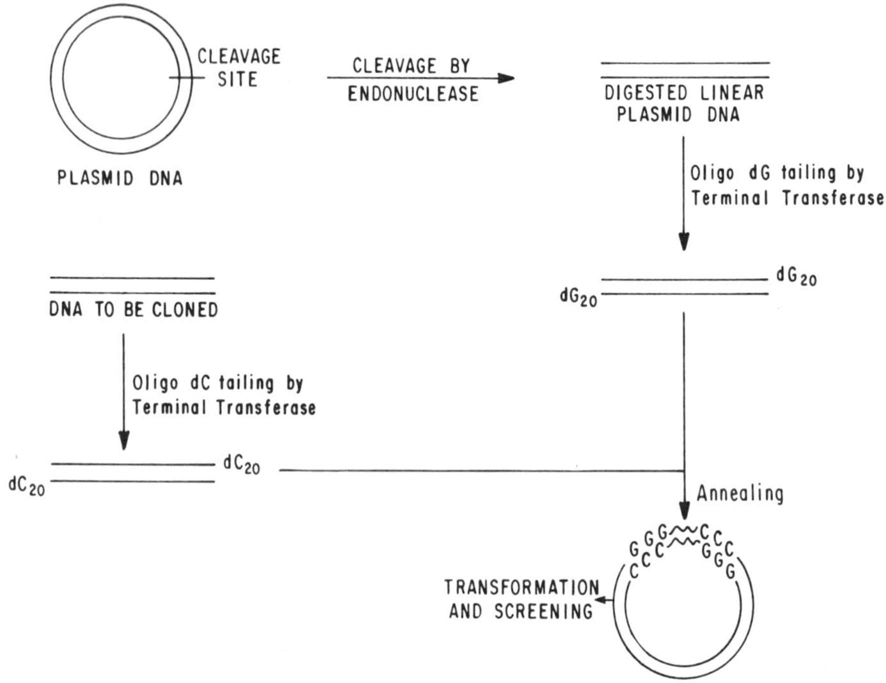

Fig. 8. Cloning of synthetic DNA in the plasmid vector by the homopolymeric dG:dC tailing technique.

project. The significance of this step becomes evident from the fact that some clones contain complete genes while others contain only fragments. The selection of the clones which contain the plasmid and produce the desired product is accomplished by a variety of methods (Fig. 10):

1. "Insertional inactivation" is the most widely used method, and it involves the insertion of a foreign DNA in the antibiotic resistance gene of plasmid, thereby causing a loss of that resistance. This method, however, only indicates that the plasmid contains foreign DNA.

2. Biological activity (an enzymatic or peptide hormone), the detection of expression of the gene product by its biological activity. For example, the clone containing specific enzyme may be detected by its specific action on the substrate. In the case of peptide hormones, the transformant containing the gene for the peptide hormone may be selected by its specific action in mouse assay.

3. Selective media, which support the growth of only those organisms that have taken up the desired gene. For example, transformants harboring the gene for histidine biosynthesis may be selected by growing a mixed population of transformants on media which does not contain histidine (Bhaduri et al., 1980).

4. Immunological detection of desired clones by radioisotope-labeled antibody specific for the product of the gene of interest (Craig and Hall, 1983).

5. Colony hybridization utilizes radioactive complementary nucleic acid probes (either DNA or RNA) which will bind with those clones containing the desired DNA sequence (Grunstein and Hogness, 1975; Doel et al., 1980).

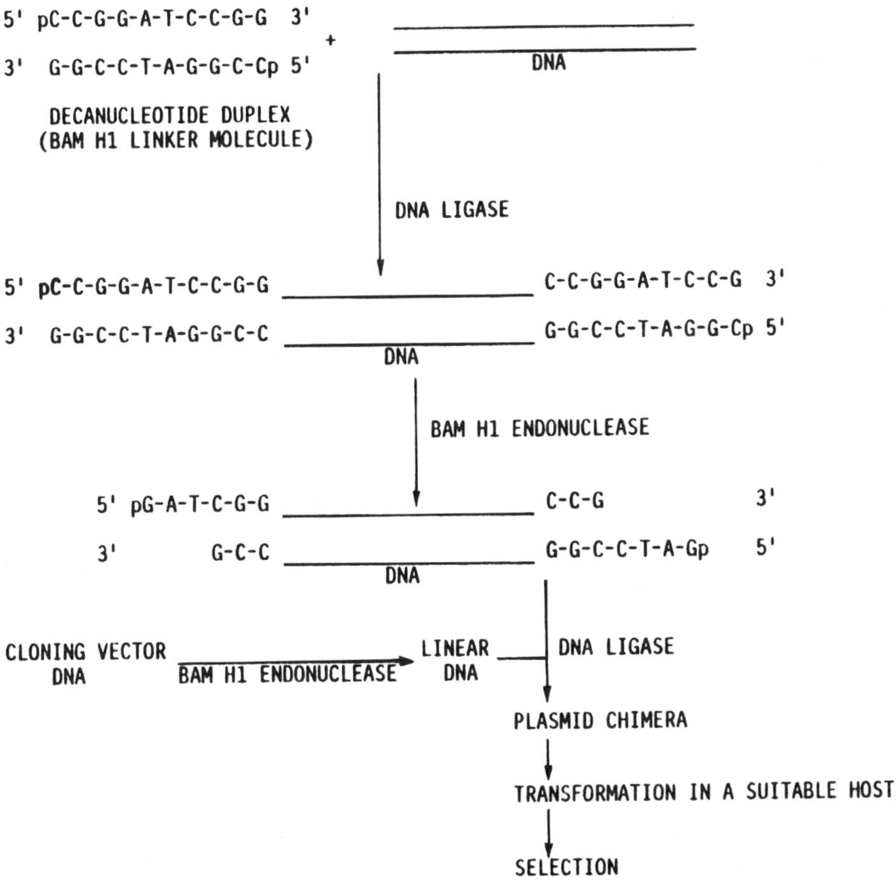

Fig. 9. Scheme for introducing cohesive ends at the termini of any duplex DNA molecule for molecular cloning.

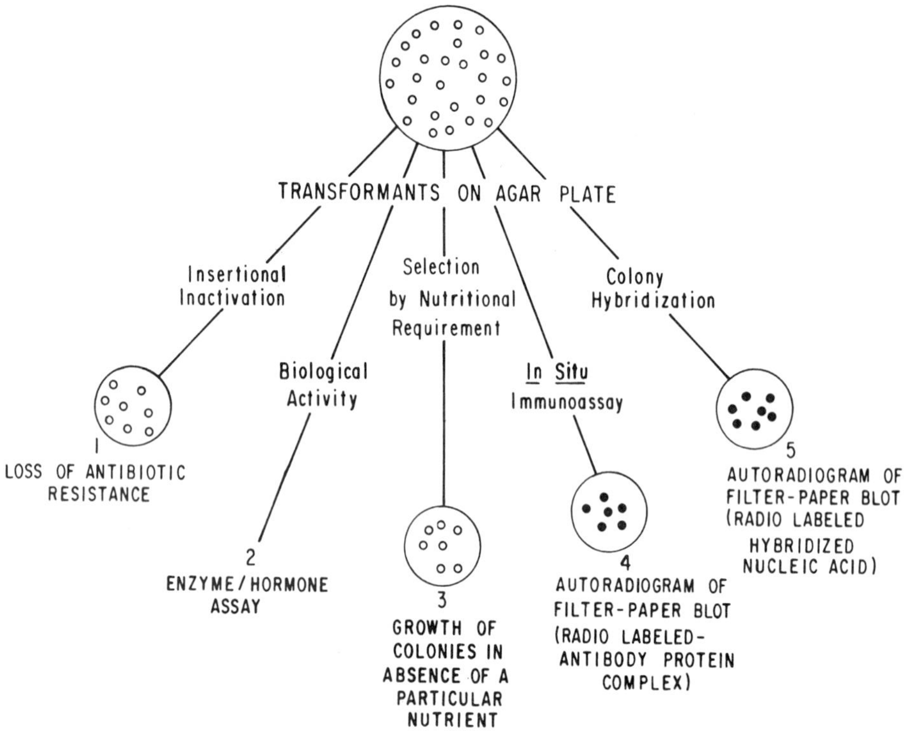

Fig. 10. The screening and selection of the desired clones include in vitro and in vivo assays and autoradiograms.

CURRENT STATUS OF RECOMBINANT DNA TECHNIQUES

A diverse range of vector systems has been developed for microbes, plants, and animals (see Table 2). These vector systems are available for their respective hosts and allow the use of rDNA techniques in other organisms (Struhl et al., 1979; Purchio and Fareed, 1979; Ream and Gordon, 1982). Useful vectors have also been developed for viruses (Old and Primrose, 1980). However, since the genetics of *E. coli* are so well defined, it is possible to achieve greater genetic manipulation within *E. coli* than with other organisms. The expression of unmodified cloned eukaryotic genes in bacteria is highly improbable, because prokaryotes appear to lack the enzymatic machinery needed to remove the intervening sequences (introns) that interrupt eukaryotic coding sequences (Goldenberg et al., 1981). Two different approaches can be used to solve this problem. One

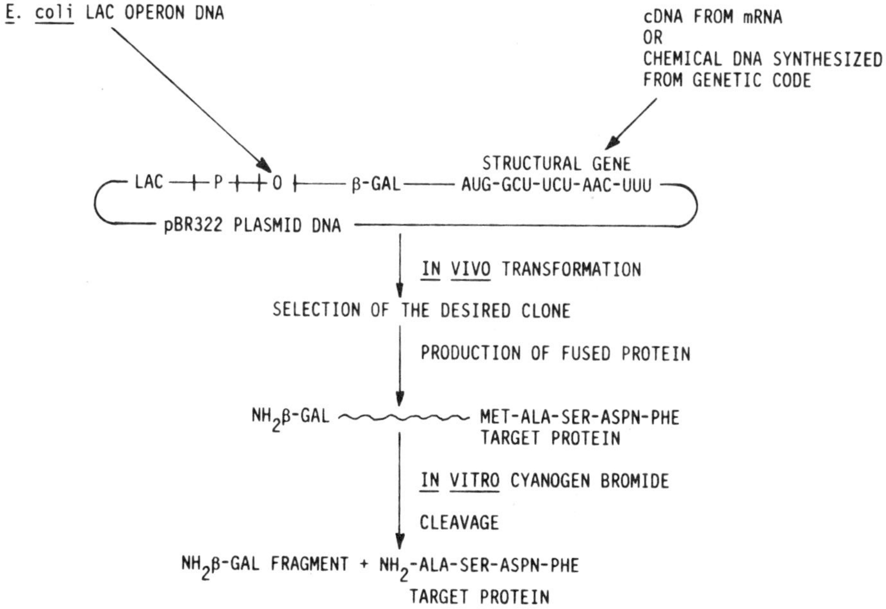

Fig. 11. Strategy for the expression of cDNA (gene) from mRNA or a chemically synthesized gene as a β-galactosidase fusion from the *lac* promoter. The active hormone can be cleaved from the hybrid protein by cyanogen bromide treatment.

is the insertion of cDNA and the other is the insertion of chemically synthesized DNA into a suitable vector. Both of these synthetic DNAs are "spliced copies" of the gene (Goldenberg et al., 1981) which can subsequently be introduced into expression-cloning vectors by standard techniques (Fig. 11).

APPLICATION OF RECOMBINANT DNA TECHNOLOGY IN THE FOOD INDUSTRY

The potential for the commercial exploitation of genetic engineering becomes more evident because of the development of the various techniques and approaches discussed previously. Although the food industry has historically been the oldest and most extensive user of biological processes for the production of its products, the use of applied genetics and modern biotechnology (rDNA technology) is currently quite limited. However, considerable research on the genetic manipulation of microorganisms for the fermentative production of such foodstuffs as cheese and related fermented dairy products, alcoholic beverages, and acetic, lactic, and citric acids has been conducted with the objective of producing strains with superior activity, greater stability, or improved product yield. Effective use of rDNA technology could enhance progress in these areas. To date, a few processes have made use of rDNA technology.

Amino Acids

Amino acids are used to fortify the human and animal diet and as flavor enhancers. Currently these amino acids are obtained by extraction of biological materials or hydrolysis of protein. A high level of amino acid production in a microbial system could be achieved by the modification of the genes by rDNA technology. It has been estimated that the market for amino acid production will increase from $1.8 billion to $2.4 billion by the year 2000 as a result of rDNA techniques (Office of Technological Assessment, 1981).

Enzymes

Commercial use of enzymes by the food and detergent industries is valued at $160 million (Office of Technological Assessment, 1981). The common enzymes used in the industry are glucoamylase, glucose oxidase, exocellobiohydrolase-1, lipase, protease, isomerase, and invertase. These enzymes are isolated from fungi or bacteria which grow at slow rates and yield small amounts of enzyme. Other enzymes such as pepsin, rennin, and papain are of plant or animal tissue origin. Microbial production of these enzymes by genetic engineering could improve their yield at a significantly lower cost. Cloning of the genes of some of these enzymes (amylase, rennin) has been reported (White et al., 1984).

Single-Cell Protein

The use of genetic engineering in the production of single-cell protein has already been implemented (Windass et al., 1980; Gelfand, 1980). Genes from *E. coli*, which are more efficient in nitrogen assimilation, have been transferred into *Methylophilus methylotrophus*. The modified *Methylophilus* demonstrated an increased carbon conversion 4–7% over its parent. The production of single-cell protein from *Saccharomyces cerevisiae* is also in the process of development (Batt and Sinskey, 1984).

Starter Cultures

The genetic manipulation of starter culture by rDNA technology could enhance the efficiency and quality of the fermented food products. Studies (Kondo and McKay, 1982; Lee et al., 1982) at the molecular genetics level in dairy fermentation have already been initiated.

Polysaccharides

Polysaccharides are used as stabilizers and texturizers. Many are derived from plants. It would be cheaper if these were produced in bacteria through genetic manipulation by rDNA technology.

Sweeteners, Flavorants, and Pigments

Aspartame (dipeptide aspartylphenylalanine), used as a substitute sweetener, can be produced in bacteria by rDNA technology. Doel et al. (1980) chemically synthesized the gene, a dodecanucleotide specifying aspartylphenylalanine, and introduced it into a plasmid and expressed the gene as multiple repeating units of the aspartame dipeptide by cloning adjacent to a controllable tryptophan promoter. Proteolytic cleavage of this molecule by thermolysin yields only aspartame. The extremely sweet peptides monellin and thaumatins are derived from plants, and their production could be achieved by rDNA technology for commercial use. At present, the flavorants inosinic acid and guanylic acid are produced by extraction from yeast; it is possible to produce these compounds in bacteria by molecular cloning. The production of natural pigment carotenoids may also be enhanced by improvising the activity of their biosynthetic pathway by rDNA technology.

Other Potentially Important Applications of Recombinant DNA Technology to the Food Industry

1. Starch saccharification to glucose via microbially derived amylase
2. Microbial conversion of food processing wastes into edible products
3. Microbial removal of toxins or objectionable components from food to make safe, edible foods

FUTURE OF RECOMBINANT DNA TECHNOLOGY IN THE FOOD INDUSTRY

The discovery of rDNA technology and the current advances have brought about in a short time a new era in biological research. Although the techniques developed in rDNA technology are for general use and also applicable to diversified systems such as bacteria, fungi, plants, and animals, further innovative techniques will be required. The application of rDNA technology in the food industry depends not only on technical feasibilities but also on economic considerations. In the final analysis, it appears that genetic manipulation by rDNA technology in the food industry should be directed toward improved nutritive yield, productivity, and quality and constitutes the most promising outfall of genetics to the food industry within the next decade.

ACKNOWLEDGMENTS

I thank David Schlessinger of Washington University Medical School, St. Louis, Mo., and Arthur J. Miller of the Eastern Regional Research Center, Philadelphia, Pa., for a critical reading of the manuscript.

REFERENCES

Batt, C. A. and Sinskey, A. J. (1984). Use of biotechnology in the production of single-cell protein. *Food Tech.* *38*:108–111.

Bhaduri, S., Kasai, T., Raskas, H. J., and Schlessinger, D. (1980). pMB9 plasmids bearing the *Salmonella typhimurium his* operon and gnd gene. *Gene* *8*:239–253.

Bolivar, F. and Backman, K. (1979). Plasmids of *E. coli* as cloning vectors. *Methods Enzymol.* *68*:245–267.

Craig, R. K. and Hall, L. (1983). Recombinant DNA technology: Application to the characterization and expression of polypeptide hormones. *Genet. Eng.* *4*:58–125.

Crea, R., Kraszewski, A., Hirose, T., and Itakura, K. (1978). Chemical synthesis of genes for human insulin. *Proc. Nat. Acad. Sci. U.S.A.* *75*:5765–5769.

Crosa, J. H. and Falkow, S. (1981). Plasmids. In *Manual of Methods for General Microbiology* (P. Gerhardt, ed.), American Society for Microbiology, Washington, D.C., pp. 266–282.

Davidson, J. N. (1969). The biosynthesis of RDA. In *The Biochemistry of Nucleic Acids*, 6th ed., Methuen, London, pp. 236–277.

Deng, G. and Wu, R. (1981). An improved procedure for utilizing terminal transferase to add homopolymers to the 3' termini of DNA. *Nucl. Acid Res. 9*:4173–4188.

Ditta, G., Stanfield, S., Corbin, D., and Helinski, D. R. (1980). Broad host range cloning system for gram negative bacteria: Construction of a gene bank of *Rhizobium melioti*. *Proc. Nat. Acad. Sci. U.S.A. 77*:7347–7351.

Doel, M. T., Eaton, M., Cook, E. A., Lewis, H., Patel, T., and Carey, N. H. (1980). The expression in *E. coli* of synthetic repeating polymeric genes coding for the poly(L-aspartyl-L-phenylalanine). *Nucl. Acids Res. 8*:4575–4592.

Gelgand, D. H. (1980). Molecular approaches to increasing carbon conversion efficiency in fermentation processes. Paper presented at the Second American Society for Microbiology Conference on Genetics and Molecular Biology of Industrial Microorganisms, University of Indiana, Bloomington, October 1980.

Goldenberg, C. J., Rosenthal, R., Bhaduri, S., and Raskas, H. J. (1981). Coordinate regulation of two cytoplasmic RNA species transcribed from early region 2 of the adenovirus genome. *J. Virol. 38*:932–939.

Grunstein, M. and Hogness, D. S. (1975). Colony hybridization: A method for the isolation of cloned DNA's that contain a specific gene. *Proc. Nat. Acad. Sci. U.S.A. 72*:3961–3965.

Harris, T. J. R. (1983). Expression of eukaryotic genes in *E. coli*. *Genet. Eng. 4*:128–185.

Helinski, D. R. (1976). Plasmid DNA replication. *Fed. Proc. 35*:2026–2030.

Helinski, D. R. (1979). Bacterial plasmids: Autonomous replication and vehicles for cloning. *Crit. Rev. Biochem. 7*:83–101.

Itakura, K., Hirose, K. T., Crea, R., Riggs, A. D., Heyneker, H. L., Bolivar, F., and Boyer, H. W. (1977). Expression in *E. coli* of a chemically synthesized gene for the hormone somatostatin. *Science 198*:1056–1063.

Kolodner, R. and Tewari, K. K. (1975). The molecular size and confirmation of the chloroplast DNA from higher plants. *Biochem. Biophys. Acta 402*:372–390.

Kondo, J. K. and McKay, L. L. (1982). Transformation of *Streptococcus lactis* protoplasts by plasmid DNA. *Appl. Environ. Microbiol. 43*:1213–1215.

Lee, L., Hansen, J. B., Jagusztyn-Krynicka, E. K., and B. M. Chassy (1982). Cloning and expression of the β-D-phosphogalactoside galactohydrolase gene of *Lactobacillus casei* in *E. coli* K-12. *J. Bacteriol. 152*:1138–1146.

Lewin, B. (1974). *Gene Expression*, Vol. 1, Wiley, New York.

Maniatis, T., Fritsch, E. F., and Sambrook, J. (1982). Molecular cloning: A laboratory manual. Cold Spring Harbor Laboratory, Cold Spring Harbor, N. Y.

Nathans, D. and Smith, H. O. (1975). Restriction endonucleases in the analysis and restructuring of DNA molecules. *Annu. Rev. Biochem. 44*:273–293.

Nirenberg, M., Caskey, T., Marshall, R., Brimacombe, R., Kellogg, D., Doctor, B., Hatfield, D., Levin, J., Rottman, R., Pestka, S., Wilcox, M., and Anderson, F. (1966). The RNA code and protein synthesis. *Cold Spring Harbor Symp. 31*:11–24.

Office of Technological Assessment (1981). *Impacts of Applied Genetics: Microorganisms, Plants, and Animals.* Office of Technology Assessment, Washington, D. C.

Old, R. W. and Primrose, S. B. (1980). *Principles of Gene Manipulation: An Introduction to Genetic Engineering,* University of California Press, Berkley.

Perbal, B. (1984). *A Practical Guide to Molecular Cloning,* Wiley, New York.

Purchio, A. F. and Fareed, G. C. (1979). Methods for molecular cloning in eukaryotic cells. *Methods Enzymol. 68*:357–375.

Ream, L. W. and Gordon, M. P. (1982). Crown gall disease and prospects for genetic manipulation of plants. *Science 218*: 854–858.

Roberts, R. J. (1981). Restriction and modification enzymes and their recognition sequences. *Nucl. Acids Res. 9*:R75–R96.

Schleif, R. F. and Wensink, P. C. (1981). *Practical Methods in Molecular Biology,* Springer-Verlag, New York, pp. 89–125.

Sherratt, D. J. (1974). Bacterial plasmids. *Cell 3*:189–195.

Struhl, K., Stinchcomb, D., Scherer, S., and Davis, R. W. (1979). High-frequency transformation of yeast: Autonomous replication of hybrid DNA molecules. *Proc. Nat. Acad. Sci. U.S.A. 76*: 1035–1039.

Watson, J. D. (1976). *Molecular Biology of the Gene,* 3rd ed., Cummings, Menlo Park, Calif.

White, T. J., Meade, J. H., Shoemaker, S. P., Koths, K. E., and Innis, M. A. (1984). Enzyme cloning for the food fermentation industry. *Food Technol. 38*:90–98.

Windass, J. D., Worlsey, M. J., Pioli, E. M., Barth, P. T., Atherton, K. T., Dart, E. C., Byron, D., Powell, K., and Senior, P. J. (1980). Improved conversion of methanol by single–cell protein by *Methylophilus methylotrophus*. *Nature 287*:396–401.

Zillig, W. K., Zechel, K., Rabussay, D., Schachner, M., Sethi, V. S., Palm, P., Heil, A., and Seifert, W. (1970). On the role of different subunits of DNA-dependent RNA polymerase from *E. coli* transcription process. *Cold Spring Harbor Symp. 35*: 47–58.

GLOSSARY

Amplification refers to the production of additional copies of a chromosomal sequence, found as either intra- or extrachromosomal (plasmid) DNA.

Exons are the remaining segment of the primary transcript that are joined together to form final mRNA.

High-copy number plasmid refers to some plasmids under relaxed replication control, which means they continue replicating in large amounts (about 1000 genomes per cell) after bacteria stop dividing.

Introns are untranslated intervening sequences of DNA that are transcribed (primary transcripts) but excised within the primary transcript by splicing together the sequences (exon) on either side.

Linkers are short synthetic oligonucleotide duplex molecules containing the recognition sequence for some restriction enzymes.

Low-copy number plasmids are maintained in bacteria under stringent replication control, which means they replicate at a ratio of 1 or 2 plasmid DNAs for every host chromosome.

Splicing (RNA splicing) describes the excisions of introns and joining of exons in finished mRNA; thus introns are spliced out, while exons are spliced together.

6

Analytical Methods in the Structure Elucidation of Fermentation Products: Low Molecular Weight Compounds

LUDGER WITTE / Gesellschaft für Biotechnologische Forschung, Braunschweig, Federal Republic of Germany

INTRODUCTION

This chapter describes analytical methods which are useful for the detection, identification, and monitoring of biotechnologically important compounds. Products of these processes are so numerous and diverse that many different analytical techniques are used. In the space allotted it is, of course, impossible to cover all the methods which have been successfully applied in solving analytical problems of biotechnological interest. Restrictions are necessary to keep the chapter down to a reasonable length.

The complexity of biological material makes component analysis, except in very specialized cases, only possible after or combined with chromatographic procedures. Thus flexible analytical techniques have been selected which work with mixtures, are useful for a quick, reliable, and sensitive estimation of known components, and are also applicable to the characterization of unknown compounds. Furthermore, the techniques illustrated use versatile equipment that is not dedicated to a single application, and methods are explained which allow the screening of a large number of components in a minimum number of chromatographic runs.

METHODOLOGY

Methods of wide applicability are liquid and gas chromatography. Instruments for these techniques are widely distributed in analytical laboratories, as the hardware is relatively cheap and the methods frequently used. The published literature in this area is manifold.

Both techniques offer high and rapid separation, results are easy to quantify, and the instruments can be combined with additional spectrometers to enhance the credibility of the analysis. Thus applications involving these two techniques are discussed, although an exhaustive treatment is impossible. Examples will be used as a guide to fundamental analytical techniques. Many books treating chromatographic methods as an analytical tool have been published; the recently available book by Poole and Schuette (1984) covers all the techniques discussed in this chapter.

The principle of separation in both gas chromatography (GC) and high-performance liquid chromatography (HPLC) is the same and relies on the different distributions of sample components between a mobile and a stationary phase. Advantages and disadvantages of each technique are determined by many factors, and several considerations must be taken into account in order to decide which method one should use. Gas chromatography analysis is in most cases cheaper, quicker, and more sensitive and has a higher separation efficiency than HPLC.

Compounds of low volatility, thermal instability, and high polarity, especially ionic molecules, are better served by HPLC analysis. However, large molecules, such as triglycerides, or extremely polar ones, such as carbohydrates, can easily be analyzed by GC after conversion to volatile derivatives. Gas chromatography columns have a much higher separation efficiency than HPLC columns, but with the latter technique the possibility of combining different stationary and mobile phases is greater.

In the following some general aspects of HPLC and GC will be discussed. The major HPLC modes are performed on solid adsorbents, ion exchange material, and reversed phases. A further method is exclusion chromatography—also called molecular sieving, gel permeation, or gel filtration—where separation depends on the molecular size.

Silica gel is the most commonly used adsorbent in liquid–solid chromatography, and the retention mechanism relies on adsorption effects. With eluent combinations, consisting of polar and nonpolar components, the retention may be caused by partitioning into a more polar liquid stationary phase produced by the eluent in situ on the column.

In cation exchange the stationary phase contains fixed anionic sites. These interact electrostatically with cationic compounds, which are thus retained. Conversely, in anion exchange the fixed sites are positively charged and anions are retained.

Reversed-phase chromatography has become more and more important in recent years. Hydrophobic interactions determine the extent of retention and this method is therefore used for the separation of nonpolar or slightly polar compounds. The more polar the compound, the more it favors the aqueous eluent and elutes faster in reversed-phase HPLC (Brown and Krstulovic, 1979). Additives of certain compounds lead to more specialized techniques. One example is ion-pairing chromatography, in which compounds, such as alkyl ammonium salts, are added to the mobile phase. There lipophilic groups interact with the nonpolar stationary reversed-phase and their ionic moiety can then interact with ionic compounds, causing greater retention of charged solutes on reversed-phase systems.

Chromatographic identificaton of compounds relies on their retention behavior and as such is not too reliable. Therefore with such simple analytical systems it is always necessary to check whether the eluted peak represents the expected compound, and its identity should be proven by a second method. This may be a chemical test, stopped-flow ultraviolet spectra, or absorbance ratios at various wavelengths. Detection in HPLC is still a problem with many biological molecules. A universal detector comparable to GC flame ionization does not exist. Structural features which result in ultraviolet absorption, fluorescence, or electrochemical activity are found only in a few biological molecules, although different members of a class of biological substances normally share a common functionality. In several cases a relatively simple derivatization method can be developed to "tag" the molecules which allows better detection with comparable sensitivity using common detectors.

Over the last few years the combination of HPLC and mass spectrometry (MS) has become a general and important technique. Problems encountered with the system are caused by the high solvent flow volumes and the necessity of a high vacuum in the mass spectrometer. Two different HPLC—MS techniques of practical use are commercially available. One of them uses a transport belt from the HPLC to the ion source of the mass spectrometer. During the transport the solvent is thermally separated in consecutive vacuum chambers and the solute is flash-vaporized from the belt into the ion source, where electron impact or chemical ionization usually occurs (McFadden, 1980; Games, 1981).

In contrast to the above system, the more recent thermospray technique (Vestal, 1984) works even with nonvolatile or thermally labile compounds. The HPLC effluent is sprayed as a supersonic jet of vapor and small droplets into the ion source. The solvent must contain a volatile buffer, usually ammonium acetate, which forms ionic adducts with the solute molecules which are analyzed by MS. Thermospray HPLC—MS seems to be an optimal extension of the moving belt system, as high flow rates and polar solvents cause no problems, and it can easily handle compounds such as carbohydrates, amino acids, peptides (Pilosof et al., 1984), nucleosides, and nucleotides (Vestal, 1984).

Gas chromatography is nowadays the most commonly applied analytical method for the separation of complex mixtures. It is applicable to a wide range of compounds, not only to those with high volatility and thermal stability but also to those not usually amenable to direct GC studies after chemical modification to volatile derivatives. Gas chromatography was first developed using packed columns, but the introduction of capillary columns has greatly enhanced the technique and these are generally always preferred. The most obvious benefits are better separation efficiency and speed of analysis with enhanced sensitivity, as high, sharp peaks provide higher concentration levels of the solutes for detection than the broad peaks resulting from packed-column GC. The recently developed flexible fused silica capillary columns coated with chemically bonded stationary phases has allowed further progress. These columns are robust, easy to handle, and inert and have improved chromatographic properties. As nearly all methods developed for packed columns are readily transferrable to capillary GC systems, this is the method of choice.

Characterization of GC-separated compounds is best performed using Kováts retention index system (Kováts, 1958). The retention of the compound is related to the retention of the homologous series of n-alkanes. The resulting values are dependent only on the stationary phase used and, to a lesser extent, on the column temperature. Column length and diameter, inlet pressure, and flow rate are not important factors and it does not matter if packed or capillary columns are used. Retention indices of the highest precision are obtained under isothermal conditions, although their graphic determination from programmed temperature GC runs result in approximate values of considerable value.

Gas chromatographic identification of components based solely on retention data is especially difficult in the analysis of complex samples. Selective detection, such as phosphorous–nitrogen detection or electron capture detection, enhances the assurance of the assignments, but unambiguous identification is impossible. Chromatography and characterization using a second column of different polarity are normally sufficient for the identification of known compounds. Two different fused silica columns can easily be introduced in one GC injection port, and if they are connected with different detectors, the required data can be obtained with a single injection. In contrast, the identification of unknowns is practically impossible.

However, the combination of GC with other analytical methods, such as infrared or mass spectrometry, can often help in such situations; GC–MS is one of the most powerful analytical techniques (Ten Noever de Brauw, 1979). Mass-spectrometric–GC detection is almost universal, yielding information on the structural details of separated components (McFadden, 1973). Mass-spectral fragmentation patterns combined with retention data allow for rapid and reliable identification, even in complex mixtures. Several small and relatively inexpensive instruments are commercially available. The technique has been widely used in mixture analysis and there exists a large quantity of relevant literature which can help solve analytical problems.

In the following section chromatographic techniques applicable to various examples of biotechnologically important classes of compounds will be considered.

ANALYSIS OF AMINO ACIDS

Amino acids, the building blocks of proteins, comprise one of the most important classes of compounds of biological and biotechnological interest. Many different techniques have been developed for their analysis over the last decades. This chapter describes several approved methods for the qualitative and quantitative estimation of these compounds.

Prior to amino acid analysis of biological samples, purification procedures are required in order to reduce or eliminate interfering substances. After ultracentrifugation or ultrafiltration, the most widely used purification step is a cation exchange clean-up on Dowex 50W resin. The material is applied in an acid medium onto a small column which adsorbs the amino acids. Washing with water separates unwanted compounds and the amino acids are retained on the resin. Their elution can be performed with 1M or 2M ammonia. After they are freeze-dried, the samples are prepared for analysis or derivatization procedures.

The classic method of amino acid analysis is ion exchange chromatography with their colorometric detection as ninhydrin derivatives. This method, developed by Moore et al. (1958), has led to the construction of automated analyzers and has remained essentially unchanged. It is still the most widely used procedure for amino acid quantification, with a detection limit in the picomole range. An example of the application of this method with biological material is given by Murayama and Shindo (1977). They determined more than 50 ninhydrine-positive compounds, including amino sugars, using a two-column chromatographic system. However, the disadvantages of amino acid analyzers are their high initial cost and the high running costs for the analysis of only one class of compounds. Thus other analytical techniques have been developed, especially those based on liquid chromatography and gas chromatography, in order to use instruments that are not dedicated to only one type of analysis.

Several approaches for amino acid analysis by high-performance liquid chromatography (HPLC) have been carried out. A rapid method for the separation of the 20 common amino acids is described by Zimmerman et al. (1977). The amino acid phenylthiohydantoins

(PTHs) are analyzed on a Zorbax ODS column in 20 min. The minimum detectable quantity of PTH derivatives is in the range of 0.5–1.0 pmol (Cunico et al., 1984) using microbore HPLC.

A popular derivatization procedure to enhance sensitivity is the treatment with o-phthaldialdehyde (OPA) in the presence of mercaptans. This leads to highly fluorescent reaction products (Umagat et al., 1982; Price et al., 1984; Konomi et al., 1984). Analysis times of approximately 15 min, including derivatization, are possible (Price et al., 1984). The lack of reactivity of secondary amino acids (proline and hydroxyproline) is a disadvantage of this method. Difficulties in quantitation are also associated with these fluorescent derivatives.

Recently another HPLC separation technique has been reported. This method allows the derivatization and analysis of amino acids in less than 20 min (Heinrikson and Meredith, 1984; Bidlingmeyer et al., 1984). The same reagent which has been used for many years with the Edman degradation method for sequencing peptides, phenylisothiocyanate, forms phenylthiocarbamyl (PTC) amino acids with primary and secondary amino acids in a single step. These derivatives can then be separated on a reversed-phase HPLC column. The strong ultraviolet absorbance of the derivatives allowed the detection of quantities as small as 1 picomol.

Various HPLC procedures have been developed to differentiate between D and L stereoisomers. In one method (Takaya et al., 1981) a racemic amino acid mixture is derivatized by reaction with the N-carboxyanhydride of an optically pure amino acid to form a mixture of diastereomeric dipeptides. These dipeptides are then separated by HPLC. Separation on a chiral stationary (Davankov and Rogozhin, 1971) or mobile phase (Tapuhi et al., 1981; Nimura et al., 1981; Hare and Gil-Av, 1979) has also been reported. To achieve enantiomer separation in the latter case standard reversed-phase columns were used with the addition of chiral metal complexes to the eluent.

A further method for the enantiomer separation of amino acids and other primary amines is precolumn derivatization with a modified OPA reagent. In this case the normal mercaptans used to form adducts which react with primary amino groups (Aswad, 1984) are replaced by the chiral sulfhydryl reagent N-acetyl-L-cysteine or N-tert-butoxycarbonyl-L-cysteine, and separation of these derivatives can then be achieved by reversed-phase HPLC.

The GC analysis of amino acids requires the synthesis of volatile derivatives. Various derivatization procedures are currently in use. Their choice depends on the amino acids to be analyzed, artifacts that may occur, and the GC column to be used.

A simple and quick derivatization method is the silylation of the amino, carboxylic, and alcoholic groups (Gehrike and Leimer, 1971).

The advantage of this technique is that the derivatization can be performed in a single step without sample transfer, evaporation steps, or the addition of other reagents. But not all amino acids form stable derivatives, and for some more than one product is found. Glycine, lysine, and all the other rarer amino acids with primary amino groups (ornithine, β-alanine, etc.) are converted into products with one or two trimethylsilyl groups at their primary amino function, depending on the derivatization conditions. Therefore this method is preferred for the determinations of the nonproblematic amino acids.

With complex mixtures of amino acids the use of retention data alone is sometimes insufficient for unequivocal identification. In this case and for the identification of unknown compounds, more reliable results can be achieved with GC–MS measurements of the samples. The mass spectra of more than 40 pertrimethylsilylated amino acids have been presented by Leimer et al. (1977b).

A more practicable derivatization technique is the esterification and acylation of amino acids. The esterification is normally performed with solutions of gaseous HCl in short-chain alcohols such as n-propanol, iso-propanol, n-butanol, and iso-butanol and several different perfluorocarboxylic acid anhydrides are used as acylating agents. A detailed derivatization procedure is described by MacKenzie and Tenaschuk (1979a,b) for the N(O,S)-heptafluorobutyryl isobutyl amino acids. The mass spectra of various similarly prepared trifluoroacetyl n-butyl esters are presented by Leimer et al. (1977a).

All derivatization procedures have the disadvantage that the rate of derivatization differs from one amino acid to another. Therefore for quantitative work an exact reproduction of the reaction conditions is always essential.

The development of chiral stationary phases, especially Chirasil-Val as an optically active polysiloxane phase of relatively high thermal stability, made possible amino acid enantiomer separation by GC (Frank et al., 1978).

Besides testing the optical purity of amino acids, another important application is possible. Addition of the unnatural enantiomer as an internal standard leads to superior quantitative results. All the problems associated with incomplete recovery or derivatization, thermal decomposition, hydrolysis of moisture-sensitive derivatives, and differing detector responses can be overcome, as the optical isomer with identical chemical properties completely compensates for these effects. The GC behavior of several suitable derivatives for this method are presented in publications by Liardon and Ledermann (1980) and Abe et al. (1983).

ANALYSIS OF AMINES

Isolation of amines from biological material is achieved by extraction of the alkalinized material with a suitable solvent (Tavakkol et al., 1985) or by the use of a cation exchanger such as Dowex 50W (Ohki et al., 1982). Loss of volatile amines during concentration steps can be avoided by conversion to hydrochlorides.

Liquid chromatographic separation methods for amines and amino acids are very similar. The same reagents for fluorometric or ultraviolet detection can be used; thus OPA can be successfully used for the derivatization of amines and analysis is performed on a reversed-phase column (Buteau et al., 1984). This method is selective for primary amines. Nakamura et al. (1984) developed an HPLC method for the stepwise fluorometric determination of primary and secondary amines. Both react with a diphenyl furanone, but only the former produce fluorescent derivatives. After their detection, a further reagent is mixed in a reaction coil wtih the eluate, which converts the furanone adducts of the secondary amines into fluorescent compounds that can then be detected with a second fluorescent monitor.

The GC analysis of amines is usually performed with suitable derivatives, as the underivatized compounds often cause problems owing to their high polarity. Adsorption problems during the analysis of nonderivatized volatile amines can be avoided by the addition of ammonia to the carrier gas (Dunn et al., 1976). Isolation of volatile amines can be performed by distillation and trapping in diluted hydrochloric acid. The hydrochlorides formed can be concentrated without loss by evaporation. Addition of a solution of sodium hydroxide allows the samples to be readily analyzed by the head-space technique (Pons et al., 1985). A further suitable derivatization procedure is their acetylation. Perfluoroacyl derivatives, easily prepared from the corresponding anhydrides, are favored owing to their excellent GC properties (Ohki et al., 1982; Tavakkol et al., 1985). These reagents also react with secondary amines and with hydroxyl groups, resulting in completely nonpolar derivatives, which can be sensitively detected by electron capture methods. The other selective detection modes which are available for the GC analysis of amines use a nitrogen-specific detector.

ANALYSIS OF CARBOHYDRATES AND RELATED COMPOUNDS

Various chromatographic methods, such as enzymatic analysis, paper chromatography, thin-layer chromatography, GC, LC, and HPLC are used in the analysis of carbohydrates. Enzymatic methods are extremely specific and therefore permit the analysis of one compound at a time. Paper and thin-layer chromatography are cheap methods, but their resolution power is low and quantitative evaluation is very limited. Liquid chromatography, reviewed by Jandera and Churáček (1974), can achieve good separations, but the method is generally very time-consuming.

Several of the most convenient methods of sugar analysis at the present time involve HPLC. Four different types of chromatography are most frequently used:

1. Chromatography on chemically bonded aminoalkyl phases ("carbohydrate columns")
2. Chromatography on silica columns dynamically coated with polyamine modifiers
3. Anion exchange chromatography of carbohydrate complexes
4. Cation exchange chromatography

Chromatography on chemically bonded aminoalkyl or "carbohydrate" phases (Linden and Lawhead, 1975; Meagher and Furst, 1976) is easy to use and elution times are short. The separation is based on interactions of carbohydrate hydroxyl groups with the amino groups of the bonded phase. Acetonitrile–water mixtures are used as the mobile phase. As water is also able to form hydrogen bonds, increasing the water content of the elution solvent decreases sugar retention and thus shortens the analysis time. Varying the amount of water allows the analysis of oligosaccharides by this method (Schwarzenbach, 1976).

Although refractometers are the most commonly used detectors, ultraviolet detection has the advantage of lower detection limits (Binder, 1980). Carbohydrates have an absorption maximum near 190 nm, but it should be noted that acetonitrile itself absorbs at slightly lower wavelengths. Impure samples and a low pH disturb the analysis and decrease resolution, as the amino groups of the bonded phase are acid sensitive. Thus the use of precolumns is recommended for protection purposes.

The deterioration of bonded amine columns during prolonged use and their prohibitive prices have been overcome by the use of conventional silica columns in combination with the addition of polyfunctional amines to the solvent mixture of acetonitrile–water (Aitzetmüller, 1978; Hendrix et al., 1981; Grimble et al., 1983).

The very high affinity of polyfunctional amines to silica results in the formation of dynamically coated "amine columns" with separation chracteristics similar to those of bonded amine columns. Concentrations of the amine in the solvent are in the range of 0.1–0.01%. This amine flow in the solvent continuously regenerates the coating of the silica, and thus the separation technique is far more tolerant of sample impurities. The effect of various amine additives was tested by Wheals and White (1979). Amine-modified silica columns separate polyalcoholic compounds in approximately the order of increasing molecular weight. Compounds with low molecular weight, particularly ethanol, cannot be resolved from the solvent.

This important product of many carbohydrate fermentations can be analyzed, together with starting material and intermediates, by cation exchange chromatography, as higher molecular weight compounds are eluted first and smaller ones later. Another advantage of this method is its greater sensitivity (Baust et al., 1983), and not only sugars but also many other carbohydrate degradation products can be determined (Bonn et al., 1984; Pecina et al., 1984). Water or 0.01 N sulfuric acid is mostly used as the mobile phase. The analyses of 2-ketogulonic acid, an important intermediate in the biotechnological production of vitamin C from sorbose, and several other by-products of this fermentation process are further examples of this technique (Anderson and Tsao, 1984). Impure samples again causes the same problems as with the amino-bonded phase and the lifetime of these columns is shorter than for the amine-modified silica system.

Applications to carbohydrate oligomer separation with cation exchange HPLC are presented by Ladisch et al. (1978) and Schmidt et al. (1981). The major analytical technique for the separation of oligosaccharides is chromatography on polyacrylamide gel. Examples have been reported where oligomers of up to 60 sugar units have been separated using Bio-Gel (John et al., 1982).

A further technique for carbohydrate characterization is anion exchange chromatography of the borate complexes (Sinner, 1976). Borate ions react with sugars to produce negatively charged sugar—borate complexes. The differences in the strengths of these complexes can be used for their separation on anion exchangers. The borate concentration and pH parameters are used for optimization of the separation. In general, reducing sugars show a greater affinity for the exchanger than nonreducing sugars. In contrast to cation exchange chromatography and to the use of chemically bonded amine phases, contaminants do not lead to a loss of separation power. The high borate molarity of the solvent continuously regenerates the borate form of the anion exchange resin.

Various color reagents that enhance the sensitivity compared with ultraviolet or refractive detection have been developed. The corrosive and dangerous reagent phenol or orcinol—sulfuric acid formerly used (Sinner, 1976) is often replaced by other dye reagents. Postcolumn derivatization with the copper(I) complex of disodium 2,2'-bicinchoninate allows for the sensitive detection of sugars at 546 nm (Sinner and Puls, 1978). This reagent reacts only with reducing carbohydrates and a heated reaction coil is needed. Aqueous ammonia solutions of copper(II) complexes form adducts with glycols, with enhanced absorption near 280 nm (Grimble et al., 1983). This has the advantage that no reaction coil is needed, as the reaction is so rapid. As all cis–cis glycols react with cuprammonium, this method detects both reducing and nonreducing sugars and it is applicable to related compounds.

Gas chromatography permits the rapid separation of sugars but requires extended and time-consuming derivatization. Quantification is often difficult because of multiple peak formation, but capillary column GC has many advantages for the analysis of very complex mixtures because of its superior separation efficiency.

There are several quick and simple derivatization procedures, although they often result in nonuniform products. In the analysis of mixtures from complex biological material, the creation of multiple peaks can lead to more complicated chromatograms which result in problems of peak resolution, identification, and quantification and lower the detection limit. Several other derivatization procedures diminish the number of products, but they are more complicated. Thus the derivatization method should only be chosen after assessing the pros and cons of each procedure.

One quick method is trifluoroacetylation (König et al., 1973). The derivatives formed have superior GC properties owing to their extreme volatility. Oligomers such as octasaccharides and glucoconjugates (Berlin et al., 1982) have been reported. Care must be taken, as these derivatives are extremely moisture sensitive.

Another rapid derivatization technique is trimethylsilylation (Sweeley et al., 1963), a procedure applicable to compounds as large as tetrasaccharides. Problems with multiple peak formation exist with this method too, although its simplicity and sensitivity often make applications possible (Chaplin, 1982). If other related compounds are to be analyzed in the same run, trimethylsilylation offers certain advantages, as carboxylic and amino functions are also derivatized. For such problems unambiguous identification by GC–MS measurements are recommended. Mass spectra of various related compounds are presented by Petersson (1970, 1972) and Dizdaroglu et al. (1977).

Preparation of acyclic derivatives is the most successful approach for reducing the number of peaks; thus better results are obtained with trimethylsilyl oximes (Petersson, 1974). The formation of anomeric mixtures is avoided, although several carbohydrates produce two peaks corresponding to the syn- and anti-oxime derivatives formed.

The most popular derivatization in carbohydrate analysis by GC is the preparation of alditol acetates. This method offers a much simpler spectrum, since the anomeric centers are removed by reduction to straight-chain alditols with a solution of sodium borohydride and consecutive acetylation with acetic acid anhydride. Detailed procedures are described by Walla et al. (1984) and Blakeney et al.

(1983). The best results of GC separation are achieved on polar stationary phases. Difficulties encountered in this method are the long analysis times required for adequate resolution. In addition, the polar phases are relatively sensitive and tend to bleed for the column. This results in an unstable baseline and a shortening of the column lifetime. Another frequent problem is the significantly lower sensitivity for amino sugars. This last effect can be overcome by using selective nitrogen detection (Whenham, 1984).

Another method for increasing sensitivity and improving unequivocal identification is the coupling of capillary GC with MS. This method offers the potential of structure elucidation and the identification of unknown components. Some disadvantages of the alditol acetate method can be overcome by silylation of the alditols (Bradbury et al., 1981). The reaction of alditols with the silylating agent is far more rapid and the conditions are not so rigorous. Additionally, good separation of the trimethylsilyl derivates is obtained on thermally stable, nonpolar silicone stationary phases.

A drawback of the alditol acetate procedure is that aldoses and ketoses afford identical alditols. Fructose, for example, results in glucitol and mannitol. To differentiate between aldoses and ketoses, a four-step derivatization has been recommended by Frank et al. (1981). Despite the complicated derivatization, only small amounts of by-products are found and the detection limit is about 1 nmol.

ANALYSIS OF ACIDIC COMPOUNDS

Acidic components of biological material are isolated by either ion exchange procedures or solvent extraction. Amberlyst A-26 can be used for ion exchange work-up (Spiteller and Spiteller, 1979). A methanol or ether solution of the material is applied to a column with the exchanger in the OH^- form and the neutral and basic components are eluted with methanol or diethyl ether. The acids can be recovered from the column with a 0.1 N solution of gaseous HCl in methanol or diethyl ether.

Solvent extraction is usually performed with ethyl acetate or diethyl ether and addition of sodium chloride to the solution improves the extraction yield. This procedure is somewhat simpler than the ion exchange work-up, but with very polar compounds the yields are not quantitative. A simplified solvent extraction procedure uses Extrelut columns (Pinkston et al., 1981). An appropriate volume of the sample is added to the column and absorbed on it. The acids can then be eluted with a suitable organic solvent.

Various HPLC separation systems have been applied to the analysis of carboxylic acids. Ion exchange chromatography gives excellent separation combined with short analysis times (Adams et al.,

1984). Dilute acids, such as 0.01 N sulfuric acid are often used as mobile phases on polystyrene-based strong cation exchange resins. The acidic compounds elute in the order of increasing pK_a values. With such systems alcohols, aldehydes, ketones, and carbohydrates are also separated (Pecina et al., 1984) which is often an advantage, as all these compounds are important in biotechnological processes as starting materials, intermediates, and products. Their analysis within a single run reduces the effort and enlarges the survey of the process events. But problems may also arise, since coelution of acids and sugars can complicate the chromatogram and make the identification of components more difficult.

Another HPLC separation method for acids uses ion-paired chromatography, in which the acids are chromatographed together with a counterion. The ion pairs have a low net electrical charge and low polarity, and good separation can be obtained with relatively nonpolar mobile phases. Quaternary ammonium counterions and chromatography on silica gel can be used (Persson and Lagerström, 1976). In reversed-phase chromatography the nonpolar parts of the counterions are absorbed on the stationary phase and can be considered as a modification toward an ion exchange column (Wahlund, 1975). The pH determines the concentration of the ionic form of the acids and it is a very important parameter for optimization of the separation. Changing the concentration of the pairing ion leads to gradient elution. Variation of the counterion type affects the separation, with more lipophilic counterions causing more acid retention on reversed phases.

A further method of separating acidic compounds on reversed-phase columns is the technique of adding acids or acidic buffers to the mobile phase. The lowered pH supresses ionization of the acidic groups and separation is based on the hydrophobic interactions of the compounds with the stationary phase (Distler, 1978).

The detection of acids is the more problematic part of the analysis. Aliphatic acids can be detected by differential refractrometry or by their ultraviolet absorption between 190 and 220 nm. Aromatic acids can be detected with high sensitivity at 280 nm. To enhance the sensitivity and selectivity ultraviolet absorbing or fluorescent derivatives can be prepared. p-Bromophenacyl (Durst et al., 1975; Mentasti et al., 1985) or pentafluorobenzyl esters (Netting and Duffield, 1984) are suitable derivatives for sensitive ultraviolet detection. With α-ketoacids a specific derivatization method has been developed. They react with o-phenylenediamine to form a single product, the quinoxalinol derivatives, which allows a sensitive fluorometric detection in the picomolar range (Kieber and Mopper, 1983).

Gas chromatography of acidic compounds without preparation of volatile derivatives is only possible in a few cases. Monocarboxylic acids, without further functional groups, can be determined nonderivatized on fused silica capillary columns (Korhonen, 1983). Short-chain fatty acids are volatile and therefore can be analyzed using the simple headspace technique (Larsson et al., 1984). This method avoids time-consuming isolation procedures, automatization enables easy treatment of a large number of samples, and good quantitative results can be obtained.

Other GC methods for analyzing acidic compounds involve derivatization procedures of which the two most commonly used are trimethylsilyl ester formation and methyl ester formation by derivatization with diazomethane. Both procedures have their advantages and disadvantages. Trimethylsilyl esters are easy to prepare and have excellent GC properties. Frequent injections of silylated material into the GC column keeps the system clean and maintains the good separation properties of polysiloxane coatings. Widely used silylating agents are N,O-bis-trimethylsilyl-trifluoroacetamide (BSTFA) and N-methyl-N-trimethylsilyl-trifluoroacetamide (MSTFA). Beside carboxylic groups, hydroxyl, phenol, and amino groups are derivatized during silylation. Many mass spectra (Petersson, 1970, 1972) and also retention indices (Tuchman et al., 1984; Tanaka et al., 1980; Tanaka and Hine, 1982) of trimethylsilylated acidic metabolites have been published. Certain compounds, such as ketoacids, form multiple derivatives and are better determined as double derivatives. Carbonyl groups are transformed into methoximes or oximes (Lancaster et al., 1973), of which some retention indices have been published (De Jong, 1982). Suitable GC derivatives of 2-ketoacids are formed from O-phenylenediamine followed by silylation to yield O-trimethylsilyl quinoxalols (Early et al., 1984). Mass spectra of these compounds have also been published (Langenbeck et al., 1977).

Methyl esters are usually prepared with diazomethane (Spiteller and Spiteller, 1979) and special care must be taken because of the hazardous properties of this reagent. Nevertheless, this methylation method is preferable, since it is a simple, rapid, and smooth procedure. In addition to carboxylic groups, phenolic hydroxyl groups and thiols react with diazomethane. This makes it impossible to distinguish between aromatic OH and methoxy groups as well as the SH or SCH_3 groups of the original molecules. By-products and artifacts may also appear with keto- and α,β-unsaturated acids (Bauer et al., 1984). Retention indices and mass-spectral data of methylated acidic compounds have been published in several papers (Spiteller and Spiteller, 1979; Pinkston et al., 1981; Bauer et al., 1984). Methyl esters of lower acids are highly volatile and may be lost during evaporation steps. This can be avoided by the preparation of esters of low volatility, such as benzyl esters (Monseur et al., 1981), which allow ready determination of formic acid.

ANALYSIS OF NUCLEOBASES, NUCLEOSIDES, AND NUCLEOTIDES

Nucleobases, nucleosides, and nucleotides are some of the most important compounds in biological systems. They are the constituents of nucleic acids, work as enzyme cofactors, and are regulatory signal molecules. Consequently the analysis of these materials and related compounds is of great interest in biological research.

In order to study the content of nucleocompounds in biological material, extraction is necessary. An important step of the work-up procedure is the rapid removal of proteins to avoid enzymatic degradation. Perchloric acid and trichloroacetic acid are commonly used for this purpose, as they lyse the cells and precipitate the proteins. After centrifugation the acidic supernatant is neutralized. Olempska-Beer and Bautz Freese (1984) reported the extraction of nucleotides using formic acid and butanol, which has the advantage of not containing ultraviolet-absorbing impurities and it can be removed by vacuum evaporation. Other additional purification steps, with losses of sensitive nucleotides, can thus be avoided. An alternative procedure is ultrafiltration, which is the preferred method for isolation from biological fluids, as it does not change the pH or introduce contamination with ultraviolet-absorbing material. Ribonucleosides are isolated by a special extraction procedure. They can be retained on a boronate column (Gehrke et al., 1978), as the vicinal hydroxy group of their sugar moiety forms a cis–diol complex. Elution is performed with dilute formic acid.

Major HPLC methods in the analysis of nucleocompounds are chromatography on ion exchange and reversed-phase columns. The latter is becoming increasingly important, since nucleobases and nucleosides can be separated. Ion-paired chromatography of the highly polar nucleotides is possible with the addition of quaternary ammonium compounds to the mobile phase (Payne and Ames, 1982). This method is an excellent alternative to ion exchange chromatography and results in better resolution and longer column life. Problems arise with preparative separations, since the ion-pairing reagent is difficult to remove from the nucleotides. In this case ion exchange systems can be used with good results (Olempska-Beer and Bautz Freese, 1984). Partisil 10-SAX is often used as an exchanger for this type of analysis.

Compounds with relatively low charge, such as nucleobases, nucleosides, and cyclic nucleotides, can be separated with conventional reversed-phase systems (Gehrke et al., 1978; Payne and Ames, 1982). Octadecyl silica columns are most commonly used and ammonium acetate is preferred as a buffer compound, since it can be removed from the sample by lyophilization. Mixtures of water with several organic solvents can also be used as unbuffered mobile phases (Ryba, 1981). A study of nucleotides and other related small molecules in biological systems involving the three important HPLC methods is presented by Payne and Ames (1982).

The GC separation of nucleocompounds requires derivatization procedures to obtain volatile derivatives. Nucleotides are difficult to analyze with GC techniques, as oxygen–phosphorus bond cleavage occurs during derivatization (Griest and Martin, 1978) and good results, especially for quantitative work, are impossible. Nucleotides should be converted to the corresponding nucleosides or nucleobases prior to GC analysis. On the other hand, nucleosides and related compounds can be determined with higher sensitivity than with HPLC methods.

Trimethylsilylation is a simple one-step derivatization procedure for nucleosides (Gehrke and Patel, 1977; Patel and Gehrke, 1977). Contamination of the sample significantly influences the derivatization. Thus biological samples should be purified or prefractionated. Mass spectra of trimethylsilylated nucleosides are well known (Pang et al., 1982) and have been used for their characterization. Likewise, GC retention data of different nucleoside derivatives have been published (Quilliam et al., 1980). Nucleobases with their high nitrogen content have been determined in the low picogram range by capillary GC using a nitrogen-specific detector (Stafford and Corse, 1982). The detection selectivity means that only simplified extraction and purification procedures are needed. Permethylated derivatives are preferred in this method, as they yield better results than the corresponding trimethylsilyl compounds. Another highly sensitive GC method involves the use of electron capture detection. Halogenated compounds can be analyzed down to very low concentrations. Using trifluoroacetylated derivatives of nucleobases and nucleosides, quantities as small as 1 pg can be detected (Ludewig et al., 1982).

A comparison of HPLC and GC methods in the analysis of nucleobases, nucleosides and nucleotides shows that HPLC techniques are applicable to all three classes of compounds without derivatization. Gas chromatography analysis is successful only with nucleobases and nucleosides and requires derivatization of the compounds, although it has the advantage of higher sensitivity.

ENANTIOMER SEPARATION

The possibility of separating optical isomers is important for amino acid analysis. Likewise, many other natural compounds exist as chiral molecules and often only one distinct enantiomer is biologically active. The inactive isomer shows no effect and in some cases even an opposite effect. Thus enantiomer separation is of great interest in the analysis of all biological compounds.

Two different modes of enantiomer separation can be used. Separation on achiral phases requires the derivatization of the enantiomers with a chiral reagent to form diastereomeric products which can than be separated. The second technique uses chiral stationary phases. Reviews of both methods using GC techniques have been published by Liu and Ku (1981, 1983).

Relatively high thermal stability siloxane phases modified with a chiral compound have been used with great success in GC enantiomer separation (Frank et al., 1977; König and Benecke, 1981). The method has been mostly applied to compounds which have a nitrogen close to the asymmetrical carbon atom. Compounds without a nitrogen at such a position can be derivatized with isopropyl isocyanate, which reacts with hydroxy and amino groups to form urea and urethane derivatives, respectively (König et al., 1982a,b). Another useful derivatization for different chiral 1,2- and 1,3-bifunctional compounds is the formation of cyclic carbonates with phosgene. Diols, hydroxy acids, and amino alcohols have been separated by this method (König et al., 1984). Likewise, the separation of enantiomer carbohydrates is possible after suitable derivatization (König et al., 1981).

Various chiral stationary phases for HPLC separation exist. Several slightly different hydantoin-based chiral stationary phases have been effectively used to separate many derivatized amino and alcoholic compounds (Pirkle et al., 1984). The completely different method of Pettersson (1984) for acids uses quinine as the chiral counterion to produce diastereomeric ion pairs which can be separated on silica HPLC columns.

ANALYSIS OF VOLATILES

Gas chromatography is the method of choice for most problems in the analysis of volatile compounds, with the most critical part being the isolation step. Particular care must be taken, especially during quantitative work. The most commonly used isolation techniques are extraction, steam distillation, vapor collection by adsorption, and headspace analysis.

Extraction seems to be a good method that avoids artifact formation and allows the determination of less volatile and nonvolatile compounds as well. This technique is usually performed using a Soxhlet apparatus and low-boiling solvents (MacLeod and Pieris, 1982), in which enrichment of the extracts by evaporation is possible without serious losses of highly volatile components. Concentration is preferably performed using a gentle stream of nitrogen to evaporate the solvent or low-temperature vacuum distillation, where the volatile compounds are collected in a trap cooled with liquid nitrogen (MacLeod and Cave, 1975). Trapping volatiles on solid adsorbents (Zladkis and Kim, 1976), such as Tenax GC (Yokouchi et al., 1981) is another isolation method, particularly if highly volatile compounds have to be collected from gaseous samples. Heat desorption transfers the sample to the GC column. This procedure is prone to artifact production with sensitive compounds, especially when working in the ppm range.

The headspace technique (Chialva et al., 1982) offers several advantages. It is a simple and rapid method with good reproducibilty, and its nondestructive character is particularly important. The sample is placed in a vial, heated to an equilibrium temperature, and then a certain volume of the vapor phase is injected into the GC column.

The choice of liquid phase greatly influences the separation. Phases often used are nonpolar methyl silicon phases such as SE30 and OV101 or polar ones such as Carbowax 20M. Many retention indices of volatiles on both phases combined with a large number of mass spectra have been published by Jennings and Shibamoto (1980). The use of such data facilitate and ensure the identification of components of complex mixtures (Shibamoto et al., 1981; Yamaguchi and Shibamoto, 1981). The recently developed chemically bonded phases allow direct injection of aqueous samples (Supelco and J&W Scientific) and in several cases no work-up is needed.

Volatile carbonyl compounds are often analyzed after their derivatization which sometimes gives better separation and increased sensitivity. Thus the 2,4-dinitrophenylhydrazones are prepared and analyzed by either GC (Hoshika and Takata, 1976) or HPLC (Lipari and Swarin, 1982). Formaldehyde can easily be detected with these methods.

MISCELLANEOUS ASPECTS

Space allows only a short review of the analytical procedures of the large variety of other biological substances. One important class of biotechnologically interesting compounds is that of vitamins. They consist of structurally different compounds and thus the analytical procedures are very diverse. Vitamins can be divided into roughly two groups: lipid-soluble and water-soluble vitamins. The lipid-soluble ones, such as carotenoids, tocopherols, calciferols, and naphtochinone compounds, can easily be extracted with organic solvents, whereas the preparation of the water-soluble vitamins is usually more complex. In many cases conversion of the vitamins into their free form is necessary. Some vitamins can be analyzed by GC:

the tocopherols (Slover and Thompson, 1981), vitamins of the K group (Bechtold and Klein, 1984), and, with some problems, the calciferols (De Vries and Borsje, 1982). Innumerable HPLC applications exist in the field of vitamin analysis. A recently published book by De Leenheer et al. (1985) covers all the GC, HPLC, and thin-layer chromatographic methods.

A considerable number of biologically interesting compounds occur as glycosides, and many compounds are metabolized by glycosylation. Saponines, phenolic glycosides, and cardiac glycosides are examples. Such compounds can be analyzed without derivatization by HPLC techniques (Winter and Herrmann, 1984; Kaizuka and Takahashi, 1983) or after derivatization by GC. Recommended derivatization methods are trimethylsilylation (Inouye et al., 1978; Julkunen-Tiitto, 1985) and trifluoroacetylation (Berlin et al., 1982). Sometimes it is easier and sufficient to analyze only the aglycon part after hydrolysis. High-performance liquid chromatography applications for phenolics, coumarins (Vande Casteele et al., 1983), and flavonoids (Vande Casteele et al., 1982) have been published.

Lipids can be analyzed by HPLC as well as by GC. Short capillary columns are recommended for the GC analysis; their use allows fast analyses with high resolution, even with high molecular weight lipids (Lercker, 1983). Fatty acids, sterols, and triglycerides can be studied within a single run. The different classes of phospholipids are easily separated by HPLC and their fatty acid profile is determined by capillary GC (Guichardant and Lagarde, 1983).

REFERENCES

Abe, I., Kuramoto, S., and Musha, S. (1983). Heliflex Chirasil-Val; GC of amino acid enantiomers. *J. High Resolut. Chromatogr. Chromatogr. Commun.* *6*:366–370.

Adams, R. F., Jones, R. L., and Conway, P. L. (1984). High-performance liquid chromatography of microbial acid metabolites. *J. Chromatogr.* *336*:125–137.

Aitzetmüller, K. (1978). Sugar analysis by high-performance liquid chromatography using silica columns. *J. Chromatogr.* *156*:354–358.

Anderson, A. W. and Tsao, G. T. (1984). Analysis of 2-keto-gulonic acid and fermentation substrates by HPLC. *Biotechnol. Bioeng.* *26*:374–376.

Aswad, D. W. (1984). Determination of D- and L-aspartate in amino acid mixtures by high-performance liquid chromatography after derivatization with a chiral adduct of o-phthaldialdehyde. *Anal. Biochem.* *137*:405–409.

Bauer, S., Neupert, M., and Spiteller, G. (1984). Characterization of artefacts produced by treatment of organic acids with diazomethane. *J. Chromatogr.* *309*:243–259.

* Baust, J. G., Lee, R. E., Rojas, R. R., Hendrix, D. L., Friday, D., and James H. (1983). Comparative separation of low-molecular-weight carbohydrates and polyols by high-performance liquid chromatography: Radial compressed amine modified silica versus ion exchange. *J. Chromatogr. 261*:65–75.

Bechtold, H. and Klein, F. (1984). Improved method for quantitative analysis of vitamin K and vitamin K 2,3-epoxide in human plasma by electron-capture gas-liquid capillary chromatography. *J. Chromatogr. 306*:333–337.

Berlin, J., Witte, L., Hammer, J., Kukoschke, K. G., Zimmer, A., and Pape, D. (1982). Metabolism of p-fluorophenylalanine in p-fluorophenylalanine sensitive and resistant tobacco cell cultures. *Planta 155*:244–250.

Bidlingmeyer, B. A., Cohen, S. A., and Tarvin, T. L. (1984). Rapid analysis of amino acids using pre-column derivatization. *J. Chromatogr. 336*:93–104.

Binder, H. (1980). Separation of monosaccharides by high-performance liquid chromatography: Comparison of ultraviolet and refractive index detection. *J. Chromatogr. 189*:414–420.

Blakeney, A. B., Harris, P. J., Henry, R. J., and Stone, B. A. (1983). A simple and rapid preparation of alditol acetates for monosaccharide analysis. *Carbohydr. Res. 113*:291–299.

Bonn, G., Pecina, R., Burtscher, E., and Bobleter, O. (1984). Separation of wood degradation products by high-performance liquid chromatography. *J. Chromatogr. 287*:215–221.

Bradbury, A. G. W., Halliday, D. J., and Medcalf, D. G. (1981). Separation of monosaccharides as trimethylsilylated alditols on fused-silica capillary columns. *J. Chromatogr. 213*:146–150.

Brown, P. R. and Krstulovic, A. M. (1979). Practical aspects of reversed-phase liquid chromatography applied to biochemical and biomedical research. *Anal. Biochem. 99*:1–21.

Buck, R. H. and Krummen, K. (1984). Resolution of amino acid enantiomers by high-performance liquid chromatography using automated pre-column derivatization with a chiral reagent. *J. Chromatogr. 315*:279–285.

Buteau, C., Duitschaever, C. L., and Ashton, G. C. (1984). High-performance liquid chromatographic detection and quantitation of amines in must and wine. *J. Chromatogr. 284*:201–210.

Chaplin, M. F. (1982). A rapid and sensitive method for the analysis of carbohydrate components in glycoproteins using gas–liquid chromatography. *Anal. Biochem. 123*:336–341. *

Chialva, F., Gabri, G., Liddle, P. A. P., and Ulian, F. (1982). Qualitative evaluation of aromatic herbs by direct headspace GC-analysis. Applications of the method and comparison with the traditional analysis of essential oils. *J. High Resolut. Chromatogr. Chromatogr. Commun. 5*:182–188.

Cunico, R. L., Simpson, R., Correia, L., and Wehr, C. T. (1984). High-sensitivity phenylhydantoin amino acid analysis using conventional and microbore chromatography. *J. Chromatogr.* *336*: 105–113.

Davankov, V. A. and Rogozhin, S. V. (1971). Ligand chromatography as a novel method for the investigation of mixed complexes: Stereoselective effects in α-amino acid copper(II) complexes. *J. Chromatogr.* *60*:280–283.

De Jong, A. P. J. M. (1982). Analysis of oxime-trimethylsilyl derivatives of organic acids on OV–1701 fused silica capillary column. *J. Chromatogr.* *233*:297–300.

De Leenheer, A. P., Lambert, W. E., and De Ruyter, M. G. M. (eds.) (1985). *Modern Chromatographic Analysis of the Vitamins*, Marcel Dekker, New York.

De Vries, E. and Borsje, B. (1982). Analysis of fat soluble vitamins. XXVII. High performance liquid chromatographic and gas–liquid chromatographic determination of vitamin D in fortified milk and milkpowder: Collaborative study. *J. Assoc. Offic. Anal. Chem.* *65*:1228–1234.

Distler, W. (1978). Trennung von Milch-, Glyoxyl-, Ameisen-, Essig- und Propionsäure mit Hilfe der Umkehrphasen-Hochdruckflüssigkeitschromatographie. *J. Chromatogr.* *152*:250–252.

Dizdaroglu, M., Henneberg, D., Neuwald, K., Schomburg, G., and von Sonntag, C. (1977). Radiation chemistry of carbohydrates, X. γ-Radiolysis of crystalline D-glucose and D-fructose. *Z. Naturforsch.* *32b*:213–224.

Dunn, S. R., Siemenhoff, M. L., and Wesson, Jr., L. G. (1976). Gas chromatographic determination of free mono-, di-, and trimethylamines in biological fluids. *Anal. Chem.* *48*:41–44.

Durst, H. D., Milano, M., Kikta, Jr., E. J., Connelly, S. A., and Grushka, E. (1975). Phenacyl esters of fatty acids via crown ether catalysts for enhanced ultraviolet detection in liquid chromatography. *Anal. Chem.* *47*:1797–1801.

Early, R. J., Tompson, J. R., McAllister, T., Fenton, T. W., and Christopherson, R. J. (1984). Branched-chain α-keto acid analysis in biological fluids: Preparative clean-up by anion-exchange and analysis by capillary gas chromatography. *J. Chromatogr.* *310*:1–10.

Frank, H., Nicholson, G. J., and Bayer, E. (1978). Enantiomer labelling, a method for the quantitative analysis of amino acids. *J. Chromatogr.* *167*:187–196.

Frank, H., Das Neves, H. J. C., and Bayer, E. (1981). Gas chromatography of monosaccharides: Formation of a single derivative for each aldose. *J. Chromatogr.* *207*:213–220.

Games, D. E. (1981). Combined high performance liquid chromatography mass spectrometry. *Biomed. Mass Spectrom.* *8*:454–462.

Gehrke, C. W. and Leimer, K. (1971). Trimethylsilylation of amino acids. Derivatization and chromatography. *J. Chromatogr.* *57*: 219–238.

Gehrke, C. W. and Patel, A. B. (1977). Gas–liquid chromatography of nucleosides. Effect of silylating reagents and solvents. *J. Chromatogr.* *130*:103–114.

Gehrke, C. W., Kuo, K. C., Davis, G. E., Suits, R. D., Waalkes, T. P., and Borek, E. (1978). Quantiative high performance liquid chromatography of nucleosides in biological materials. *J. Chromatogr.* *150*:455–476.

Griest, W. H. and Martin, T. W. (1978). Phosphorus–oxygen bond cleavages during trimethylsilyl-derivatization of condensed polyphosphates and related nucleotides. *J. Chromatogr.* *148*: 405–412.

Grimble, G. K., Barker, H. M., and Taylor, R. H. (1983). Chromatographic analysis of sugars in physiological fluids by post-column reaction with cuprammonium: A new and highly sensitive method. *Anal. Biochem.* *128*:422–428.

Guichardant, M. and Lagarde, M. (1983). Phospholipid analysis and fatty acid content in platelets by the combination of high-performance liquid chromatography and glass capillary gas-liquid chromatography. *J. Chromatogr.* *275*:400–406.

Hare, P. E. and Gil-Av, E. (1979). Separation of D and L amino acids by liquid chromatography: Use of chiral elutants. *Science* *204*:1226–1228.

Heinrikson, R. L. and Meredith, S. C. (1984). Amino acid analysis by reversed-phase high-performance liquid chromatography: Precolumn derivatization with phenylisothiocyanate. *Anal. Biochem.* *136*:65–74.

Hendrix, D. L., Lee, R. E., Baust, J. G., and James, H. (1981). Separation of carbohydrates and polyols by a radially compressed high-performance liquid chromatographic silica column modified with tetraethylenepentamine. *J. Chromatogr.* *210*: 45–53.

Hoshika, Y. and Takata, Y. (1976). Gas chromatographic separation of carbonyl compounds as their 2,4-dinitrophenylhydrazones using glass capillary columns. *J. Chromatogr.* *120*:379–389.

Inouye, H., Uobe, K., Hirai, M., Masada, Y., and Hashimoto, K. (1976). Studies on monoterpene glucosides and related natural products. XXXI. Gas chromatography and gas chromatography–mass spectrometry of iroid and secoiroid glucosides. *J. Chromatogra.* *118*:201–216.

Jandera, P., and Churáček, J. (1974). Ion-exchange chromatography of aldehydes, ketones, ethers, alcohols, polyols and saccharides. *J. Chromatogr.* *98*:55–104.

Jennings, W. and Shibamoto, T. (1980). *Qualitative Analysis of Flavor and Fragrance Volatiles by Glass Capillary Gas Chromatography*, Academic, New York.

John, M., Schmidt, J., Wandrey, C., and Sahm, H. (1982). Gel chromatography of oligosaccharides up to DP 60. *J. Chromatogr.* *247*:281–288.

Julkunen-Tiitto, R. (1985). Chemotaxonomical screening of phenolic glycosides in northern willow twigs by capillary gas chromatography. *J. Chromatogr.* *324*:129–139.

Kaizuka, H. and Takahashi, K. (1983). High-performance liquid chromatographic system for a wide range of naturally occurring glycosides. *J. Chromatogr.* *258*:135–146.

Kieber, D. J. and Mopper, K. (1983). Reversed-phase high-performance liquid chromatographic analysis of α-keto acid quinoxalinol derivatives. Optimization of technique and application to natural samples. *J. Chromatogr.* *281*:135–149.

König, W. A. and Benecke, I. (1981). Gas chromatographic separation of enantiomers of amines and amino alcohols on chiral stationary phases. *J. Chromatogr.* *209*:91–95.

König, W. A., Bauer, H., Voelter, W., and Bayer, E. (1973). Gaschromatographie und Massenspektrometrie trifluoroacetylierter Kohlenhydrate. *Chem. Ber.* *106*:1905–1919.

König, W. A., Benecke, I., and Bretting, H. (1981). Gaschromatographische Trennung enantiomerer Kohlenhydrate an einer neuen chiralen stationären Phase. *Angew. Chem.* *93*:688–690.

König, W. A., Francke, W., and Benecke, I. (1982a). Gas chromatographic enantiomer separation of chiral alcohols. *J. Chromatogr.* *239*:227–231.

König, W. A., Benecke, I., and Sievers, S. (1982b). New procedure for gas chromatographic enantiomer separation. Application to chiral amines and hydroxy acids. *J. Chromatogr.* *238*: 427–432.

König, W. A., Steinbach, E., and Ernst, K. (1984). Phosgene—A versatile reagent for enantiomer separation by capillary gas chromatography. *J. Chromatogr.* *301*:129–135.

Konomi, H., Hayashi, T., Takehana, Y., and Arima, M. (1984). Rapid and sensitive amino acid analysis of human collagens using high-performance liquid chromatography. *J. Chromatogr.* *311*: 375–379.

Korhonen, I. O. O. (1983). Simultaneous gas chromatographic determination of aliphatic C_2–C_{20} n-carboxylic acids and their methyl esters using SE–30 and OV–351 quartz capillary columns. *Chromatographia* *17*:70–74.

Kováts, E. (1958). Gas-chromatographische Characterisierung organischrr Verbindungen Teil 1: Retentionsindices aliphatischer Halogenide, Alkohole, Aldehyde und Ketone. *Helv. Chim. Acta* *41*:1915–1932.

Ladisch, M. R., Heubner, A. L., and Tsao, G. T. (1978). High-speed liquid chromatography of cellodextrines and other saccharide mixtures using water as the eluent. *J. Chromatogr.* *147*:185–193.

Lancaster, G., Lamm, P., Scriver, C. R., Tjoa, S. S., and Mamer, O. A. (1973). Quantitative analysis of branched-chain α-keto acids as their trimethylsilylated oximes. *Clin. Chim. Acta 48*: 279–285.

Langenbeck, U., Möhring, H.-U., Hinney, B., and Spiteller, M. (1977). Quinoxalinol derivatives of aliphatic 2-oxocarboxylic acids. Infra red and mass spectra of the O-trimethylsilylated compounds. *Biomed. Mass Spectrom.* *4*:197–202.

Larsson, L., Sällström-Baum, S., and de la Cochetiere-Collinet, M.-F. (1984). A two-step extraction procedure for concentrating acidic organic volatiles in aqueous solution prior to gas chromatographic head-space analysis, as exemplified by short-chain fatty acids produced by *Bacillus cereus*. *J. Microbiol. Methods* *2*:9–14.

Leimer, K. R., Rice, R. H., and Gehrke, C. W. (1977a). Complete mass spectra of N-trifluoroacetyl-n-butyl esters of amino acids. *J. Chromatogr.* *141*:121–144.

Leimer, K. R., Rice, R. H., and Gehrke, C. W. (1977b). Complete mass spectra of the per-trimethylsilylated amino acids. *J. Chromatogr.* *141*:355–375.

Lercker, G. (1983). Short capillary columns in the analysis of lipids. *J. Chromatogr.* *279*:543–548.

Liardon, R. and Ledermann, S. (1980). GC behaviour of N(O,S)-perfluoroacyl D,L-amino acid alkyl esters on Chirasil-Val stationary phase. *J. High Resolut. Chromatogr. Chromatogr. Commun.* *3*:475–477.

Linden, J. C. and Lawhead, C. L. (1975). Liquid chromatography of saccharides. *J. Chromatogr.* *105*:125–133.

Lipari, F. and Swarin, S. J. (1982). Determination of formaldehyde and other aldehydes in automobile exhaust with an improved 2,4-dinitrophenylhydrazine method. *J. Chromatogr.* *247*: 297–306.

Liu, J. H. and Ku, W. W. (1981). Determination of enantiomeric N-trifluoroacetyl-L-prolyl chloride amphetamine derivatives by capillary gas chromatography/mass spectrometry with chiral and achiral stationary phases. *Anal. Chem.* *53*:2180–2184.

Liu, R. H. and Ku, W. W. (1983). Chiral stationary phases for the gas–liquid chromatographic separation of enantiomers. *J. Chromatogr.* *271*:309–323.

Ludewig, M., Dörffling, K., and König, W. A. (1982). Electron-capture capillary gas chromatography and mass spectrometry of trifluoroacetylated cytokinins. *J. Chromatogr.* *243*:93–98.

McFadden, W. (ed.) (1973). *Techniques of Combined Gas Chromatography Mass Spectrometry: Applications in Organic Analysis*, Wiley, New York.

McFadden, W. H. (1980). Liquid chromatography/mass spectrometry systems and application. *J. Chromatogr. Sci. 18*:97–115.

MacLeod, A. J. and Cave, S. J. (1975). Volatile flavor components of eggs. *J. Sci. Food Agric. 26*:351–360.

MacLeod, A. J. and Pieris, N. M. (1982). Analysis of the volatile essential oils of *Murraya koenigii* and *Pandanus latifolius*. *Phytochemistry 21*:1653–1657.

MacKenzie, S. L. and Tenaschuk, D. (1979a). Quantitative formation of N(O,S)-heptafluorobutryryl isobutyl amino acids for gas chromatographic analysis. II. Acylation. *J. Chromatogr. 173*:53–63.

MacKenzie, S. L. and Tenaschuk, D. (1979b). Quantitative formation of N(O,S)-heptafluorobutyryl isobutyl amino acids for gas chromatographic analysis. I. Esterification. *J. Chromatogr. 171*:195–208.

Meagher, R. B. and Furst, A. (1976). Reversed-phase high-pressure liquid chromatography of normal rat urinary carbohydrates. *J. Chromatogr. 117*:211–215.

Mentasti, E., Gennaro, M. C., Sarzanini, C., Baiocchi, C., and Savigliano, M. (1985). Derivatization, identification and separation of carboxylic acids in wines and beverages by high-performance liquid chromatography. *J. Chromatogr. 322*:177–189.

Monseur, X., Walravens, J., Dourte, P., and Termonia, M. (1981). Determination of volatile carboxylic acids in animal wastes by $(GC)^2$ of their benzyl esters. *J. High Resolut. Chromatogr. Chromatogr. Commun. 4*:49–53.

Moore, S., Spackman, D. H., and Stein, W. H. (1958). Chromatography of amino acids on sulfonated polystyrene resin. An improved system. *Anal. Chem. 30*:1185–1190.

Murayama, K. and Shindo, N. (1977). Recommended method for the analysis of amino acids in biological materials. *J. Chromatogr. 143*:137–152.

Nakamura, H., Takagi, K., Tamura, Z., Yoda, R., and Yamamoto, Y. (1984). Stepwise fluorometric determination of primary and secondary amines by liquid chromatography after derivatization with 2-methoxy-2,4-diphenyl-3(2H)-furanone. *Anal. Chem. 56*:919–922.

Netting, A. G. and Duffield, A. M. (1984). High-performance liquid chromatographic separation of fatty acids as pentafluorobenzyl esters. *J. Chromatogr. 336*:115–123.

Nimura, N., Toyama, A., Kasahara, Y., and Kinoshita, T. (1982). Reversed-phase liquid chromatographic resolution of underivatized D,L-amino acids using chiral eluents. *J. Chromatogr. 239*:671–675.

Ohki, T., Saito, A., Yamanaka, N., Ohta, K., Sakakibara, J., Niwa, T., and Maeda, K. (1982). Gas chromatographic-mass spectrometric analysis of amine metabolites in urine. *J. Chromatogr.* *228*:51–57.

Olempska-Beer, Z. and Bautz Freese E. (1984). Optimal extraction conditions for high-performance liquid chromatographic determination of nucleotides in yeast. *Anal. Biochem.* *140*:236–245.

Pang, H., Schram, K. H., Smith, D. L., Gupta, S. P., Townsend, L. B., and McCloskey, J. A. (1982). Mass spectrometry of nucleic acid constitutents. Trimethylsilyl derivatives of nucleosides. *J. Org. Chem.* *47*:3923–3932.

Patel, A. B. and Gehrke, C. W. (1977). Derivatization and chromatography of nucleosides and nucleotides. *J. Chromatogr.* *130*:115–128.

Payne, S. M. and Ames, B. N. (1982). A procedure for rapid extraction and high-pressure liquid chromatographic separation of the nucleotides and other small molecules from bacterial cells. *Anal. Chem.* *123*:151–161.

Pecina, R., Bonn, G., Burtscher, E., and Bobleter, O. (1984). High-performance liquid chromatographic elution behaviour of alcohols, aldehydes, ketones, organic acids and carbohydrates on a strong cation-exchange stationary phase. *J. Chromatogr.* *287*:245–258.

Persson, B.-A. and Lagerström, P.-O. (1976). Ion-pair partition chromatography in the analysis of drugs and biogenic substances in plasma and urine. *J. Chromatogr.* *122*:305–316.

Petersson, G. (1970). Mass spectrometry of aldonic and deoxyaldonic acids as trimethylsilyl derivatives. *Tetrahedron* *26*:3413–3428.

Petersson, G. (1972). Mass spectrometry of hydroxy dicarboxylic acids as trimethylsilyl derivatives. Rearrangement fragmentations. *Org. Mass Spectrom.* *6*:565–576.

Petersson, G. (1974). Gas-chromatographic analysis of sugars and related hydroxy acids as acyclic oxime and ester trimethylsilyl derivatives. *Carbohydr. Res.* *33*:47–61.

Pettersson, C. (1984). Chromatographic separation of enantiomers of acids with quinine as chiral counter ion. *J. Chromatogr.* *316*:553–567.

Pilosof, D., Kim, H.-Y., Vestal, M. L., and Dyckes, D. F. (1984). Direct monitoring of sequential enzymatic hydrolysis of peptides by thermospray mass spectrometry. *Biomed. Mass Spectrom.* *11*:403–407.

Pinkston, D., Spiteller, G., von Henning, H., and Matthaei, D. (1981). High-resolution gas chromatography-mass spectrometry of the methyl esters of organic acids from uremic hemofiltrates. *J. Chromatogr.* *223*:1–19.

Pirkle, W. H., Ho Myun, M., and Bank, B. (1984). A rational approach to the design of highly effective chiral stationary phases. *J. Chromatogr.* *316*:585–604.

Pons, J.-L., Rimbault, A., Darbord, J. C., and Leluan, G. (1985). Gas chromatographic–mass spectrometric analysis of volatile amines produced by several strains of *Clostridium*. *J. Chromatogr.* *337*:213–221.

Poole, C. F. and Schuette, S. A. (1984). *Contemporary Practice of Chromatography*, Elsevier, New York.

Price, S. J., Palmer, T., and Griffin, M. (1984). High-speed assay of amino acids using reversed-phase liquid chromatography. *Chromatographia* *18*:62–64.

Quilliam, M. A., Ogilvie, K. K., Sadana, K. L., and Westmore, J. B. (1980). Gas chromatographic retention data for silyl and acyl derivatives of nucleosides. *J. Chromatogr.* *196*:367–378.

Ryba, M. (1981). Reversed phase liquid column chromatography of pyrimidine and purine derivatives. I. Unbuffered binary aqueous organic mobile phases on octadecylsilica. *J. Chromatogr.* *219*:245–254.

Schmidt, J., John, M., and Wandrey, C. (1981). Rapid separation of malto-, xylo- and cello-oligosaccharides (DP 2–9) on cation-exchange resin using water as eluent. *J. Chromatogr.* *213*:151–155.

Schwarzenbach, R. (1976). A chemically bonded stationary phase for carbohydrate analysis in liquid chromatography. *J. Chromatogr.* *117*:206–210.

Shibamoto, T., Kamiya, Y., and Mihara, S. (1981). Isolation and identification of volatile compounds in cooked meat: Sukiyaki. *J. Agric. Food Chem.* *29*:57–63.

Sinner, M. (1976). Separation of methyl ethers of xylose, glucose and some other sugars by liquid chromatography. *J. Chromatogr.* *121*:122–130.

Sinner, M. and Puls, J. (1978). Non-corrosive dye reagent for detection of reducing sugars in borate complex ion-exchange chromatography. *J. Chromatogr.* *156*:197–204.

Slover, H. T. and Thompson, Jr., R. H. (1981). Chromatographic separation of the stereoisomers of α-tocopherol. *Lipids* *16*:268–275.

Spiteller, M. and Spiteller, G. (1979). Trennung und Charactersierung saurer Harnbestandteile. *J. Chromatogr.* *164*:253–317.

Stafford, A. E. and Corse, J. (1982). Fused-silica capillary gas chromatography of permethylated cytokinins with flame-ionization and nitrogen–phosphorus detection. *J. Chromatogr.* *247*:176–179.

Sweeley, C. C., Bentley, R., Matika, M., and Wells, W. W. (1963). Gas–liquid chromatography of trimethylsilyl derivatives of sugars and related substances. *J. Am. Chem. Soc.* *85*:2497–2507.

Takaya, Y., Kishida, Y., and Sakakibara, S. (1981). Determination of the optical purity of amino acids by HPLC. Modification of the Manning and Moore procedure. *J. Chromatogr.* *215*:279–287.

Tanaka, K. and Hine, D. G. (1982). Compilation of gas chromatographic retention indices of 163 metabolically important organic acids, and their use in detection of patients with organic acidurias. *J. Chromatogr.* *239*:301–322.

Tanaka, K., Hine, D. G., West-Dull, A., and Lynn, T. B. (1980). Gas-chromatographic method of analysis for urinary organic acids. I. Retention indices of 155 metabolically important compounds. *Clin. Chem.* *26*:1839–1846.

Tapuhi, Y., Miller, N., and Karger, B. L. (1981). Practical considerations in the chiral separation of dns-amino acids by reversed-phase liquid chromatography using metal chelate additives. *J. Chromatogr.* *205*:325–337.

Tavakkol, A. and Wilson, J. M. (1985). Gas chromatography/mass spectrometry of bacterial amines. *Biomed. Mass Spectrom.* *12*:359–363.

Ten Noever de Brauw, M. C. (1979). Combined gas chromatography–mass spectrometry: A powerful tool in analytical chemistry. *J. Chromatogr.* *165*:207–233.

Tuchman, M., Bowers, L. D., Fregien, K. D., Crippin, P. J., and Krivit, W. (1984). Capillary gas chromatographic separation of urinary organic acids. Retention indices of 101 urinary acids on a 5% phenylmethyl silicone capillary column. *J. Chromatogr. Sci.* *22*:198–202.

Vande Casteele, K., Geiger, H., and Van Sumere, C. F. (1982). Separation of flavonoids by reversed-phase high-performance liquid chromatography. *J. Chromatogr.* *240*:81–94.

Vande Casteele, K., Geiger, H., and Van Sumere, C. F. (1983). Separation of phenolics (benzoic acids, cinnamic acids, phenylacetic acids, quinic acid esters, benzaldehydes and acetophenones, miscellaneous phenolics) and coumarins by reversed-phase high-performance liquid chromatography. *J. Chromatogr.* *258*:111–124.

Vestal, M. L. (1984). High-performance liquid chromatography–mass spectrometry. *Science* *226*:275–281.

Wahlund, K.-G. (1975). Reversed-phase ion-pair partition chromatography of carboxylates and sulphonates. *J. Chromatogr.* *115*:411–422.

Walla, M. D., Lau, P. Y., Morgan, S. L., Fox, A., and Brown, A. (1984). Capillary gas chromatography–mass spectrometry of carbohydrate components of *Legionellae* and other bacteria. *J. Chromatogr.* *288*:399–413.

Wheals, B. B. and White, P. C. (1979). In situ modification of silica with amines and its use in separating sugars by high-performance liquid chromatography. *J. Chromatogr.* *176*:421–426.

Whenham, R. J. (1984). Sensitive assay for amino sugars using capillary gas chromatography with nitrogen-selective detection. *J. Chromatogr.* *303*:380–385.

Winter, M. and Herrmann, K. (1984). Analysis of hydroxycinnamic acid esters and their glucosides by reversed-phase high-performance liquid chromatography after polyamide separation. *J. Chromatogr.* *315*:243–251.

Yamaguchi, K. and Shibamoto, T. (1981). Volatile constitutents of green tea, Gyokuro (*Camelia sinensis* L. var *Yabukita*). *J. Agric. Food Chem.* *29*:366–370.

Yokouchi, Y., Fujii, T., Ambe, Y., and Fuwa, K. (1981). Determination of monoterpene hydrocarbons in the atmosphere. *J. Chromatogr.* *209*:293–298.

Zimmerman, C. L., Appella, E., and Pisano, J. J. (1977). Rapid analysis of amino acid phenylhydantoins by high-performance liquid chromatography. *Anal. Biochem.* *77*:569–573.

Zladkis, A. and Kim, K. (1976). Column eluation and concentration of volatile compounds in biological fluids. *J. Chromatogr.* *126*: 475–485.

7

Fermentation Systems and Processes

EDWARD E. BJURSTROM / Fluor Technologies Inc., Irvine, California

INTRODUCTION

Biotechnology has become something of a "catch-all" for any process whose steps involve living material or material that was once alive. In the broadest sense this includes such diverse industries as beer brewing, food packaging, the production of pharmaceuticals, enzyme manufacturing, and blood processing. Biotechnology has also become closely associated with the field of genetic engineering and its application to the human health care market. Usually the portion of a process that identifies it as a biotechnological process is a fermentation step. Fermentation has been used for thousands of years in the production of basic foodstuffs such as beer, wine, bread, and cheese. In modern times fermentation has been used to produce a wide variety of industrial chemicals as well as food and health care products.

THE FERMENTATION PROCESS

Fermentation is the process where feed materials are converted to desired products by the action of specific microorganisms. Feed streams frequently consist of mixtures of simple carbohydrates such as glucose and various nutrient salts dissolved in water. The nutrient salts are requirements of the particular microorganisms being used and provide necessary elements for proper cellular functions. The carbohydrate material acts as a carbon source for the organism and provides necessary energy for cellular growth and the production of products. Nitrogen is also required for the production of proteins and is often added to the feed material in the form of ammonium hydroxide. Other feed components which may be added, depending on the specific microorganism's requirements, include vitamins, antibiotics, and oxygen in the form of compressed air. Vitamins are usually added to optimize organism growth and shorten the overall fermentation cycle time. Antibiotics are often used in small-scale and developmental studies to reduce the possibility of contamination from extraneous organisms in fermentations involving organisms that have antibiotic resistance. Antibiotics are seldom used, however, in commercial-scale fermentations owing to their comparatively high cost and the need for their complete removal from final products. It is generally preferable to rely on sterilization procedures and fermenter design for controlling system contamination.

The liquid feed to the fermenter becomes the fermentation medium in which the selected organism grows. Aerobic fermentations require oxygen, which is usually supplied by sparging compressed air directly into the liquid pool within the fermenter. Anaerobic fermentations are carried out in the absence of air. Aerobic fermentations generally have shorter cycle times and can produce complex products such as proteins more efficiently than anaerobic fermentations. As a result, most commercially important fermentation processes are aerobic. The obvious exception is the anaerobic fermentation of yeasts to produce ethanol for beverage and fuel use.

All feeds to the fermenter, including air feeds, must be sterilized to avoid the introduction of foreign organisms. If foreign organisms are allowed to infect the fermenter, they will usually outgrow the desired organism, consume media components, produce undesirable by-products, and even kill the production organism.

The liquid medium is most often sterilized using steam heat. Any media components subject to heat degradation should be filter-sterilized separately using a 0.2-μm sterile filter. This type of filter is sometimes referred to as an absolute filter and retains even the smallest bacteria. After being filter-sterilized, the heat-sensitive media is combined with the cooled heat-sterilized media.

Before charging sterile media to the fermenter, the fermenter itself and all feed piping must be sterilized. This is accomplished by steaming the feed piping and the fermenter until all metal in the system has reached at least 120°C. The system is held at that condition for a minimum of 30 min and then cooled by flooding with sterile air. The sterile air is produced by passing compressed air through sterile filters. The air required by aerobic fermentations is also filter-sterilized. This has proven to be the most economical approach for sterilizing the large volumes of air required by most aerobic fermentations.

Once the fermenter and its feed piping have been properly sterilized, the fermentation media can be transferred. The media components discussed earlier are mixed in a batching tank. The mixture is then transferred to a batch sterilization tank or sterilized on the way to the fermenter in a continuous sterilizer. Once the transfer to the fermenter is complete, the media is inoculated with a pure culture of the desired organism and fermentation begins.

Fermentation can be accomplished using either a batch or continuous system. Historically, batch fermentation in a mechanically agitated or stirred vessel has been the system of choice owing to its flexibility and relatively simple operation. Continuous fermentation can achieve higher overall productivity and for some products is currently being used as the most efficient production method. This area is being intensively studied and continuous systems will likely be used increasingly often in the future. Currently, however, the vast majority of fermentation production facilities are based on batch systems. For this reason the following discussion of fermenter operation will be based on batch fermentation. Alternate fermentation systems will be discussed later in the chapter.

Once the batch fermenter is inoculated, the fermentation proceeds through a characteristic cycle involving up to five stages (Fig. 1). The first stage is a lag period which begins at inoculation and ends with the onset of measurable organism growth. During this period the organism is adapting to the new environment of the fermenter and no growth occurs. The fermenter is inoculated using a "seed culture" of the production organism. The seed culture is prepared starting from an inoculation vial containing less than 1 ml of original stock culture stored at cryogenic temperatures. This first culture is grown in a laboratory shake flask and used to inoculate a small fermenter, which in turn is used to inoculate larger fermenters. This process is continued until the production volume is reached. The ratio of the fermenter volume to the inoculant volume can be as small as 10:1 for slow-growing organisms or as high as 50:1 or even 100:1 for fast-growing organisms. The media used to produce the seed culture is designed to optimize the growth of cells. This is a natural requirement for the efficient production of seed culture but often adds to the lag period in the production fermenter. The media in the production fermenter is designed to optimize the production of the product and may be quite different from the seed culture media (unless the cell mass *is* the product, as in the case of single-cell protein). The organism spends the lag period adjusting to the differences between the seed media and the production media. This can involve adjustments in the organism's metabolism and internal enzyme systems for growth using the production media as opposed to the seed media. Unfortunately, this process takes time which is

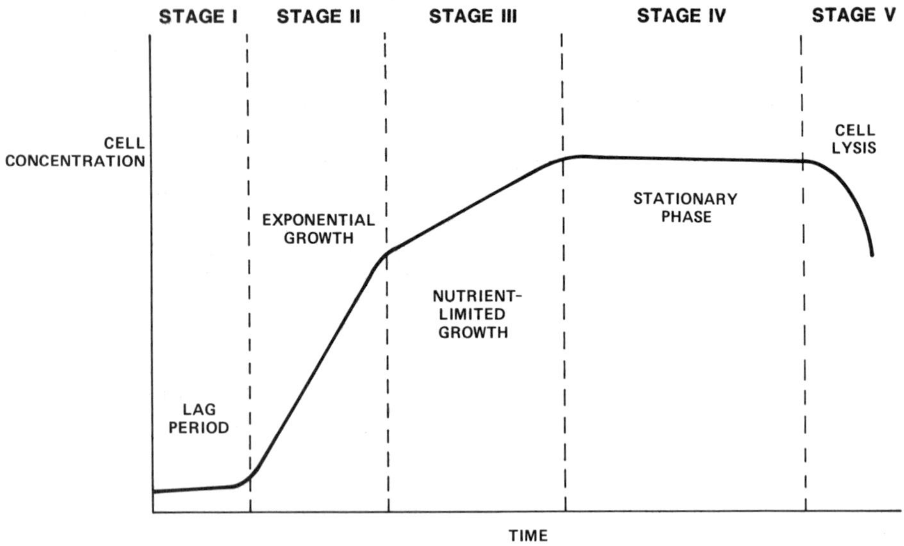

Fig. 1. Fermentation cycle of a batch fermenter.

lost from a production standpoint. The lag period can be minimized by keeping the fermenter warmed to its normal production temperature. Once the fermentation begins, the metabolic heat generated by the organisms must be removed by cooling to maintain the proper temperature.

The second stage shown in Figure 1 is exponential growth. This occurs immediately after the lag period when growth has started and all required nutrients are present in excess, including oxygen, which is a key nutrient for aerobic fermentations. As soon as one of the required nutrients is present in only limited amounts, the growth pattern shifts to a nutrient-limited rate. Most often this occurs in aerobic fermentations when the potential oxygen uptake rate of the mass of cells in the fermenter begins to exceed equipment's capability to transfer oxygen. As discussed earlier, the oxygen requirement of the system is supplied by sparging compressed air into the liquid within the fermenter. Unfortunately, oxygen is sparingly soluble in the waterlike solutions which generally make up the fermentation broth (Kappli and Fiechter, 1981). For a given fermentation, the ability to transfer oxygen from an air bubble into the bulk liquid of the fermenter, thus making it available to the organism, is determined by the agitation and aeration rates. At some point in the fermentation, as the organism multiplies, the cell mass begins to consume the oxygen dissolved in the bulk liquid faster than the agitation and aeration systems can replenish it. As a result, the level of dissolved oxygen decreases to a new equilibrium corresponding to a lower than exponential growth rate. In practice this occurs over a reasonably short period of time, such as 1–2 hr.

The last two stages of the fermentation cycle shown in Figure 1 may or may not occur, depending on the specific organism involved and the nature of the product. If the product is purely growth associated, then the fermenter should be harvested when the cell density reaches a maximum. In such a case the stationary phase would never be reached. If the product is non-growth-associated, it would be produced during a stationary phase after the cells had grown to a predetermined density. Generally some shift in the way the fermenter is operated causes growth to cease and product production to start. Product production may be induced by a number of methods, including the addition of a chemical, a change in temperature or pH, or a sudden shift in nutrient availability. Batch fermentations can be operated as either true batches or fed batches. Fed batch operation involves feeding nutrients to the fermenter during the fermentation cycle and lends itself well to intentionally changing the availability of a key nutrient to halt growth and induce production of a non-growth-associated product. Fed batch operation will be discussed in more detail under alternate fermentation systems. The final stage in the fermentation cycle is cell lysis. This is normally not reached in production fermenters, as uncontrolled lysis or cell breakup releases many intracellular proteins into the broth, resulting in severe product recovery problems. Cells do have a finite cycle in a batch fermenter where the concentrations of toxic by-products build up and result in cell lysis or death. To avoid extra by-product contamination, the fermenter must be harvested before this occurs.

Fermenter harvest is simply the removal of the whole broth from the fermenter, usually to a hold tank. Fermentation usually stops immediately, as the hold tank is not aerated or fed with nutrients. It may, however, be agitated to keep the broth homogeneous and the cells suspended to provide a consistent feed to the product recovery operations. The harvest tank is often chilled to 40–50°F to prevent protein product degradation.

Product recovery and purification can involve a wide spectrum of operations, depending on the specific product and intended use. Product recovery usually involves the gross treatment of product-bearing streams, such as the removal of whole cells and volume reduction. Product purification takes place after recovery and primarily involves the removal of by-products and contaminants. Some of the common methods of fermentation product recovery and purification are listed in Table 1. Figure 2 is a summary of the usual steps found in a fermentation-based production process.

Table 1. Product Recovery and Purification Methods

Operation	Primarily used for recovery	Primarily used for purification
Homogenization	X	
Flocculation	X	
Coagulation	X	
Centrifugation	X	
Ultrafiltration	X	X
Precipitation	X	X
Extraction		X
Chromatography		X

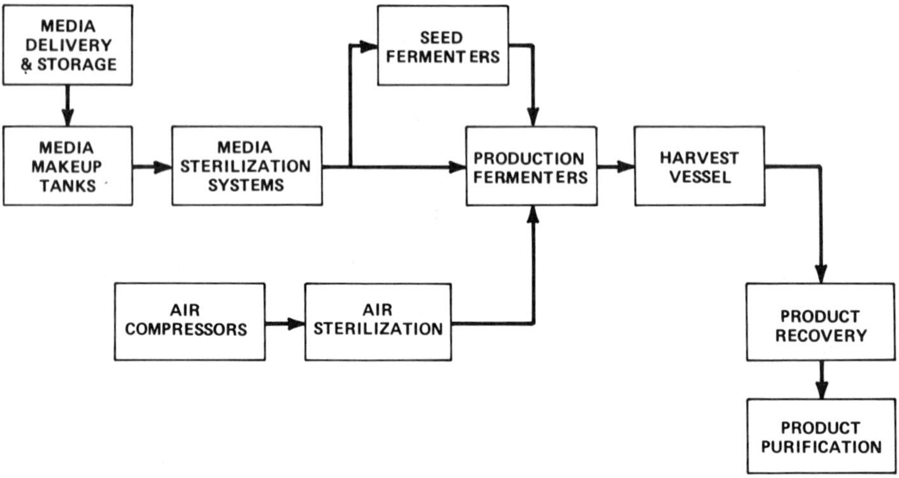

Fig. 2. Steps of a fermentation-based production process.

FERMENTATION PROCESSING IN THE FOOD INDUSTRY

The opening comments of this chapter pointed out that man's first use of fermentation, literally thousands of years ago, involved the production of food. Today fermentation is still widely used in the food industry. This section will review some of the more common applications and examine how genetic engineering techniques may impact these areas in the future.

The most well-known use of fermentation in the food industry is the batch production of alcoholic beverages. This is an anaerobic system where the presence of air is detrimental to the process. Yeast fermentation to produce alcohol is a relatively slow process in which the product alcohol is produced during organism growth. Usually operated as a true batch, the organism grows until the concentration of alcohol reaches a critical level (e.g., 12–14% for wine). This inactivates or kills the yeast organism and fermentation ceases. The alcohol is actually produced as a by-product or waste from the anaerobic metabolism of sugar by the yeast organism. In the case of beer and wine the clarified whole broth is the product. Distillation is required to produce the higher alcohol concentration found in liquors such as brandy and whiskey. This is why these concentrated alcoholic beverages are called distilled spirits. This process is a good example of the use of fermentation to produce a chemical product (ethanol) which can be recovered by fairly rigorous methods such as distillation. Most of the recovery and purification techniques listed in Table 1 are geared to recover more sensitive fermentation products such as proteins that would be destroyed by excessive heat.

Another group of well-known products produced by fermentation include amino acids. Amino acids are the building blocks of proteins and are essential for proper metabolic function in all animals and human beings. Humans and animals can synthesize many of the required amino acids, but not all of them. The amino acids labeled essential are the ones that the human body cannot synthesize at a rate that is sufficient to meet the body's needs, if at all. They are therefore essential components of the human diet. Half of these essential amino acids are commonly produced by fermentation methods and used as food additives or supplements (Considine, 1982).

Many microorganisms have been found that can synthesize amino acids in large quantity from a simple carbon source such as sugar and nitrogen (supplied as ammonium hydroxide). Amino acid fermentations are aerobic and generally conducted in a batch or fed batch operation. The product amino acids are secreted into the broth. Product recovery and purification are accomplished by first separating the cells from the broth and then concentrating the product through evaporation and precipitation. Ion exchange chromatography is also frequently used as a purification step. The highest production volume amino acid, glutamic acid, is produced via fermentation. It is not an essential amino acid but is used as a common flavor enhancer in the form of monosodium glutamate (MSG).

Enzymes are another class of food-related products produced in part by fermentation systems. They are a class of proteins that act to catalyze a variety of chemical reactions, including many involved in the metabolism of living systems. As such, enzymes play a vital role in the food chain from production through utilization. Enzyme complexes or systems are generated by living cells and so have three main sources; they can be produced by extraction from animal tissue or plant material or by fermentation of microbial cells.

Fermentations to produce enzymes are aerobic and are commonly run in batch or fed batch systems. The product enzyme may be secreted into the broth as an extracellular enzyme or may be retained within the organism as an intracellular enzyme. This will affect the way the fermentation is operated, as well as the steps required for product recovery and purification. If the product is extracellular and non-growth-associated, its concentration may be independent of the microbial cell concentration. In this case the fermenter would be operated to maximize the product. If the product is intracellular or growth associated, the product concentration will be a function of the cell concentration. The fermenter should then be operated to optimize the cell concentration and the production of the product enzyme.

Aerobic fermentation has also been traditionally used to culture cell mass for direct consumption by human beings and animals. An example is torula yeast produced by culturing *Candida utilis*. This product has been produced on a commercial scale since World War II and is used primarily as a nutritional supplement. Over the last 15 years there has been a great deal of interest in the production of single-cell protein for consumption as an alternate protein source. Prior to the rise in world oil prices, single-cell protein grown on methanol was thought to be a partial low-cost answer to the world food shortage. Today single-cell protein grown on methanol cannot effectively compete with soy protein in the United States; however, the need to produce single-cell protein at the lowest possible cost by taking advantage of economies of scale led to the successful scale-up of the continuous-draft tube air-lift fermenter. This fermenter configuration will be examined in the section on alternate fermenter designs.

Today recombinant DNA techniques have been successfully employed in the production of human and animal health care products. These have generally been high-value, low-volume materials and constitute a natural area where recombinant DNA techniques would first be used. As time goes on, however, recombinant organisms will increasingly be used in the production of the larger-volume, lower-cost products typical of the food industry. The first food area likely to be impacted by recombinant DNA is the production of enzymes. Rennin, a key enzyme in the manufacture of cheeses, is usually obtained by tissue extraction from the fourth stomach of a cow. This enzyme has been targeted for production via recombinant microorganisms by several genetic engineering companies. Another enzyme system receiving a great deal of attention is cellulase. Cellulase enzymes convert cellulose (the main structural material of wood and woody materials) to fermentable sugars which can be converted to fuel alcohol or edible proteins.

FERMENTER SYSTEM DESIGN AND OPERATION

Previous sections have described the process of fermentation along with examples of its role in the food processing industry. This section will focus on the design details of fermenter systems and their operation.

The design of a fermentation system revolves around the following four key parameters:

1. Maintenance of aseptic conditions
2. Oxygen transfer
3. Heat transfer
4. Instrumentation and control requirements

The real challenge of fermenter system design is to simultaneously satisfy the requirements of each of these areas. Aseptic conditions refer to the normal operating state of the fermenter, where only a pure culture of the production organism grows. As discussed previously, all feeds to the fermenter must be sterilized, as well as all feed piping and the fermenter itself. The system design must prevent any intrusion of foreign or extraneous organisms after the fermenter has been sterilized. This has a far-reaching impact on the design and affects everything from valve selection to the type of surface finish required on the process equipment. Notice that aseptic does not mean sterile. Sterility refers to the total absence of microorganisms; asepsis refers to the control or prevention of organisms entering a system. *Sanitary* is another term often used in conjunction with the subject of sterility. A system that has a sanitary design is one that can be easily cleaned, usually by simple flushing. Any system that will be sterilized in conjunction with normal operations should incorporate a sanitary design. If organic material from previous operations remains in a niche or crevice that cannot be cleaned, it can build up an insulating layer that may prevent adequate sterilization. For example, even though the metal of the system (the piping and equipment) may reach sterilization temperatures, material trapped in the crack of a poorly made weld may not reach the same temperature at all and escape sterilization. When the next batch of media is placed in the system and fermentation begins, any contaminating organisms in that material buildup could work their way out of the crack and begin multiplying in the fermenter. Microorganisms are very small, with bacteria being on the average 1-2 μm in diameter and yeast approximately 10 μm in diameter. Very little space is required for an organism and enough organic material to provide an insulating layer.

A sanitary design is one that seeks to minimize or eliminate all surface imperfections or irregularities. The material of choice is 316 stainless steel. All welds must be ground smooth and all surfaces in contact with the process should be polished to a mirrorlike finish. The vessel should be designed to drain completely. Unfortunately the cleanability of the fermenter is complicated by the vessel internals. This is especially true for large-production fermenters, where internal heat exchange is necessary to meet the heat transfer requirements. All aerobic fermenters also have an air sparger and an agitation system. A typical stirred batch fermenter is shown in Figure 3; it incorporates a ring sparger for the introduction of air, a top-mounted agitator, baffles, and a helical cooling coil. The design, fabrication, and installation of these internal components must be done in a way that minimizes bolting and the creation of areas where material could accumulate.

If a fermenter is properly cleaned and sterilized, maintaining aseptic conditions becomes a matter of preventing contamination from an external source. The points where contamination could enter the fermenter are designated in Figure 4 and basically consist of all the places where the vessel shell is pierced. It is important that each such area be carefully designed to prevent this from happening. First, the fermenter is usually operated under pressure, so if there are any small leaks in the system, it will be from the fermenter outward, and not into the fermenter. The agitator shaft enters the fermenter through a seal that allows the shaft to turn while still keeping the vessel under pressure. For a fermenter this seal must be a double mechanical design supplied with a sterile lubricant such as clean steam condensate. The harvest valve on the bottom of the fermenter is kept closed during the fermentation

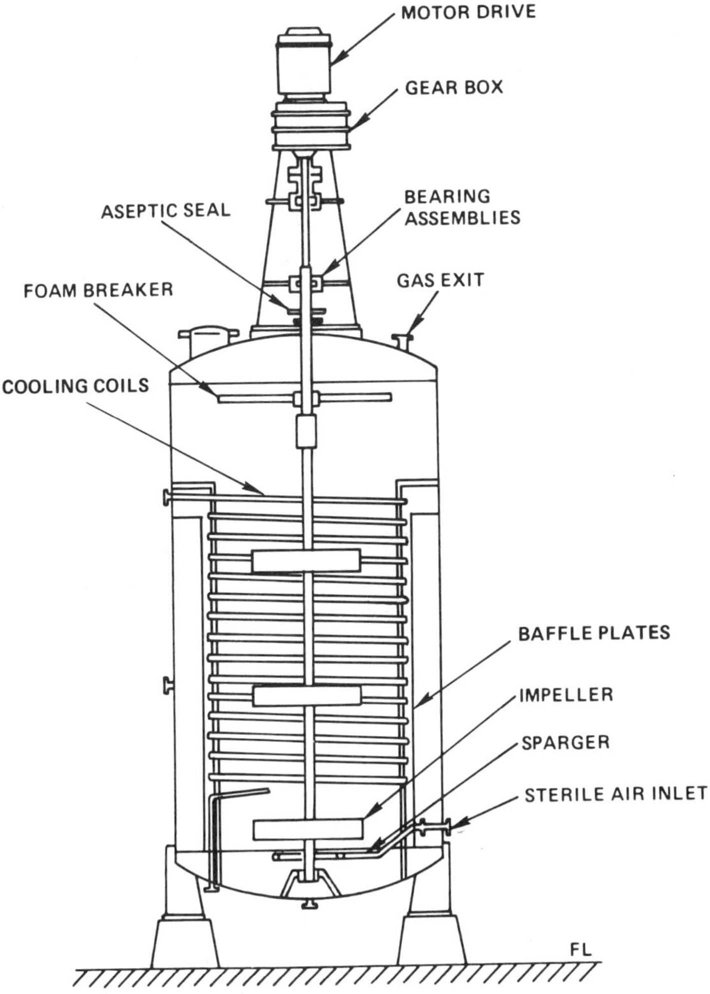

Fig. 3. Stirred batch fermenter design.

and is opened only to remove, or "harvest", the broth from the fermenter. This valve should be a flush-seating valve, which means that in the closed position the valve seats flush with the inside vessel wall and leaves no dead space or stagnant pocket which would be hard to clean or sterilize. The valve should also be under steam pressure during the fermentation run to provide added protection against contamination. This is called a steam seal and is desirable on any line connected to the fermenter that is not used during the fermentation run. The sample port design is very similar to the harvest valve and should include a flush-seating valve. Steam is also connected to this valve to form a steam seal, as well as to sterilize residual material left in the interior of the valve after each use. Instrument ports are usually made using a standard Ingold fitting. The instruments are loaded into these fittings before the fermenter is sterilized so the portion of the instrument probe projecting into the fermenter is sterilized along with the fermenter.

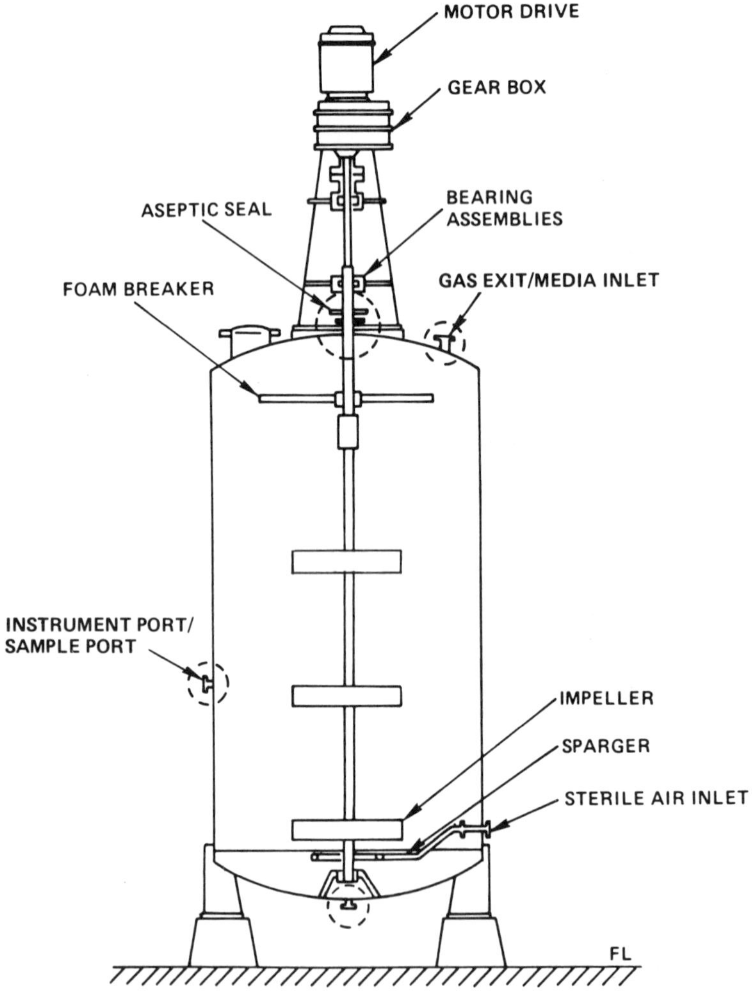

Fig. 4. Potential points for the introduction of contamination in a fermenter.

The probes are screwed tightly into place and sealed with double O-rings. The inlet media and inoculation lines must be sterilized before sterile media are transferred through them and should not be a problem as long as the initial cleaning and sterilization are done properly. If the line will not be used during the fermentation, the inlet valve at the fermenter should be closed and put under a steam seal. The exhaust gas line is used during the run to carry away excess oxygen and nitrogen sparged into the fermenter, as well as by-product gas such as carbon dioxide generated by the growing microorganisms. This exhaust gas line must be designed so that any liquid that condenses out of the gas after leaving the fermenter does not collect and drain back into the fermenter, possibly carrying contamination with it. The line must be sloped away from the fermenter as soon after leaving it as possible. For this the line should first rise vertically from the fermenter and then turn and slope away. This vertical section must be sterilized with the fermenter and often includes a separator such as a cyclone to knock back entrained liquid to the fermenter before it has a chance to become contaminated.

The next key parameter in setting the design of a fermentation system is the required level of oxygen transfer, that is, the problem of transferring oxygen molecules from an air bubble through the bulk liquid in the fermenter and into the microorganism. There are a number of diffusional and boundary layer forces that resist this transfer; however, the rate-limiting resistance is almost always the liquid film around the air bubble (Fig. 5). The oxygen transfer rate is therefore proportional to this resistance, measured as a transfer coefficient called K_L, and the total area through which the transfer occurs, namely, the surface area a of all the bubbles in the fermenter. Oxygen transfer in fermentation systems is usually discussed in terms of the lumped parameter K_La, as both the transfer coefficient and the bubble surface area are very difficult to measure independently. The oxygen transfer rate (OTR) can be calculated by the following equation:

$$\mathrm{OTR} = K_L a(C^* - C_L) \qquad (1)$$

where C^* is the equilibrium dissolved oxygen concentration, that is, the theoretical amount of dissolved oxygen in the fermentation broth, and C_L is the actual, measurable concentration of dissolved oxygen in the broth. The difference between the potentially dissolved oxygen and the actual dissolved oxygen concentrations, $C^* - C_L$, is the driving force for the transfer. The actual dissolved oxygen in an operating fermenter is less than the theoretical or equilibrium value because the organisms are consuming it. As long as the organisms

GENERAL EQUATION:

NUTRIENTS + CARBON SOURCE + O_2 $\xrightarrow[\text{CELLS}]{}$ PRODUCTS + BY–PRODUCTS + HEAT

BARRIERS TO MASS TRANSFER:

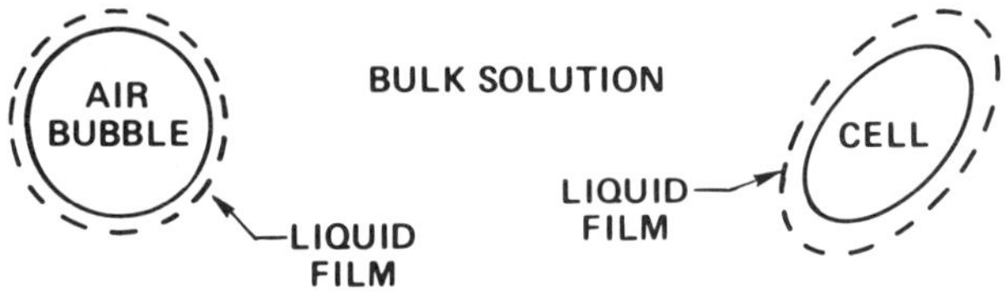

Fig. 5. The liquid film surrounding the air bubble is almost always the rate-limiting resistance factor in oxygen transfer.

in the fermenter have the potential to consume oxygen at an equal or faster rate than it can be transferred, the oxygen transfer rate will be equal to the oxygen uptake rate of the organisms. The oxygen uptake rate can be easily calculated from the difference between the oxygen concentration in the compressed air being fed to the fermenter and the oxygen concentration in the exit gas. The oxygen uptake rate is a good indication of how well the fermentation operation is progressing. Usually not all of the oxygen in the air sparged into the fermenter is transferred; in fact, removal of more than 50% is unusual. A high oxygen concentration in the gas throughout the fermenter is desirable to keep the transfer rate as high as possible.

The ability to transfer oxygen is often the parameter that limits production in aerobic fermentation systems. In theory, the higher the oxygen transfer capability, the higher the productivity. The fundamental factors which determine the oxygen transfer in a given system have been briefly discussed. Inspection of Eq. (1) will help to identify how these factors may be influenced. First, notice that the driving force $C^* - C_L$ is concentration dependent. This is difficult to signficantly affect unless air enriched in oxygen is used, which is unfortunately an expensive way to enhance oxygen transfer. Another approach to increasing the driving force for oxygen transfer is to operate the fermenter under increased pressure conditions. A higher pressure directly increases the solubility of oxygen in the broth. The solubility of other gases in the system is increased as well. Recall that one of the common by-products produced in fermentation systems is CO_2 gas. The levels of dissolved CO_2 must not be allowed to rise too high or it will act as a poison to the microorganisms and negatively affect the fermentation. This limits the usefulness of operating fermentation systems at pressures much above 3–5 atm.

The other term in Eq. (1) which determines oxygen transfer is K_La. As discussed, this is a lumped term made up of the transfer coefficient K_L and the surface area a of the bubbles in the system. The term K_L is a function of many variables, including the physical properties of the fermentation broth. The factors that determine K_L for a given system are not well understood and involve some controversy in the literature; however, a discussion of this subject is outside the scope of this chapter. The factors affecting the bubble surface area are much more straightforward and give significant insight on the design of fermentation systems. The obvious desire is to maximize the surface area. This can usually be accomplished by maximizing the quantity of bubbles and minimizing their size. Bubble size and number are determined by the power input to the broth through the agitator to break the bubbles up and the air flow rate through the system. As a result, maximizing oxygen transfer involves optimizing the power input and air flow rate.

The primary function of the agitator in an aerobic fermenter is to provide the power required to disperse the sparged air and increase its holdup time in the liquid. The most common agitator design for fermentation applications uses a Rushton turbine (flat-blade turbine) as shown in Figure 6 for an impeller. The ratio of the outside diameter of the impeller to the inside diameter of the fermentation vessel is generally 0.3–0.4. If multiple impellers are used, they should be placed roughly evenly over the working volume of the fermenter. The bottom impeller should be set approximately one impeller diameter from the bottom of the vessel. Agitators can be

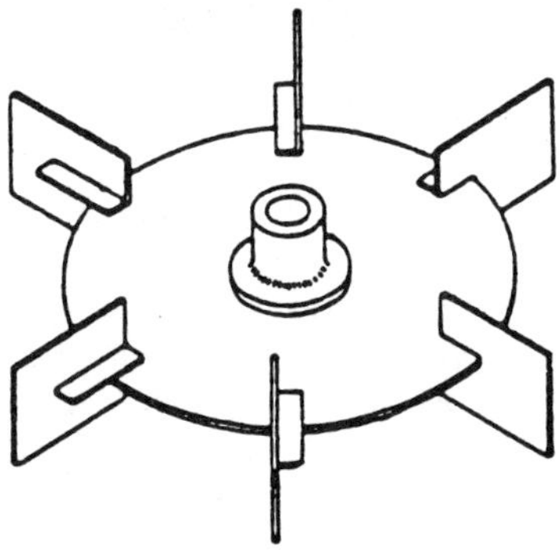

Fig. 6. Rushton turbine.

either top entering or bottom entering, with roughly equal advantages and disadvantages to each type of design. The power delivered to the fermentation broth by the agitator is determined by both the diameter of the impeller and the speed of rotation. The power input is discussed in terms of power per unit volume, such as watts per liter or horsepower per 1000 gal.

The other factor which determines the surface area of the bubbles in the system is the air flow rate. It naturally follows that if more air flows through the fermenter, more air bubbles will be present at any given time. As was discussed earlier, enough air must flow through the system so that the oxygen concentration in the exit gas is at least 50% of the concentration in the inlet air stream. Most often the air flow rate is higher than this minimum. Air flow is often reported as the ratio of the air volume fed, to the volume of ungassed broth in the fermenter per minute (VVM). Flow rates of 1.0 VVM in stirred batch systems are not uncommon. The air is introduced to the fermenter through a ring sparger placed directly below the bottom impeller. The outside diameter of the sparging ring is usually slightly less than the outside diameter of the bottom impeller (Rautzen et al., 1977). This arrangement introduces the air directly into the high-shear mixing zone of the bottom impeller, which immediately disperses the air into fine bubbles. As these air bubbles rise through the fermenter they tend to coalesce into larger bubbles. Multiple impellers are required to redisperse the air.

Oxygen transfer is one of the main factors limiting production in aerobic fermentations owing to the practical considerations involved in designing agitation and aeration systems. High oxygen transfer rates could be achieved through high agitation rates. Unfortunately this requires large and expensive motors and a high consumption of electricity. If large air flow rates are used to increase oxygen transfer, large air compressors would be required. Excessively high air flow rates also reduce production efficiency by reducing the available volume for liquid in the fermenter. Fermenter volume is typically occupied by three elements, the liquid broth, the gas holdup in the system, and a cap of stable foam that rides on the surface of the liquid.

In a highly agitated and aerated system (i.e., the gas holdup is large) the actual volume of ungassed liquid broth may be only 50–60% or even less of the total fermenter volume. The rest of the volume would be occupied by a combination of free gas and foam. However, even in systems where the aeration rates are modest, ungassed liquid volumes rarely exceed 70–75% of the total fermenter volume. These practical limitations for stirred batch systems have been one of the driving forces for developing alternate fermenter designs.

The third key parameter in the design of fermentation systems is the required level of heat transfer. All organisms generate heat as a by-product of metabolic activity. This metabolic heat has been shown to be proportional to the amount of oxygen consumed by the microorganism according to the following simple relationship (Cooney, 1968):

$$Q_m = 0.12M_{O_2} \tag{2}$$

The heat generated by the microorganism, Q_m, has units of kilocalories per liter per minute; the mass of oxygen consumed, M_{O_2}, has units of millimoles of oxygen per liter per minute. There are other sources of heat which must be removed from the fermenter, but none are as significant as the metabolic heat, which typically accounts for over 90% of the total heat load. The only other heat source that is usually accounted for is the heat generated by the power input to the fermenter liquid through the agitator.

An efficient heat removal system must be provided for proper operation of a fermenter, as the temperature should deviate by no more than 1°C for optimum production. Small fermenters (under 2000 liters) can be provided with adequate heat transfer through a simple vessel jacket. The difficulty arises when systems are scaled up. The heat generated is proportional to the volume of the system and therefore scales up according to the cube of the vessel diameter. The surface area of the vessel (i.e., the available area for heat transfer through a cooling jacket) scales up only according to the square of the vessel diameter. For volumes of about 2000 liters a cooling jacket may become inadequate, depending on the oxygen consumption. At this point the cooling jacket must be supplemented or replaced by some internal heat transfer surface area such as a cooling coil or cooling panel. The internal heat transfer equipment increases the difficulties of properly cleaning and sterilizing the fermenter. If a large amount of surface area is required, its configuration must be carefully designed to avoid disturbing the vessel mixing patterns and negatively affecting the oxygen transfer in the system. Use of external heat exchange, such as a shell and tube exchanger, is often proposed as an alternate solution that avoids this problem while easily providing the required surface area. Unfortunately, this would require pumping the broth in a loop from the fermenter through the exchanger and back again. A very large circulating stream would be necessary to meet the heat removal requirements and avoid violating the 1°C temperature variation limit on the system. A larger temperature difference in the circulating loop would reduce the flow, but this usually results in high organism death rates.

External heat exchange has proved to be difficult in actual practice. Often severe problems of contamination are experienced as a result of the pumping requirement; it is very difficult to aseptically pump a large stream. The practical limitations relating to heat transfer have also been a factor in the development of alternate fermentation systems. As organisms are developed with higher oxygen requirements, it will be easier to develop systems that can supply the required oxygen than ones that can remove the resultant heat generated. If it has not already happened, in the not too distant future heat transfer will replace oxygen transfer as the production-limiting factor in aerobic fermentation.

The final key parameter in the design of fermentation systems is the instrumentation and control requirements. Fermentation systems are very complex and involve the interaction of many variables in a dynamic system. Computer control has become an industry standard for new fermentation facilities. Existing facilities, some built more than 30 years ago, continue to be operated with little or no instrumentation, using very rudimentary control methods. This is due to the high cost of retrofitting an existing facility with modern instrumentation. Over the years the operation of these existing facilities has been improved and developed to the point where high efficiency has been achieved; however, this has involved a process of trial and error worked out over the course of years for a given product. As long as the established procedure is followed, known average results are achieved.

The advent of genetic engineering has placed tremendous emphasis on developing a much more scientific approach to fermenter operation. As the science of microbiology has advanced, it has become more important and useful to know how every stage of an organism's growth and metabolism relates to the real goal of product formation. This new emphasis has developed simultaneously with the mushrooming capability of the computer-linked process control area. As a result, process development, once accomplished over the course of years, can be achieved in a matter of months. Computer-linked systems capable of on-line analysis and feedback control can execute sophisticated control algorithms for optimizing fermenter operations. Some of the commonly monitored parameters and controlled variables are listed in Table 2.

The most important monitored parameter is the exit gas composition. This stream should be monitored at least semicontinuously by a mass spectrometer (Buckland and Fastert, 1982). As discussed earlier, the composition of this stream provides essential information for calculating the oxygen uptake of the organisms in the system. All of the controlled variables are important, but several warrant special attention. The dissolved oxygen in the fermentation broth was discussed earlier in relation to the system oxygen transfer. It should be kept as low as is practical to enhance the driving force for oxygen transfer but should not generally be allowed to go to

Table 2. Summary of Fermenter Parameters

Monitored parameters	
	Inlet air pressure
	Inlet air temperature
	Inlet air composition
	Cooling water supply temperature
	Cooling water return temperature
	Broth turbidity
	Broth fluorescence
	Exit gas composition
Controlled variables	
	Inlet air flow rate
	Agitator speed
	Vessel pressure
	Substrate composition
	Substitute feed rate
	Dissolved oxygen in broth
	Vessel temperature
	Cooling water flow rate
	pH
	Foam

zero. If it does, many organisms shift their metabolic cycle accordingly and can begin producing excessive quantities of by-products (Buckland, 1984). An example of this is the yeast *Saccharomyces cerevisiae.* Under aerobic conditions the cells metabolism works to maximize cell mass. Under anaerobic conditions (i.e., dissolved oxygen equal to zero) the production of ethanol is maximized. The pH of a fermentation system is also very important and should be kept within a narrow range identified as optimum for each organism and process. Generally, bacterial fermentations are run at or near neutral pH, while yeast fermentations are optimized at more acidic conditions such as pH 5.0. Most fermentations require the continuous addition of small amounts of base to neutralize the organic acids produced as a natural result of cellular metabolism.

The final controlled variable listed in Table 2 is foam. Fermentation broths tend to foam to one degree or another. For some fermentations it is not a serious problem and for others it can be a very serious, production-limiting problem. Foam is generated by surface-active agents released into the broth by the growing organisms. These surface-active agents are proteins, polypeptides, and fatty acids. A certain amount of foam is unavoidable and may even enhance oxygen transfer (Bjurstrom, 1985), but excessive amounts will occupy fermenter volume and thus significantly reduce the available working volume for the production of product. Also, if foam is left uncontrolled, it will sometimes fill the fermenter and begin flowing out of the exit gas line. This creates an obvious cleanup problem and can lead to contamination of the fermenter, depending on the design of the vent gas system and how carefully the cleanup is done. The foam generated in the fermenter can be controlled by either a mechanical foam breaker or the addition of chemical antifoam agents. A thorough discussion of this subject is given by Phillips et al. (1960) and Hall et al. (1973).

The information obtained by monitoring the fermenter and controlling key variables at fixed points can be used by a process-linked computer to calculate parameters indicating system performance (oxygen uptake rate, overall mass transfer rate, system heat balance, etc.) as well as estimating techniques for the cell growth rate, mass concentration, and carbon utilization rate. Target values of these parameters can be preestablished and used in control algorithms to adjust system variables to give the desired performance. This approach provides more successful fermenter runs, more consistent results, and higher average product yields.

FERMENTER SCALE-UP

The successful commercialization of any new process depends heavily on scale-up from the pilot plant to the production facility. This topic necessarily encompasses a process in its entirety, from media preparation through product recovery and purification. Fermenter scale-up, as well as the scale-up of the recovery and purification techniques in a biotechnological process, can be very interesting as well as challenging; however, the scope of this chapter will restrict the following discussion to fermentation systems only.

The basic goal of scale-up is the successful translation of an acceptable level of production efficiency from a small scale to a larger scale. Production efficiency can be measured in terms of the final product concentration in the broth, the yield on substrate, the fermentation cycle time, or any combination of these parameters. If the environment created in the small fermenter could be duplicated in the larger fermenter, the scale-up would be perfect. Unfortunately, a term as ambiguous as *environment* must be used to include all the real factors that influence fermentation systems on scale-up, including nutrient availability, oxygen transfer, heat transfer, mixing effects, and physical and mechanical limitations. These complexities and the risk exposure involved in industrial production facilities require that scale-up be based on pilot plant data. The minimum size of a fermenter that should be used as a scaling basis is 500 liters, with 2000 liters or larger as a preferred scaling basis. This is not meant to be a rigid rule but, rather, a guideline based on a variety of factors. Fermenters smaller than 500 liters tend to have relatively high surface aeration effects and are generally close to being ideally mixed systems (Humphrey et al., 1971). Also, the effect of the static head of liquid in small fermenters is negligible compared to large systems. Finally, as indicated in the discussion on heat transfer, fermenters in the range of 1000–2000 liters begin requiring an internal heat transfer surface, which influences agitation and mixing within the fermenter.

Historically, fermenters were not always scaled up according to a rational scheme. The approach was frequently based on geometric similarity, where the ratio of the height to the diameter of the fermenter was maintained on scale-up to the larger system. However, this does not provide consistent results owing to the many parameters in a fermenter system that scale differently on the basis of linear dimensions. For example, the volume of the system will scale on the basis of the cube of the diameter, whereas surface areas scale up according to the square of the diameter. The impeller diameter will scale directly, always being 30–40% of the vessel diameter. The maximum shear rate will always increase on scale-up, as it is a function of the tip speed of the impeller; however, the average shear rate will usually decrease on scale-up (Midler and Finn, 1966). Scale-up based strictly on similar geometries provides no guarantee of the process result at the larger scale.

A variety of rational scale-up techniques have been developed over the years, including ones based on constant impeller tip speed, constant agitator power per unit volume, and constant aeration rate per unit volume. However, the most widely accepted scale-up technique today is based on maintaining a constant K_La. The factor K_La is representative of the oxygen transfer capability of the equipment in a system under given conditions. For example, for a given organism at a given system pressure, the equipment (agitator, fermenting vessel, and aeration system) will provide a certain oxygen transfer level based on K_La. The factor K_La is used as a design basis because it is determined by the efficiency and capability of the mechanical system. In scaling up a particular fermentation process, pilot plant data are usually available. The pilot plant fermenter K_La is determined and used as a target value for designing the larger system. A generally accepted scale-up correlation for K_La is (Aiba et al., 1973):

$$K_L a = A(P/V)^b v_s^c \tag{3}$$

where P/V is the power input per unit volume, v_s is the superficial gas velocity, A is a constant determined by the organism involved, and the exponents b and c are considered to fall in the ranges of 0.6–0.77 and 0.2–0.67, respectively (Toshida, 1982; Wang et al., 1979).

Equation (3) states that oxygen transfer as represented by K_La is dependent on the power added to the system through the agitator and the air flow through the fermenter. As discussed earlier, practical limitations must be considered. There is a limit to how large a mechanical agitator can be made. Heat transfer requirements begin to be a problem in very large fermenter systems, as internal cooling coils become crowded, affecting mixing patterns. The superficial velocity v_s of the air moving through the system can also become a problem. It is calculated by dividing the air flow through the system by the vessel cross-sectional area. The air flow scales up by the cube power. The cross-sectional area scales up by the square power. The superficial velocity therefore becomes larger as the system is scaled up. This is why the theoretical limit, where air moves through the system so fast that it blows all the liquid out through the vent gas line, is of concern only for large-scale systems. It is because of these practical limits on stirred batch systems that alternate fermenter configurations have been so extensively investigated. The next section will give a brief review of this area.

ALTERNATE FERMENTER CONFIGURATIONS

The stirred batch system has been the predominant fermenter configuration, primarily because of its ability to meet the needs of a wide range of processes. However, as process requirements become more diverse, alternate configurations have become more useful. The modern literature on fermentation systems often refers to fermenters as bioreactors, especially in discussions involving alternate fermenter designs. In terms of definition, a true stirred batch fermenter is one that has all of the required media in place at the start of the fermentation run. The system is inoculated with the production culture and then agitated and aerated until the culture grows to some predetermined level. The broth is then harvested or removed from the fermenter.

A common variation is the fed batch fermenter. This really involves a variation in the way the fermenter is operated rather than in its configuration. After the system is inoculated and while the culture is growing, a feed stream of some key nutrient is added to the fermenter. This type of operation provides an additional control variable that can be effectively used to limit or enhance growth rates, influence product production, or shift the organism into or out of a stationary phase. This is still considered a batch system, as the entire contents of the fermenter are removed or harvested as a batch. For this type of operation the fermenter volume increases over the course of the run.

An additional variation that allows a system originally designed to operate as a batch fermenter to be used as a continuous fermenter involves the withdrawal of a "product" stream while the fermenter is being run in a "fed batch" mode. The product withdrawal rate should equal the feed rate to keep the system at a constant volume. This type of continuous fermenter is defined as a chemostat. Chemostats are often used in the laboratory to study the effects of continuous culture on microorganisms. This is especially important for recombinant organisms because of their tendency to revert to the nonrecombinant form after a certain number of generations. This lack of stability with respect to reversion is the main reason why recombinant organisms are not normally used in continuous fermentation systems.

Industrial systems are much more sophisticated than the laboratory chemostat; however, this simple device illustrates most of the advantages and disadvantages of continuous fermentation, regardless of scale. Generally, continuous fermenters have a higher overall productivity compared to batch systems. Even though they tend to operate at lower cell concentrations than the maximum in a batch fermenter, they more than make up for this by operating for much longer periods. Every organism is different, but generally bacterial fermentations have a batch cycle time of 1–2 days, while yeast and mycelial fermentations can have batch cycle times of several days to a week or longer. By comparison, a continuous fermentation system should have a minimum run time of 30 days, and preferably 90–120 days. Generally, smaller equipment is required by a continuous system to produce the same amount of product as a batch system. The equipment tends to be better utilized and the system as a whole is more efficient. One disadvantage of the continuous system's long run time is the increased susceptibility to contamination by foreign organisms. The careful design of a continuous fermentation system from the standpoints of sterility and the maintenance of asepsis is critical to the success of the process. Two additional problems particular to continuous fermentation are organism washout and loss of unused substrate to the product stream. Organism washout occurs when the rate of substrate feed and product withdrawal removes the organism from the fermenter faster than it can replace itself through its normal growth rate. Generally, the fermenter is a well-mixed system. As whole broth is withdrawn, a certain number of cells are removed from the system. In a continuous fermenter, these cells can only be replaced by the growth of the cells that remain. Therefore, the product withdrawal rate must be carefully balanced with the organism growth rate to avoid washout. This also sets the volumetric feed rate of the substrate if constant volume operation is to be maintained. The organism growth rate then becomes the factor that limits productivity in the system and can represent a serious limitation for non-growth-associated products. Loss of unused substrate to the product stream occurs when the feed and product withdrawal points are too close together. Channeling of substrate from inlet to outlet reduces yield and complicates the product recovery operations. Fortunately the feed rate is usually small compared to the fermenter volume, so if the feed and withdrawal points are far enough apart, this problem should not occur.

To this point we have reviewed alternate fermenter operation. The remainder of the discussion will cover alternate fermenter designs as grouped into the following four categories:

1. Air-lift fermenters
2. Modified stirred and hybrid systems
3. Immobilized cell bioreactors
4. Cell recycle systems

The air-lift is a tower fermenter that relies solely on the compressed air sparged into the liquid to provide the needed power for oxygen transfer. Figure 7 illustrates the basic configuration. Air is sparged into a central draft tube containing baffles and coils or tubes for heat transfer. As the air rises in the central draft tube, the baffles slow the rise velocity and break up coalesced bubbles. The design of the draft tube must balance the need for continuously breaking up the bubbles and controlling their velocity to provide good oxygen transfer with the need to disengage the gas from the liquid at the top of the draft tube. In actual practice, good oxygen transfer rates are achieved at the expense of less than complete gas disengagement. As the air bubbles rise in the draft tube, the displaced liquid flows downward in the annular space, creating a circulating pattern. The main advantages of the air-lift fermenter are the low-shear mixing characteristics, relatively low energy requirements, and the absence of rotating shafts which require aseptic

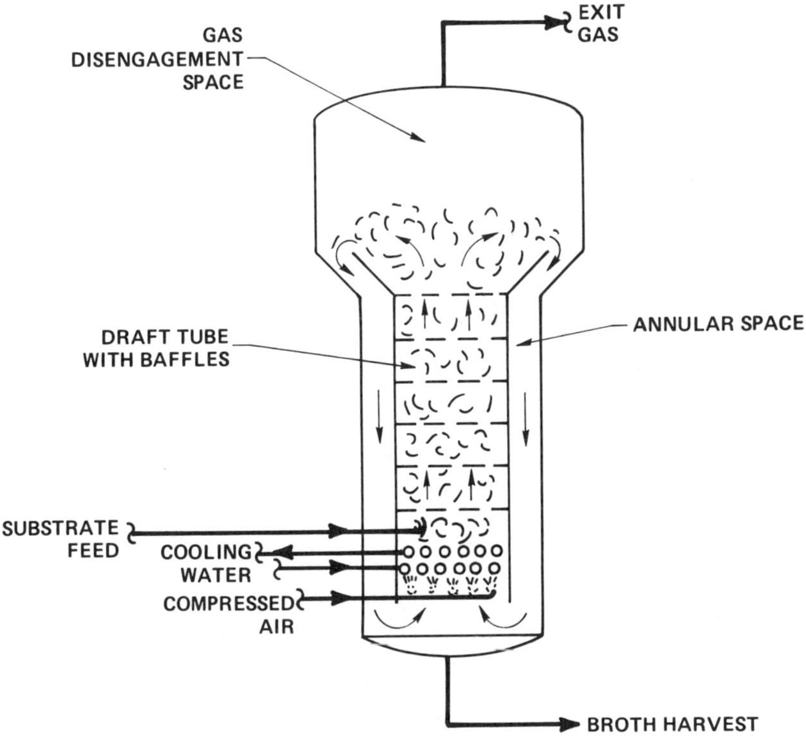

Fig. 7. Basic configuration of an air-lift fermenter.

seals. Air-lift fermenters can be operated in a batch mode or as a continuous system with properly placed feed and withdrawal ports. However, unless special design features are added, this type of fermenter cannot be operated in a fed batch mode, as the hydraulics of the system depend on maintaining a realtively constant liquid volume. Careful consideration must also be given to the effects on the organism of cycling between nutrient-rich and nutrient-poor areas; for example, the dissolved oxygen concentration in the draft tube will be much higher than that in the annular space. This fermenter has been scaled up to very large commercial sizes for producing single-cell protein in bulk quantities. These are some of the world's largest fermenters, with reported liquid capacities of over 10^6 liters per fermenter (Senior and Windess, 1980).

There have been a variety of modified stirred batch fermenters and hybrid designs incorporating the characteristics of stirred batch, tower, and air-lift fermenters. These have included mechanically agitated tower fermenters, tower fermenters with multiple draft tubes that develop complicated liquid circulation patterns, and air-lift fermenters that incorporate a mechanical agitator in the central draft tube instead of baffles for bubble dispersion (Margaritis and Wallace, 1984). Other fermenter configurations designed to mimic the liquid circulation within the air-lift type are variously called loop reactors, jet loop reactors, and plunging jet reactors. Each of these fermenter types represents an attempt to improve on the efficiency of the stirred batch and air-lift fermenters, but usually at the cost of flexibility and adaptability. None of these fermenters have been scaled up to the operating commercial level of either the stirred batch or air-lift types.

The next category of fermenter types is the immobilized cell bioreactor. In this design whole cells are immobilized or trapped in or on a solid matrix and held within the fermenter. These systems are by definition almost continuous in nature, where the feed material flows into the fermenter and product material is withdrawn. The key design requirement is that feed or nutrient material flow easily through the solid matrix to the cells and that product and by-product materials flow easily back out through the solid matrix. The product must be extracellular and preferably non-growth-associated. Usually rapid organism growth clogs the solid matrix and hinders the free flow of nutrients and products into and out of the system.

The most useful immobilized cell bioreactor configurations appear to be the fluidized bed system and the hollow fiber or membrane bioreactor. The fluidized bed system involves trapping the organism within a solid particle or on the surface of a particle. These particles are then held in the fermenter as a fluid bed. Feed material flows into the fluid bed section and product liquid is withdrawn. Multiple beds or long residence times are used to ensure the economic conversion of feed to product (Fig. 8). This is required to avoid withdrawing significant amounts of unconverted feed material with the product stream.

The hollow fiber or membrane bioreactor consists of a conventional bundle, or cartridge, of ultrafiltration or microfiltration hollow fiber membranes. In normal cartridge construction each end of the bundle of fibers is encased in a block of resin. This isolates what is normally referred to as the retentate side of the membrane from the permeate side of the membrane (Fig. 9). Ultrafiltration membranes are rated in terms of their molecular weight cutoff, which can be anything from 10,000 to 300,000. A membrane with a molecular weight cutoff of 100,000 is porous to substances with a molecular weight of 100,000 or less and retains most larger molecules. The membrane for a hollow fiber bioreactor must be selected on the basis of the size of the product molecule. Microporous membranes are rated in terms of microns. A 0.2-μm filter will retain even the

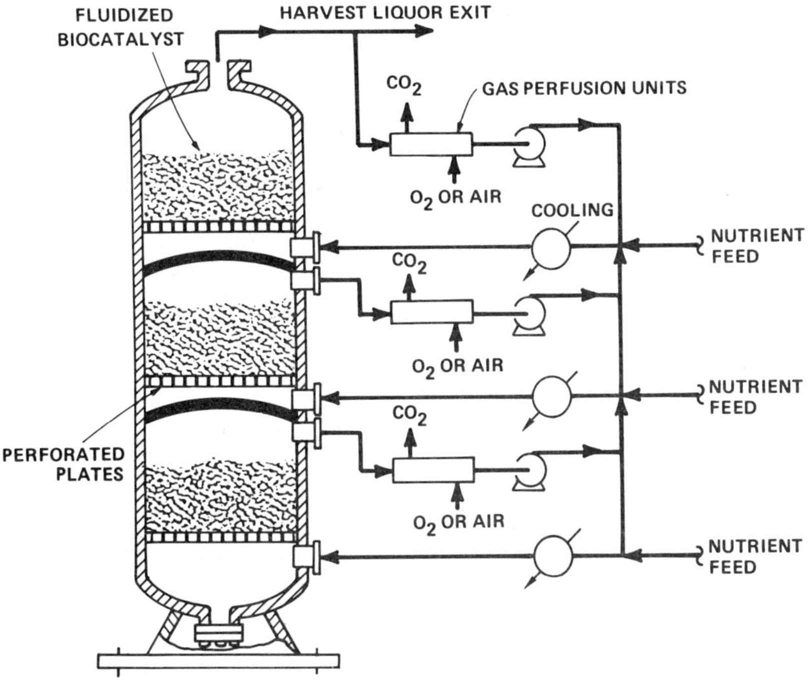

Fig. 8. Fluidized bed system.

smallest bacteria but will allow macromolecules to pass through freely. The permeate side of the cartridge of hollow fibers is inoculated with the organism of interest and the cells lodge in the void spaces of the membrane structure. Feed material is introduced on the retentate or tube side of the membrane and must pass through the membrane to be used by the trapped cells. The product and by-products must then pass back through the membrane to exit the system. Again, staged units or long residence times must be used to maximize the yield of feed material.

Both fluid bed and hollow fiber systems can achieve high cell densities, depending on the design of the solid support system. When this is combined with continuous operation, these systems have the potential of very high productivity. These systems also avoid the problem of organism washout as the cells are permanently held with the fermenter. The main difficulties in developing these systems have been the restrictions on organism growth, product secretion, and nutrient availability. Another factor that has been a serious hindrance to the development of these systems is the supply and

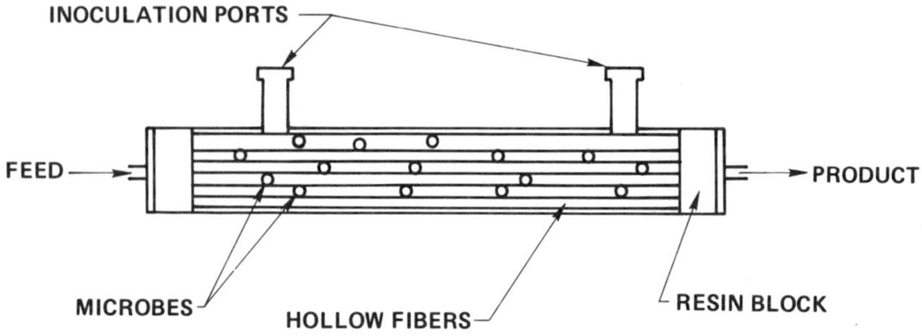

Fig. 9. Hollow fiber bioreactor cartridge.

removal of gaseous components such as oxygen and carbon dioxide. Currently the most successful applications of immobilized systems have been the production of ethanol by immobilized yeast and the production of various products by immobilized mammalian cells (Roy, 1983). Mammalian cell culture or tissue culture is particularly well suited to immobilized cell fermentation, being a very slow-growing system that usually secretes product proteins. Also, tissue culture typically requires very low amounts of dissolved oxygen and produces by-product gases at a comparably low rate.

The final category of alternate fermenter types is cell recycle systems. This design incorporates the initial separation of whole cells from the fermenter broth either within the fermenter itself or as an operating part of the fermentation system. Once the cells are separated, all or some are recycled back to the fermenter while the clarified broth containing the product goes on to recovery and purification operations. Cell recycle systems were developed as an improved approach to continuous fermentation. The problem of organism washout is eliminated and the cell density in the system can be controlled independent of the growth rate.

The two fundamental approaches used to accomplish cell separation are centrifugation and filtration. These are the usual techniques used to separate cells from fermentation broth, but their use in a cell recycle system creates some special requirements principally related to maintaining aseptic conditions. The main difficulty is ensuring that the returning cell concentrate has not been contaminated by foreign organisms. The design of the separating system should use only sanitary piping, valving, and equipment. It is important to remember that to be sanitary, the system must be cleanable and, as part of a fermentation system, must also prevent the intrusion of foreign organisms. Piping and valving systems are available that can accomplish this, but some difficulties exist with available centrifugation and filtration equipment. Unless the equipment is carefully designed, maintained, and properly operated, the cell recycle stream going back to the fermenter can be easily contaminated. Recent advances in the design of hermetically sealed centrifuges and ceramic microporous filters have reduced some of the problems of contamination and cleanability. It is best to avoid the use of pumps, as these tend to be a common point of contamination as well as a source of high shear forces which may lyse or destroy the recycled cells. For this reason some proposed cell "recycle systems" actually have filtration equipment located within the fermenting vessel. The cells are then simply retained in the fermenter and only clarified broth is drawn off. Centrifugation has been successfully used on a commercial scale to recycle yeast cells to a fermenter in the production of fuel ethanol by continuous fermentation. Bacterial contamination of this yeast fermentation is eliminated as the bacteria, which are much smaller than the yeast cells, are continuously washed out of the system with the supernatant flow from the centrifuges. Only the larger yeast cells are captured by the centrifuge and recycled back to the fermenter.

Cell recycle systems have not been widely used due to several limitations other than the problem of system contamination. First, the production organism itself is subjected to a certain amount of cycling in going from the fermenter to the separating device and back again. This is a particular problem with aerobic fermentations where the organism's oxygen requirement could not be met in the separation system. During the time these organisms spend in an oxygen-depleted environment, metabolic shifts occur which result in the production of excessive by-products and reduction in the overall yield of desired product. For this reason the successful applications of cell recycling tend to be with anaerobic fermentation and fermentations of organisms with low oxygen requirements. Another problem associated with cycling the organisms through the separation system is the dynamic forces put upon the cells. The system must be designed to keep the liquid shear forces well below what is required to lyse the cells. Different kinds of organisms will vary greatly in their sensitivity to shear forces and must be evaluated on an individual basis.

REFERENCES

Aiba, S., Humphrey, A. E., and Millis, N. F. (1973). *Biochemical Engineering*, Academic, New York, pp. 182–183.

Bjurstrom, E. (1985). Biotechnology, fermentation and downstream processing. *Chem. Eng. 92*:126–158.

Buckland, B. C. (1984). The translation of scale in fermentation processes: The impact of computer process control. *Biotechnology 10*:875–882.

Buckland, B. C. and Fastert, H. (1982). Analysis of fermentation exhaust gas using a mass spectrometer. In *Computer Applications in Fermentation Technology*, London: Society of Chemical Industry, London, pp. 119–126.

Considine, D. M. (ed.) (1982). *Foods and Food Production Encyclopedia*, Van Nostrand Reinhold, New York, pp. 27–32.

Cooney, C. L. (1968). Measurement of heat evolution and correlation with oxygen consumption during microbial growth. *Biotechnol. Bioeng. 11*:269–281.

Hall, M. J., et al. (1973). Foams and foam control in fermentation systems. *Prog. Ind. Microbiol. 12*:171–234.

Humphrey, A., et al. (1971). Effects of surface aeration on scale-up procedures for fermentation processes. *Ind. Eng. Chem. Process Res. Dev. 10*:190–196.

Kappli, O. and Fiechter, A. (1981). A convenient method for the determination of oxygen solubility in different solutions. *Biotechnol. Bioeng. 23*:1897–1901.

Margaritis, A. and Wallace, J. (1984). Novel bioreactor systems and their applications. *Biotechnology* 5:447–453.

Midler, M., Jr. and Finn, R. K. (1966). A model system for evaluating shear in the design of stirred fermenters. *Biotechnol. Bioeng. 8*:71–84.

Phillips, K., et al. (1960). Effect of antifoam agents in oxygen transfer in deep tank fermentations. *J. Biochem. Microbiol. Technol. Eng. 2*:81–91.

Rautzen, R., Benz, G., and Dickey, D. (1977). Design and scale up of agitators for gas dispersion in fermentors. Paper presented at the Engineering Foundation Converence on Mass Transfer and Scale Up of Fermentors, Henniker, New Hampshire.

Roy, T., et al. (1983). Microbial hollow fiber bioreactors. *Trends Biotechnol. 1*:135–139.

Senior, P. J. and Windass, J. (1980). The ICI single cell protein process. *Biotechnol. Lett. 2*:205–210.

Wang, D., Cooney, C., Demain, A., Dunnill, P., Humphrey, A., and Lilly, M. (1979). *Fermentation and Enzyme Technology*, Wiley, New York, p. 185.

Yoshida, F. (1982). Aeration and mixing in fermentation. *Annu. Rep. Ferment. Processes. 5*:1–34.

8

Bioprocess Control

KARL A. BAYER / University of Agriculture,
Vienna, Austria

INTRODUCTION

Biotechnology utilizes microorganisms and/or biocatalysts to carry out special syntheses and conversions. The origins of biotechnological engineering were significantly influenced by chemical engineering; however, during the last few years biotechnology has emerged as a field in its own right, concentrating on specific problems such as process control, reactor design, and downstream processing. The following considers the main differences between biotechnological and pure chemical engineering.

Complexity and Reproducibility of Bioprocesses

The driving force behind bioprocesses is the microbial cell, which has the genetic potential to synthesize a variety of enzymes, depending on its metabolic demands. Microbial cells produce their own catalysts. The flexibility of a cell's metabolism is much more pronounced in wild-type strains than in industrial strains, which are selected on the basis of special metabolic activities. The microbial cell has an easily controlled and highly interactive metabolism.

However, the reproducibility of bioprocesses suffers from complexity of the reactions involved and the numerous factors affecting cell metabolism. The genetic stability and reproducibility of microorganisms must also be considered.

Bioprocesses and Environmental Conditions

Since bioproduct formation is carried out by the microbial cell, it is a function of the cell's growth processes. Depending on the mode of enzyme synthesis involved, one can distinguish between primary and secondary metabolites. Primary metabolites are essential to microbial growth and reproduction and thus comprise the enzymes synthesized. Primary metabolite production is therefore mostly growth-associated. Secondary metabolites are those that are not essential to microbial growth and reproduction. Zähner (1979) described their formation as reflecting the "scope of the evolution" of the microorganism. Secondary metabolite formation is non-growth-associated (trophophase to idiophase). Because of the cell's genetic potential, secondary metabolite formation is strongly influenced by environmental conditions and the evolutionary stages of the culture. Malek (1976) called this important set of factors the cell's "physiological state." Malek's interpretation substantially facilitates the understanding of biotechnological processes. Different physiological states will also be manifested by morphological variations of the culture. As already noted in the Introduction, microorganisms are characterized by their ability to easily adapt to changing environmental conditions. Therefore the production of secondary metabolites clearly requires the maintenance of certain environmental conditions.

Compared to chemical engineering, biochemical reactions are carried out under relatively mild conditions, which have to be monitored exactly within certain ranges. The facts as considered above confirm the importance of process control in biochemical engineering.

THE TASK OF BIOPROCESS CONTROL

The metabolic functions of microorganisms are in principal genetically determined. The activation of various metabolic pathways depends largely on the environmental conditions at the time. Therefore the primary task of process control in general is to monitor the environmental conditions which have been evaluated as optimal.

Industrial Production

Monitoring plays a much more important role in industrial production than in research work. The aim of industrial work is to prepare an economically marketable product. This is usually achieved by a process whose behavior is well known under certain conditions. The process itself is often poorly understood, especially in the production of secondary metabolites. Process control is carried out via the classical parameters: temperature, oxygen partial pressure, pH, respiratory quotient, and agitation speed. The mode of cultivation, that is, by fed batch operation or the supplementation of nutrients at special phases of culture evolution, also plays a fundamental role in product formation. Applying well-defined conditions guarantees certain product yields.

Research

In research work, the tasks of process control are different from those in industrial production, where, as a rule, processes are viewed as "black boxes." The rational optimization of a process, however, will depend primarily on one's insight into the process and the metabolic interactions involved. By enhancing the number of parameters a substantially better knowledge of the process can be attained. Progress can be made by identifying those parameters of physiological relevance and formulating the kinetics of product formation. From these data one can determine the possibilities of interfering with the process from outside and define a control strategy. In contrast to its role in industrial applications, process control in research is directed toward data acquisition. The data obtained on an industrial scale are utilized mainly to evaluate set points.

Process Automation

Another area of application of process control in biotechnology is in process automation, which concerns upstream and downstream processing and partly the fermentation process itself. Upstream processing includes nutrient preparation and sterilization; downstream processing deals mainly with product recovery, for example, centrifugation, sedimentation, chromatography, and ultrafiltration. In process control mainly the technique of sequencing is applied. Some of these unit operations are classical chemical engineering procedures and they can be applied in biotechnology without modification.

The fermentation process itself is too complex for the application of sequence control. As will be outlined later, a great obstacle to increasing the degree of automation is a pronounced lack of sensors, resulting in insufficient knowledge of the process. A process control system must also carry out various aspects of data processing, such as providing graphical displays and printouts of the results. Since these operations represent the state of the art of computer technology, they will not be treated in more detail.

SPECIFIC PROBLEMS IN BIOPROCESS CONTROL

As already stated earlier, bioprocesses are significantly different from purely chemical processes. The microbial cell and its products constitute the basis of any bioprocess. *Escherichia coli* has the genetic potential to synthesize more than 1000 enzymes, which are formed according to the cell's metabolic demands and environmental conditions. Under optimal conditions the bioprocess is completely regulated and all metabolites are produced in optimal quantities. The biotechnologist is not very concerned with these aspects, and an overproducing system with weak control mechanisms, which can easily be shunted, would be more interesting.

Mechanisms of Metabolic Regulation

On the biochemical level cell metabolism is regulated mainly by enzyme synthesis and enzyme activity.

Enzyme Synthesis

Enzyme synthesis is a coarse metabolic regulator, acting at the transcription level (i.e., information transfer from DNA to mRNA) or at the translation level (i.e., information transfer from mRNS to proteins). The regulation of bacteria is primarily limited to transcription owing to the short lifetime of their mRNA. Phenomenologically enzyme synthesis is regulated via induction and repression. Each microbial cell possesses a set of enzymes, independent of actual environmental conditions, catalyzing the main routes of metabolism (constitutive enzymes). Many of the catabolic enzymes are inductive; their synthesis is stimulated by the metabolites. Repression occurs mainly in anabolism; the enzyme synthesis is repressed by a surplus of end-products.

Enzyme Activity

Enzyme activity is the fine regulator of metabolic pathways. In contrast to enzyme synthesis, enzyme activity is controlled by the following mechanisms.

Feedback Inhibition

The end-product of synthesis has an inhibitory effect on one of the initial enzymes of the feedback chain. Overproduction can result from the elimination of this mechanism. The lysine production of *Corynebacterium glutamicum* has been increased extensively by the inhibition of dihydropicolinate synthetase. A general stragegy for countering the effects of inhibition is to lower the concentration of the inhibitor. Auxotrophic mutants are used to avoid further depreciation of the desired product. If essential substances are supplied in limiting concentrations, their continuous consumption will lead to the elimination of feedback inhibition.

Energy Charge

The energy charge (EC) regulates enzyme activity. A high EC will inhibit the enzymes involved in the catabolic pathways and stimulate the enzymes of the anabolic pathways.

Enzyme Degradation

Enzyme activity may be regulated by enzyme degradation; for example, *Saccharomyces cerevisiae* tryptophan synthetase is degraded by a specific protease at the transition from the exponential to the stationary phase.

Enzyme Modification

The glutamine synthetase production of *E. coli* is inhibited to 80–90% if the medium is supplemented with NH_4^+. There exist two forms of this enzyme: The active one, glutamine synthetase A, is transformed by adenylation into the inactive form, glutamine synthetase B. The adenylating enzyme, adenylate transferase, is stimulated by glutamine and inhibited by α-ketoglutarate. The inhibition of glutamine synthetase results from an increase of the glutamine level caused by the addition of NH_4^+.

The selection of microbial regulation principles as presented above gives greater insight into the problems of bioprocess control, but the know-how of classical control engineering cannot be transferred to bioprocess control. A single biochemical reaction, corresponding to a single loop in control engineering, is regulated not only by the metabolites involved, but superior mechanisms, like EC or catabolite repression, also take part in the regulation. The processes in a microbial cell cannot be viewed separately; only with the generally less complex enzyme-catalyzed processes can a system analytical approach be applied.

A logical approach to improving a bioprocess would be to increase one's knowledge of it and determine key parameters. As was already stated above, the possibilities of influencing a process in a particular direction are very small. Regulation mostly takes place on the molecular level. In this case interfering with the process from outside is practically impossible, and sensors to control key parameters are rarely available. An exception is the regulation of glutamate synthetase by the addition of NH_4^+. In the production of secondary metabolites, the problems are manifold.

Returning to the control of bioprocesses, it must be pointed out that the complexity of the process has to be considered. The approach to new control strategies, namely, combining various parameters and generating new ones, points to the use of computer technology.

Sensors

As already outlined, a fundamental approach to gain better insight into bioprocesses is to increase the quantity and quality of data acquisition.

The bioprocess has a dynamic behavior. The appropriate sensors should be able to provide information about the dynamics and status of the process. Thomanetz et al. (1982) evaluated the degradation of adenosine triphosphate (ATP) of *E. coli* from thermodynamic data: 2.5×10^6 molecules of ATP are transformed per second, indicating high bioprocess reaction rates.

As Malek (1976) emphasized in his treatment of the physiological state, the formation of various products can be closely correlated with specific evolutionary phases of the microorganism. The characterization of various phases implies the acquisition of numerous parameters and their quantification in well-defined frameworks, thus confronting the control engineer with almost unsolvable problems. Also, as of yet, there is no solution to the problem of on-line biomass measurement.

Classical bioprocess control is carried out with instruments taken from chemical engineering. The task of the biotechnologist is to monitor complex, interactive processes with rather simple equipment. Depending on the application, in industry or in research, specific tasks have to be fulfilled. Industrial control tasks involve monitoring a well-defined process by means of a few parameters of generally little physiological relevance. Product analysis is done mainly off-line. With the evolution of genetic engineering, industry is encountering more and more genetically manipulated microorganisms. Since these strains have lost much of their physiological flexibility, maintenance of exact, predetermined environmental conditions is essential. From this point of view, industry will require sophisticated sensor systems too.

In research the lack of physiologically relevant transducers is much more pronounced. On-line analysis is desirable because of the dynamic behavior of bioprocesses. The availability of appropriate transducers is drastically lessened by the necessity of working under aseptic conditions. The operation of a series of probes is limited to chemical engineering or to septic fermentations. The measurement of dissolved oxygen under aseptic conditions is a classic example of the kinds of problems the biotechnologist must solve. The membrane of the electrode is significantly modified by steam sterilization. Drifting is observed in long-term experiments and recalibration is problematic. Since many transducers cannot be implemented in situ, by-pass measurements and sampling via membranes have recently gained in importance.

Different Parameters

State Variables

State variables provide information on the process status. Sensors capable of transmitting process-specific signals are rare. Usually process control is limited to classical parameters, from which many manipulated parameters can be derived. Some common state variables are as follows:

pH, CO_2 partial pressure, and O_2 partial pressure
O_2 and CO_2 in exhaust gas
Pressure, power consumption, volume (weight), density of mash, air supply, and foam
Product formation and biomass

Manipulated Variables

Manipulated variables are the decisive elements of a control system. They offer the possibility of influencing the process from outside. In classical process control the following parameters are controlled:

Temperature, aeration rate, feed rate of nutrients, precursors, acid, base, and antifoam
Agitation and volume (weight)

These parameters reflect the similarity of biochemical and chemical process control.

Quality Coefficients

Bioprocesses are characterized by a high degree of interaction. Therefore the state variables per se are not able to provide physiologically relevant information on the bioprocess. The signals collected have to be transformed and combined with others to yield process-specific coefficients. A process computer is helpful in this area. The following are examples of such variables:

O_2 consumption rate (QO_2)
CO_2 production rate (QCO_2)
Respiratory quotient (RQ)
Substrate consumption rate (Q_S)
Product formation rate (P)
Calorimetric and material balancing
Yields (Y)
e.g. biomass produced/substrate consumed ($Y_{X/S}$)
biomass produced/oxygen consumed ($Y_{X/O}$)
product produced/substrate consumed ($Y_{P/S}$)

product produced/oxygen consumed ($Y_{P/O}$)
product produced/biomass produced ($Y_{P/X}$)
Yield in relation to the amount of ATP produced from the energy source (Y_{ATP})

Bioprocess Monitoring Parameters and Recent Developments

Physical Parameters

Temperature. Fermentation behavior follows the Arrhenius plot, that is, there is a correlation between temperature and the reaction kinetics. The sensors are commonly resistance thermometers. Measurement of the heat evolution during fermentation by dynamic calorimetry (Cooney et al., 1968; Bayer and Führer, 1982) can be utilized to evaluate the physiological state of the culture.

Weight. Nowadays the volume of fermentation vessels and the addition of nutrients and other reactants are evaluated by weight measurement. The measurements are based on the fact that certain materials alter their resistance with changing pressure, that is, the piezoresistive effect. Here we have

$$\frac{dR}{R} = \frac{d\rho}{\rho} + \frac{dl}{l} + \frac{dF}{F}$$

where dR/R is the change in resistance, ρ is the specific resistance of the material, l is the length of the material, and F is the cross-sectional area of the material.

Density. A convenient method of density determination is the flexural resonator technique (Kratky et al., 1969). A U-shaped glass tube (the flexural resonator) is filled with a certain volume of the liquid sample and vibrated. The liquid alters the natural frequency of the resonator and the period of oscillation can be correlated with the density of the liquid:

$$\rho = A(T^2 - B)$$

where ρ is the density of the tested liquid, T is the period of oscillation, and A and B are equipment coefficients. A flow-type flexural resonator is also available.

The measurement of other parameters such as agitation speed and power consumption and flowmetering represent the state of the art in chemical engineering and will not be treated here.

Chemical Parameters

pH and Ion-Selective Electrodes. A high degree of sophistication has been reached in pH metering, even under aseptic conditions. The growth of microorganisms on the glass membrane, however, can be troublesome. Besides pH electrodes, there exist a large variety of ion-selective electrodes (Camman, 1977). Only a few of them are applicable to fermentation technology (e.g., CO_2 electrode). For example, the application of the NH_4^+ electrode is very restricted due to the fact that measurements can only be performed under alkaline conditions (pH > 12).

Dissolved Oxygen. The measurement of dissolved oxygen (DO) is very important; it provides information on the amount of oxygen available to the cell. The O_2 is reduced at the cathode (Ag or Pt), and at the anode (Pb) ions are formed:

$$\frac{1}{2}O_2 + H_2O + 2e \longrightarrow 2OH^-$$

$$\text{Metal} \longrightarrow \text{metal} + 2$$

These equations show that a current proportional to the partial pressure of oxygen is generated. Interfering substances are separated by special membranes. The measured current I depends on the number of electrons transferred (n), the Faraday constant (F), the area of the cathode (A), the permeability of the membrane (P_m), the thickness of the membrane (b), and the partial pressure of oxygen (pO_2):

$$I = nF\left(\frac{P_m}{b}\right)pO_2$$

The determination of I is significantly influenced by the characteristics of the membrane. Hydrophilic membranes facilitate the formation of a water film and hydrophobic ones lead to the adherence of gas bubbles. Since sterilization modifies the characteristics of the membrane, recalibration is necessary.

Another technique for determining the dissolved oxygen is the tubing method (Aiba et al., 1973). A carrier gas is flowed through a Teflon tube mounted in the fermentation mash; the gas becomes saturated with oxygen to a degree that corresponds to the O_2 partial pressure. The oxygen content of the carrier gas is then determined in a paramagnetic oxygen analyzer.

Dissolved Carbon Dioxide. Carbon dioxide, one of the endproducts of oxidation, plays an important role in cell metabolism (Mudgett, 1980). Although this fact is well known, few attempts have been made to measure the dissolved CO_2. Carbon dioxide sensors available on the market are simple pH electrodes mounted in a H^+/HCO_3^- buffer and separated from the liquid sample by a $CO_2(HCO_3^-)$-permeable membrane. The HCO_3^- ions penetrating the membrane give rise to pH variations, which are recorded. The Ingold Company (Bühler and Bücher, 1981) markets a sterilizable pCO_2 electrode. The membrane consists of a silicon layer mounted on a nylon net. After sterilization a solution with a known pCO_2 is injected from the outside to calibrate the electrode. As in the determination of the pO_2, the pCO_2 may also be evaluated by the tubing method.

Exhaust Gas Analysis. Besides the gases dissolved in the mash, O_2 and CO_2 are also determined in the exhaust gas, either by mass spectrometry or in specific O_2 and CO_2 analyzers.

Mass spectrometer. In mass spectrometry molecules are ionized in a high vacuum by electron bombardment and then separated according to mass number. Mass spectrometric analysis is carried out rapidly and up to 30 fermenters can be simultaneously monitored on-line (Buckland and Fastert, 1981). Headspace analysis with hydrocarbons may lead to difficulties in interpretation.

Oxygen analyzers. The operation of these instruments is based on the paramagnetic behavior of oxygen, which depends highly on the temperature. The magnetic susceptibility of diamagnetic materials is inversely proportional to the temperature, and that of paramagnetic materials is inversely proportional to the square of the temperature.

A sensor consisting of a zirconium oxide cell was recently brought on the market. Oxygen is ionized at 800°C in this cell, generating a current proportional to the oxygen content.

Carbon dioxide analyzers. Determination of CO_2 in exhaust gas is done by infrared spectrometry or by measuring thermal conductivity. The CO_2-containing gases absorb infrared radiation and this absorbed energy alters the conductivity of an electrical resistor.

For the measurement of thermal conductivity a constant flow of gas passes a heated wire and the amount of heat removed is measured. Carbon dioxide is detected because of its significantly lower thermal conductibility compared to that of N_2, O_2, or CO.

In fermentation technology infrared spectrometry is well established.

Biological Parameters

This group of parameters consists of those aiding in the quantitative determination of metabolites or end-products.

Fluorescence. In biotechnology the phenomenon of fluorescence can be applied in the following fields.

Fluorometry. This technique is based on the determination of NADH or NADPH. These two compounds show absorption at 360 nm and a fluorescence maximum at 460 nm. Since NADH is mainly responsible for H_2 transfer, monitoring its concentration can provide valuable information on the physiological state of the culture. Changes in substrate or oxygen consumption can be detected. As long as oxygen or substrate limitation can be excluded, the NADH detected can be correlated with the biomass formed. Einsele and Puhar (1980) utilized a fluorometric probe to evaluate the mixing behavior of fermenters, K_La, mechanisms of substrate uptake, the redox potential of growing microorganisms, growth rates of cell cultures, and carbon limitations of fed batch cultures.

Fluorescence quenching. Molecular O_2 causes fluorescence quenching. An Austrian company (AVL, Graz) has developed a sensor based on this principle, called the optode. A fluorescence signal is emitted into the culture liquid and reflected; its reduction after reflection is proportional to the oxygen partial pressure in the culture liquid. The probe can undergo sterilization in situ and equilibrates rapidly and oxygen is not consumed during the measuring operation. On the other hand, it has all the problems associated with membrane sensors.

For completeness, laser flow microfluorometry must be mentioned. Microorganisms are marked with various fluorophores and separated in a jet stream. Laser tracing is used to detect cytological characteristics.

ATP. Based on the central position of the adenylates in the metabolic pathways, many attempts have been made (Karl, 1980) to characterize the physiological state of a culture by ATP determination. Usually the bioluminescence technique (McElroy, 1947; Levin et al., 1964) is applied.

As already mentioned, metabolic regulation at the adenylate level is very rapid; up to 2.5×10^6 molecules of ATP per second can be converted to adenosine diphosphate and phosphate. Thomanetz et al. (1982) tried to correlate ATP and activated sludge content. They found 0.2–2.0 mg of ATP per gram of activated sludge dry matter! Although at first sight ATP seems to be a valuable parameter in fermentation control, its potential in control strategy is actually rather limited. For the moment the on-line analysis of ATP is practically impossible.

Enzyme-Bound Sensors. Enzyme-bound transducers offer the most specific probes in process analysis. Since sterilization in situ is not possible, bypass analysis has to be done.

Enzyme electrodes. These sensor systems are generally considered as "transducer-bound enzymes" (Bowers and Carr, 1980). A layer of enzymes is mounted on a semipermeable membrane that gives rise to definite chemical and physical changes of various substrates; these are then converted into electrical signals. The specificity of the sensor is determined mainly by the action of the enzymes and, to a lesser extent, by the membrane. The glucose electrode is a typical probe of this type:

$$\text{Glucose} + O_2 \xrightarrow[]{\text{glucose oxidase}} \text{gluconolactone} \longrightarrow \text{glucuronic acid} + H_2O_2$$

The decrease in the oxygen content is measured and is well correlated with glucose concentration under certain conditions. In recent years about 40 enzyme-bound electrodes have been developed (Mor, 1981).

To demonstrate the scope of possible applications, the cephalosporin electrode will be described (Bender and Blume, 1980). Cephalosporin C is degraded by cephalosporinase, isolated from *Enterobacter cloacae,* and a proportional amount of liberated H^+ ions is determined with a simple pH electrode. Except for the isolation and immobilization of the enzyme, the sensor is quite simple. Measurements can be carried out in 5 min. The probe worked well during several weeks.

Microbial electrodes. These sensors in principal are identical to the enzyme electrodes, except, instead of enzymes, entire microorganisms are fixed on a layer. Fundamental work in the development of these sensors has been done by Karube et al. (1977) and Hikuma et al. (1979).

Kobos and Pyon (1981) have developed an electrode for the determination of nitrilotriacetic acid. It is degraded in four steps to glycerate by decarboxylation and deamination. A proportional amount of ammonia is produced and then detected with an ammonia electrode. The enzymes involved in the various reaction steps were isolated from *Pseudomonas* sp.

Enzyme thermistors. This sensor system works in principal like a calorimeter. The heat liberated during biochemical reactions can be measured very accurately. The high specificity of the system is gained through combinations with various enzymes. The method was worked out by a Swedish group (Danielsson et al., 1981). The analyses of about 35 different substances have been carried out, mainly in clinical applications.

Affinity Sensors. The design of affinity sensors (Schultz and Sims, 1979) is similar to the radioimmunoassay technique. The metabolites are determined by optical methods. Concanavalin A (ConA) has binding sites for carbohydrates (glucose, saccharose, maltose) and is immobilized on a glass fiber-optic carrying the exciting light. The measuring chamber contains FITC (fluorescein-marked dextran) bound to ConA. The presence of sugars displaces the FITC, which results in an increase in fluorescence. Although the method is rather complicated compared to other glucose assays, it is an interesting strategy.

Process-Characterizing Parameters

The potential of single variables to characterize a bioprocess may be very limited. Combinations of single variables will lead to the creation of new parameters of significantly increased physiological relevance.

Respiration. Respiratory activity is currently the most frequently applied parameter for the evaluation of the physiological state of biomass. Respiratory activity is usually characterized by the following terms:

Specific oxygen uptake rate, QO_2 (in mmoles of O_2 per gram per hour)
Specific CO_2 production rate, QCO_2 (in millimoles of CO_2 per gram per hour)
Respiratory quotient ($RQ = QCO_2/QO_2$)

Based on the general equation for microbial growth,

$$\text{C source} + \text{N source} + O_2 \longrightarrow \text{biomass} + \text{(end)products} + \text{heat}$$

biomass was evaluated by material balancing (Zabriskie et al., 1976; Cooney et al., 1977) and modifications thereof (Humphrey, 1973; Nyiri et al., 1974; Hampel et al., 1976, 1977; Wang et al., 1977, 1979; Swartz and Cooney, 1979; Nanba et al., 1981).

A problem that arises in designing a control strategy based on oxygen consumption is the fact that the specific oxygen demand (ml O_2/g biomass) is not a linear function of the growth rate. In our experiments this phenomenon was accounted for by empirical equations.

Another phenomenon observed in our laboratories (Bayer and Meister, 1982) that has to be considered occurs when the substrate feed is controlled by O_2 consumption. If substrate is fed pulsewise, O_2 consumption may increase 1.5-fold due to an accelerated substrate uptake. With *Candida intermedia* specific carbohydrate uptake rates up to 100 mg/g per gram yeast dry matter per minute were detected. The substrate is metabolized after accumulation. In wastewater technology this phenomenon is known as adsorption. The peak oxygen uptake closely following the substrate pulse may lead to elevated biomass estimations. Similar effects were reported by Leegwater et al. (1982) with *Klebsiella aerogenes*.

Calorimetry. According to the balanced equation given above, the amount of heat produced in biochemical reactions is apt to give some insight into a bioprocess. The heat generated in an aerobic fermentation is due mainly to phosphorylation of substrate-bound and respiration-bound reactions and biosynthesis. According to the estimations of Forrest and Walker (1971), 71% of the available ATP-bound energy is consumed in protein synthesis, of which 75% is lost in the form of thermal energy. In the synthesis of lipids 67% of the energy was lost, and in the synthesis of polysaccharides 77% was lost. These facts demonstrate the physiological relevance of the amount of heat produced in a fermentation.

Considering various publications, calorimetry was rarely utilized as a control parameter in bioprocessing. One of the reasons may be that measurements were mainly carried out in bypass and not in situ. Bypass operation leads to nutrient and O_2 limitations, the system is not homogeneous, and wall growth often occurs.

Our own experiments applied the technique of dynamic calorimetry, described by Cooney et al. (1968). The fermenter vessel itself is used as a measuring cell. Temperature control is set off for a certain period of time (e.g., 5 min) and the increase in temperature is recorded. To minimize the influence of environmental factors, the vessel is insulated and the air entering the fermenter is isothermally vapor-saturated. Effects of agitation and heat dissipation are also considered. The application of dynamic calorimetry shows close correlations ($r = .99$) between the heat evolution, O_2 consumption, and biomass productivity of *Candida intermedia* (Bayer and Führer, 1982).

Since heat is derived mainly from phosphorylation of the respiratory chain and synthesis, deviations of the metabolism (e.g., uncoupling of ATP and biomass production) can be deduced from variations of the ratio of heat produced to the amount of O_2 consumed.

Owing to the periodical measurement of heat evolution (the minimum interval is about 7 minutes), calorimetry is not suitable for online control. Mass spectrometry measurements can, however, be carried out every few seconds. Based on these facts, calorimetry will always be assigned a superior control function in a control strategy.

To prove the aptitude of respiration and calorimetry as control parameters, defined amounts of substrate (saccharose or the full medium) were pulsed to the culture under steady state conditions (Table 1). The response times of the two parameters under steady-state conditions and after the substrate pulses were evaluated. Deviations from the normal reaction course can already be detected after 1 min.

Table 1. Effect of Substrate Pulses on the Behavior of *C. intermedia*

Time (min)	Decrease in O_2 in exhaust air (% abs)		Increase in temperature (dynamic calorimetry)	
	Steady state	Pulse	Steady state	Pulse
0	0	0	0	0
1	0.2	0.3	0.18	0.23
2	0.5	0.9	0.35	0.44
3	0.7	1.2	0.52	0.67
4	—	1.5	0.71	0.88
5	—	1.7	0.90	1.13
6	—	1.6	1.08	1.34
7	—	1.5	1.21	1.57

Recent Developments in Sensor Systems

Control of chemical engineering shows a distinct trend toward the use of microelectronics (microsensors). These devices send out a direct electrical signal. An example of this technology is the CHEMFET, where the metallic gate contact has been replaced by a chemical-sensitive coating and a reference electrode. If palladium is used as the coating material, the compound is sensitive to H_2 and NH_3.

The CHEMFET, also known as the enzyme transistor, has been used in studies of enzymatic activities by a Swedish group (Winquist et al., 1980). For example, urea and creatinine were analyzed via the NH_3 liberated by deaminases, and $NAD(P)^+/NAD(P)H$-coupled reactions were analyzed via the amount of H_2 liberated by dehydrogenases.

Another sensor system, consisting of piezoelectric crystals, is currently being studied. Piezoelectric crystals have been used in the trace amount analysis of various gases. The operation of the probe is based on the finding that the frequency of the crystal decreases when certain compounds adsorb onto its surface. The Mosbach group (Chemical Center, Lund, Sweden, now the Federal Technical University in Zurich) investigated the adsorption of enzymes as active layers.

Recently Mosbach et al. (1983) also reported on another sensor system, ellipsometry. The principle of this method is based on measuring changes of the polarization angle when polarized light is reflected at a surface. These changes are a function of the properties of the surface, for example, the presence of a layer of biomolecules.

The trend in microtechnique has led to the development of complete sensor systems, like the microgas chromatograph, made by Microsensor Technology of Fremont, California. Data on the carrier gas and sample channels, valves, and thermal conductivity are integrated on a $7.5 \times 7.5\ cm^2$ chip; the results of up to 370 samples may be stored.

STATUS, TRENDS, AND DEVELOPMENTS IN PROCESS CONTROL

Conventional (Analog) Control

Biotechnologists have gained their experience in process control from chemical engineering. The main control loops of a standard fermentation are temperature, pH, agitation, volume, and level control. These signals are converted by single loop operation, using different transfer elements for control, such as P (proportional), PI (proportional integral), and PID (proportional integral differential) algorithms and delay elements. Single-loop structures offer the advantage that the process probably will not fail completely upon failure of a single control unit.

Computer-Aided Process Control

The application of computers offers a new area in the field of process control. The bioprocess has many structural elements that operate highly interactively. Classical process control design does not have the potential to fully meet the special demands of the bioprocess. The rapid evolution of computer technology is able to fulfill the requirements of the biotechnologist almost perfectly. Nowadays cheap micro- and minicomputers with appropriate peripheral equipment are available which satisfy the demands of bioprocess control. Depending on the degree of process knowledge, the computer is an aid in the acquisition and statistical treatment of data, the graphical and numerical display of results, and in process control through modeling and process optimization.

The evolution of bioprocess control closely follows that of chemical engineering. In the chemical industry today a high degree of computerization has been attained. By the appropriate distribution of digital controls, production units of different locations may work together as a single unit. Depending on the course of production, process control is carried out at different levels and is hierarchically structured. Considering the recent developments in this field, the term *process management* should be used instead of *process control.* Computerized control systems of thousands of loops represent the state of the art in control engineering. From a purely control engineering standpoint, the treatment of chemical processes is much easier than that of bioprocesses, because chemical processes exhibit less interactivity. This facilitates monitoring and modeling, which is the main reason for the advanced computerization of chemical engineering compared to that of biotechnology.

Concepts of Computer-Aided Fermentations

The principles of a computer-coupled fermenter are shown in Figure 1. The systems elements will be treated in the order of signal flow.

The fermenter sends out analog signals which are transferred to the digital computer via interfaces. The computer aspects of data management (data reduction, data storage, graphical display) and process monitoring are handled through set points determined by the software.

Before a process control system can be determined, all the tasks required must be thoroughly discussed and defined. In case only data acquisition is to be done, a single computer with the capacity to sample a given number of probes in an appropriate period of time is sufficient. If monitoring is required, the possibility of computer failure must be taken into account to avoid the breakdown of the entire system; hierarchically structured software and hardware will largely prevent failures. Since nowadays microcomputers are available for relatively low prices, it is economically possible to have one monitor one or two fermenters. Microcomputers perform local control tasks and send the acquired data to a master computer for further treatment. Upon failure of one microcomputer, only that part of the plant will have to be shut down. In this way software design and modifications are facilitated and operations are simplified. The following section discusses the various elements of a process control system.

The Computer

Besides controlling all peripheral devices, the computer transforms various raw data into process-relevant variables and is able to "make decisions" about the fermentation in progress according to logical operations (AND, NOT, OR, etc.). Presently the demands of the biotechnologist for computer hardware are rather low due to the shortage of sensors and insufficient knowledge about bioprocesses. Therefore, in the current literature the application of rather simple personal computers for process control is frequently

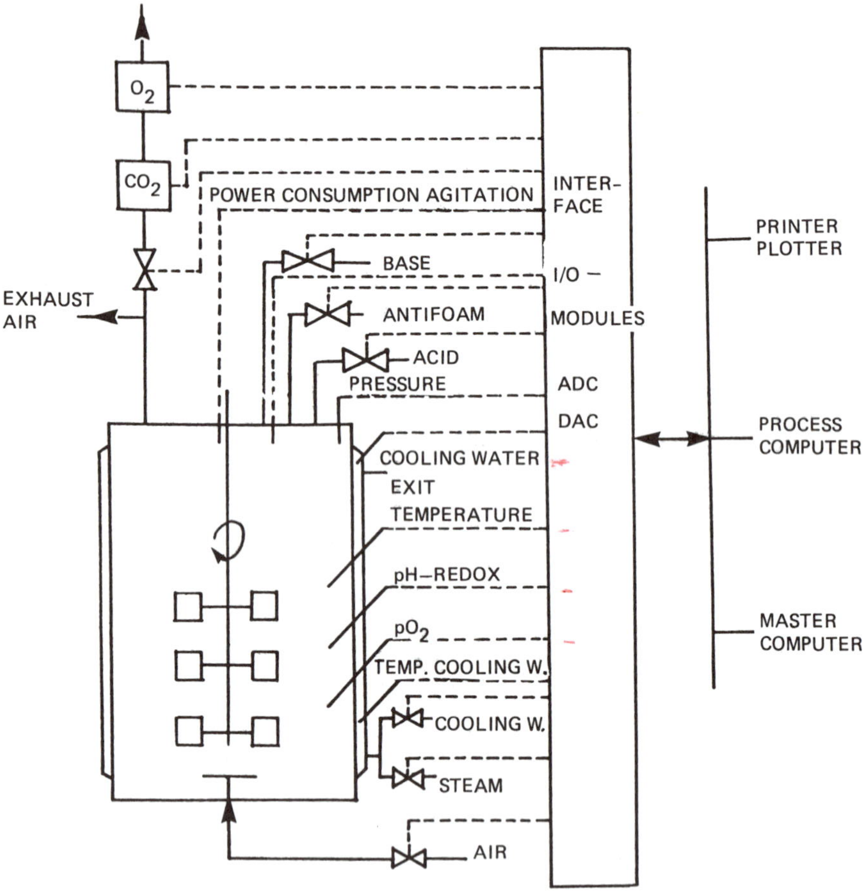

Fig. 1. Principles of a computer-coupled fermenter.

described. According to our experience these computers often do not entirely meet the conditions of an industrial process control system (e.g., reautostart, easily programmable input/output hardware, etc.). Only a few manufacturers are able to offer complete systems, and the setup available is mainly a question of price.

The ideal setup for a process control system consists of one or more systems specifically designed for data acquisition and monitoring and a master computer for mathematical and statistical treatment.

The following criteria must be considered in the selection of a process computer:

- Easy programming in higher languages
- Availability of various input–output cards and simple programming
- Multitasking (i.e., the ability to run several operations independently of each other in the same program)
- Autostart and insensitivity to noise potentials
- A 16-bit central processing unit

Given the demands of bioprocess control, our laboratory chose a MACSYM (Analog Devices).

Interfaces

An interface provides the coupling between the digital computer and the real-time process. This includes, for example, analog-to-digital conversion (ADC), synchronization of asynchronous operating devices, data storage, control of data transfer, transfer of control commands, and hardware adaptation. Generally a distinction is made between parallel or serial and synchronous or asynchronous data transfer.

In independently working process control systems, the IEC-bus (IEEE 488) is standardly used. Data transfer is executed asynchronously and in parallel. Many measuring devices are already equipped with an IEC-bus output and can be directly integrated into the process control system. The quality of an interface is also determined by its signal resolution. An 8-bit ADC has a resolution of 2^{-8} ($=4\times10^{-3}$), and the 12-bit ADC a resolution of 2^{-12} ($=2.4\times10^{-4}$). With the 12-bit ADC, the accuracy of the measuring instrument plays a more decisive role in the result than the resolution of the ADC. Interfaces are usually equipped with a single ADC of high resolution, and the signals of various measuring points are multiplexed. Semiconductor multiplexers are generally preferred.

From our own experience, more care has to be taken in the selection of the interfaces than in that of the computer itself when the interfaces are not provided by the computer manufacturer. Small companies are usually not in a position to keep all ICs in stock that have already been removed from the market.

Interface hardware performance is also a decisive factor in the flexibility of a control system; nonprofessionals should be able to carry out modifications of the input–output configuration.

The remaining peripheral equipment of the computer, such as printers, plotters, and memory, consists of standard devices, which are marketed by various companies.

Computer Tasks

Data Management

The importance of data acquisition is emphasized by the fact that progress in bioprocessing is to a large extent determined by the accumulation of process knowledge and application of sophisticated process control.

The analog signals collected have to be digitized (ADC) and subsequently transformed into corresponding chemical or physical units, usually by statistical methods. In cases where the correlation is not linear, polynomials may be set up:

$$M = f(u) = a_0 + a_1 u + a_2 u^2 + . . . + a_n u^n$$

Errors are minimized by the least-squares method and the coefficients stated as optimum can be evaluated.

In measurement value treatment, systematic errors, such as arise from hysteresis or stochastics, may occur. Their elimination is known as digital filtering. A simple method was described by Bernard et al. (1980) in which the measured values are averaged and the peak values ignored. A more sophisticated method involves the Kalman filter. The Kalman filter is actually a dynamic model; a few parameters are measured and the others are estimated by means of the model. Svercek et al. (1974) used the Kalman filter technique to simulate continuous cultures. Another group (Bellgardt et al., 1984) used the same method to evaluate the biomass formed by *S. cerevisiae* in fed batch culture. In the past application of the Kalman filter technique has often led to problems because of the shortage of parameters needed to characterize the physiological state. All parameters calculated in the model were derived solely from respiration, which resulted in many uncertainties of the estimated parameters. Besides the respiration, Bellgardt and co-workers (1984) analyzed the amount of ethanol produced and glucose consumed and were thus able to significantly increase the certainty of the model.

Another method for deriving a mathematical function from a series of measured values is the application of spline algorithms (Späth, 1978). An interpolation polynomial is set up from the measured values; with increasing numbers of measured values, the polynomial will oscillate significantly. The solution of this problem is to set up lower-degree polynomials for certain areas of the abscissa, resulting in a polygon bond with fewer oscillations but with discontinuities, known as spline functions.

Another problem of data acquisition is the enormous amount of data resulting from the computer's high scanning rate; data reduction is essential. Usually values that do not deviate from the preceding one are stored in long intervals. When significant variations arise, data storage is amplified.

Process Control

Sequencing. The various unit operations in upstream and downstream processing follow a certain scheme that is easily monitored by sequence control units. In case the fermentation plant has already been computerized, these operations will naturally be executed by the computer; if not, small microprocessor-based control units on the market in the last few years can be used. They are free programmable with a minimum of 12 digits of input–output and feature the logical operators AND and OR. They are battery buffered and the program will not be lost in the case of current failures. The price of such a unit is from $450 upwards. Their application in fermentation control is rather limited, since they cannot execute arithmetic operations.

Set Point Control. In set point control (SPC) analog control has been retained in its function to a great extent; the computer only submits the set points, which were fixed by the software, to each control unit. Monitoring is carried out by the controller itself. Owing to dual hardware installation, the system is expensive, but it has the advantage that, in the case of computer failure, the fermentation is controlled by the single controllers. On the other hand, the operator is very limited in influencing the mode of control. Set point control is preferred in starting computer control, since the software is rather simple.

Direct Digital Control. In direct digital control (DDC) signals generated by the computer and its peripheral devices are directly used to control various actors according to the software. In contrast to set point control, only single hardware installation is necessary. The systems are usually cheaper than conventional (relay-based) ones. The break-even point is about 30 loops (Smith, 1981).

Direct digital controllers work discontinuously. The data are collected periodically and signal output is also periodic. Because of the high frequency of these operations, digital control is quasi continuous.

As already mentioned, the hierarchical structure facilitates software design and the security of a control system. Local tasks are executed by single microcomputers. As in conventional control, in the case of failures only parts of the plant will be shut down. Direct digital control offers the possibilities of applying various control strategies, like P, PI, and PID, by software, independent of local controllers.

Finally, it should be emphasized that the layout of a computer-based control system is much easier than conventional ones, because the detailed design is defined by the software. However, the savings gained by the simplified layout are usually offset by the expenses for the software.

Software

Software provides the intelligent connection between man and the machine. It enables the solution of specific problems in process control. About 20 years ago knowledge of computer hardware was much more essential than it is today. Owing to the availability of higher programming languages and the tremendous evolution of hardware, machine peculiarities and memory capacity are only second in importance to software development. Hardware is getting more powerful and decreasing in price and the integration density of ICs is doubling every 1.5 years (Moor's law), resulting in easier programming and fewer restrictions in software design through limited hardware functions.

The software support for the control of bioprocesses has greatly increased in recent years. Software design should consider ease of use and flexibility in programming language. Several languages are tailored to process control, like C and PEARL, but they are not very commonly used in bioprocess control. Although it has its disadvantages, BASIC is more apt to be used in bioprocess control because of its ample diffusion that results from its availability. In bioprocess control program modifications and adaptations are often necessary, and the user should be able to carry them out with BASIC programs without further problems.

Software should be structured and modularly designed and modern hardware configurations must meet the user's demands. In practice, the software is often obscure so as to avoid the need for a copyright. Such programs naturally grow with each modification, with additions rather than alterations being made for new program packages. Eventually such programs become susceptible to failure.

The attempt to standardize software design in recent years has developed into a new discipline, called software engineering. General standards of software development have been established. Creativity, an absolute necessity in software design, should fit within a certain framework, without restricting the quality of the software. Software development is similar to modeling. The first step is problem analysis. In systems analysis the demands are specified and the suitability of the hardware tested; then the layout of the system, comprising the mode of data processing, is set up. The next step is designing the layout of the components. During the implementation period, programming is carried out and tested and the user introduced. The following gives some examples of software concepts applied to biotechnology.

Meiners (1982) adapted the HIPO (Hierarchal Input Process Output) System, originally developed by IBM, to control about 20 fermenters. He emphasized the need of hierarchical and functional software structures. This need should be evident from the fact that process control consists of two different elements: real-time processing and data treatment, often executed off-line. The principal differences between these two tasks are also considered in system configuration. The trend in process control is to install specific functional systems for each task.

The author's lab utilizes in part a real-time processing system (MACSYM 350) connected to a standard computer system (e.g., PDP 11) for data processing. Having successfully achieved the control of two and three laboratory fermenters, we are now planning control of a pilot plant, including downstream processing. The software support system for the above-mentioned configuration was provided by the Austrian steel company Voest Alpine. They have developed a software package, called CORES, which can be easily adapted to bioprocess control. Considering the price of microcomputers, the hardware configuration of Meiners (1982) could also be easily adapted to a hierarchical system.

Besides software simplifications, hierarchical structures are advantageous in the startup of the system. Although HIPO provides many benefits in software development, reticular structures, loops, and parallel processes are difficult to design in this system. Jeffris et al. (1976) describes a configuration consisting of a process computer link up to a time-sharing computer. The pilot computing tasks, namely, data processing, operator services, and communications, could be fulfilled by file structuring. Owing to its file structuring methodology, the system may be easily expanded to several process computers. This program structure has been applied by Siebert and Hustede (1982) to control a citric acid plant, which will be described in more detail later on.

Modeling and Simulation

The goal of modeling is process simulation and therefore optimization on a theoretical basis. In computer-based process control models are the vehicles ("software") of the control strategies. Process control is inherently dependent on the model, taking into account the actual data acquired. Optimal control algorithms may be integrated, eventually leading to on-line optimization. A comprehensive treatment of modeling and simulation have been published by Roels and Kossen (1978) and Blanch and Dunn (1974).

The problems of bioprocess modeling are mainly centered on the inherent characteristics of bioprocesses, that is, the physiological state, the lack of sensors, and the process dynamics. The trend in modeling is clearly toward structured models. Increased knowledge in bioprocessing will thus facilitate progress in modeling in this field.

Optimization

Process optimization may be carried out on a theoretical basis by the application of models. Muzychenko et al. (1974) tried to model continuous cultures by evaluating the process parameters from batch cultures: Growth was described by Monod kinetics and the transients were calculated by Pontryagin's maximum principle. The model demonstrated the inapplicability of Monod kinetics to specific growth conditions and lacks experimental verification.

Successful optimization through modeling requires experimental verification, acquired through the application of iterative methods. The following optimization steps have been evaluated on the basis of experimental data and verified. Iterative methods help finding the direction and magnitude of each optimization step. A rather general strategy is given by the following equation:

$$x^{i+1} = x^{i} + h^{i}d^{i}$$

where x^{i+1} is the value of the proceeding step, h^i is a constant, and d^i is a vector assigning the direction of optimization.

Many of these optimization methods were published during World War II. Since their application requires many arithmetical calculations, these methods have gained in importance with the evolution of digital computers. A few examples of optimization strategies in fermentation technology follow.

A Hungarian group (Nyeste et al., 1981; Veres et al., 1981) minimized (optimized) the doubling time of *Hansenula anomala* by the application of a modified Simplex method to half the original value. Unden and Heden (1973) tried to optimize the growth of *Methylomonas methanolica* via pH and temperature, using Powell's method (Powell, 1964) combined with that of Hooke and Jeeves (1961). A set of directing vectors was used to search for new environmental conditions. Hooke and Jeeves used the concept of prefixed searching. The optimization procedure was not successful: No sensors were available to detect growth inhibition or the microorganisms did not exhibit significant response to environmental changes.

The optimization of purely chemical processes, such as the maximization of the oxygen transfer rate via dynamic k_La measurements, has been more successful (Corrieu et al., 1976; Nyeste et al., 1979). Another method frequently applied in the chemical industry is the method of steepest ascent (Box and Wilson 1951). Schröder and Weide (1974) maximized the growth rate of *Candida guilliermondii* by optimizing nutrient composition. Constantinides et al. (1970) applied Pontryagin's maximum principle to optimize penicillin production. By working out a temperature profile, they attained a 15% increase in yield. As these authors emphasized, elucidation of the optimal conditions for a single parameter is not sufficient to satisfy the demands of an optimization program. Increased knowledge of the kinetics and physiological phenomena is absolutely necessary for further progress in this field.

Finally, a valuable method in multifactorial experimental design should be mentioned. Biotechnologists are often faced with problems of multifactorial optimization, as, for example, in media composition. Nutrient media may consist of up to 60 components, making multifactorial optimization impossible. Plackett and Burman (1946) have published a method to eliminate variables of lesser relevance to arrive at a set of four to six variables.

Practical Realization of Computer-Aided Process Control

Computer control in citric acid production as described by Siebert and Hustede (1982) was chosen here as a case study for various reasons. The fundamental biochemical pathways of the process are generally understood. Starting from saccharose or glucose, pyruvate is formed via glycolysis and the pentose phosphate cycle. The pathway then proceeds to acetyl coenzyme A and oxaloacetate, which are synthesized to citric acid. The mechanism of citric acid secretion cannot be fully explained yet. Röhr and Kubicek (1981) consider the accumulation and release of citrate to be stimulated by a specific physiological state of the mycelium which is due to environmental conditions.

In the past citric acid production was mostly controlled empirically. To gain insight into the process and analyze its kinetics, the amount of instrumentation in production fermenters was increased. The following data were acquired on-line:

Exhaust gas analysis (O_2, CO_2) variables
Energy consumption (electrical power, cooling water) variables
Process variables (temperature, pH, pO_2, redox reactions)
Aeration (flow rate, pressure, temperature) variables

Data acquisition was carried out with the aid of a microcomputer (HP 9825A). According to on-line and off-line analyses, the following equations of citric acid production were obtained:

1. $C_{12}H_{22}O_{11} + H_2O \longrightarrow C_6H_{12}O_6 + C_6H_{12}O_6$

   saccharose → glucose + fructose

2. $C_6H_{12}O_6 + \frac{1}{2} O_2 \longrightarrow C_6H_{12}O_7$

   glucose → gluconic acid

3. $C_6H_{12}O_6 + 6O_2 \longrightarrow 6CO_2 + 6H_2O$

glucose, fructose

4. $C_6H_{12}O_6 + NH_4^+ + 12(A) \longrightarrow C_6H_{12}O_4N(A)_{12} + 2H_2O$

glucose, fructose ash mycelium

5. $C_6H_{12}O_6 + 1.5\ O_2 + H_2O \longrightarrow C_6H_8O_7 + 6CO_2$

fructose citric acid

6. $6C_6H_{12}O_7 + 10.5\ O_2 \longrightarrow 5C_6H_8O_7 + 6CO_2$

gluconic acid citric acid

From these equations carbohydrate consumption and citrate production were estimated.

On-line data acquisition is a significant tool in the control of citric acid production. Measurement of respiration is a valuable parameter for estimating biochemical activities during fermentation. Kinetic models detect deviations from the desired yield. In this manner the entire citric acid plant was computerized.

Data acquisition and monitoring are carried out by a HP 9825 A process computer coupled to a HP 9845 S computer, which is mainly used for the mathematical treatment of the collected data. Both computers are programmed in BASIC. Maximum flexibility and ease of operation of the hardware require adequate software, provided by the file-oriented program structure developed by Jeffris (1977). Instrument specification, calibration, and so forth, are stored in data files that are accessible for each program. Special communication programs simplify modifications and provide information on the fermentation in progress.

The application of on-line computer control in citric acid production has led to a significant enhancement in yield and improved reproducibility. The work of Siebert and Hustede (1982) has proved that, once the fundamentals of a process are understood, computer-aided control is a valuable tool in optimization.

REFERENCES

Aiba, S., Humphrey, A. E., and Millis, N. F. (eds.) (1973). *Biochemical Engineering*, Academic, New York.

Bayer, K. and Führer, F. (1982). Computer coupled calorimetry in fermentation. *Process Biochem. 17*: 42.

Bayer, K. and Meister, G. (1982). Hyperkinetic nutrient uptake by *C. intermedia*. *Eur. J. Appl. Microbiol. Biotechnol. 15*: 36–40.

Bellgardt, K. H., Meyer, H. D., Kuhlmann, W., and Thoma, M. (1984). On-line estimation of biomass and fermentation parameters by a Kalman filter during a cultivation of *Saccharomyces cerevisiae.* Third International Congress on Biotechnology, Munic, September 1984.

Bender, R. and Blume, G. (1980). *Cephalosporinbestimmung mittels einer Enzymelktrode II. Rotenburger Symposium 1980.* (R. M. Lafferty, ed.), Springer-Verlag, Vienna.

Bernard, A., Cordonnier, M., and Lebeault, J. M. (1980). An approach to on-line optimization of biomass production in continuous processes. In *Advances in Biotechnology* (M. Mou-Young, C. W. Robinson, and C. Vezina, eds.), Pergamon, Toronto, p. 407.

Blanch, H. W. and Dunn, I. J. (1974). Modelling and simulation in biochemical engineering. *Adv. Biochem. Eng. 3*:127.

Bowers, L. D. and Carr, P. W. (1980). Immobilized enzymes in analytical chemistry. *Adv. Biochem. Eng. 15*:89.

Box, G. E. P. and Wilson, K. B. (1951). On the experimental attainment of optimum conditions. *J. R. Stat. Soc. 13*:1–38.

Buckland, R. C. and Fastert, H. (1981). Analysis of fermentation exhaust gas using a mass spectrometer. Symposium on Computer Application in Fermentation Technology, Manchester.

Bühler, H. and Bücher, R. (1981). The use of pH, PO_2, PCO_2-electrodes in fermentation. Symposium on Computer Application in Fermentation Technology, Manchester.

Cammann, K. (1979). *Das Arbeiten mit ionenselektiven Elektroden,* Springer-Verlag, Berlin.

Constantinides, A., Spencer, J. L., and Gaden, Jr., E. L. (1970). Optimization of batch fermentation processes. I. Development of mathematical models for batch penicillin fermentations. II. Optimum temperature profiles for batch penicillin fermentations. *Biotechnol. Bioeng. 12*:803, 1081.

Cooney, C. L., Wang, D. I. C., and Mateles, R. I. (1968). Measurement of heat evolution and correlation with oxygen consumption during microbial growth. *Biotechnol. Bioeng. 11*:269.

Cooney, C. L., Wang, H. Y., and Wang, D. I. C. (1977). Computer aided material balancing for prediction of fermentation parameters. *Biotechnol. Bioeng. 19*:55.

Corrieu, G., Lalande, M., Peringer, P., Jarrot, C., and Almanza, R. (1976). Détérmination du coéfficient de transfert d'oxygène dans un fermenteur à partir du bilan gazeux d'une culture microbienne. *Rev. Ferment. Ind. Aliment. 30*:125–131.

Danielsson, B., Mattiasson, B., and Mosbach, K. (1981). Enzyme thermistor devices and their analytical applications. *App. Biochem. Bioeng. 3*:97–143.

Einsele, A. and Puhar, E. (1980). On-line Erfassung von Fluoreszenz and Kohlendioxidpartialdruck in Bioreaktoren. *Acta Biotechnol.*

Forrest, W. W. and Walker, D. J. (1971). The generation and utilization of energy during growth. In *Advances in Microbial Physiology* (Rose and Wilkinson, eds.), Academic, London.

Hampel, W., Wöhrer, W., Bach, H. P., and Röhr, M. (1976). Automatic Anaylsis of Fermentation Parameters. Fifth International Fermentation Symposium, Berlin.

Hampel, W., Bach, H. P., and Röhr, M. (1977). Low cost data acquisition and analysis with on-line desk calculators. In *GBF Workshop Computer Application in Fermentation Technology* (R. P. Jeffris III, ed.), Verlag Chemie, Wernheim.

Hikuma, M., Suzuki, H., Yasuda, T., Karube, I., and Suzuki, S. (1979). Amperometric estimation of BOD by using living immobilized yeasts. *Eur. J. Appl. Microb. Biotechnol.* *8*:289–297.

Hooke, R. and Jeeves, T. A. (1961). Direct search solution of numerical and statistical problems. *J. Assoc. Comput. Mach.* *8*:212–29.

Humphrey, A. E. (1973). Rationale for and principles of computer coupled fermentation systems. The First European Conference on Computer Process Control in Fermentation, Dijon.

Jeffris, R. P. (1977). Software and file structures for computer coupled pilot fermentation plants. In: Workshop Computer Application in Fermentation Technology (R. P. Jeffris, ed.), Verlag Chemie, Weinheim, p. 21.

Jeffris, R. P., Winter, H., and Vogelmann, H. (1976). Digital filtering for automatic analysis of cell density and productivity. In *Workshop Computer Application in Fermentation Technology* (R. P. Jeffris III, ed.), Verlag Chemie, Wernheim.

Karl, D. M. (1980). Cellular nucleotide measurements and applications in microbial ecology. *Microb. Rev.* *44*:739–796.

Karube, I., Matsunaga, T., Mitsuda, S., and Suzuki, S. (1977). Microbial electrode BOD sensors. *Biotechnol. Bioeng.* *19*: 1535–1547.

Kobos, R. K. and Pyon, H. Y. (1981). Application of microbial cells as multistep catalysts in potentiometric biosensing electrodes. *Biotechnol. Bioeng.* *23*:627–633.

Kratky, O., Leopold, H., and Stabinger, H. (1969). Dichtemessung an Flüssigkeiten und Gasen auf 10^{-6} g/cm^3 bei 0,6 cm^3 Präparatvolumen. *Z. Angew. Phys.* *4*:273.

Leegwater, M. P. M., Neijssel, O. M., and Tempest, D. W. (1982). Aspects of microbial physiology in relation to process control. *J. Chem. Technol. Biotechnol.* *32*:92–99.

Levin, G. V., Clendenning, J. R., Chapelle, E. W., Heim, A. H., and Rocek, E. (1964). A rapid method for detection of microorganisms by ATP assay. *Bioscience* *14*:37–38.

McElroy, W. D. (1947). The energy source for bioluminescence in an isolated system. *Proc. Nat. Acad. Sci. U.S.A. 33*:342–345.

Forrest, W. W. and Walker, D. J. (1971). The generation and utilization of energy during growth. In *Advances in Microbial Physiology* (Rose and Wilkinson, eds.), Academic, London.

Malek, I. (1976). Physiological state of continuously grown microbial cultures. In *Continuous Culture*, Vol. 6 (A. C. R. Dean, D. C. Ellwood, C. G. T. Evans, and J. Melling, eds.), Ellis Horwood, Chichester, p. 23.

Meiners, M. (1982). Data structures in the analysis of biochemical processes. *Comput. Chem. Eng. 6*:59.

Mor, J. R. (1981). A review of instrumental analysis in fermentation technology. Symposium on Computer Application in Fermentation Technology, Manchester.

Mosbach, K., Mandenius, C. F., and Danielsson, B. (1983). New biosensor devices. *Proc. Biotechnol. 83*.

Mudgett, R. E. (1980). Controlled gas environments in industrial fermentations. *Enzyme Microb. Technol. 2*:273.

Muzychenko, L. A., Mascheva, L. A., and Yaklovelva, G. V. (1974). Algorithm for optimal control of microbiological synthesis. *Biotechnol. Bioeng. Symp. 4*:629–645.

Nanba, A., Hirota, F., and Nagai, S. (1981). Microcomputer-coupled baker's yeast production. *J. Ferment. Technol. 59*:383–389.

Nyeste, L., Veres, A., Szigeti, L., Kurucz, I., Pungor, E., and Hollo, J. (1979). A mini-computer controlled fermentation system. *Abh. Akad. Wiss. DDR Abt. Math. Naturwiss. Technol. 3N*:347–358.

Nyeste, L., Szigeti, L., Veres, A., Pungor, E., Kurucz, I., and Hollo, J. (1981). Automated fermentation equipment. II. Computer–fermenter system. *Biotechnol. Bioeng. 23*:405–417.

Nyiri, K. L., Jefferis, R. P., and Humphrey, A. E. (1974). Application of computers to the analysis and control of microbiological processes. *Biotechnol. Bioeng. Symp. 4*:613–628.

Nyiri, K. L., Toth, G. M., Krishnaswami, C. S., and Parmenter, D. V. (1976). Assessment of on-line computer operations with fermenters. Fifth International Fermentation Symposium, Berlin.

Plackett, R. L. and Burman, J. P. (1946). The design of multifactorial experiments. *Biometrika 33*:305.

Powell, M. J. D. (1964). An efficient method of finding the minimum of a function of several variables without calculation derivatives. *Comput. J. 7*:155.

Roels, J. A. and Kossen, N. W. F. (1978). On the modelling of microbial metabolism. In *Progress in Industrial Microbiology*, (M. J. Bull, ed.), Elsevier, Amsterdam, p. 95.

Röhr, M. and Kubicek, C. P. (1981). Regulatory aspects of citric acid fermentation by *Aspergillus niger*. *Process Biochem.* *16*:34.

Schröder, K. D. and Weide, H. (1974). Optimization of growth conditions for yeasts. *Biotechnol. Bioeng. Symp.* *4*:713–720.

Schultz, J. S. and Sims, G. (1979). Affinity sensors for individual metabolites. *Biotechnol. Bioeng. Symp.* *9*:65–71.

Siebert, D. and Hustede, H. (1982). Citronensäure-Fermentation—Biotechnologische Probleme und Möglichkeiten der Rechnersteuerung. *Chem. Ing. Techn.* *54*:659.

Smith, R. J. (1981). Computers for fermentation. What else can we do? Symposium on Computer Application in Fermentation Technology, Manchester.

Späth, H. (1978). *Spline-Algorithmen zur Konstruktion glatter Kurven und Flächen*, R. Oldenbourg Verlag, Munichen.

Svercek, W. Y., Elliott, R. F., and Zajic, J. E. (1974). The extended Kalman filter applied to a continuous culture model. *Biotechnol. Bioeng.* *16*:827–846.

Swartz, J. R. and Cooney, Ch. L. (1979). Indirect fermentation measurements as a basis for control. *Biotechnol. Bioeng. Symposium* Nr. 9, p. 95.

Thomanetz, E., Sperandio, A., and Bardtke, D. (1982). Ist ATP ein geeigneter Biomasseparameter für belebte Schlämme? *Gas Wasserfach Wasser Abwasser* *123*:96, 147.

Unden, G. A. and Heden, C. G. (1973). An approach to on-line continuous culture optimization. The First European Conference on Computer Process Control in Fermentation, Dijon.

Veres, A., Nyeste, I., Kurucz, L., Kirchknopf, L., Szigeti, L., and Hollo, J. (1981). Automated fermentation equipment. I. Program-controlled fermenter. *Biotechnol. Bioeng.* *23*:391–404.

Wang, H. Y., Cooney, C. L., and Wang, D. I. C. (1977). Computer-aided baker's yeast fermentations. *Biotechnol. Bioeng.* *19*:69–86.

Wang, H. Y., Cooney, Ch. L., and Wang, D. I. C. (1979). On-line gas analysis for material balances and control. *Biotechnol. Bioeng. Symposium* Nr. 9, p. 13.

Winquist, F., Danielsson, B., Lundtröm, I., and Mosbach, K. (1980). Über die Verwendung von Wasserstoff- und Ammoniak-empfindlichen Pd-MOS-Einheiten in der biochemischen Analyse. II. In *Rotenburger Symposium*, (R. M. Lafferty, ed.), Springer-Verlag, Vienna.

Zabriskie, D. W., Armiger, W. B., and Humphrey, A. E. (1976). Applications of computer to the indirect measurement of biomass concentration and growth rate by component balancing. In *Workshop on Computer Application in Fermentation Technology*, (R. P. Jeffris III, ed.), Verlag Chemie, Wernheim, p. 59.

Zähner, M. (1979). What are secondary metabolites? *Folia Microbiol.* *24*:435–443.

9

Animal Cell Culture Methods

HERMANN W. D. KATINGER / University of Agriculture, Vienna, Austria

RUDOLF F. BLIEM / Cambridge Life Sciences, Cambridge, England

INTRODUCTION

Within a decade animal cell culture has evolved from a peripheral research discipline, in which most of the activity was directed toward its development as a basic research tool and in which general commercial applications were still largely a matter of adventurous speculation, to an area of industrial development attracting multimillion dollar investments.

Currently the major focus of attention is on the direct production of a wide variety of protein-based cellular substances useful as human therapeutics (Katinger and Bliem, 1983, Griffiths, 1985).

Parallel developments in recombinant DNA technology have considerably foreshortened the industrial application of animal cells (Bebbington, Hentschel, 1985). Although the industrial feasibility of recombinant DNA technology is still limited to the expression and elevated synthesis of a given protein in a foreign cell, it is realistic to speculate on the recombination of whole metabolic chains of nonproteinaceous substances.

Animal vaccines were the first industrial cell culture products; foot-and-mouth disease virus (FMDV) vaccine was routinely produced on 1000-liter levels in baby hamster kidney cells by the beginning of the 1970s. Although animal cell technology has found its first significant commercial application in the production of pharmaceuticals, other cell culture applications are rapidly approaching commercial usefulness, particularly for the agricultural and food industries. Cell culture techniques will provide the materials for diagnostic kits (Gatz et al., 1983) and for the basis for new test systems (Borenfreund et al., 1983; Ekwell, 1983), and above all it will revolutionize animal breeding (Mapletoft, 1984; Brackett et al., 1983).

This brief introduction to the methods of animal cell culture is intended to give some idea of the potential usefulness of this technology and to introduce the reader to some methodological principles, required skills, materials, and equipment.

Basic terms have been defined within their practical context and, although some typical methods are briefly described, the reader is referred to manuals for details of protocols and general theoretical aspects. In keeping with the orientation of this book, particular attention has been paid to technological aspects, highlighting some typical problem areas and current issues and trends. It is hoped that this chapter will thus not only provide a concept of what cell culture means in practice but also illustrate why it has received so much attention and investment in recent years.

METHODS AND TERMINOLOGY

Introduction

Animal cells are typically 10–50 μm in size, highly compartmentalized, and surrounded by only a fragile membrane. Within the three-dimensional body tissue the cells do not exist as independent units but, rather, rely for their functional activities on their environment, that is, both on cell-to-cell contact and on molecules supplied systemically. Taken from this complex habitat and placed in the relatively crude environment of the culture, the cells can hardly be expected to perform with the same efficiency and specificity as in the body. However, our knowledge in this field is increasing at an enormous pace, resulting in constant improvements in culture conditions (Jakoby and Pastan, 1979; Kuchler, 1977; Freshney, 1984).

In Vitro Growth Characteristics

Animal cells fall broadly into two growth types: those that require solid supports for growth and those that grow freely in suspension. Both types, however, follow the same well-known growth pattern observed with microbial cultures: an initial lag phase followed by a logarithmic growth phase, a stationary phase, and a death phase. The lag phase may last days or even weeks. Having obtained the maximum growth rate in suitable growth medium, the cells may divide with a culture doubling time of 12–48 hr, varying between cell types and culture conditions. The cells can be maintained in the stationary phase for months, given suitable environmental conditions. Critical culture parameters are pH, ionic strength, O_2 and nutrient supply, and temperature. The maintenance energy of a stationary cell is, by definition, lower than the energy required for growth, so that the medium, particularly the serum requirements are reduced during this phase and product formation thus becomes more economic (Jakoby and Pastan, 1979; Kuchler, 1977; Freshney, 1984).

Initiation of a Cell Culture

The term *animal cell cultures* will, for practical purposes, be used to denote both human and animal cell cultures. Other terms follow the definitions proposed by the American Tissue Culture Association (Schaeffer, 1984).

The range of cell types which can be satisfactorily isolated from animal tissues or fluids and cultured over a number of generations is continually increasing. In principle, the procedure for the initiation of a cell culture follows the flow diagram in Figure 1.

The source material for cell cultures has traditionally been explanted tissue. Cells derived from tumor or embryonic tissue usually exhibit better growth characteristics than those derived from nontumorous adult tissue. However, research into the identification and isolation of cell growth factors is continually reducing such source limitations; for example, with the identification of interleukins, it has recently become possible to maintain long-term cultures of normal lymphocytes (Paul et al., 1981).

A prerequisite for any successful cultivation is a sound knowledge and skill in aseptic handling techniques. This principle must already be applied in the manipulation of the original source material, be it tissue or fluid. Microbial contamination is more often a problem with human tissues, as these are often only available after having passed through the histology or pathology laboratories. Also, the tissue may be contaminated during the operation itself, as is the case with urinary or colon samples. If there is any indication that the tissue may be heavily contaminated, it is best discarded.

The tissue is transported to the culture laboratory in nutrient medium containing a high concentration of antibiotics, where it may be surface sterilized (e.g., with 5% H_2O_2) before being cut into fragments a few millimeters in diameter. These fragments are washed free of blood residues and then macerated with proteolytic enzymes (commonly crude trypsin), possibly in combination with a chelating agent such as EDTA. This treatment disaggregates the tissue cells and results in a cell suspension. The single cells are filtered free of tissue fragments, centrifuged, and taken up in serum-containing medium. The serum both inactivates the proteolytic activity and provides essential but as yet largely undefined growth factors. This cell suspension is then inoculated at a density of 10^5–10^6 cells/ml into a culture flask. For economic reasons, disposable plastic

TISSUE EXPLANT

CUT

WASH FREE OF BLOOD

DISAGGREGATE

CENTRIFUGE

CELL SUSPENSION

IN NUTRIENT MEDIUM

CELL COUNT

INOCULATE

CULTIVATE

Fig. 1. Flow chart for the initiation of a cell culture.

culture flasks are replacing traditional glass culture bottles. For the initiation of culture it is usual to use flat-bottom (Roux-type) culture flasks; a wide variety of speciality ware is commercially available. The cells will first adhere to the culture surface and then begin to multiply. This initial, growing culture is termed primary culture (Freshney, 1984).

The described procedure follows a standard pattern, to which there are many modifications; for example, the cells can be isolated in situ by perfusing an organ (e.g., kidney) with the proteolytic enzyme solution.

Subcultivation

Depending on their specific growth characteristics, the primary cells will multiply several times to form a more or less densely packed cell layer(s). Much of cell culture still remains an art and relies on empirical skill. This skill must be called upon to assess a primary culture and the appropriate time to subcultivate.

Subcultivation involves flooding the culture surface with a trypsin solution (or other proteolytic enzymes, as required) and decanting the enzyme solution before the cells begin to dissociate from the culture surface. This is followed by a short incubation in the presence of the residual enzyme solution, which effects the release of the cells from their growth surface. The enzyme residue will release the cells from the surface. The cells are then resuspended in fresh serum-containing nutrient medium and inoculated into fresh flasks at a concentration of about 10^5 cells/ml, or some $1-5 \times 10^4$ cells/cm^2 of growth surface (Freshney, 1984).

The ensuing cultures are then repeatedly subcultured in the same manner; the culture is now referred to as a *cell line*, and a single subculture is a *passage*. Consecutive numbering of passages is used to vaguely indicate the age of a cell line, although the culture doubling number provides a more valid indication. Normal cell lines can be subcultured only for a finite number of passages before exhibiting signs of degeneration and senescence. Cells may be selected for certain properties from a cell culture; the ensuing culture is the term *cell strain*.

On the average, a normal cell can be expected to multiply 50–100 times. However, cell degeneration, characterized by decreased growth and loss of specific cell function, is a gradual process. "Normal" cells, which are characterized by a diploid set of chromosomes, senescence, and various morphological and functional parmeters, can undergo a process broadly described by the term *transformation*. One result of such a transformation is that the cell may be rescued from senescence and become a *continuous cell line*, that is, the line can be subcultivated indefinitely. This characteristic is of major technological importance. Although this phenomenon of transformation and its technological implications will be discussed in more detail below, it should be noted at this point that transformation is basically the result of genetic aberration. It can be initiated by physical (γ-rays, ultraviolet light), chemical (carcinogens, oncogens, etc.), or viral (oncogenic viruses) agents or take place spontaneously. The aberration may take place in vivo, resulting in tumor formation, or in vitro, described as *in vitro transformation*.

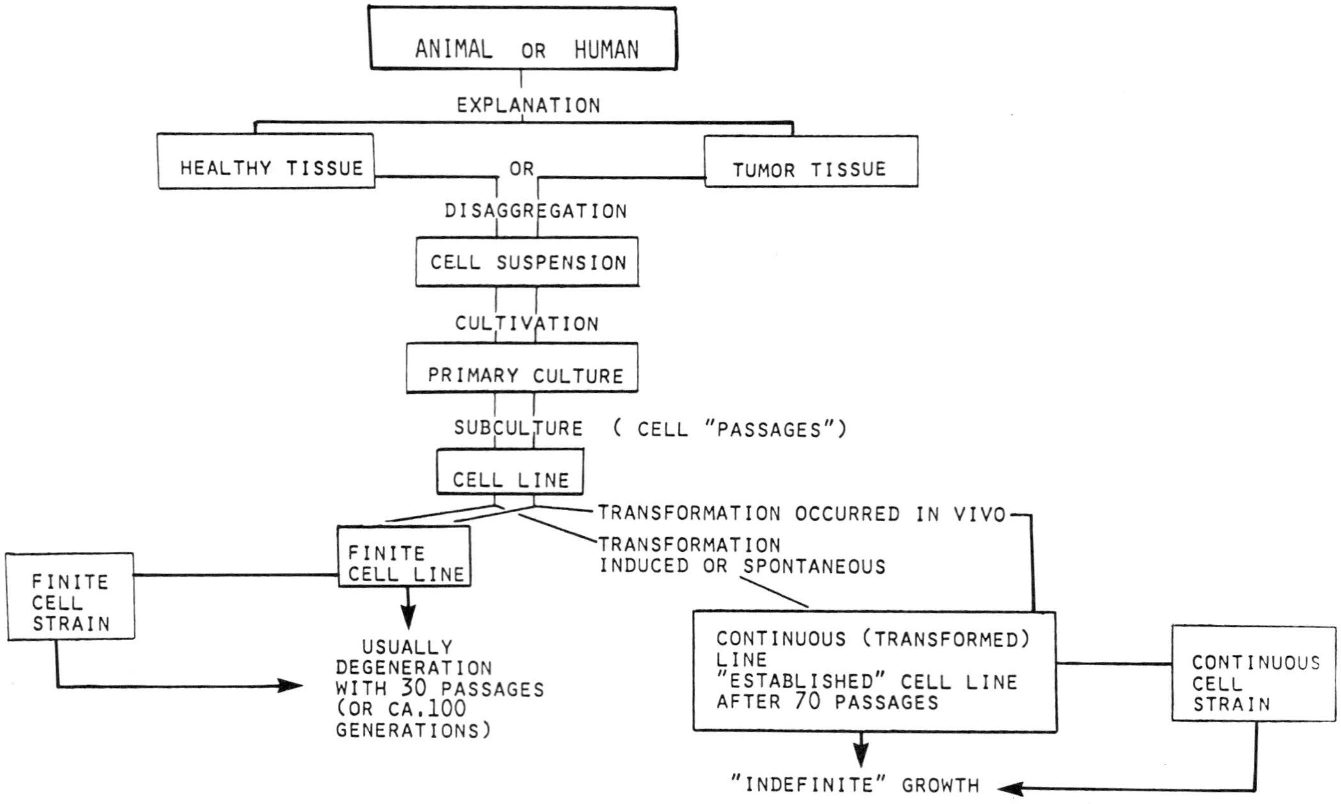

Fig. 2. Critical steps in establishing a cell culture.

A cell line may thus be derived from normal or tumor tissue, which may result in a finite or continuous cell line. On the other hand, cells in culture can be transformed and thus also provide a continuous cell line (Jakoby and Pastan, 1979; Kuchler, 1977; Freshney, 1984). Figure 2 summarizes the critical steps in establishing a cell culture from normal or tumor-derived tissue.

TRANSFORMATION

Introduction

In vitro transformation has been defined by the American Tissue Culture Association (Schaeffer, 1984) as follows:

> A heritable change, occurring in cells in culture, either intrinsically or from treatment with chemical carcinogens, oncogenic viruses, irradiation, etc., and leading to the acquisition of altered morphological, antigenic, neoplastic, proliferative, or other properties. This expression is distinguished from "in vitro neoplastic transformation" in that the alterations occurring in the cell population may not always include the ability of the cells to produce tumors in appropriate hosts. The type of transformation should always be specified in any description.

The general technological advantage of transformation lies in its effects on cell growth. Major limitations restricting the use of normal animal cells on an industrial scale result from their finite life span, their relatively poor growth rates, and their high serum requirements (commonly 5–10% fetal calf serum, current list price about £100 per liter).

It is in these limitations that transformation can introduce major improvements, such as (1) the immortalization of a cell line, thereby securing a continuous producer culture; (2) an increase in the growth rate of a culture, and (3) a reduction in the required level of costly serum in the growth and maintenance media (Jakoby and Pastan, 1979; Kuchler, 1977; Freshney, 1984). It is also common for cells to become less anchorage dependent following transformation. Although the acquisition of suspension-type characteristics represents a major technological advantage, a complete change from an anchorage-dependent culture to one displaying full suspension-type characteristics through in vitro transformation is a rare event.

The resulting changes in cell growth are relatively independent of cell specificity; however, the effects on specific cell functions can be dramatic, often resulting in total loss of specific characteristics. Transformation often results in the dedifferentiation of the cells with respect to their production of specific biologicals. On the other hand, transformation has also been found to induce the production of certain products, for example, the currently highly valued tissue plasminogen activator (Dano et al., in press; Gronow, Bliem, 1983).

To date, transformed cell lines have only been approved for the commercial production of veterinary vaccines (e.g., BHK21 cells for FMD vaccine production) but not for human therapeutics. Although the definition of the American Tissue Culture Association distinguishes *transformation* from *neoplastic transformation*, the general phenomenon is still strongly associated with oncogenesis. It is this association that has to date prevented the authorities from clearing the way for the industrial use of transformed cells for human use (Bliem, 1986; Wilson, 1984).

Transformation and Oncogenesis

Oncogenesis is now widely accepted as a multistep process exhibiting various characteristic parameters throughout the development of oncogenesis, until ultimately the stage of neoplasia arrives. This final stage is characterized by the cells' ability to form tumors in test animals (Zimmerman and Little, 1983). Therefore oncogenesis and transformation have only process steps in common, but transformation is not the same as oncogenicity. This distinguishing fact was emphasized at a 1984 U.S. Food and Drug Administration (FDA) workshop on biologicals in Bethesda, Maryland.

The process of oncogenesis has been broadly subdivided into two steps, an initiating step and a completing step. Initiation is thought to be an absolute requirement involving mutational events in as yet unknown genes, while completion involves subsequent alterations that result in the tumorigenic state.

In the experimental model, the cells are immortalized with the initiation step and exhibit few phenotypic characteristics of malignant cells; only with the completing step do the cells then acquire the characteristics typical of malignancy, the most critical being the ability to form tumors.

In recent years a number of viral genes, oncogenes, have been identified which initiate these steps. Some of these oncogenes are thought to be derived from normal cellular genes, termed proto-oncogenes. These gene sequences can be employed to selectively induce transformation, as opposed to random mutation by chemical carcinogens. Furthermore, they can be quantified, allowing for both improved experimental control and cell- and product-oriented quality control. The current efficiency of transformation using rat oncogenes lies around several colonies per 10^5 rat cells, with a 100-fold lower efficiency using human cells; (D. A. Spandidos, personal communication), although transformation efficiency appears to vary with cells (for example see Sager, 1983).

Table 1. Conclusions Drawn from the 1984 FDA Workshop in Bethesda, Maryland, on the Risks Posed by the Use of Abnormal Cells and the Contamination of New Products (by F. Robbins, President of the Institute of Medicine)

Cell transformation is not the same as oncogenicity.
All cells contain proto-oncogenes
Active oncogenes are present in some cell lines.
It is possible to transfect cells in vitro and in vivo, but the complete genome is normally required and in large quantity. Human cells are fairly resistant to transfection.
In most biologicals it is possible to reduce the levels of residual DNA, and so forth, to below those likely to induce biological changes.
Most of the DNA present would be in forms not likely to be oncogenic.
The human body possesses a major protective capacity to deal with contaminants.

Attitudes of Regulatory Authorities

The U.S. Food and Drug Administration (FDA) is probably the single most influential authority referred to by the pharmaceutical industry on the topic of tumor-derived cells for the production of biologicals. Currently the FDA is considering recommendations compiled at a 1984 workshop (FDA, 1984) which would clear the way to using transformed and tumor-derived cells lines. The recommendations are summarized in Table 1. Robbins, President of the Institute of Medicine, concluded at this meeting that there were no insurmountable barriers to the introduction of new and useful products in the field of drugs and biologicals. He emphasized the need to lower prices for vaccines and that it was therefore very important not to overregulate and invent problems, thereby restricting the industry. Furthermore, abnormal cells were an important part of the production methods used and their use could be pursued with safety; continued realistic risk assessment would not only safeguard the public but also allow them to reap the benefits of the new technologies in the form of new drugs and other products.

It is the policy of the FDA to use risk-versus-benefit criteria to evaluate new production methods (Wilson, 1984). Therefore, it is generally felt that the FDA, under pressure from both the scientific and industrial quarters, will soon accept these recommendations (see further Bliem, 1986).

FACILITIES AND MATERIALS

Basic Laboratory Requirements

The basic layout for a cell culture laboratory comprises at least seven functional areas subdivided into three or more rooms. The main functions provided for in a cell culture laboratory are aseptic handling, incubation, washing, sterilization, equipment and medium preparation, storage, and biochemical operations (Freshney, 1984).

Aseptic Handling

This should preferably be carried out in a separate custom-designed clean room comprising a laminar-flow cabinet, a refrigerator, a water bath, some shelving, an incubator, and an inverted microscope.

Incubator

If only very small numbers and volumes of cultures are handled, a 1- to 2-m^3 CO_2 incubator will suffice. However, this will soon become limiting, so incorporation of a separate incubator room is highly recommended in the initial design.

Washing, Sterilization, and Preparation

Equipment washing, sterilization (autoclave, filtration), drying, and media and equipment preparation can be carried out within the same room, although preferably these functions are allocated to a separated clean room.

Storage

Material and equipment stocks fall into four groups with respect to storage temperature: room temperature, 4°C, −30°C, and −196°C (liquid nitrogen). The −30°C deep-freezer and the liquid nitrogen tanks are best kept within a 4°C cold-room. Adequate stocks of both equipment and materials are essential at any time, so storage areas should not be underestimated in the initial design.

Biochemical Operations

Biochemical operations usually require standard biochemical laboratory facilities. These should be housed in a separate laboratory area.

Growth Vessels

Cell culture-derived biologicals currently represent low volume—high cost products. There is therefore no strict delineation between the laboratory and the technical scale or between the technical and the industrial scale in terms of media volumes per culture. However, for the purpose of didactic presentation and based on current production levels of FMD vaccine, interferon, and plasminogen activator, an attempt has been made to describe working scales in terms of culture volumes. Thus in the laboratory single culture volumes rarely exceed the liter level. Up to 100 liters might be described as technical or pilot scale, and beyond this lies the industrial scale. Wellcome Laboratories (England) routinely operate an 8000-liter Rushton-type fermenter for their Namalva-Interferon production. This currently represents the largest growth propagator, although an expansion scheme is already being considered.

The two main growth types of animal cells, anchorage-dependent growth and growth in free suspension, form the basis for the design concepts of growth propagators. Cells can be grown on solid supports, ranging from Petridishes to metal plates of several square meters. The laboratory favorite for routine operations is a Roux-type glass or plastic flask with a surface area ranging from 25 to about 180 cm^2. A variety of disposable culture dishes satisfy most requirements down to less than 1 cm^2. On the other hand, utilizing the full inside surface of a roller bottle provides up to 2000 cm^2 of growth surface. Figure 3 depicts some of the possible choices of scale-up beyond this (Spier, 1980; Stand et al., 1984; Glacken et al., 1983; Ku et al., 1981; Katinger and Scheirer, 1982; Spier and Griffiths, 1985). Recent developments have also shown promising results through the entrapment or encapsulation of cells in gel material (Nilsson et al., 1983; Damon Corp.). The technical disadvantages of a stationary growth propagator are those typical of any heterogeneous system, that is, poor process control and scale-up characteristics when compared to homogeneous suspension systems. Although suspension characteristics make for easier process control, anchorage-dependent cell cultures do provide some advantages. Two main advantages are that these cells can often be maintained in a stationary phase for longer periods than suspension cells, and with reduced serum requirements. Furthermore, the supernatant medium contains less cellular debris, thereby reducing the demands on the clarification process.

However, cells can be grown on microcarriers, which can in turn be held in liquid suspension, thus offering the advantages of a homogeneous system yet satisfying the requirements of anchorage-dependent cells for solid growth supports (Reuveny, 1983). Figure 4 shows human embryonic cells grown on microcarriers. An alternative to microcarriers has been demonstrated in the growth of cells in aggregate forms, which are cultivated in suspension. In this form the cells provide each other with an anchorage point for growth. However, this method requires that aggregate growth can be halted at a defined stage. This difficulty still impedes the general application of this technique (R. Bliem, unpublished results).

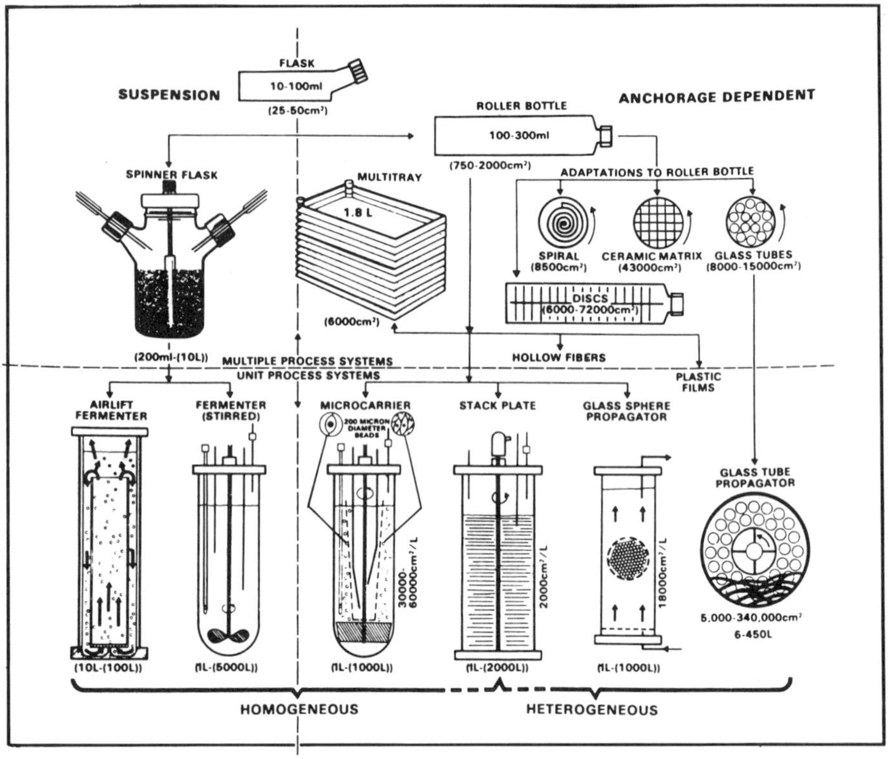

Fig. 3. Possible culture scale-up versions. (From Griffiths, B., 1983. *Lab Practice 12*:11.)

Suspension-type cells are more frequently found among lymphocyte derivatives, the monoclonal antibody-producing hybridoma cells presenting the most popular example. Figure 5 shows the basic measurement and control requirements for the suspension cultivation of animal cells, illustrated on an air-lift reactor (Katinger and Scheirer, 1982).

Media

Cell culture media have a defined basal composition of salts, amino acids, vitamins, various growth factors, and serum supplement (Jakoby and Parstan, 1979; Kuchler, 1977; Freshney, 1984). Much of the early work in cell culture research was devoted to developing appropriate media, so that we now have an established group of defined media compositions forming the basis for modifications, which are often quite specific to a given laboratory strain.

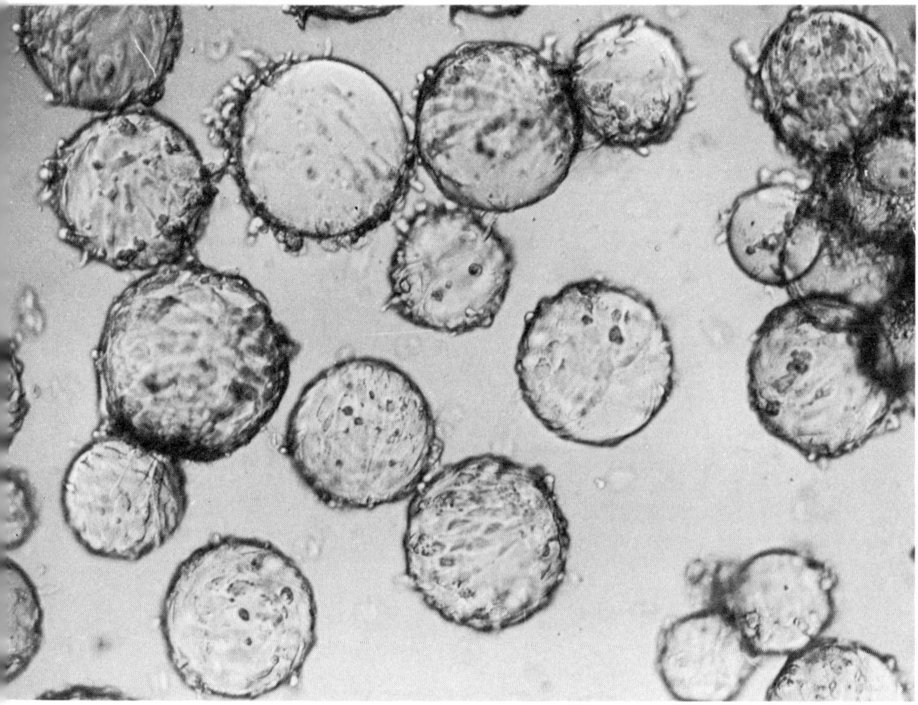

Fig. 4. Human embryonic cells grown on microcarriers.

The serum, although still an essential growth component for most culture media, is undesirable on both economic and technical grounds. The reasons can be summarized as follows. Serum is commonly added at 1–10% vol/vol to the basal defined medium. The culture thus contains on the order of 0.5–5 mg/ml protein, which constitutes an excess of serum protein of some 100–1000 times the desired cell culture protein (current status). The desired product must then be isolated and sufficiently purified from the bulk of the added serum protein. Currently the products upon which industry has focused its major efforts are human proteins, while the sera used in the production process are of bovine origin. Serum comprises more than 100 proteins, and even residues of bovine protein can give rise to antigenic reactions in humans.

Therefore the protein products destined for human therapeutics are subjected to isolation procedures which ensure their purification free of nonhuman contaminants. However, product yields also decrease with the complexity of the purification process, which results in decreased production economics. In addition, serum quality

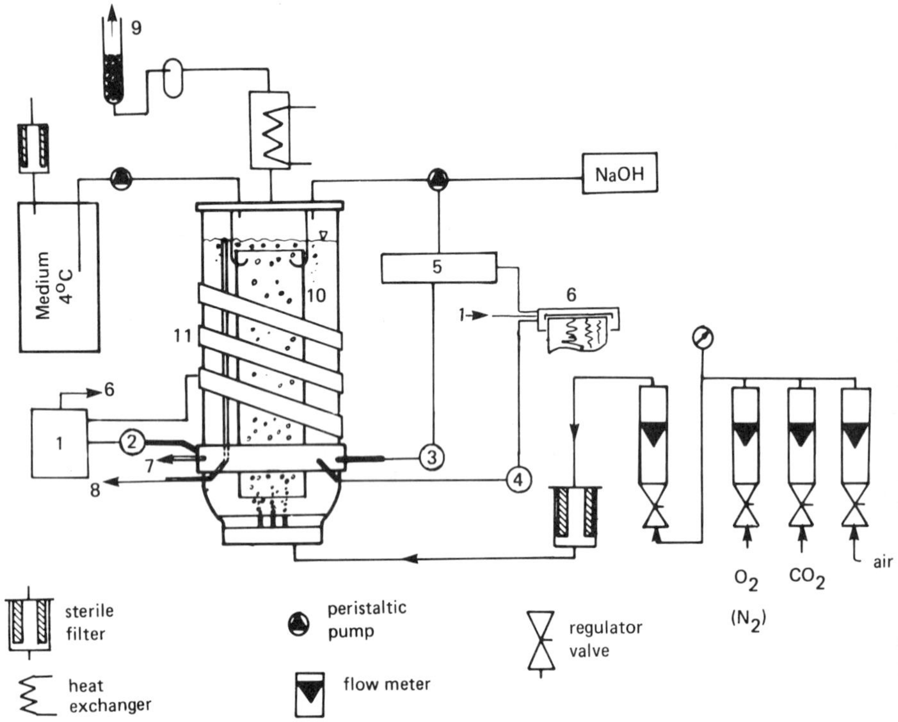

Fig. 5. Basic measurement and control requirements for the suspension cultivation of animal cells in an air-lift reactor. 1, temperature controller; 2, temperature sensor; 3, pH electrode and meter; 4, dissolved oxygen electrode and meter; 5, titrator; 6, printer; 7, sample port; 8, medium effluent; 9, gas exhaust through acid-lock; 10, draft tube; 11, heater belt.

varies between batches and cannot be controlled. Some processes now use cheaper serum types, the cheapest source being adult bovine serum purchased directly from a slaughterhouse. However, manipulation costs are still significant, particularly considering the unreliability of the source and the demands on the final product. Furthermore, sterile filtration does not sufficiently isolate viruses or mycoplasma contaminants, so that γ-irradiation becomes essential. Much effort is therefore currently being devoted to developing serum replacements (Murakami, H., et al.).

TECHNOLOGICAL DEMANDS AND CONCLUSION

Animal Cell Technology for the Production of Therapeutics

Traditionally, complex therapeutic biologicals such as hormones, enzymes, and similarly active agents are extracted from animal or human tissues or body fluids or they are produced by microbial technology. In the mid-1970s pressures were increasing on industry to seek novel biologicals, with only a limited supply of human and animal raw materials and increasingly high production costs. Alternative technologies were thus essential. Table 2 summarizes the demands placed on such an alternative technology.

It was hoped by many in the pharmaceutical and veterinary industries that animal cell technology could satisfy these requirements

Table 2. Demands on Alternative Technology

Advantageous product characteristics:

- Identical to product of traditional technology, if latter already on the market
- Homologous and nonantigenic
- Free from pyrogen contamination

Essential product characteristics:

- High clinical efficacy
- Long-term stability
- Free from hazardous materials (e.g., oncogenic polynucleotides or proteins)

Essential production characteristics:

- Reliable and economic raw materials
- Efficient process control
- Possibilities of process scale-up

within the next decade, thereby offering a follow-up technology for current and intended product lines. With a short interlude offered by microbial recombinant DNA technology, this hope is now becoming reality, as evidenced by several industrial operations—Namalva-Interferon, Wellcome; plasminogen activator in Mouse-L and CHO cells, Genentech; monoclonal antibody production in hybridomas, various companies worldwide; vaccines, Wellcome (see also Spier and Horaud, 1985).

Although the product-oriented applications of animal cell culture are currently taking the stage, a variety of other applications are in development. As already indicated in the Introduction, animal breeders will benefit through such measures as the determination of the sex of an embryo to fertilization, the precise determination of ovulation in cows using simple test methods, and the in vitro fertilization and frozen storage of embryos with a view to possible transplantation into surrogate mother animals (Gatz et al., 1983; Mapletoft, 1984; Brackett et al., 1983). Another important area of development is the use of cell cultures as replacements for test animals. These few examples are merely intended to illustrate the possible range of applications through which animal cell technology will soon receive a valuable position in the food-related industries.

REFERENCES

Bebbington, C., Hentschel, C. (1985). The expression of recombinant DNA products in mammalian cells. *Trends in Biotech.*, Vol. 3:314–317.

Bliem, R. (1986). Products from transformed cell lines: the stance of WHO and FDA. ESMct '85 meeting report. *Trends in Biotech.*, Vol. 4:1–2.

Borenfreund, E., Shopsis, C., Borrero, Ö., and Sathe, S. (1983). In vitro alternative irritancy assays: comparison of cytotoxic and membrane transport effects of alcohols. *Ann. N. Y. Acad. Sci. 407*:416–419.

Brackett, B. G., Seidel, G. E., and Seidel, S. M. (eds.). (1983). *New Technologies in Animal Breeding*, Academic, New York.

Dano, K., Andreasen, P. A., Grondahl-Hansen, J., Kristensen, P., Nielsen, L. S., Skriver, L. Plasminogen Activators and Cancer. *Adv. Cancer Res.* (in press).

Ekwall, B. (1983). Correlation between cytotoxicity in vitro and LD_{50}-values. Proceedings of The First CFN Symposium: LD_{50} and Possible Alternatives, Sept. 1981. *Acta Pharmacol. Toxicol. Suppl. 52*:80–99.

Freshney, R. I. (1984). *Culture of Animal Cells. A Manual of Basic Techniques*, Liss, New York.

Gatz, R. L., Young, B. A., Facklam, T. J., and Scantland, D. A. (1983). Monoclonal antibodies: Emerging product concepts for agriculture and food. *Biotechnology 1*:337–341.

Glacken, M. W., Fleischaker, R. J., and Sinskey, A. J. (1983). Mammalian cell culture: Engineering principles and scale-up. *Trends Biotechnol. 1*:102–108.

Jakoby, W. B. and Pastan, I. H. (eds.) (1979). Cell culture. *Methods Enzymol. 58*:3–613.

Katinger, H. W. D. and Bliem, R. (1983). Production of enzymes and hormones by mammalian cell culture. In *Advances in Biotechnological processes*, Vol. 2 (A. Mizrahi and A. L. van Wezel, eds.), Liss, New York, pp. 62–95.

Katinger, H. W. D. and Scheirer, W. (1982). Status and development on animal cell technology using suspension culture techniques. *Acta Biotechnol. 2*:3–41.

Ku, K., Kuo, M. J., Delente, B. S., Wildi, B. S., and Feder, J. (1981). Development of a hollow-fiber system for large-scale culture of cells. *Biotech. Bioeng. 23*:79–95.

Kuchler, R. J. (1977). *Biochemical Methods in Cell Culture and Virology*, Dowden, Hutchinson, and Ross, Stroudsburg, A.

Mapletoft, R. J. (1984). Embryo transfer technology for the enhancement of animal reproduction. *Biotechnology*, pp. 149–160.

Murakami, H., Yamane, I., Barnes, D. W., Mather, J. P., Hayashi, I., Sato, G. H. (1985). Proceedings of the international symposium on growth and differentiation of cells in defined environment. Copublished by Springer-Verlag, Heidelberg, and Kodansha, Tokyo.

Nilsson, K., Scheirer, W., Merten, O. W., Östberg, L., Liehl, E., Katinger, H. W. D., and Mosbach, K. (1983). Entrapment of animal cells for production of monclonal antibodies and other biomolecules. *Nature 302*:629–630.

Paul, W. E., Sredni, B., and Schwartz, R. H. (1981). Long term growth and cloning of non-transformed lymphocytes. *Nature 294*:697.

Reuveny, S. (1983). Microcarriers for culturing mammalian cells and their applications. In *Advances in Biotechnological Processes*, Vol. 2 (A. Mizrahi and A. L. van Wezel, eds.), Liss, New York, pp. 2–32.

Sager, R., Tanaka, K., Lau, C. C., Ebina, Y., Anisowicz, A. (1983). Resistance of human cells to tumorigenesis induced by cloned transforming genes. *Proc. Natl. Acad. Sci. U.S.A.*, Vol. 80:7601–7605. Genetics.

Schaeffer, W. I. (1984). Usage of vertebrate, invertebrate and plant cell, tissue and organ culture terminology. *In Vitro 20*:19–24.

Spandidos, D. A., and Wilkie, N. M. (1984). Malignant transformation of early passage rodent cells by a single mutated human oncogene. *Nature 310*:469–475.

Spier, R. (1980). Recent developments in the large scale cultivation of animal cells in monolayers. In *Advances in Biochemical Engineering*, Vol. 14 (A. Fiechter, ed.), Springer-Verlag, Berlin, pp. 120–156.

Spier, R. E., Griffiths, J. B. (eds.) (1985). *Animal Cell Biotechnology*, Vol. 1 and 2. Academic Press, London, New York.

Spier, R. E., Horaud, F. (1985). The biotechnological future for animal cells in culture. In: *Animal Cell Biotechnology*, Vol. 2 (R. E. Spier, J. B. Griffiths, eds.), Academic Press, New York, pp. 432–459.

Strand, J. M., Quarles, J. M., and McConnel, S. (1984). A modified matrix perfusion–microcarrier bead cell culture system. II. Production of human (β)-interferon in a matrix perfusion system. *Biotech. Bioeng. 36*:508–512.

Wilson, T. (1984). FDA loosens restraints on cell substrates. *Biotechnology 2*:842.

Zimmerman, R. J. and Little, J. B. (1983). Characteristics of human diploid fibroblasts transformed in vitro by chemical carcinogens. *Cancer Res. 43*:2183–2189.

10

Methods in Plant Tissue Culture

ROBERT J. GRIESBACH / U.S. Department of Agriculture, Beltsville, Maryland

INTRODUCTION

Plant somatic cell genetics involves tissue culture technology which is based upon two principles of plant development: (1) Auxin hormones in general promote undifferentiated growth and (2) cytokinin hormones usually sitmulate differentiated growth. By varying the ratio and concentrations of these two types of hormones, it is possible to switch from one mode of growth to another. For example, a leaf placed on a tissue culture medium which promotes undifferentiated growth will form an amorphous mass of actively divided cells called callus. The callus, when transferred to a different medium which stimulates differentiation, will develop small meristems and eventually shoots.

Tissue culture technology could have a tremendous impact in both basic and applied science. This technology has now been used in propagation, embryo culture, haploid production, germ plasm preservation, mutant production, hybridization or cell fusion, developmental studies, and metabolic studies, including secondary metabolites.

HISTORY

The first attempt at plant tissue culture began in 1902, when Haberlandt placed the epidermal, pith parenchyma, and palisade cells of monocotyledons in culture. The culture medium contained various sugars, inorganic salts, and amino acids. None of the cells, however, divided. The first successful attempt at tissue culture was made in 1904, when Hannig, using similar media, was able to grow whole plants from embryos.

During the next two decades, work centered around improving embryo culture techniques. It was found that several complex additives, like yeast extract, coconut milk, and peptone, greatly stimulate growth. In 1934, White placed excise tomato root tips in culture. When yeast extract was added to the medium, the roots were able to divide and grow indefinitely.

In 1936, Brown and Gardener found that tumors, similar to the tumors induced by crown gall bacteria, could be mimicked by exogenous auxin applications. This information was quickly applied to tissue culture. In 1939, Gautheret, Nobecourt, and White each independently demonstrated that the auxin indoleacetic acid, when incorporated into culture media, stimulated the production of undifferentiated callus. This was the first time hormones were added to tissue culture media. In 1956, Miller and others discovered that the active ingredient in coconut milk and yeast extract, which promoted growth in culture, was another class of hormones, the cytokinins. Skoog and Miller further reported in 1957 that the auxin/cytokinin balance was very important for the growth of cells in culture. If the auxin level was relatively high and the cytokinin level relatively low, undifferentiated callus growth occurred. High levels of cytokinin relative to auxin induced the appearance of differentiated shoots. Thus, it was now possible to regenerate a whole plant from a single undifferentiated cell.

A further advance came in 1964 when Guha and Maheshwari placed datura anthers in culture. From these anthers embryoids formed which developed into haploid plants. Tissue cultures of haploid plants was a major advance for genetic studies.

In 1971 Takebe et al. demonstrated that it was possible to regenerate whole plants from protoplasts. Protoplasts are wall-less plant cells usually produced by incubating tissue in crude, fungal, cellulolytic preparations. The first somatic hybrid plant was produced in 1972, when Carlson and colleagues fused protoplasts from two tobacco species and regenerated the hybrid cell into a whole plant.

In 1974 Zaenen et al. discovered that a plasmid (Ti plasmid) in *Agrobacterium tumefaciens* was responsible for inducing the tumors in crown gall-infected plants. Through the use of mutants, Ooms et al. (1981) demonstrated there were genes on the Ti plasmid which effected the plant's auxin—cytokinin balance. One gene controlled auxin metabolism and another cytokinin metabolism. In 1983 the first example of the expression of a foreign protein in a plant cell was demonstrated by Fraley and others. They inserted into the Ti plasmid a gene for kanamycin resistance. Petunia and tobacco cells infected with this hybrid Ti plasmid were resistant to kanamycin.

In 1984 Horsch et al. reported that the transformed cells were regenerated into whole plants and that the kanamycin-resistant gene was inherited as a single-gene dominant trait. Genetic engineering was no longer a dream.

UNDIFFERENTIATED CALLUS GROWTH

The first step in initiating an actively growing callus culture involves sterilizing the explant. The explant can come from almost any tissue. For example, cultures have been established from flower petals, roots, stems, leaves, ovaries, stamens, and so on. Very few tissues fail to respond to media designed to stimulated callus growth. The most common chemical for sterilizing the explant is the active ingredient in household bleach, sodium hypochlorite. Typical concentrations which are used range from 2 to 30% vol/vol of a commercial preparation. Commercial bleach is approximately 5% sodium hypochlorite. The length of treatment usually varies from 2 to 30 min. After the hypochlorite treatment the explant is washed in sterile water. A typical protocol for petunia leaves involves a 25-min treatment with 20% commercial bleach followed by three washes in sterile water (Gamborg and Wetter, 1975).

For explants that are difficult to sterilize several modifications can be made. A wetting agent like Tween 20 can be added to the hypochlorite solution. The addition of 1% Tween 20 allows the bleach to make greater contact with the explant. Another modification can be a 15-sec dip in 70% ethanol either before or after the hypochlorite treatment. Ethanol pretreatment can remove waxes and other resins which prevent complete contact between the bleach and the explant. Posttreatment with ethanol can kill microorganisms which were not affected by the hypochlorite. Another modification involves placing the explant under a mild vacuum during the hypochlorite and wash incubations. This treatment may eliminate fungal contaminants which are inside the tissue (e.g., underground tubers). A surface sterilization treatment would not kill the fungi.

Once the explant is sterilized, it is usually placed on a solid culture medium. Callus growth then occurs at the points of contact between the medium and the explant. A greater degree of growth occurs at cut surfaces. At these surfaces unknown substances form which stimulate cell division. In addition, a high ratio of surface area to volume is beneficial, for it facilitates both gas and nutrient exchange (Yeoman, 1973).

The basis of almost all tissue culture media is a mixture of macro- and microelements (see Table 1). Several factors are important in the mineral composition (Uchimiya and Murashige, 1976). The ratio of nitrogen supplied as nitrate or ammonium can be critical for growth. For example, high concentrations of ammonium (7 mM)

Table 1. Chemical Composition of Several Widely Used Tissue Culture Media

	White (1934)	Murashige and Skoog (1962)	Gamborg et al. (1968)
$CaCl_2$-$2H_2O$	—	440	150
$CoCl_2$-$2H_2O$	—	0.025	0.025
$CuSO_4$-$5H_2O$	—	0.025	0.025
$FeSO_4$-$7H_2O$	2.5	27.8	27.8
Na_2SO_4	200	—	—
$Ca(NO_3)_2$ $4H_2O$	300	—	—
H_3BO_3	1.5	6.2	3
KH_2PO_4	26.5	170	150
KI	0.75	0.83	0.75
KNO_3	80	1900	3000
M_gSO_4-$7H_2O$	720	370	500
$MnSO_4$-$4H_2O$	7	22.3	10
Na_2MoO_4-$2H_2O$	—	0.25	0.25
NH_4NO_3	—	1650	—
$ZnSO_4$-$7H_2O$	3	8.6	2
$(NH_4)_2SO_4$	—	—	134
KCl	65	—	—
Inositol	—	100	100
Nicotinic acid	0.5	0.5	1
Pyridoxine HCl	0.1	0.5	1
Thiamine	0.1	0.1	10
Sucrose	20	30 g	20 g
Glycine	3	2	—
Cysteine	1	—	—
Ca-panthothenate	1	—	—
Na_2EDTA-$2H_2O$	—	37.3	37.3

inhibited the growth of rice callus. Media containing 7 mM ammonium and 28 mM nitrate was optimal (Ching et al., 1975). In soybeans a shift from 40 mM to 20 mM ammonium was an essential step in triggering the differentiation of cultured cells (Christianson et al., 1983). Other minerals can be equally important. The ratio of potassium to magnesium and levels of calcium can change the friability of callus (Yoshida and Watanabe, 1971). In general, however, the total salt concentration is more important than the ions present. For example, *Phalaenopsis* orchid callus will not grow on full-strength M and S salts (Murashige and Skoog, 1962) but will grow very well on either half- or quarter-strength salts (Hölters, 1983).

Explants will not grow on a medium composed of only inorganic compounds. Besides a carbon source, which is usually sucrose, vitamins, organic growth stimulants, and hormones are usually required. Many of the organic growth stimulants are complex extracts such as yeast extract, conconut milk, peptone, casein hydrolysate, and potato water. These extracts usually supply amino acids and several unknown compounds essential for growth. In many cases callus growth can be initiated on a basal medium lacking these complex organic supplements, but for sustained growth the supplements must be added.

The most typical vitamins which are added to basal media are thiamine, inositol, nicotinic acid, and pyridoxine. High concentrations of any vitamin can have less desirable effects. For example, high thiamine concentrations can decrease callus friability (Reiner and White, 1956).

The most important supplement for callus growth is the plant hormones (Bayless, 1977). Undifferentiated growth requires a high ratio of auxin to cytokinin. There are three widely used auxins: indoleacetic acid (IAA), napthyleneacetic acid (NAA), and 2,4-dichlorophenoxyacetic acid (2,4-D). The weakest auxin is IAA and the strongest is 2,4-D. Besides an auxin, a low concentration of cytokinin is usually required for callus growth. The typical cytokinins used in tissue culture are kinetin, 6-benzylaminopurine (BAP), dimethylallylaminopurine (2iP), and zeatin. Many combinations can be successful (Fonnesbech, 1972). For instance, tobacco callus grows well on medium containing 3 mg/liter IAA and 0.3 mg/liter kinetin, while petunia callus can be induced to grow on medium containing 2 mg/liter 2,4-D and 0.25 mg/liter kinetin.

Once an actively growing, friable callus culture has been established, liquid suspension cultures can be initiated. Liquid suspension cultures result when callus is agitated in liquid. Once the cells become adapted to this environment, they will grow as small, 5- to 10-cell aggregates. The growth rate of liquid suspension cultures is much faster than for solid callus cultures (Street, 1973).

Protoplasts are plant cells which are lacking a cell wall. The presence of a cell wall can make many genetic and biochemical studies impossible, for the cell wall is a very effective barrier against the uptake of large molecules. In the past it was very difficult to isolate large quantitites of viable protoplasts. Protoplasts, however, can now be quite easily obtained in massive numbers. The reason for this is the commercial availability of crude cellulytic enzyme preparations. Protoplasts can be produced by incubating either differentiated tissue like a leaf or undifferentiated tissue like callus in a mixture of cellulase and macerase. These enzymes digest the cell wall (cellulose) and surrounding pectins and hemicellulose. Typical cellulase concentrations range from 75 to 200 units of activity per milliliter, while typical macerase concentrations range from 20 to 60 units of activity per milliliter. Other enzymes such as pectinase, hemicellulase, driselase, and rhozyme are also used on occasion. There are many different crude enzyme mixtures commercially available (Gamborg and Wetter, 1975).

Enzyme-digested tissue is usually cleared of large debris through filtration through 100-μm sieves. The resulting protoplast suspension is then cleared of cellular debris by differential centrifugation. In some instances the protoplast suspension is adjusted to a final concentration of 20% sucrose. Under these conditions the viable protoplasts will float during centrifugation. In other instances the protoplasts are placed on a step gradient of either sucrose, Ficoll, or Percoll. During centrifugation the protoplasts will band at their density. The purified protoplasts are then washed free of enzymes by centrifugation and plated in a tissue culture medium which induces callus formation. Within 1 or 2 days a cell wall reforms and the new cells undergo their first cell division (Butenko, 1979).

DIFFERENTIATION OR MORPHOGENESIS

Plants can be regenerated from either undifferentiated callus or a differentiated explant. The regeneration of shoots from undifferentiated tissue cultures is one of the most difficult aspects of plant tissue culture. In general, it is easier to generate shoots from a differentiated explant like a leaf than from callus.

There are many environmental, physiological, and genetic factors which affect the differentiation of tissue cultures. In wheat, a twofold difference in the percentage of shoot regeneration existed between cultivars (Lazar et al., 1983). In addition, there were no statistically significant correlations between callus initiation, callus growth rate, and morphogenesis. This suggests that different genes are involved in each response. In the pea 16 genotypes were tested for their morphogenetic potential. Only two genotypes were capable of regenerating plants from callus which was 6 months old (Malmberg, 1979).

Aside from the genetic effects, the physical environment is very important in regeneration. The most important physical factors are light and temperature. In most instances the culture medium contains all the elements essential for continued growth. Photosynthesis is not necessary for growth; however, low levels of photosynthesis can influence both growth and morphogenesis. In tobacco light was essential for shoot initiation (Thorpe and Murashige, 1970), while in *Anthurium* light inhibited morphogenesis (Pierik et al., 1979). In most instances low light, around 1000 lx, is required for regeneration. The photoperiod is also important. In some species, like cauliflower, a short day (9 hr) is required for regeneration (Margara, 1969), while in other species, like tobacco, a long day (16 hr) is essential (Murashige and Nakano, 1968). Continuous light can, however, strongly inhibit differentiation in almost all species. For example, geranium callus, when cultured in continuous light, did not turn green or initiate buds (Pillai and Hildebrandt, 1969). The quality of the light can effect regeneration. In lettuce as little as 5 min of 660-nm light at 2.5 W/m^2 each day could double the number of shoots produced (Kadkade and Seibert, 1977).

Temperature can also be critical in regeneration. Callus cultures are generally grown at 25°C. This temperature is usually not optimum for morphogenesis. In many species a 2- to 4-week cold temperature pretreatment can improve morphogenesis. For example, in begonia temperatures below 15°C and above 9°C stimulate shoot production (Hilding and Welander, 1976). In phalaenopsis temperatures above 25°C stimulated reproductive growth of inflorescence nodes, while temperature between 20 and 25°C stimulated vegetative growth (Tanaka and Sakanishi, 1978). Temperature can also effect media composition. At high temperatures (24°C), asparagus shoot regeneration required a 10-fold increase in cytokinin over low temperatures (17°C) (Narayanaswamy, 1977). The opposite was true for lettuce, which required higher cytokinin concentrations at low temperatures (Goloff et al., 1979).

Morphogenesis is generally dependent upon the size of the callus or explant. The larger the explant, the better the regenerative capacity (Narayanaswamy, 1977). The source of the explant is also important in regeneration. In general, explants which are enriched for meristematic cells, such as embryos, tend to have a higher regenerative capacity. In the petunia shoot regeneration is easily obtained from the leaves but is not possible from the petals. Not all species respond in the same manner, for in the chrysanthemum the opposite is true: It has not been possible to regenerate shoots from chrysanthemum leaves; plants have, however, been obtained from the petals (Bush et al., 1976).

The age of the explant is another important factor. For instance, young echeveria leaves were capable of only regenerating roots, whereas mature leaves regenerated shoots (Raju and Mann, 1970). A similar situation exists for callus regeneration. The older the callus, the lower the regenerative capacity. For example, tobacco pith is composed of cells approximately half of which are diploid and half of which are tetraploid. After 1 year in culture the cell population was composed of 26% tetraploids, 20% octaploids, and 54% aneuploids. After 6 years in culture the population was composed of 100% aneuploids. The euploid cultures had a higher morphogenetic potential than the aneuploid cultures (Murashige and Nakano, 1967).

The tissue culture medium used to induce morphogenesis usually has a high ratio of cytokinin to auxin. Unlike the general hormone requirements for callus induction, morphogenesis requires a very specific hormone balance which can even be cultivar dependent. For instance, leaves of *Petunia hybrida* cv. Pink Magic produced shoots on a medium containing 1 mg/liter NAA and 2 mg/liter BAP, while leaves of *P. hybrida* cv. Dancy Lady Pink did not produce shoots on this medium but did on one containing 2 mg/liter zeatin (R. Griesbach, unpublished results).

There are two morphogenetic pathways. One pathway involves the organization of meristematic areas within the regenerating tissue. These areas then proceed to grow, divide, and form shoots. The other pathway involves embryongenesis. Under the appropriate conditions small embryolike structures can form. These embryoids can then be stimulated to develop like normal embryos. A switch from a very high-auxin medium (2 mg/liter 2,4-D) to a very low-auxin medium (0.2 mg/liter 2,4-D) can in some instances trigger the formation of embryoids (Gamborg and Eveleigh, 1968).

There are now over 50 species in which procedures have been developed for regenerating protoplasts into whole plants. In addition, there are hundreds of species in which techniques have been worked out for regenerating plants from undifferentiated callus and thousands of species where whole plants can be produced from cultured differentiated tissue. A quote from Torrey (1977) is appropriate: "Lack of success in culturing a tissue is usually attributable to lack of trying."

BIOCHEMISTRY AND GENETICS OF SOMATIC CELLS

There are two major advantages in using cultured cells in metabolic studies. First, one can obtain a uniform population of undifferentiated, heterotropic cells in culture (Parke and Carlson, 1979). When using whole plants or tissues in studies, one is forced to work with a mixed population of differentiated cell types. Cells are variously programmed for photosynthesis, water uptake, gas exchange, nutrient movement, continued growth, or physical support. All these different cell types make it almost impossible to determine the underlying biochemical basis for most phenomena.

The second advantage in using cultured cells is that both the physical and chemical environments can be controlled and defined (Parke and Carlson, 1979). All of the nutrients and growth regulators must be supplied for continued cell growth. Transport phenomenon, differentiation, and cellular associations can affect the distribution and perception of both nutrients and genetic regulator signals in whole plants, as well as the response of organs and cells to these signals and chemicals.

Cultured cells, even though they do not reflect any specific developmental state found within the whole plant, can still be helpful in elucidating some biosynthetic pathways (Ludden and Carlson, 1980). For example, the comparison of the behavior of mutant cells with that of normal cells allows a more thorough characterization of a given biochemical event. Cultured carrot cells, for example, which were resistant to 5-methyltryptophan, have been selected and compared with normal wild-type cells (Widholm, 1977). By adding intermediates of the tryptophan biosynthetic pathway to the culture medium, it was determined that 5-methyltryptophan inhibits the production of anthranilic acid. The enzyme anthranilate synthetase then was isolated from the 5-methyltryptophan-resistant cell lines and characterized. The resistant phenotype was due to a lack of feedback inhibition. Further studies comparing the defective enzyme from several different mutants with the normal enzyme will allow one to characterize the mechanism involved in feedback inhibition. It would be difficult, if not impossible, to study this type of enzyme activity without the use of mutants. Many of the steps in the flavonoid biosynthetic pathway have also been elucidated using cultured cells.

In vitro anthocyanin synthesis in *Helianthus tuberosus* L. cell cultures was stimulated by a nutrient medium containing kinetin. In addition, high light intensity, low temperature, and media rich in phosphates and inorganic nitrogen were essential for the in vitro production of cyanidin 3,5-diglucoside (Ibrahim et al., 1971). Likewise, high light intensity was essential for the in vitro production of cyanidin 3-rutinoside in *Heplopappus gracilis* L. cell cultures (Fritsh and Griesbach, 1975; Hahlbrock and Griesbach, 1979). By feeding radioactive precursors to cultured, dimethylsulfoxide-permeabilized *Haplopappus* cells, it was concluded that within the cytoplasm l-phenylalanine is deaminated to cinnamic acid, which is then hydroxylated to p-coumaric acid on some membrane. Activation of p-coumaric acid to the coenzyme A thiol ester and condensation of the coenzyme A thiol ester with 3-malonyl-coenzyme A to produce naringenin occur free in the cytoplasm. Hydroxylation of naringenin to produce dihydroquercetin takes place on some membrane again. Further studies (Gerats, et al., 1982; Hrazdina et al., 1978; Jonsson et al., 1982a,b) using protoplasts isolated from flower petals have indicated that the glucosylation of dihydroquercetin and the methylation of the anthocyanidin take place free in the cytoplasm. The final product is then transported into the vacuole, where it accumulates.

When the flavonoid biosynthetic pathway of cultured cells was compared with the pathway found in cells in vivo, interesting results were obtained. Both cyanadin and delphinidin are produced in cultured rose cells, while in intact petal cells only cyanadin is produced (Ibrahim et al., 1971). The difference between cyanadin and delphinidin is in the number of hydroxyl groups, delphinidin having one more. These data suggest the presence of an additional hydroxylation gene which is active in the in vitro cultured cells and inactive or nonfunction in the in vivo cells.

One must be careful in correlating the gene activity of cultured cells with the activity of those genes in differentiated tissues and organs. Many genes in whole plants are expressed only in specific tissues or organs. An important part of plant development involves repressing unneeded genes. Genetic repression can be quite strong and in some instances irreversible. This developmental trait can make it difficult to characterize many biochemical pathways, for few cells within differentiated tissue contain all of the needed genes for a given pathway in an active, functional state. The use of undifferentiated cultured cells can overcome this difficulty because cultured cells usually are under weak genetic regulation. An example of this weak regulation is seen in the fact that environmental factors can change gene expression in cultured cells. In the case of anthocyanin biosynthesis, a slight change in the concentration or type of hormone, light intensity, or even temperature can change the expression of the genes involved in this pathway (Fritsh and Griesbach, 1975; Ibrahim et al., 1971).

Mutations and chromosome aberrations accumulate over time in callus culture (Larkin and Scowcroft, 1981). These genetic changes may be caused by one of two processes. First, the tissue culture cycle itself may induce the variation. It is well known that many of the chemicals like 2,4-D which are included in tissue culture media are mutagenic. Second, tissue culture releases cells from a specific developmental fate. Spontaneous mutations are occurring continually as developmentally predetermined cells undergo division to reach their differentiated state. Deleterious mutations in those genes which are not expressed in the differentiated state will tend to accumulate over time. When this differentiated tissue is placed in culture, additional deleterious mutations will tend to accumulate in those genes which are not expressed in the cultured state. Therefore it is not all surprising if genetic variation is obtained in plants regenerated from cultured cells. For example, 5% of the plants regenerated from 30-day-old tobacco callus expressed variant leaf colors, shapes, and sizes. After 255 days in culture the frequency of variants rose to 40% (Barvier and Dulieu, 1980). The genetype can also be important in genetic stability during culture. For instance, the oat cultivar Lodi produced twofold fewer variants than the cultivar Tippecanoe during the same period in culture (McCoy et al., 1982).

Cultured cells are under little genetic regulation and have relatively short generation time; thus a wide array of variants can be isolated. A number of amino acid auxotrophs have been selected in both tobacco and carrot cell cultures. Tobacco cells have also been selected which are able to grow in the absence of cytokinin hormones (Meins, 1983). These habituated cells are, however, not true genetic mutants, for the habituation occurs at very high rates and is regularly reversible. In addition, the altered phenotype is not transmitted sexually. This nongenetic variation has been termed epigenetic. Epigenetic variation may be produced through a number of different processes. The migration of transposable elements, for example, is known to reversibly alter the expression of both structural and regulatory genes. Epigenetic variation, even though reversible, can be quite stable. It raises the possibility that many of the so-called mutants which have been isolated in cell cultures are produced through changes in gene expression and not through changes in the gene itself.

GENETIC MANIPULATION

Tissue culture can be very important in gene transfer (Kleinhofs and Behki, 1977; Lurquin and Kado, 1979). It is possible to modify the genetic makeup of a single cell and then regenerate a whole plant with the modified phenotype from that modified cell (Morton et al., 1978). There are numerous methods for introducing foreign genetic material into plant cells. Methods are now available for creating somatic hybrids by fusing protoplasts. In this manner hybrid plants can be created from sexually incompatible species. Techniques are also available to create cells called cybrids, which are a type of hybrid in which only the organellar or cytoplasmic genomes are in a hybrid state, and not the nuclear genome. Additional technology exists for introducing foreign genes into host cells through the microinjection of protoplasts, the chemically induced uptake of DNA, nuclei, chromosomes or organelles by protoplasts, the use of the Ti plasmid from *Agrobacterium* as a DNA vector, and the use of artificially created lipid vesicles in cell fusion (Griesbach, 1984).

Tissue-cultured cells can be used effectively to produce new genetic variability; however, care must be taken in selecting the most appropriate means for producing or introducing specific types of variation (Sybenga, 1983). We now have an abundance of biotechnology but still lack the basic understanding of plant development, physiology, and genetics required to apply this technology to plant improvement.

REFERENCES

Barbier, M. and Dulieu, H. (1980). Effets génétiques observés sur des plantes de tabac regénérées à partir de cotylédons par culture in vitro. *Ann. Amelior. Plant. 30*: 321–344.

Bayless, M. (1977). The effect of 2,4-D on growth and mitosis in suspension cultures of *Daucus*. *Plant Sci. Lett. 8*: 99–103.

Brown, N. and Gardener, F. (1936). Galls produced by plant hormones, including a hormone extracted from *Bacterium tumefaciens*. *Phytopathology 26*:708–713.

Bush, S., Carle, E., and Langhans, R. (1976). Plantlets from petal, petal epidermis and shoot tips of the peridinal chimera *Chrysantheumu morifolium*. *Am. J. Bot. 63*:729–737.

Butenko, R. (1979). Cultivation of isolated protoplasts and hybridization of somatic cells. *Int. Rev. Cytol. 59*:323–372.

Carlson, P., Smith, H., and Dearing, R. (1972). Parasexual interspecific plant hybridization. *Proc. Nat. Acad. Sci. U.S.A. 69*:2292–2294.

Christianson, M., Warnick, D., and Carlson, P. (1983). A morphogenetically competent soybean suspension culture. *Science 222*:632–634.

Ching, C., Chu, W., San, S., Chen, E., Chu, Y., Yin, C., and Yun, B. (1975). Establishment of an efficient medium for anther culture of rice through comparative experiments on nitrogen sources. *Sci. Sin. 18*:559–668.

Fonnesbech, M. (1972). Growth hormones and propagation of *Cymbididum in vitro*. *Physiol. Plant. 27*:310–316.

Fraley, R., Rogers, S., Horsch, R., Sanders, P., Flick, J., Adams, S., Bittner, M., Brand, L., Fink, C., Fry, J., Galluppi, G., Goldberg, S., Hoffman, N., and Woo, S. (1983). Expression of bacterial genes in plant cells. *Proc. Nat. Acad. Sci. U.S.A. 80*:4803–4807.

Fritsh, H., and Grisebach, H. (1975). Biosynthesis of cyanidin in cell cultures of *Haplopappus*. *Phytochemistry 14*:2437–2442.

Gamborg, O. and Eveleigh, D. (1968). Culture methods and detection of gluconases in suspension cultures of wheat and barley. *Can. J . Biochem. 46*:417–421.

Gamborg, O. and Wetter, L. (1975). *Plant Tissue Culture Methods*, National Research Council, Canada, Saskatchewan.

Gamborg, O., Miller, R., and Ojima, K. (1968). Nutrient requirements of suspension cultures of soybean root cells. *Exp. Cell Res. 50*:151–158.

Gautheret, R. (1939). Sur la possibilité de réaliser la culture indéfinie des tissus de tubercules de carotte. *C. R. Acad. Sci.* *208*:188–121.

Gerats, A., de Vlaming, P., Doodeman, M., Al. E., and Schram, A. (1982). Genetic control of the conversion of dihydroflavonols into flavonols and anthocyanins in flowers of *Petunia hybrida*. *Annu. Rev. Plant Physiol.* *32*:277–266.

Goloff, A., Black, D., Romano, J., and Lawrence, R. (1979). Selective induction of adventure shoot and/or root morphogenesis in cultured lettuce leaf explants. *In Vitro* *19*:19.

Griesbach, R. (1984). An introduction to somatic cell genetics. *HortScience* *19*:367–371.

Guha, S. and Maheshwari, S. (1964). *In vitro* production of embryos from anthers of *Datura*. *Nature* *204*:497.

Haberlandt, G. (1902). Culturversuche mit isolierten Pflanzenzellen. *Sitzungsber. Kaiser Akad. Wiss.* *111*:69–92.

Hahlbrock, K. and Grisebach, H. (1979). Enzymic controls in the biosynthesis of lignin and flavonoids. *Annu. Rev. Plant Physiol.* *33*:609–650.

Hannig, E. (1904). Zur Physiologie pflanzlicher Embryonen. *Bot. Z.* *62*:45–80.

Hilding, A. and Welander, T. (1976). Effects of some factors on propagation of *Begonia* x *hiemalis in vitro*. *Swed. J. Agric. Res.* *6*:191–199.

Hölters, J. (1983). Möglichkeiten der vegetativen Vermehrung von *Phalaenopsis*. *Orchidie* *34*:78–82, 119–122, 208–210, 231–236.

Horsch, R., Fraley, R., Rogers, S., Sanders, P., Lloyd, A., and Hoffmann, N. (1984). Inheritance of functional foreign genes in plants. *Science* *223*:496–498.

Hrazdina, G., Wanger, G., and Siegelman, H. (1978). Subcellular localization of enzymes of anthocyanin biosynthesis in protoplasts. *Phytochemistry* *17*:53–56.

Ibrahim, R. K., Thakur, M. L., and Permanand, B. (1971). Formation of anthocyanins in callus tissue cultures. *Lloydia* *34*:175–182.

Jonsson, L. M., Aarsman, M. E., Schram, A. W., and Bennink, G. J. (1982a). Methylation of anthocyanins by cell-free extract of flower buds of *Petunia hybridia*. *Phytochemistry* *21*:2457–2459.

Jonsson, L. M., Donker-Koopman, W. E., Uitslager, P., and Schram, A. W. (1982b). Subcellular localization of anthcyanin methyltransferase in flower of *Petunia hybrida*. *Plant Physiol.* *72*:287–290.

Kadkade, P. and Siebert, M. (1977). Phytochrome regulated organogenesis in lettuce tissue culture. *Nature* *270*:49–50.

Kleinhofs, A. and Behki, R. (1977). Prospects for plant genome modification by non-conventional methods. *Annu. Rev. Genet.* *11*:79–102.

Larkin, P. and Scowcroft, W. (1981). Somaclonal variation—A novel source of variability from cell cultures for plant improvement. *Theor. Appl. Gelet.* *60*:197–214.

Lazar, M., Collins, G., and Vian, W. (1983). Genetic and environmental effects on the growth and differentiation of wheat somatic cell cultures. *J. Hered.* *74*:353–357.

Ludden, P. and Carlson, P. (1980). Use of plant cell cultures in biochemistry. In *Biochemistry of Plants*, Academic, New York, pp. 55–90.

Lurquin, P. and Kado, C. (1979). Recent advances in the insertion of DNA into high plant cells. *Plant Cell Environ.* *2*:251–256.

McCoy, T., Phillips, R., and Rines, H. (1982). Cytogenetic analysis of plants regenerated from oat tissue cultures: High frequency of partial chromosome loss. *Can. J. Genet. Cytol.* *24*:37–50.

Malmberg, R. (1979). Regeneration of whole plants from callus culture of diverse genetic lines of *Pisum sativum*. *Planta 146*: 243–244.

Marton, L., Nagy, F., Gupta, K., and Maliga, P. (1978). 5-Budr resistant tobacco cells incorporating the analogue into DNA. *Plant Sci. Lett.* *12*:333–341.

Margara, J. (1969). Etude des facteurs de la néoformation de bourgeons en culture chez le choufleur. *Ann. Physiol. Veg.* *11*:95–112.

Meins, F. (1983). Heritable variation in plant cell culture. *Annu. Rev. Plant Physiol.* *34*:327–346.

Miller, C., Skoog, F., Okumura, F., Saltza, F., and Strong, F. (1956). Isolation, structure and synthesis of kinetin, a substance promoting cell division. *J. Am. Chem. Soc.* *78*:1375–1380.

Murashige, T. and Nakano, R. (1967). Chromosome complement as a determinant of the morphogenetic potential of tobacco cells. *Am. J. Bot.* *54*:963–970.

Murashige, T. and Nakano, R. (1968). The light requirement for shoot initiation in tobacco callus cultures. *Am. J. Bot.* 55:710.

Murashige, T. and Skoog, F. (1962). A revised medium for rapid growth and bioassays with tobacco tissue cultures. *Physiol. Plant* *15*:473–497.

Narayanaswamy, S. (1977). Regeneration of plants from tissue cultures. In *Applied and Fundamental Aspects of Plant Cell, Tissue and Organ Culture* (J. Reinert and Y. Baja, eds.), Springer-Verlag, Berlin, pp. 179–206.

Nobecourt, P. (1939). Sur la pérennite et l'augmentation de volumes des cultures de tissu végétaux. *C.R. Soc. Biol.* *130*:1270–1271.

Ooms, O., Hooykaas, P., Moolenaar, G., and Schileroort, R. (1981). Crown gall plant tumours of abnormal morphology, induced by *Agrobacterium* carrying mutated octapine Ti plasmids. *Gene* *14*:33–50.

Parke, D. and Carlson, P. (1979). Somatic cell genetics of higher plants: Appraising the application of bacterial systems to higher plant cells in culture. In *Phsiological Genetics*, Academic, New York, pp. 196–237.

Pillai, S. and Hildebrandt, A. (1969). Induced differentiation of geranium plants from undifferentiated callus *in vitro*. *Am. J. Bot. 50*:52–58.

Pierik, R., van Leeuwan, L., and Rigter, G. (1979). Regeneration of leaf explants of anthurium *in vitro*. *Neth. J. Agric. Sci. 27*:221–226.

Raju, M. and Mann, H. (1970). Regenerative studies in the detached leaves of *Echeveria elegans*: Anatomy and regeneration of leaves in sterile culture. *Can. J. Bot. 48*:1887–1891.

Reinert, J. and White, P. (1956). The cultivation *in vitro* of tumor tissues and normal tissues of *Picea*. *Physiol. Plant 9*:117–189.

Skoog, F. and Miller, C. (1957). Chemical regulation of growth and organ formation in plant tissues cultured *in vitro*. *Symp. Soc. Exp. Biol. 11*:118–130.

Street, H. (1973). Cell suspension cultures—Techniques. In *Plant Tissue Culture* (Street, ed.), University of California Press, Los Angeles, pp. 59–97.

Sybenga, J. (1983). Genetic manipulation in plant breeding: Somatic vs. generative. *Theor. Appl. Genet. 66*:179–201.

Takebe, I., Labib, G., and Melchers, G. (1971). Regeneration of whole plants from isolated mesophyll protoplasts of tobacco. *Naturwissenschaften 58*:318–320.

Tanaka, M. and Sakanishi, Y. (1978). Clonal propagation of phalaenopsis through leaf tissue culture. *Am. Orchid Soc. Bull. 46*:733–735.

Thorpe, T. and Murashige, T. (1970). Some histological changes underlying shoot initiation in tobacco callus cultures. *Can. J. Bot. 48*:277–285.

Torrey, J. (1977). Cytodifferentiation in cultured cells and tissues. *HortScience 12*:138–139.

Uchimiya, H. and Murashige, T. (1976). Influence of the nutrient medium on the recovery of dividing cells from tobacco protoplasts. *Plant Physiol. 57*:424–429.

White, P. (1934). Potentially unlimited growth of excised tomato root tips in a liquid medium. *Plant Physiol. 9*:585–600.

White, P. (1939). Potentially unlimited growth of excised plant callus in an artificial nutrient medium. *Am. J. Bot. 26*:59–64.

Widholm, J. (1977). Selection and characterization of amino acid analog resistant plant cells cultures. *Crop Sci. 17*:597–600.

Yeoman, M. (1973). Tissue callus cultures—Techniques. In *Plant Tissue Culture* (Street, ed.), University of California Press, Los Angeles, pp. 31–58.

Yoshida, F. and Watanabe, H. (1971). Effects of mineral nutrients on chlorophyll contents, friability and yield of cultured tobacco callus. *Bull. Fac. Agric. Tamagawa Univ.* *11*:3–13.

Zaenen, I., Larebeke, N., Teuchy, H., Montagu, M., and Shell, J. (1974). Super coiled DNA in crown-gall inducing *Agrobacterium* strains. *J. Mol. Biol.* *56*:109–127.

11

Immobilization of Microbial and Cultured Plant Cells

DIETRICH KNORR / University of Delaware,
Newark, Delaware

INTRODUCTION

Immobilization has been characterized as a technique that confines a catalytically active enzyme or cell within a reactor system and prevents its entry into the mobile phase which carries the substrate and product (Rosevear, 1984). Biocatalysts can be immobilized by confinement within a porous membrane (i.e., gel entrapment, membrane reactor, interfacial membrane) or by attachment to a solid surface (i.e., inner surface of a porous structure, outer surface of a carrier by adsorption or covalent bond). Physical entrapment in a porous matrix is the most flexible and most popular approach employed for whole cell immobilization (Freeman, 1984; Klein and Vorlop, 1983). According to Freeman (1984), a process designed for the efficient entrapment of whole cells should allow for the following:

1. High retention of cell *viability*. The biological activity of the entrapped cells should not be impaired by the immobilization conditions.
2. The *porosity* of the formed gel should be uniform and controllable. Free exchange of substrates, products, cofactors, gases, and so forth, is essential for efficient performance of the immobilized cells.
3. The gel obtained should retain good mechanical, chemical, and biological *stability*. It should not be easily degraded by enzymes, solvents, pressure changes, or shearing forces.
4. The gel should be composed of reasonably priced components and the process should be amenable to ready scale-up.

Table 1. Some Advantages of Immobilized Microbial or Plant Cell Reactors over Traditional Batch Fermentation

Reuse of biocatalysts (due to entrapment)
Maintenance of stable and active biocatalysts (due to separation of cell growth and metabolite production, due to entrapment)
Accelerated reaction rates (due to high cell densities and elimination of nonproductive cell growth phases)
High volumetric productivity (due to continuous process and removal of desired metabolites and metabolic inhibitors, etc.)
Improved process control (due to continuous process, product separation, removal of metabolic inhibitions)
Improved product recovery (due to physical separation of biocatalyst and desired products within the reactor)
Increased possibilities for secondary metabolite formation (due to cell aggregation)
Improved efficiency of production (due to reuse of biocatalysts, recycling of cofactors and coenzymes, high reaction rates, removal of inhibitors)

Immobilization provides various advantages over traditional batch fermentation processes with freely suspended cells (Table 1), including maintenance of stable and active biocatalysts over long periods of time, accelerated reaction rates, high volumetric productivity, and improved product recovery.

MICROBIAL CELLS

Biochemical processing using immobilized microbial cells is a relatively new approach to biocatalysis (Venkatsubramanian, 1979). However, despite this fact, several semicommercial and commercial processes are already in operation (Klibanov, 1983; Knorr and Sinskey, 1985; Nagashima et al., 1983; Samejima et al., 1985; Mattiasson, 1983; Venkatsubramanian, 1979).

Immobilization of Microbial Cells

The following categorization of methods for the immobilization of microbial cells has been provided by Klein and Wagner (1983):

1. Physical crosslinking (flocculation)
2. Covalent crosslinking
3. Adsorption on insoluble matrices
4. Covalent binding to insoluble matrices
5. Physical entrapment in porous materials
6. Encapsulation

Klein and Wagner (1983) also classified immobilization methods for whole cells with respect to the type of bonding in the catalyst, differentiating between bonding (secondary bonding, i.e., adsorption, flocculation; covalent bonding, i.e., carrier bonding, crosslinking) and physical entrapment (i.e., entrapment, encapsulation).

The above categorization deals with the state of the immobilized biocatalyst. Using the route along which the biocatalysts have been prepared, Klein and Wagner (1983) suggested four categories: (1) carrier-free immobilization, (2) immobilization of a given biomass onto a preformed carrier, (3) immobilization of a given biomass in the course of carrier preparation, and (4) immobilization by growth of immobilized cells. The first category includes compartmentalization of cells by adsorption (i.e., flocculation, pelletization, use of flocculating aids) or covalent crosslinking (i.e., direct chemical crosslinking of cells with bivalent coupling reagents such as glutaraldehyde) with each other. Immobilization onto a preformed carrier requires that rather large cell entities adhere to the outer and inner surfaces of the carrier, with reasonable stability against washout. Here attachment can be achieved by adsorption or covalent bonding using porous carriers, including hollow fiber membranes. The third category provided by Klein and Wagner (1983) includes entrapment and encapsulation, which will be discussed in more detail below. Growth of immobilized cells within the biocatalyst is done by either incubation of freshly prepared biocatalysts under suitable growth conditions or reactivation of the biocatalyst after a certain degree of deactivation for both one-step and multistep enzyme systems. Guidelines for the characterization of immobilized biocatalysts have been developed by the European Federation of Biotechnology (Anonymous, 1983).

Entrapment of Microbial Cells

Entrapment methods are based on the inclusion of cells within a rigid network to prevent the cells from diffusing into the surrounding medium, while still allowing mass transfer of nutrients and metabolites (Durand and Navarro, 1978). Entrapment in polymeric carriers has been classified into polymeric networks from oligomeric precursors (i.e., epoxy resins, polyurethane networks from polycondensation, photocrosslinking oligomers) and polymeric networks from long-chain prepolymers (Klein and Wagner, 1983). This last group requires subcategorization and has been organized into precipitation (i.e., cellulose, cellulose triacetate), gelation (i.e., gelatin, agar, κ-carrageenan, collagen), inotropic gelation (i.e., alginates, chitosan), and covalent crosslinking using, for example, albumin, collagen, gelatin as polymers and glutaraldehyde as crosslinking agent (Chibata and Tosa, 1981; Durand and Navarro, 1978; Klein and Wagner, 1983). Numerous matrices have been employed for entrapment and have been summarized in the above-mentioned reviews. Recent examples of polymer matrices are given in Table 2, which indicates that calcium alginate and polyacrylamide are the most commonly used polymers.

Calcium alginate gel provides a mild and simple immobilization procedure but has the disadvantage of being unstable in the presence of various complexing anions such as phosphate (Paul and Vignais, 1980; Dainty et al., 1986; Klein and Wagner, 1983). Freeman and Aharonowitz (1981) showed that cell damage generally caused by the acrylamide monomer was avoided when *Streptomyces clavuligerus* cells were suspended in a solution of preformed, linear, water-soluble polyacrylamide chains partially substituted with acylhydrazide groups. The prepolymerized backbone was then crosslinked by stoichiometric amounts of dialdehydes. Comparison of various gel systems (Tuli et al., 1985) showed that agar was more effective than polyacrylamide for *Lactobacillus casei* entrapment and lactic acid production. In addition, the highest activity of an entrapped methanogenic population was found in agar gel as compared to collagen or polyacrylamide (Karube et al., 1980). Comparison of polyacrylamide, foam particles of bovine serum albumin, calcium alginate, and κ-carrageenan revealed highest L-tryptophan production by *Escherichia coli* entrapped in the κ-carrageenan matrix (Langrene et al., 1984). Calcium alginate gel-entrapped methanogenic bacterium cells were found to be active for a longer period of time than freely suspended ones (Scherer et al., 1981) and activities of immobilized cells generally were reported to be about 60–80% (Vorlop and Klein, 1983; Bang et al., 1983; Matsunaga et al., 1983). A threefold increase in the half-life of patulin production was found for κ-carrageenan-entrapped *Penicillium urticae* as compared to freely suspended ones (Deo and Gaucher, 1983). Comparison of numerous polymers resulted in high ethanol production from *Saccharomyces cerevisiae* cells in calcium alginate gel, carrageenan gel, agar gel, and silica sol (Samejima et al., 1984). Immobilization of *Rhizopus nigricans* in polyacrylamide resulted in loss of ability to 11α-hydroxylate progesterone, while agar gel- and alginate gel-entrapped cells proved capable of hydroxylation, with agar gels displaying faster rates and higher yields (Maddox et al., 1981).

Table 2. Recent Examples of Entrapment of Microbial Cells in Polymer Matrices

Polymer matrix	Organism	Product or conversion	References
Calcium alginate	*Mycobacterium*	Ethylene oxide	De Bont et al. (1983)
	Nitrosomonas europaea	NH_4^+ to NO_2^-	Van Ginkel et al. (1983)
	Saccharomyces cerevisiae, Saccharomyces ovarum, Zymomonas mobilis	Ethanol	McGhee et al. (1982), Linko et al. (1984)
	Methanogenic population	Methane	Karube et al. (1980)
	Saccharomyces cerevisiae	Ethanol	Williams and Munnecke (1981), Samejima et al. (1984)
	Methanosarcina barkeri	Methanole to methane	Scherer et al. (1981)
	Kluyveromyces marxianus	Inulin to fructose	Bajpai and Margaritis (1985)
	Pichia etchellsii	Cellobiose to glucose	Jain and Ghose (1984)
	Pachysolen tannohilus	D-Xylose to ethanol	Slininger et al. (1982)
	Kluyveromyces marxianus	Whey to ethanol	Marwaha and Kennedy (1984)
	Lactobacillus bulgaricus, Lactobacillus pentosus, Lactobacillus helveticus	Lactic acid	Linko et al. (1984)

Table 2. Recent Examples of Entrapment of Microbial Cells in Polymer Matrices (Continued)

Polymer matrix	Organism	Product or conversion	References
κ-Carrageenan	*Klyveromyces marxianus*	Whey to ethanol	Marwaha and Kennedy (1984), King and Zall (1983)
	Zymomonas mobilis	Ethanol	Jain et al. (1985a,b)
	Penicillium chrysogenum	Penicillium G	Deo and Gaucher (1984)
	Serratia marcescens	L-Isoleucine	Fujimura et al. (1984), Wada et al. (1980)
	Penicillium urticae	Patulin	Jones et al. (1983), Deo and Gaucher (1983)
	Tolypocladium inflatum	Cyclosporin A	Foster et al. (1983)
	Escherichia coli	L-Tryptophan	Langrene et al. (1984), Klein et al. (1984)
	Rhodopseudomonas capsulata	Hydrogen	Francou and Vignais (1984)
	Corynebacterium glutamicum	Glutamate	Kim and Ryu (1982)
	Saccharomyces cerevisiae	Ethanol	Wang and Hettwer (1982), Marwaha and Kennedy (1984)
Chitosan	*Escherichia coli*	Tryptophan	Vorlop and Klein (1983)
	Pseudomonas sp.	L-Tyrosine	Stöcklein et al. (1983)

	Clostridum butyricum	Hydrogen	Matsunaga et al. (1980)
Agar	*Rhizopus nigricans*	11α-Hydroxyprogesterone	Maddox et al. (1981)
	Thermophilic population	Methane	Matsunaga et al. (1983)
	Lactobacillus casei	Lactic acid	Tuli et al. (1985)
Collagen	*Brevibacterium flavum*	Glutamic acid	Constantinides et al. (1981)
	Clostridium butyricum	Hydrogen	Matsunaga et al. (1980)
	Methanogenic microorganism	Methane	Karube et al. (1980)
Polyacrylamide	*Aspergillus niger*	Citric acid	Horitsu et al. (1985)
	Saccharomycopsis lipolytica	Citric acid	Maddox and Kingston (1983)
	Streptomyces fradiae	Protease	Kokubu et al. (1981)
	Escherichia coli	L-Tryptophan	Bang et al. (1983)
	Lactobacillus casei	Lactic acid	Tuli et al. (1985)
	Saccharomyces formosensis	Ethanol	Furusaki et al. (1983)
	Escherichia coli	L-Tryptophan	Langrene et al. (1984)
	Methanogenic microorganism	Methane	Karube et al. (1980)
	Corynebacterium dismutans	Alanine	Sarkar and Myaudon (1983)

Immobilized growing cells were found to grow very well in κ-carrageenan gels and increased in cell concentration from 3×10^3 to 6×10^7 cells per milliliter of gel at the initial state to 5×10^9 to 4×10^{10} cells per milliliter of gel at steady state using continuous fluidized bed and packed column reactors (Wada et al., 1979). The maximum population of κ-carrageenan-entrapped *Serratia marcescens* cells increased to five times that of free cells when the diffusion barrier to oxygen transport created by the gel matrix was overcome by the supply of pure oxygen (Fujimura et al., 1984).

Stability of Immobilized Microbial Cells

Half-lives of immobilized microbial cells from various studies have been summarized by Durand and Navarro (1978) and range from 5 to 140 days. Recent data on the duration of biocatalyst stability (or the duration of the experiment) in continuous processes are given in Table 3, with a maximum of over 6 months (Nagashima et al., 1984). Also, the heat stability of immobilized microbial cells has been found to be higher than that of freely suspended cells (Durand and Navarro, 1978).

Coentrapment Procedures and Cofermentation Processes

According to Hahn-Hägerdahl (1984), coimmobilization composed of two biocatalytic species should be compared to a mixed-culture fermentation and should have all the advantages of immobilized preparations. Immobilization of β-D-glucosidase on conconavalin-A-Sepharose and coentrapment of the immobilized enzyme with *Zymomonas mobilis* in calcium alginate gel spheres both effectively converted cellobiose to ethanol in batch as well as in continuous-flow fermentation systems (Lee et al., 1983). Lee et al. (1983) also observed a markedly reduced susceptibility to inhibition by high substrate concentrations using β-glucosidase and *S. cerevisiae* cells in calcium alginate gels for the conversion of cellobiose in ethanol. The coimmobilized preparation was found superior to a combination of separately immobilized biocatalysts, which reached conversions of 80 and 40%, respectively (Hahn-Hägerdahl, 1984). Hartmeier (1984) reached approximate methanol yields when using *S. cerevisiae*, β-galactosidase, and β-glucosidase. Coentrapment of Sepharose-immobilized β-glucosidase and *Talaromyces emersonii* cells in calcium alginate gel also resulted in an effective conversion of cellobiose (Kierstan et al., 1982). Simultaneous saccharification and fermentation of cellulose to ethanol using *Penicillium funiculosum* cellulase and gel-immobilized *Saccharomyces uvarum* has been reported (Deshpande et al., 1983). The advantages of such a cofermentation system are increased ethanol yields, due to removal of end-product inhibition, and elimination of the need for a separate reactor, which reduces the cost of ethanol production.

Continuous Immobilized Microbial Cell Reactors

Some examples of continuous immobilized microbial cell reactors as available in the literature have been summarized in Table 3. Most of these data have been collected on laboratory- or pilot plant-scale reactors. However, industrial application of immobilized microbial cell reactors has also been reported (Klein and Wagner, 1983). As is evident from Table 3, ethanol production has received the most attention and calcium alginate is the most commonly used polymer for entrapment procedures.

Productivity of continuous reactor systems was reportedly superior to batch fermentation using either free or immobilized cells (Krouwel et al., 1983; Inloes et al., 1983; Kim and Ryu, 1982; McGhee et al., 1984). For example, production of high-quality beer with a low content of diacetyl precursors within 1 day was achieved in a packed column reactor, as compared to a conventional batch fermentation of about 8 days, representing a twofold increase in productivity per reaction volume (Onaka et al., 1985). It is interesting to note that Prevost et al. (1985) found higher lactic acid production rates when *Lactobacillus bulgaricus* and *Streptococcus thermophilus* were entrapped in separate calcium alginate beads as compared to coimmobilized biocatalysts.

The mechanical properties, especially mechanical stability (i.e., compression behavior), of biocatalysts have been stressed as an important engineering aspect of scale-up procedures (Klein and Wagner, 1983); however, only limited information is available as of yet. A comparison of the physical stability of calcium alginate beads in an air-lift reactor versus a stirred tank reactor revealed higher stability in the air-lift reactor (Kloosterman and Lilly, 1985). A "drum reactor" was reported (Tanaka et al., 1983) to be ideal for the reaction of immobilized cells, since it provided little mechanical stress to the biocatalysts. The kinetic performance of the biocatalyst is of key importance to reactor performance (Klein and Wagner, 1983; Klein et al., 1984; Tanaka et al., 1984a; Karkare et al., 1985). However, as Radovich (1985) suggests in an excellent review, the influence of interparticle and intraparticle mass transfer in the performance of immobilized living cells has not been thoroughly examined in the literature and much work is needed on the development of reactor design equations which account for the mass transfer effects.

Table 3. Examples of Continuous, Immobilized Microbial Cell Reactors

Organism	Immobilization method	Reactor
Saccharomyces cerevisiae	"Synthetic sponge"	Rotating disk
Acetobacter aceti	Cordierite (ceramic)	Pulsed flow (fixed bed)
S. cerevisiae, S. uvarum	Porous support particles	Fluidized bed, circulating bed
S. cerevisiae	Pectin gel	"Horizontal reactor"
Brevibacterium ammoniagenes	Radiation copolymerization	Drum reactor
Penicillium chrysogenum	κ-Carrageenan	Fluidized bed
Penicillium urticae	Carrageenan	Stirred tank
Tolypocladium inflatum	Carrageenan	Airlift
Corynebacterium glutamicum	κ-Carrageenan	Air-stirred
Streptomyces cattleya	Cellite particles	Bubble column
Escherichia coli	Hollow fiber membrane	Hollow fiber membrane
S. cerevisiae	Alginate/micronisized silica	Crossflow
Clostridium beijerinckii	Ca-alginate	Packed bed
S. uvarum	Gelatin	Packed bed
S. cerevisiae	Alginate	Fluidized bed
S. cerevisiae	Dialysis membrane	Stirred tank
Aspergillus terreus	Ca-alginate	Column
Arthrobacter simplex	Ca-alginate	Air-lift

Product or conversion	Biocatalyst stability or duration of experiment	References
Ethanol	—	De Borghi et al. (1985)
Acetic acid	—	Ghomidh et al. (1982)
Ethanol	113 days	Black et al. (1984)
Ethanol	30 days	Navarro et al. (1984)
NADP	90 hr	Tanaka et al. (1983)
Penicillin G	16 days	Deo and Gaucher (1984)
Patulin	440 hr	Jones et al. (1983)
Cyclosporin	18 days	Foster et al. (1983)
Glutamate	30 days	Kim and Ryu (1982)
Thienamycin	240 hr	Arcuri et al. (1983)
Protein	23 days	Inloes et al. (1983)
Ethanol	270 hr	Chotani and Constantinides (1984)
Isopropanol, butanol	290 hr	Krouwel et al. (1983)
Ethanol	—	Mohite and SivaRaman (1984)
Ethanol	6 months	Nagashima et al. (1984)
Ethanol	—	Kyung and Gerhardt (1984)
Itaconic acid	2 weeks	Kautola et al. (1985)
Dehydrogenation	—	Kloosterman and Lilly (1985)

Table 3. Examples of Continuous, Immobilized Microbial Cell Reactors

Organism	Immobilization method	Reactor
Lactobacillus bulgaricus, *Streptococcus thermophilus*	Ca-alginate	Stirred tank
S. cerevisiae	Polyacrylamide	Stirred tank
S. cerevisiae	Ca-alginate	Packed column
Yeast	Ca-alginate	Packed column
S. uvarum	Ca-alginate	Packed column
Bacillus sp.	Polyacrylamide	Air-bubbled
Hansenula polymorpha	Polyacrylamide	Modified ultrafiltration unit
S. cerevisiae	κ-Carrageenan	"Fluidized slurry"
S. cerevisiae	Ca-alginate	Column
Leuconostoc aenos	Ca-alginate	Packed bed

CULTURED PLANT CELLS

The basis of cellular theory (Schleiden, 1838; Schwann, 1839) was postulated about 150 years ago and the principles of cell culture were formulated at the beginning of the century (Haberlandt, 1902; Gautheret, 1983). Meanwhile the feasibility of plant tissue culture for the improvement of plant food functionality and nutritional quality has been well established (Chaleff, 1984; Sharp et al., 1984; Teutonico and Knorr, 1984, 1985a). Also, a large variety of secondary metabolites useful for the food industry have been isolated from cultured plant cells (Nickel, 1980; Sahai and Knuth, 1985) and the commercial production of at least one metabolite has been achieved (Curtin, 1983).

Product or conversion	Biocatalyst stability or duration of experiment	References
Yogurt	—	Prevost et al. (1985)
Fructose, gluconic acid	—	D'Souza and Nadkarni (1980)
Ethanol	20 days	Lee et al. (1983)
Ethanol	12 days	McGhee et al. (1984)
Beer	—	Onake et al. (1985)
Bacitracin	10 days half-life	Morikawa et al. (1980)
Oxidation	6–30 hr half-life	Couderc and Baratti (1980)
Ethanol	—	Karkare et al. (1985)
Ethanol	1000 hr	Samejima et al. (1984)
Wine	15 days	Spettoli et al. (1984)

Until recently one limiting factor to the development of the large-scale production of metabolites was production costs, with a previous estimation suggesting that only products valued at more than $500 or even $1000 per kilogram were worth producing via plant tissue culture (Brodelius, 1984; Curtin, 1983; Goldstein, 1983; Sahai and Knuth, 1985). However, current estimates indicate that technical advances, especially the development of continuous biocatalytic processes, can enable the production of plant metabolites in a price range of $20 to $50 per kilogram (Curtin, 1983; Sahai and Knuth, 1985). This makes the development of immobilized plant cell reactors for biocatalytic processes an essential part of the scale-up of plant cell culture systems.

Table 4. Various Polymers Used for Plant Cell Immobilization

Polymer	Gelling mechanism
Agar, agarose (carrageenan)	Thermal
Alginate, carrageenan, chitosan[a]	Ionotropic
Gelatin	Crosslinking with glutaraldehyde
Polyacrylamide	Radical polymerization of acrylamide and bisacrylamide
Alginate–chitosan, chitosan–alginate, or chitosan–carrageenan	Ionotropic, polyelectrolyte complex formation
Prepolymerized polyacrylamide	Crosslinking with dialdehyde

[a]With low molecular weight counterions.
Source: Brodelius (1984), Brodelius and Mosbach (1983), Knorr (1985a), Knorr and Teutonico (1985), Knorr et al. (1985), Vorlop and Klein (1983).

Immobilization of Cultured Plant Cells

Polymers commonly used for the immobilization of plant cells are summarized in Table 4.

Entrapment techniques have been used almost exclusively to immobilize plant cells (Table 5). They can be classified in three general groups (Brodelius and Mosbach, 1982; Vorlop and Klein, 1983): (1) gel formation by ionic crosslinking of a charged polymer (ionotropic); (2) gel formation by cooling of a heated polymer (thermal); and (3) gel formation by chemical reaction (crosslinking, radical polymerization).

Ionotropic gelation with a charged polyelectrolyte, such as alginic acid as the polyanion and calcium ions as low molecular weight multivalent counterions, as well as chitosan and polyphosphate, alginic acid, or κ-carrageenan as the high molecular weight counterion for polyelectrolyte complex formation have received much attention (Brodelius, 1984; Knorr, 1985a,b; Vorlop and Klein, 1983; Knorr and Teutonico, 1985). The unique properties of chitosan, including its polycationic nature, offer a wide variety of applications (Vorlop and Klein, 1983; Rha et al., 1985).

Cross-sectional views of part of a chitosan gel globule and a chitosan–alginate gel capsule are shown in Figure 1.

Table 5. Examples of Cultured Plant Cell Immobilization

Plant species	Immobilization method/polymer	Product	References
Amaranthus tricolor	Chitosan[a]	Oxalate	Knorr and Tuetonico (1985)
Asclepias syriaca	Chitosan[a]	Proteases	Miazga and Knorr (1985)
Catharanthus roseus	Agarose[a]	Ajmalicine isomers	Felix et al. (1981)
	Alginate[a]	Ajmalicine isomers	Brodelius et al. (1979)
	Alginate, agarose, agar, carrageenan[a]	Ajmalicine isomers	Brodelius and Nilsson (1983)
Capsicum frutescens	Polyurethane foam[b]	Capsaicin	Lindsey et al. (1983)
Daucus carota	Alginate[a]	Digoxin	Brodelius et al. (1979)
	Alginate[a]	5 β-Hydroxygitoxigenin	Veliky and Jones (1981)
Glycine max	Hollow fiber[a]	Phenolics	Shuler (1981)
Solanum aviculare	Covalent linkage/phenylene oxide	Steroid glycerols	Jirku et al. (1981)
Lavandula vera	Urethane prepolymers[a]	Pigments	Tanaka et al. (1984a)
	Agar, alginate, κ-carrageenan[a]	Pigments	Nakajima et al. (1985)

[a] Entrapment.
[b] Adsorption.

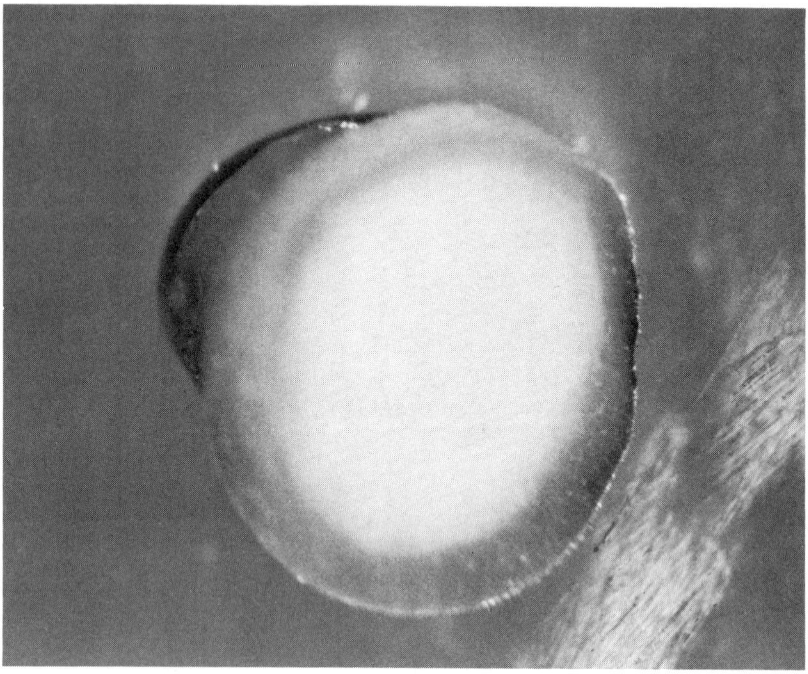

A

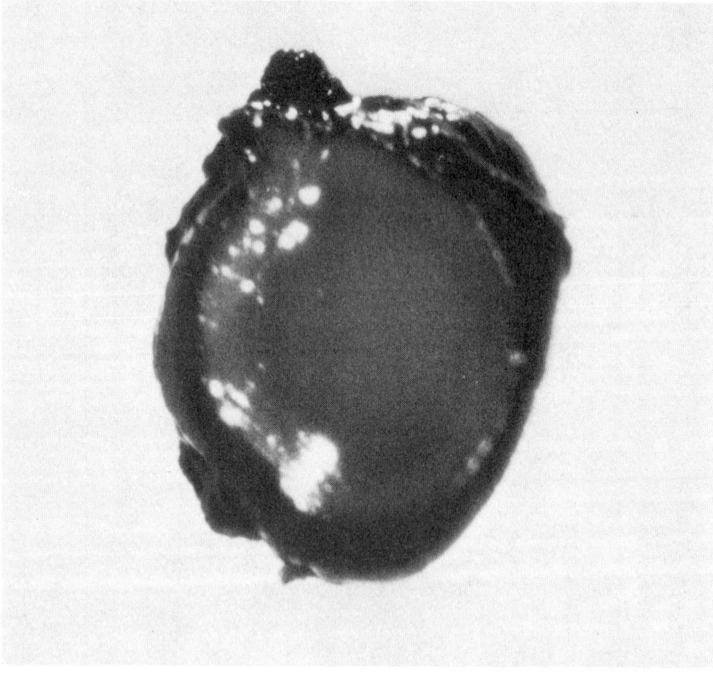

B

Fig. 1. Cross-sectional view of part of (A) a chitosan gel globule with a solid core and (B) a chitosan–alginate capsule with a liquid core and interphasic membrane.

Viability and Stability of Immobilized Plant Cell Systems

Effects of polymers used for cultured plant cell entrapment on their viability, plasmolysis, respiration, cell growth, and cell division are presented in Table 6. Plant cells in chemically prepared gel systems (gelatin, polyacrylamide) appeared to be dead after immobilization, while cells entrapped in various polysaccharides remained viable (Brodelius, 1983). This is of key importance, since one of the aims of selecting immobilization methods which are gentle and nontoxic is to provide viable immobilized cells. Stability of immobilized plant cell systems for over 7 months has been reported (Sahai and Knuth, 1985; Nakajima et al., 1985). High viability of plant cells was reported (Lindsey, et al., 1983) when plant cells were retained in polyurethane foam particles over a 21-day period. Increased stability of isolated protoplasts from *Vicia faba* and *Daucus carota* obtained by immobilization has been demonstrated with calcium alginate gels (Linse and Brodelius, 1984; Schnabl et al., 1983). This

Table 6. Effects of Polymers Used for Cultured Plant Cell Entrapment on Viability, Plasmolysis, Respiration, Cell Growth, and Cell Division

Polymer	Viability after immobilization	Plasmolysis	Respiration	Cell growth	Cell division
Agar	+	+	+	+	N.D.
Agarose	+	+	+	+	+
Alginate	+	+	+	+	+
κ-Carrageenan	+	+	+	+	N.D.
Chitosan	+	N.D.	N.D.	N.D.	N.D.
Gelatin	–	+	–	–	N.D.
Polyacrylamide	–	–	–	–	N.D.

Source: Knorr et al. (1985), with permission of the Institute of Food Technologists.

entrapment offers the possibility of increasing cell turgor of protoplasts and for studying membrane transport and cellular functions of wall-less cells under conditions where internal pressure has built up over a long period of time. This is of major importance, since Schnabl et al. (1983) questioned the validity of data obtained from nonentrapped, turgorless cells. In addition, isolated protoplasts, lacking plant cell walls, are very sensitive to mechanical stress, unstable, and only useful for short-term experiments.

Immobilized Plant Cell Reactors

Scale-up has been identified as crucial to the success of plant biotechnology (Curtin, 1983; Sahai and Knuth, 1985). Batch and continuous reactors using freely suspended cells have been developed for the production of secondary metabolites (Fowler, 1983; Furuya et al., 1984; Sahai and Shuler, 1982, 1984; Schmauder and Koblitz, 1979; Schmauder et al., 1984; Tanaka et al., 1983) and have been successful on a large scale in at least one case (Curtin, 1983). In addition, much of the reported work concentrated on immobilized cell reactors (Table 7) because of the various advantages of immobilized systems outlined in Table 1. An organization of immobilized plant cell reactors in gel-entrapped and membrane systems has been provided by Shuler et al. (1984) and a distinction between batch-type and continuous systems also seems useful. A simplified organization of immobilized plant cell reactors is provided in Table 8.

Batchtype fermentation processes have been identified as expensive processes in terms of both capital investment and production cost (Sahai and Knuth, 1985), while gel-entrapped systems have been generally considered as less expensive to initiate than membrane reactors (Shuler et al., 1984). On the other hand, membrane reactors are considered to provide better control over reactor fluid dynamics and flow distribution and they are also potentially reusable, since old cells can be flushed out and fresh cells can be pumped into the system (Sahai and Knuth, 1985; Sculer et al., 1984). The reactor types considered most promising are packed bed, fluidized bed, and hollow fiber membrane reactors (Prenosil and Pedersen, 1983; Sahai and Knuth, 1985).

Permeabilization of Immobilized Plant Cells

Many of the desired plant metabolites are stored within the producing cells, requiring release or extraction of these products. Although spontaneous release of products normally stored within the cell vacuoles has been observed in immobilized cells (Brodelius, 1984), release of intracellularly stored products is usually induced by

Table 7. Duration of Experiments with Gel-Entrapped Plant Tissue Culture Systems

Polymer	Plant species	Reactor	Duration of experiments	References
Agar	*Catharanthus roseus*	Batch	5–14 days	Brodelius and Nilsson (1983)
	Lavandula vera	Batch	3 weeks	Nakajima et al. (1985)
Agarose	*Catharanthus roseus*	Batch	1 day	Felix et al. (1981)
		Batch	5–14 days	Brodelius and Nilsson (1983)
Alginate	*Morinda citrofolia*	Batch	22 days	Brodelius et al. (1979)
	Catharanthus roseus	Recirculating packed column	90 hr	Brodelius et al. (1979)
	Daucus carota	Semicontinuous column	30 days	Veliky and Jones (1981)
	Lavandula vera	Batch	7 months	Nakajima et al. (1985)
κ-Carrageenan	*Catharanthus roseus*	Batch	5–14 days	Brodelius and Nilsson (1983)
	Lavandula vera	Batch	3 weeks	Nakajima et al. (1985)
Chitosan	*Amaranthus tricolor*	Batch	5 days	Knorr and Teutonico (1985)
	Asclepias syriaca	Batch	4 days	Miazga and Knorr (1985)

Table 8. Organization of Immobilized Plant Cell Reactors

Reactor type	References
Gel-entrapped systems	
Batch reactors	
Shake flasks	See Table 7
Continuous reactors	
Continuous stirred	Markkanen et al. (1984)
Air-lift	Markkanen et al. (1984)
Fluidized bed	Morris et al. (1983), Prenosil and Pedersen (1983)
Packed bed	Brodelius et al. (1979), Veliky and Jones (1981)
Membrane systems	
Continuous reactors	
Tubular membrane	Shuler (1981), Prenosil and Pedersen (1983), Shuler et al. (1985), Jose et al. (1983)
Multimembrane	Shuler et al. (1985)
Flat plate	Shuler et al. (1984)

Source: Knorr et al. (1985), with permission of the Institute of Food Technologists.

permeabilization of cell membranes with chemicals or by temperature treatment of the cell cultures. Various methods for permeabilization of plant cells are available, including toluene treatment (Lerner et al., 1978); dimethyl sulfoxide (DMSO) treatment, the most commonly used one (Brodelius, 1984); a treatment with dissolved chitosan (Young et al., 1982; Knorr and Teutonico, 1985); freeze–thaw treatment (Felix et al., 1981); and, most recently, treatment based on the high ionic strength of the extraction medium (Tanaka et al., 1985). Although procedures such as DMSO treatment are effective, they require treatment with the permeabilizing agent over a given period of time, removal of the permeabilizing agent, and subsequent washing of the cells. These steps are time-consuming, complicated continuous processes, can result in losses of plant metabolites produced during treatment and washing, and can add to the risk of microbial contamination of the cell cultures, already an issue of major concern in plant tissue culture procedures.

A combined immobilization–permeabilization process involving the "controlled release" of the permeabilizing agent from the polyelectrolyte(s) matrix used in the entrapment of the plant cell cultures has been designed (Knorr and Teutonico, 1985). Cell cultures of amaranth (*Amaranthus tricolor*) and common milkweed (*Asclepias syriaca* L.) were used to examine the effect of chitosan on the release of oxalate and protein, respectively (Knorr, 1985a; Miazga and Knorr, 1985). The data indicate that chitosan was effective in significantly ($p < .05$) increasing the release of oxalate, a low molecular weight plant metabolite, as well as proteins, high molecular weight substances. Although the mechanisms by which chitosan, a polycationic biopolymer (Knorr, 1984, 1985b), increases cell permeability is not clear (Young and Kauss, 1983), our results suggest that chitosan concurrently serves as an immobilizing and permeabilizing agent for cultured plant cells.

A simplified comparison of secondary plant metabolites production through batch fermentation, continuous immobilized, or continuous immobilized–permeabilized processes is presented in Figure 2 and suggests major advantages of the immobilized process and the immobilized–permeabilized process over the batch fermentation process. These include improved product recovery and productivity due to physical separation of plant cells from the fermentation medium and elimination of the nonproductive phases of a batch cycle by delinking growth and product formation functions, respectively (Sahai and Knuth, 1985), as well as other advantages already presented in Table 1.

Summary and Needs in Immobilized Microbial and Cultured Plant Cells Research

Many immobilization methods have been developed for microbial cells. There have been excellent reviews on the subject (Mattiasson, 1983; Venkatsubramanian, 1979; Klein and Wagner, 1983), useful classifications of immobilization methods have been provided (Klein and Wagner, 1983; Radovich, 1985), and guidelines for the characterization of biocatalysts have been developed (Anonymous, 1983). In addition, extensive work has been carried out on continuous immobilized systems and their performance (Radovich, 1985). The main challenges for future work include the need for scaling up existing laboratory-scale reactors and processes. Here the performance of polymer matrices (i.e., the structure–function relationship

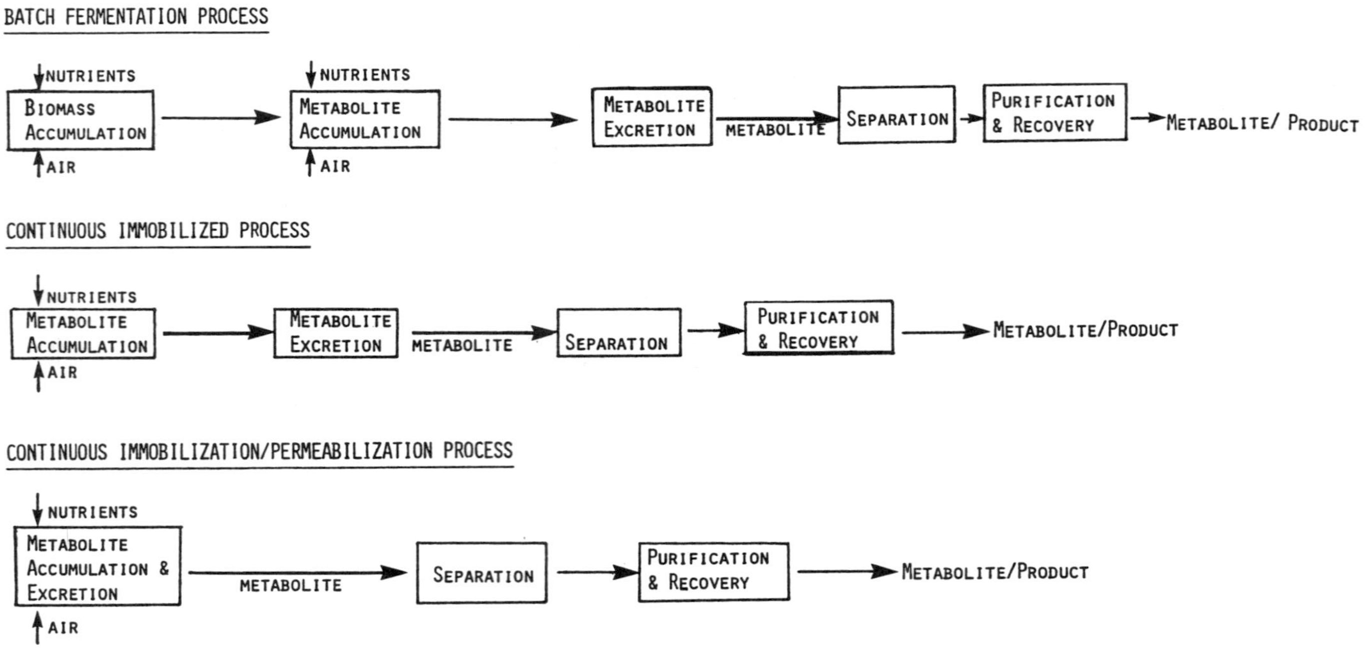

Fig. 2. Simplified flow charts for the production of secondary metabolites through batch fermentation, continuous immobilized, or continuous immobilized–permeabilized plant tissue culture processes (Knorr et al., 1985, with permission of the Institute of Food Technologists).

of polysaccharides) needs to be better understood and optimized, intra- and interbiocatalyst reactions need to be explored further, inter- and intraparticle mass transfer in the performance of immobilized microbial cells must be examined more thoroughly, and, finally as Radovich (1985) stated, much work is needed to bring the design of immobilized cell reactors up to the level of sophistication found in the design of heterogeneous catalytic reactors.

Advances have been made in utilizing immobilized plant cell systems for the production of useful chemicals, and much work is being carried out on improving immobilized plant biocatalysts (Brodelius, 1984; Knorr et al., 1985; Sahai and Knuth, 1985; Shuler et al., 1984) to make the production of natural food components and processing aids via plant tissue culture attractive and economically feasible (Sahai and Knuth, 1985). However, almost all the work reviewed in this report has been performed on a laboratory scale. Consequently, there are numerous future challenges to meet in this rapidly expanding area of plant biotechnology. The most crucial requirement is the already mentioned need for scale-up development. Here essential target areas are mass transfer problems, including nutrient-, metabolite-, by-product-, and gas transport and improvement of reactor design.

To achieve these goals, a better understanding of all critical mass transfer and environmental factors (and their interactions) involved in the production of plant metabolites from immobilized cells is of key importance and studies on the interrelationships between gel type, structure and stability, and plant cell productivity and viability seem essential. Optimization of polymer matrix properties can only be achieved if we gain more insight into the structure–function relationship of the gel systems and the effects of gel components on plant cell performance, such as "copolymerization" of chitosan with polyanionic polymers (Knorr et al., 1985). Questions on why spontaneous leakage can occur in gel-entrapped cells (Brodelius, 1984; Knorr, 1985a) or on microenvironmental effects, such as decreased water activity and oxygen deficiency, on the metabolic behavior of immobilized cells (Mattiasson and Hahn-Hägerdahl, 1982) must be addressed in order to improve and perfect immobilization–permeabilization processes.

Systems are needed for the continuous recovery and identification of desired metabolites produced in immobilized plant cell reactors. The increased use of dense gases as extractants (i.e., supercritical carbon dioxide) or the development of two-phase systems and adsorbent cultures needs to be intensified (Bisson et al., 1983; Knoop and Biederbeck, 1983; Stahl, 1982). In addition, the application of affinity chromatography and high-performance liquid chromatography (Bjurstrom, 1985) in plant metabolite purification and recovery is noteworthy, as well as the potential use of biosensors (Smit and Rechnitz, 1984) for plant metabolite identification.

ACKNOWLEDGMENTS

Valuable comments were provided to drafts of this chapter by J. Berlin, R. A. Teutonico, and K. D. Vorlop.

This work was supported in part by the National Sea Grant College Program under Grant No. NA83AA-D-00017, Project No. R/N-9.

REFERENCES

Arcuri, E. J., Nichols, J. R., Brix, T. S., Santamarina, V. G., Buckland, B. C., and Drew, S. W. (1983). Thienamycin production by immobilized cells of *Streptomyces cattleya* in a bubble column. *Biotechnol. Bioeng.* *25*:2399–2411.

Anonymous (1983). Guidelines for the characterization of immobilized biocatalysts. *Enzyme Microb. Technol.*, *5*:304–307.

Bajpai, P. and Margaritis, A. (1985). Improvement of inulinase stability of calcium alginate immobilized *Kluyveromyces marxianus* cells by treatment with hardening agents. *Enzyme Microb. Technol.* *7*:34–36.

Bang, W., Behrendt, U., Lang. S., and Wagner, F. (1983). Continuous production of L-tryptophan from indole and L-serine by immobilized *Escherichia coli* cells. *Biotechnol. Bioeng.* *25*:1013–1025.

Bisson, W., Beiderbeck, R., and J. Reichling (1983). Die Produktion ätherischer Öle durch Zellsuspensionen der Kamille in einem Zweiphasensystem. *Planta Med.* *47*:164–168.

Bjurstrom, E. (1985). Biotechnology: Fermentation and downstrem processing. *Chem. Eng.* *92*:126–158.

Black, G. M., Webb, C., Matthews, T. M., and Atkinson, B. (1984). Practical reactor systems for yeast cell immobilization using biomass support particles. *Biotechnol. Bioeng.* *26*:134–141.

Brodelius, P. (1983). Production of biochemicals with immobilized plant cells: Possibilities and problems. *Ann. N.Y. Acad. Sci.* *413*:383–393.

Brodelius, P. (1984). Immobilized viable plant cells. *Ann. N.Y. Acad. Sci.* *434*:382–393.

Brodelius, P. and Mosbach, K. (1982). Immobilized plant cells: General aspects. *J. Chem. Technol. Biotechnol.* *32*:330–337.

Brodelius, P. and Nilsson, K. (1983). Permeabilization of immobilized plant cells resulting in release of intracellularly stored products with preserved viability. *Eur. J. Appl. Microbiol. Biotechnol.* *17*:275–280.

Brodelius, P., Deus, B., Mosbach, K., and Zenk, M. H. (1979). Immobilized plant cells for the production and transformation of natural products. *FEBS Newslett.* *103*:93–97.

Chaleff, R. S. (1984). Isolation of agronically useful mutants from plant cell cultures. *Science 219*:676–682.

Chibata, I. and Tosa, T. (1981). Use of immobilized cells. *Annu. Rev. Biophys. Bioeng. 10*:197–216.

Chotani, G. K. and Constantinides, A. (1984). Immobilized cell cross-flow reactor. *Biotechnol. Bioeng. 26*:217–220.

Constantinides, A., Bhattia, D., and Vieth, W. (1981). Immobilization of *Brevibacterium flavum* cells on collagen for the production of glutamic acid in a recycle reactor. *Biotechnol. Bioeng. 23*:899–916.

Couderc, R. and Baratti, J. (1980). Immobilized yeast cells with methanol oxidase activity: Preparation and enzymatic properties. *Biotechnol. Bioeng. 22*:1155–1173.

Curtin, M. E. (1983). Harvesting profitable products from plant tissue culture. *BioTechnology 1*:649–657.

Dainty, A. L., Goulding, K. H., Robinson, P. K., Simpkins, I., and Trevan, M. D. (1986). Stability of alginate-immobilized algal cells. *Biotechnol. Bioeng. 28*:210–216.

deBont, J. A. M., van Ginkel, C. G., Tramper, J., and Luyben, K. C. A. M. (1983). Ethylene oxide production by immobilized *Mycobacterium Pyl* in a gas–solid bioreactor. *Enzyme Microb. Technol.* 5:55–59.

De Borghi, M., Converti, A., and Parisi, F. (1985). Continuous alcohol fermentation in an immobilized cell rotating disk reactor. *Biotechnol. Bioeng. 27*:761–768.

Deo, Y. M. and Gaucher, G. M. (1983). Semi-continuous production of the antibiotic patulin by immobilized cells of *Penicillium urticae*. *Biotechnol. Lett.* 5:125–130.

Deo, Y. M. and Gaucher, G. M. (1984). Semi-continuous and continuous production of penicillin-G by *Penicillium chrysogenum* cells immobilized in κ-carrageenan beads. *Biotechnol. Bioeng. 26*:285–295.

Deshpande, V., SivaRaman, H., and Mala, R. (1983). Simultaneous saccharification and fermentation of cellulose to ethanol using *Penicillium funiculosum* cellulase and free or immobilized *Saccharomyces uvarum* Cells. *Biotechnol. Bioeng. 25*:1679–1684.

D'Souza, S. F. and Nadkarni, G. B. (1980). Continuous conversion of sucrose to fructose and gluconic acid by immobilized yeast cell multi-enzyme complex. *Biotechnol. Bioeng. 22*:2179–2189.

Durand, G. and Navarro, J. M. (1978). Immobilized microbial cells. *Process Biochem. 13*(9):14–23.

Felix, H., Brodelius, P., and Mosbach, K. (1981). Enzyme activites of the primary and secondary metabolism of simultaneously permeabilized and immobilized plant cells. *Anal. Biochem. 116*:462–470.

Foster, B. C., Coutts, R. T., Pasutto, F. M., and Dossetor, J. B. (1983). Production of cyclosporin A by carrageenan-immobilized *Tolypocladium inflatum* in an airlift reactor with external loop. *Biotechnol. Lett.* 5:693–696.

Fowler, M. W. (1983). Commercial application and economic aspects of mass plant cell culture. In *Plant Biotechnology* (S. H. Mantell and H. Smith, eds.), Cambridge University Press, Cambridge, pp. 3–37.

Francou, N. and Vignais, P. M. (1984). Hydrogen production by *Rhodopseudomonas capsulata* cells entrapped in carrageenan beads. *Biotechnol. Lett.* *6*:639–644.

Freeman, A. (1984). Gel entrapment of whole cells and enzymes in cross-linked, prepolymerized polyacrylamide hydrazide. *Ann. N.Y. Acad. Sci.* *434*:418–426.

Freeman, A. and Aharonowitz, Y. (1981). Immobilization of microbial cells in crosslinked, prepolymerized, linear polyacrylamide gels: Antibiotic production by immobilized *Streptomyces clavuligerus* cells. *Biotechnol. Bioeng.* *23*:2747–2759.

Fujimura, M., Kato, J., Tosa, T., and Chibata, I. (1984). Continuous production of L-arginine using immobilized growing *Serratia marcescens* cells: Effectiveness of supply of oxygen gas. *Appl. Microbiol. Biotechnol.* *19*:79–84.

Furusaki, S., Seki, M., and Fukumura, K. (1983). Reaction characteristics of an immobilized yeast producing ethanol. *Biotechnol. Bioeng.* *25*:2921–2928.

Furua, T., Yoshikawa, T., Orihara, Y., and Oda, H. (1984). Studies on the culture conditions for *Panax ginseng* cells in jar fermentors. *J. Nat. Prod.* *47*:70–75.

Gautheret, R. J. (1983). Plant tissue culture: A History. *Bot. Mag. Tokyo* *93*:393–410.

Ghommidh, C., Navarro, J. M., and Durand, G. (1982). A study of acetic acid production by immobilized *Acetobacter* cells: Oxygen transfer. *Biotechnol. Bioeng.* *24:605–617.*

Goldstein, W. E. (1983). Large-scale processing of plant cell culture. *Ann. N.Y. Acad. Sci.* *431*:394–408.

Haberlandt, G. (1902). Culturversuche mit isolierten Pflanzenzellen. *Sitzungsber. Akad. Wiss. Wien Math. Naturwiss. Kl. Abt.* *3*:69–92.

Hahn-Hägerdahl, B. (1984). An enzyme co-immobilized with a microorganism: The conversion of cellobiose to ethanol using β-glucosidase and *Saccharomyces cerevisiae* in clacium alginate gels. *Biotechnol. Bioeng.* *26*:771–774.

Hartmeier, W. (1984). Co-immobilizates: New biocatalysts for fermentation technology. *Process Biochem.* *19*:40–42.

Horitsu, H., Adachi, S., Takashi, Y., Kawai, K., and Kawano, Y. (1985). Production of citric acid by *Aspergillus niger* immobilized in polyacrylamide gels. *Appl. Microbiol. Biotechnol. 22*: 8–12.

Inoles, D. S., Smith, W. J., Taylor, D. D., Cohen, S. N., Michaels, A. S., and Robertson, C. R. (1983). Hollow-fiber membrane bioreactors using immobilized *E. coli* for protein synthesis. *Biotechnol. Bioeng. 25*:2653–2681.

Jain, D. and Ghose, T. K. (1984). Cellobiose hydrolysis using *Pichia etchellsii* cells immobilized in calcium alginate. *Biotechnol. Bioeng. 26*:340–346.

Jain, V. K., Toran-Diaz, I., and Baratti, J. (1985a). Preparation and characterization of immobilized growing cells of *Zymomonas mobilis* for ethanol production. *Biotechnol. Bioeng. 27*:273–279.

Jain, V. K., Toran-Diaz, I., and Baratti, J. (1985b). Continuous production of ethanol from fructose by immobilized growing cells of *Zymomonas mobilis*. *Biotechnol. Bioeng. 27*:613–620.

Jirku, V., Macek, T., Vanek, T., Krumphanzl, V., and Kubanek, V. (1981). Continuous production of steroid glycoalkaloids by immobilized plant cells. *Biotechnol. Lett. 3*:447–451.

Jones, A., Berk, D., Lesser, B. H., Behie, L. A., and Gaucher, G. M. (1983). Continuous production of patulin by immobilized cells of *Penicillium urticae* in a stirred tank reactor. *Biotechnol. Lett. 5*:785–790.

Jose, W., Pederson, H., and Chin, C. (1983). Immobilization of plant cells in a hollow fiber reactor. *Ann. N.Y. Acad. Sci. 413*:409–412.

Karkare, S. B., Dean, Jr., R. C., and Venkatasubramanian, K. (1985). Continuous fermentation with fludized slurries of immobilized microorganisms. *BioTechnology 3*:247–251.

Karube, I., Kuriyama, S., Matsunaga, T., and Suzuki, A. (1980). Methane production from wastewaters by immobilized methanogenic bacteria. *Biotechnol. Bioeng. 22*:847–857.

Kautola, H., Vahvaselkä, M., Linko, Y.-Y., and Linko, P. (1985). Itaconic acid production by immobilized *Aspergillus terreus* from xylose and glucose. *Biotechnol. Lett. 7*:167–172.

Kierstan, M., McHale, A., and Coughlan, M. P. (1982). The production of ethanol from cellobiose using immobilized β-glucosidase co-entrapped with yeast in alginate gels. *Biotechnol. Bioeng. 24*:1461–1463.

Kim, H. S. and Ryu, D. D. Y. (1982). Continuous glutamate production using an immobilized whole-cell system. *Biotechnol. Bioeng. 24*:2167–2174.

King, V. A. E. and Zall, R. R. (1983). Ethanol fermentation of whey using polyacrylamide and kappa-carrageenan entrapped yeasts. *J. Gen. Appl. Microbiol.* *29*:379–393.

Klein, J. and Vorlop, K. D. (1983). Immobilized cells. In *Foundations of Biochemical Engineering* (H. W. Blanch, E. T. Papoutsakis, and G. Stephanopoulos, eds.), American Chemical Society, Washington, D. C., pp. 377–392.

Klein, J. and Wagner, F. (1983). Methods for the immobilization of microbial cells. *Appl. Biochem. Bioeng.* *4*:11–51.

Klein, J., Vorlop, K. D., and Wagner, F. (1984). The implication of reaction kinetics and mass transfer on the design of biocatalytic processes with immobilized cells. *Ann. N.Y. Acad. Sci.* *434*: 437–449.

Klibanov, A. M. (1983). Immobilized enzymes and cells as practical catalysts. *Science* *219*:722–727.

Kloosterman, J. and Lilly, M. D. (1985). An airlift loop reactor for the transfromation of steroids by immobilized cells. *Biotechnol. Lett.* 7:25–30.

Knoop, B. and Beiderbeck, R. (1983). Adsorbens-Kultur-ein Weg zur Steigerung der Sekundärstoff/Produktion in pflanzlichen Suspensionskulturen. *Z. Naturforsch.* *38c*:484–486.

Knorr, D. (1984). Use of chitinous polymers in food: A challenge for food research and development. *Food Technol.* *38*(1):85–97.

Knorr, D. (1985a). Chitosan gels for entrapment of cultured plant cells. In *Chitin and Chitosan* (R. Muzzarelli, ed.), Plenum, New York (in press).

Knorr, D. (1985b). Utilization of chitinous polymers in food processing and biomass recovery. In *Biotechnology of Marine Polysaccharides* (R. R. Colwell, E. R. Pariser, and A. J. Sinskey, eds.), Hemisphere Publishing, Washington, D. C., pp. 313–332.

Knorr, D. and Sinskey, A. J. (1985). Biotechnology in food production and processing. *Science* *229*:1224–1229.

Knorr, D. and Teutonico, R. A. (1985). Chitosan as immobilizing and permeabilizing agent for cultured *A. tricolor* cells. *J. Agric. Food Chem.* (submitted).

Knorr, D., Miazga, S. M., and Teutonico, R. A. (1985). Immobilization and permeabilization of cultured plant cells. *Food Technol.* *39*(10):139–142.

Kokubu, T., Karube, I., and Suzuki, S. (1981). Protease production by immobilized mycelia of *Streptomyces fradiae*. *Biotechnol. Bioeng.* *23*:29–39.

Krouwel, P. G., Groot, W. J., Kossen, N. W. F., and van der Laan, W. F. M. (1983). Continuous isopropanol-butanol-ethanol fermentation by immobilized *Clostridium beijerinckii* cells in a packed bed fermenter. *Enzyme Microb. Technol.* 5:46–54.

Kyung, K. H. and Gerhardt, P. (1984). Continuous production of ethanol by yeast "immobilized" in a membrane-contained fermentor. *Biotechnol. Bioeng.* *26*:252–256.

Langrene, S., Silsil, S., and Le Gottic, F. (1984). Entrapment of L-tryptophan producing *Escherichia coli* in different matrices: Activity of immobilized cells. *Enzyme Microb. Technol.* *6*:81–84.

Lee, J. M., Woodward, J. (1983). Properties and application of immobilized β-D-glucosidase co-entrapped with *Zymomonas mobilis* in calcium alginate. *Biotechnol. Bioeng.* *25*:2441–2451.

Lee, T. H., Ahn, J. C., and Ryu, D. D. Y. (1983). Performance of an immobilized yeast reactor system for ethanol production. *Enzyme Microb. Technol.* 5:41–45.

Lerner, H., Ban-Basset, D., Reinhold, L., and Poliakoff-Mayber, A. (1978). Induction of "pore" formation in plant cell membranes by toluene. *Plant Physiol.* *61*:213–217.

Lindsey, K., Yoeman, M. M., Black, G. M., and Mavituna, F. (1983). A novel method for the immobilization and culture of plant cells. *FEBS Lett.* *155*:143–146.

Linko, P., Stenroos, S. -L., Linko, Y. -Y., Koristinen, T., Harju, M., and Heikonen, M. (1984). Applications of immobilized lactic acid bacteria. *Ann. N.Y. Acad. Sci.* *434*:406–417.

Linse, L. and Brodelius, P. (1984). Immobilization of plant protoplasts. *Ann. N.Y. Acad. Sci.* *434*:487–490.

McGhee, J. E., St. Julian, G., Detroy, R. W., and Bothast, R. J. (1982). Ethanol production by immobilized *Saccharomyces cerevisiae, Saccharomyces uvarum* and *Zymomonas mobilis*. *Biotechnol. Bioeng.* *24*:1155–1163.

McGhee, J. E., Carr, M. E., and St. Julian, G. (1984). Continuous bioconversion of starch to ethanol by calcium-alginate immobilized enzymes and yeasts. *Cereal Chem.* *61*:446–449.

Maddox, I. S. and Kingston, P. J. (1983). Use of immobilized cells of the yeast, *Saccharomycopsis lipolytica,* for the production of citric acid. *Biotechnol. Lett.* 5:795–798.

Maddox, I. S., Dunnill, P., and Lilly, M. D. (1981). Use of immobilized cells of *Rhizopus nigricans* for the 11α-hydroxylation of progesterone. *Biotechnol. Bioeng.* *23*:345–354.

Markkannen, P., Idman, T., and Kanppinen, V. (1984). Growth and carodenolide production by *Digitalis panata* in different fermenter types. *Ann. N.Y. Acad. Sci.* *434*:491–495.

Marwaha, S. S. and Kennedy, J. F. (1984). Ethanol production from whey permeate by immobilized yeast cells. *Enzyme Microb. Technol.* *6*:18–22.

Matsunaga, T., Karube, I., and Suzuki, S. (1980). Some observations on immobilized hydrogen-producing bacteria: Behavior of hydrogen in gel membranes. *Biotechnol. Bioeng.* *22*:2607–2615.

Matsunaga, T., Karube, I., and Suzuki, A. (1983). Methane production from organic acid rich wastewaters by immobilized thermophilic methane producing bacteria. *Enzyme Microb. Technol.* 5:441–444.

Mattiasson, B. (1983). *Immobilized Cells and Organelles,* Vols. 1 and 2, CRC Press, Boca Raton, Fla.

Mattiasson, B. and Hahn-Hägerdahl, B. (1982). Microenvironmental effects on metabolic behavior of immobilized cells. A hypothesis. *Eur. J. Appl. Microbiol. Biotechnol. 16*:52–55.

Miazga, S. M. and Knorr, D. (1985). Use of cultured common milkweed (*Asclepias syriaca* L.) cells for protease production. (unpublished manuscript).

Mohite, U. and SivaRaman, H. (1984). Continuous conversion of sweet sorghum juice to ethanol using immobilized yeast cells. *Biotechnol. Bioeng. 26*:1126–1127.

Morikawa, Y., Karube, I., and Suzak, S. (1980). Continuous production of bacitracin by immobilized living whole cells of *Bacillus* sp. *Biotechnol. Bioeng. 22*:1015–1023.

Morris, D., Smart, N. J., and Fowler, M. W. (1983). A fluidized bed vessel for the culture of immobilized plant cells and its application for the continuous production of fine cell suspensions. *Plant Cell Tissue Organ Culture. 2*:207–216.

Nagashima, M., Azuma, M., and Noguchi, S. (1983). Technology developments in biomass alcohol production in Japan: Continuous alcohol production with immobilized microbial cells. *Ann. N.Y. Acad. Sci. 413*:457–468.

Nagashima, M., Azuma, M., Noguchi, S., Inuzuka, K., and Samejima, H. (1984). Continuous ethanol fermentation using immobilized yeast cells. *Biotechnol. Bioeng. 26*:992–997.

Nakajima, H., Sonomoto, K., Usui, N., Sata, N., Yamada, T., Tanaka, A., and Fukin, S. (1985). Entrapment of *Lavandula vera* cells and production of pigments by entrapped cells. *J. Biotechnol. 2*:107–117.

Navarro, A., Marangoni, H., Plaza, I. M., and Callieri, D. (1984). Horizontal reactor for the continuous production of ethanol by yeasts immobilized in pectin. *Biotechnol. Lett. 6*:465–470.

Nickel, L. G. (1980). Products. In *Plant Tissue Culture as a Source of Biochemicals* (E. J. Staba, ed.), CRC Press, Boca Raton, Fla., pp. 235–269.

Onaka, T., Nakamishi, K., Inoue, T., and Kubo, S. (1985). Beer brewing with immobilized yeast. *BioTechnology 3*:467–470.

Paul, F. and Vignais, P. M. (1980). Photophosphoylation in bacterial chromatophores entrapped in alginate gel: Improvement of the physical and biochemical properties of gel beads with barium as gel-inducing agent. *Enzyme Microb. Technol.* *2*:281–287.

Prenosil, J. G. and Pedersen, H. (1983). Immobilized plant cell reactors. *Enzyme Microb. Technol.* *5*: 323–331.

Prevost, H., Diries, C., and Rousseau, E. (1985). Continuous yoghurt production with *Lactobacillus bulgaricus* and Streptococcus *thermophilus* entrapped in Ca-alginate. *Biotechnol. Lett.* *7*:247–252.

Radovich, J. M. (1985). Mass transfer effects in fermentations using immobilized whole cells. *Enzyme Microb. Technol.* *7*:2–10.

Rha, C. K., Rodriquez-Sanchez, D., and Kienzle-Sterzer, C. (1985). In *Biotechnology of Marine Polysaccharides* (R. R. Colwell, E. R. Parisier, and A. J. Sinskey, eds.), Hemisphere Publishing, Washington, D.C., pp. 283–311.

Rosevear, A. (1984). Immobilized biocatalysts—A critical review. *J. Chem. Technol. Biotechnol.* *34B*:127–150.

Sahai, O. P. and Knuth, M. (1985). Commercializing plant tissue culture processes: economics, problems and prospects. *Biotechnol. Prog.* *1*:1–9.

Sahai, O. P. and Shuler, M. L. (1982). On the non-ideality of chemostat operation using plant cell suspension cultures. *Can. J. Bot.* *60*:692–700.

Sahi, O. P. and Shuler, M. L. (1984). Multistage continuous culture to examine secondary metabolite formation in plant cells: Phenolics from *Nicotiana tabacum*. *Biotechnol. Bioeng.* *26*:27–36.

Samejima, H., Nagashima, M., Azuma, M., Noguchi, S. and Inizuka, K. (1985). Semi-commercial production of ethanol using immobilized microbial cells. *Ann. N.Y. Acad. Sci.* *434*:394–405.

Sarkar, J. M. and Mayaudon, J. (1983). Alanine synthesis by immobilized *Corynebacterium dismutans* cells. *Biotechnol. Lett.* *5*:201–206.

Scherer, P., Kluge, M., Klein, J., and Sahm, H. (1981). Immobilization of the methanogenic bacterium *Methanosarcina barkeri*. *Biotechnol. Bioeng.* *23*:1057–1065.

Schleiden, M. J. (1838). Beiträge zur Phytogenesis. *Müller Arch. Anat. Physiol.*, pp. 137–176.

Schmauder, H. P., Döbel, P., and Gröder, D. (1984). Charakterisierung von *Nigella damascena* Zellkulturen in Airlift-Fermentoren. *Biochem. Biophysiol. Pflanzen* *179*:611–622.

Schnabl, H., Youngman, R. J., and Zimmerman, U. (1983). Maintenance of plant cell membrane integrity and function by the immobilization of protoplasts in alginate matrices. *Planta* *158*:392–397.

Schwann, T. (1839). *Mikroskopische Untersuchungen über die Übereinstimmung in der Struktur und Wachstum der Thiere und Pflanzen*, Oswalds, Berlin.

Sharp, W. R., Evans, D. A., and Ammirato, P. V. (1984). Plant genetic engineering: Designing crops to meet food industry specifications. *Food Technol. 38*:112–120.

Shuler, M. L. (1981). Production of secondary metabolites from plant tissue culture—Problems and prospects. *Ann. N.Y. Acad. Sci. 369*:65–79.

Shuler, M. L., Pyne, J. W., and Hallsby, G. A. (1984). Prospects and problems in the large scale production of metabolites from plant cell tissue cultures. *J. Am. Oil Chem. Soc. 61*:1724–1728.

Shuler, M. L., Hallsby, G. A., Pyne, J. W., and Cho, T. (1985). Bioreactors for immobilized plant cell cultures (unpublished).

Slininger, P. J., Bothast, R. J., Black, L. T., and McGhee, J. E. (1982). Continuous conversion of D-xylose to ethanol by immobilized *Pachysolen tannophilus*. *Biotechnol. Bioeng. 24*:2241–2251.

Smit, N. and Rechnitz, G. A. (1984). Leaf based biocatalytic membrane electrodes. *Biotechnol. Lett. 4*:209–213.

Spettoli, P., Nuti, M. P., Pal, A., Peruffo, B., and Zamorani, A. (1984). Malolactic fermentation and secondary product formation in wine by *Leuconostoc* genus cells immobilized in a continuous-flow reactor. *Enzyme Eng. 434*:461–464.

Stahl, E. (1982). Komprimierte Gase zur Gewinnung von Naturstoffen. *Fette Seifen Anstrichmitt 84*:444–451.

Stöcklein, W., Eisgruber, A., and Schmidt, H. L. (1983). Conversion of L-phenylalanine to L-tyrosine by immobilized bacteria. *Biotechnol. Lett. 5*:703–708.

Tanaka, H., Matsumura, M., and Veliky, I. A. (1984a). Diffusion characteristics of substrates in Ca-alginate gel beads. *Biotechnol. Bioeng. 26*:53–58.

Tanaka, H., Sonomoto, K., and Fukui, S. (1984b). Application of living cells immobilized by prepolymer methods. *Ann. N.Y. Acad. Sci. 434*:479–482.

Tanaka, H., Nishuijima, F., Suwa, M., and Iwamoto, T. (1983). Rotating drum fermentor for plant cell suspension cultures. *Biotechnol. Bioeng. 25*:2359–2370.

Tanaka, H., Hirao, C., Semba, H., Tozawa, Y., and Ohmomo, S. (1985). Release of intracellularly stored 5'-phosphodiesterase with preserved plant cell viability. *Biotechnol. Bioeng. 27*:890–892.

Teutonico, R. A. and Knorr, D. (1984). Plant tissue culture: Food applications and the potential reduction of nutritional stress factors. *Food Technol. 38*(2):120–127.

Teutonico, R. A. and Knorr, D. (1985a). Improvement of nutritional quality of food plants through tissue culture techniques. *Food Technol.* *39*(4):49–60.

Tuli, A., Sethi, R. P., Khanna, P. K., and Marwaha, S. S. (1985). Lactic acid production from whey permeate by immobilized *Lactobacillus casei*. *Enzyme Microb. Technol.* *7*:164–168.

Van Ginkel, C. G., Tramper, J., Luyben, K. C. A. M., and Klapwijk, A. (1983). Characterization of *Nitrosomonas europaea* immobilized in calcium alginate. *Enzyme Microb. Technol.* *5*: 297–303.

Veliky, I. A. and Jones, A. (1981). Bioconversion of gitoxigenin by immobilized plant cells in a column bioreactor. *Biotechnol. Lett.* *3*:551–556.

Venkatsubramanian, K. (1979). *Immobilized microbial cells. Am. Chem. Soc. Symp. 106.*

Vorlop, K. D. and Klein, J. (1983). In *Enzyme Technology* (R. M. Lafferty, ed.), Springer-Verlag, Berlin. pp. 219–235.

Wada, M., Kato, J., and Chibata, I. (1979). A new immobilization of microbial cells. *Eur. J. Appl. Microbiol. Biotechnol.* *8*: 241–247.

Wada, M., Uchida, T., Kayto, J., and Chibata, I. (1980). Continuous production of L-isoleucine using immobilized growing *Serratia marcescens* cells. *Biotechnol. Bioeng.* *22*:1175–1188.

Wang, H. Y. and Hettwer, D. J. (1982). Cell immobilization in κ-carrageenan with tri-calcium phosphate. *Biotechnol. Bioeng.* *24*:1827–1838.

Williams, D. and Munnecke, D. M. (1981). The production of ethanol by immobilized yeast cells. *Biotechnol. Bioeng.* *23*:1813–1825.

Young, D. H. and Kauss, H. (1983). Release of calcium from suspension-cultured *Glycine max* cells by chitosan, other polycations and polyions in relation to effects on membrane permeability. *Plant Physiol.* *73*:698–702.

Young, D. H., Köhle, H., and Kauss, H. (1982). Effect of chitosan on membrane permeability of suspension cultured *Glycine max* and *Phaseolus vulgaris* cells. *Plant Physiol.* *70*:1449–1454.

THREE

Modification and Bioconversion of Raw Materials

12

Technology for the Development of New Breeding Lines and Plant Varieties for the Food Industry

DAVID A. EVANS and ROBERT J. WHITAKER / DNA Plant Technology Corporation, Cinnaminson, New Jersey

INTRODUCTION

Progress in the past several years has helped establish tissue culture techniques as valuable tools for the development of new crops. This is an outgrowth of the first commercialization of tissue culture, which was the use of shoot tip propagation as an alternative to conventional vegetative propagation. When applied to ornamental plants or to estate crops such as oil palm, tissue culture could be used for rapid, consistent reproduction of elite or difficult-to-propagate genotypes. The value of cloning is, however, limited to those cash crops or ornamentals in which each individual organism is valuable. Hence cloning would not be useful for field crops such as corn or wheat.

However, several tissue culture techniques have been perfected in recent years that could have commercial application to a wide range of food crops. These methods can be used to develop novel variation that has a genetic basis and can be transmitted through seed in a predictable manner. Somaclonal and gametoclonal variations may be used to introduce nonspecific variation into food crop species using standardized plant regeneration methods. While the full genetic nature of this variation has not been firmly established, new plant varieties have already been developed via somaclonal variation. Anther culture or gametoclonal variation can be used as an adjunct to conventional breeding. The high-frequency production of homozygous dihaploid breeding lines of crop species, particularly when anthers of F_1 hybrids are used, has led to the development of new plant varieties. Development of haploid plants has already been exploited extensively in China. Cellular and molecular genetics offer a more precise method of introducing useful genetic changes but require additional basic research before widespread application is possible.

Secondary product synthesis is an area in which cell cultures themselves produce useful chemicals for the food industry. With techniques of genetic manipulation, some cultures have already been identified that accumulate higher concentrations of chemicals than the intact plant. The application of all these newly developed technologies should result in significant new advances in the development of agricultural products.

CLONAL PROPAGATION

Innumerable plant species can be propagated in vitro (Murashige, 1978). In most cases clonal propagation is achieved by placing sterilized shoot tips or axillary buds onto a culture medium that is sufficient to induce the formation of multiple buds. Shoot tip clonal propagation has already been used to commercially propagate a large number of marketable ornamentals (see Oglesby, 1978). Murashige (1974) has described a three-stage procedure that normally requires alteration of culture medium or growth conditions between stages. Stage 1 pertains to the establishment of tissue in vitro. Stage 2 is most important, as it requires production of multiple shoots. Stage 3 must result in root formation and conditioning of propagules prior to transfer to the greenhouse. High light intensity is important in stage 3 (Murashige, 1978). In many species the media and culture conditions are not altered between stages 1 and 2 (Murashige, 1978).

Advantages of cloning for plants are the speed of plant multiplication and the quality and uniformity of plants produced. In many species propagation in vitro is considerably faster than in conventional species. Ferns, bromeliads, orchids, and ornamental trees can all be propagated more rapidly in vitro in controlled environments than using conventional propagation methods. For example, nearly all economically important orchids, except *Paphiopedilum*, are easily cloned in vitro (Murashige, 1974). Orchids have traditionally been difficult to mass-propagate using conventional methods.

While cell culture has already been demonstrated to be commercially important for the propagation of ornamentals, cell culture may also be useful to propagate certain food crops:

1. In plants with seed viability problems, breeding or parent lines can be regenerated *in vitro*. Somatic embryos produced in

tissue culture could be directly planted into the field using systems already developed for pregerminated seed or transplants.

2. Mutated plants can also be propagated in vitro. Albino mutants or other genetic lines useful in cellular genetics can be maintained in vitro.

3. Parents used in a breeding program also can be propagated in vitro. Male sterile mutants have been used to produce commercial F_1 hybrids in a number of crop species. Normally restorer lines must be used to maintain and propagate the male sterile mutant. This procedure requires a series of sexual crosses with subsequent selection among all progeny for the male sterile types. Unless genetic markers are used, the selection must be completed on mature plants. This selection is particularly time-consuming when the male sterile parent line is under nuclear genetic control. In some species it is possible to maintain male sterile parent lines and preserve the male sterile character using in vitro propagation to allow for consistent hybrid seed production.

4. When advanced breeding lines have been identified, it is important to propagate as many seeds or plants as possible to permit variety release. At this point tissue culture may be used in conjunction with other asexual methods to propagate clonal lines for seed production. Such an approach was used in Ecuador to establish elite clones of pyrethrum (*Chrysanthemum cinerariaefolium*) for commercial production (Levy, 1981).

5. In some cases cultivated crops, particularly cash crops, where each individual plant is valuable, may be cloned using tissue culture. For example, varieties for greenhouse crop production or for tropical estate crops can be propagated in vitro using shoot apices.

In crops where male sterility is unavailable, production of hybrid seed is expensive. In crosses between divergent varieties hybrid seed cannot be propagated sexually without genetic segregation in the F_2 population. Genetic segregation in the F_2 population is inversely correlated with relatedness of the parental lines. Hybrid plants could be propagated using large-scale in vitro propagation. Such hybrids may be cheaper to produce than hybrids originating from seed produced by hand pollination. A business analysis of the economics of propagation of hybrids should consider the cost of transplanting regenerated hybrid plants to the field as opposed to directly seeding the field with F_1 hybrid seed. Unless plants can be regenerated very inexpensively or are in a species in which transplants are commonly used, F_1 hybrid in vitro propagation is not profitable.

In certain crops and ornamentals it has also been economically useful to develop in vitro techniques to produce virus-eradicated plants. This can be accomplished by regenerating plants from a virus-free plant. Meristems are generally free of virus infection owing to the lack of vascular differentiation in the meristem that impairs intercellular movement of viruses and the active metabolism of mitotic cells that precludes viral infection. In order to take advantage of virus-free cells, the smallest possible meristem explant should be cultured. On the other hand, small explants do not regenerate or produce roots as well as large meristems. These two factors must be balanced to identify optimal explant size. Genetic stability as measured by phenotypic and chromosomal stability is usually preserved in plants recovered from cultured meristems.

Heat treatment is commonly used to inactivate the virus prior to culturing meristems. In many cases, using 34–36°C will result in inactivation of the virus without deleterious effects on the plant. About one-half of the known plant viruses, particularly small spherical viruses, can be inactivated with thermotherapy (Hu and Wang, 1983). Heat treatment during donor plant growth can result in successful use of larger meristem explants than from unheated plants (Mullin et al., 1974). In some species heat treatment is essential for successful virus elimination. In *Chrysanthemum* 98.5% of the progeny from heat-treated plants were virus free, while only 15% of apices from room-temperature grown plants were virus free (Hollings et al., 1972). Heat treatment can also be applied by incubating tissue cultures at elevated temperatures (Walkey and Cooper, 1975).

Viruses have been eliminated using meristem culture from a number of economical species. These species include the elimination of mottle virus from strawberry, potato virus X from potato, mosaic virus from cassava, and cauliflower mosaic virus from cauliflower (Quak, 1977). Virus-free plants produced by meristem culture have resulted in significant increases in yield when compared to virus-infected plants (Walkey and Cooper, 1975). Results have been particularly favorable in the potato (Gregorini and Lorenzi, 1974), where the yield of virus-free potatoes is 60% higher than in infected plants. Virus-free plants, though, are not resistant to reinfection. As expected, field-grown plants often become reinfected with virus. Stock plants should be maintained to reproduce virus-free plants.

Plants regenerated from callus may also be free of viral infection. Callus tissue is similar to meristematic tissue, as cell mitosis is rapid and vascular differentiation is incomplete. In callus or cell suspension cultures viral infection may be completely eliminated via repeated subculture. Plants regenerated from uninfected leaf tissue may also be used to recover virus-free plants. Murakishi and Carlson (1976) regenerated tobacco plants from dark-green uninfected islands of a tobacco mosaic virus-infected leaf. Approximately 50% of regenerated plants were virus free.

SOMACLONAL VARIATION

In contrast to shoot tip propagation, which faithfully produces clones, evidence has accumulated suggesting that regeneration of plants from callus, leaf explants, or plant protoplasts results in recovery of somaclonal variants (Reisch, 1983). Regeneration of plants from callus culture has been associated with recovery of aneuploid plants, sterile plants, and morphological variants. The observation that in both potato (Shepard, 1982) and sugarcane (Larkin and Scowcroft, 1981) somaclonal variants were resistant to diseases suggests that production of this variability in regenerated plants could prove agriculturally useful.

The phenotypic variability recovered in regenerated plants probably reflects both preexisting cellular genetic differences and tissue culture-induced variability. Skirvin and Janick (1976) systematically compared plants regenerated from callus of five cultivars of *Pelargonium* spp. Plants obtained from geranium stem cuttings in vivo were uniform, whereas plants from in vivo root and petiole cuttings and plants regenerated from callus were quite variable. Changes were observed when regenerated plants were compared to parent plants for plant and organ size, leaf and flower morphology, essential oil constituents, fasciation, pubescence, and anthocyanin pigmentation. Long-term cell cultures result in tissue culture-induced variability with regard to chromosome number that is expressed in both callus and plants regenerated from callus (D'Amato, 1977). This results in regeneration of aneuploid plants that are commercially useless in sexually propagated species. On the other hand, aneuploidy may not interfere with the productivity of asexually propagated crops such as sugarcane and potato.

Plants regenerated from callus of sugarcane have been examined in detail. A wider range of chromosome numbers ($2n = 71-300$) has been observed in plants regenerated from sugarcane callus (Heinz et al., 1977) than in parent lines. These clones of regenerated sugarcane were examined for disease resistance. Resistance to three diseases (eye-spot disease, Fiji disease, and downy mildew) was observed in some plants regenerated from a susceptible sugarcane clone (Heinz et al., 1977). One regenerated line was simultaneously resistant to both Fiji disease and downy mildew. These lines have been incorporated into a conventional breeding program.

Plants regenerated from mesophyll protoplasts of potato have also been analyzed. Although a detailed genetic analysis has not been published, it is apparent that regenerated clones are highly variable. There is evidence that some of the variability is due to chromosomal rearrangements (Shepard, 1982). As in sugarcane, lines have been identified that are resistant to diseases (late blight and early blight) to which the parent line, Russet Burbank, is susceptible (Shepard, 1982).

Evans and Sharp (1983) made the first detailed genetic evaluation of the plants regenerated from cell culture of a sexually propagated crop plant, the tomato, and provided evidence for the recovery of single-gene changes using somaclonal variation. This discovery demonstrates that the biotechnological tool of somaclonal variation can result in stable changes in the genetic traits of tissue culture-regenerated plants. Several of these single-gene changes of the tomato have been mapped. For example, one of these variants has been localized to a specific region on the long arm of chromosome number 10. Among the variants of tomato observed with this procedure were changes in fruit color, plant architecture, and characteristics to improve the ease of mechanical harvesting. This new tool provides scientists with the ability to develop new breeding lines for the generation of improved varieties for food and industrial products from existing varieties within a reasonable time frame. This compresses the time required for the modification of existing varieties.

GAMETOCLONAL VARIATION

Haploid plants derived from male or female gametes have value in plant breeding, as they greatly reduce the time for obtaining homozygous breeding lines. Doubled haploids, when integrated into a conventional breeding program, have resulted in the rapid development of new varieties. Kasha and Reinberg (1980) have reported that use of doubled haploids reduced the time for the release of a new variety of barley from 12 to 5 years. Haploid plants can also be used for genetic analysis. Using an *Aurea* mutant, Burk (1970) demonstrated that single-gene heterozygous diploid plants produce a 1:1 ratio of the two haploid parental types following anther culture. In *Nicotiana*, haploids have been used to analyze the number of genes controlling disease resistance (Nakata and Kurihara, 1972) and nicotine production (Nakamura et al., 1974), as well as to aid in the analysis of mutants induced in vitro (Chaleff, 1981) and of somatic hybrids (Schieder, 1978).

Haploid plants have been obtained in crop species using conventional breeding methods, anther culture, immature ovule culture, or pollen culture. As the haploid plants produced by each method are desirable, the method with the highest frequency of haploid production should be used.

Haploid plants arise frequently following interspecific hybridization, and haploids produced this way have been integrated into breeding programs in barley, potato, and tobacco. In each of these species haploids are produced following fertilization of a cultivated crop with a wild relative. In barley, haploids are produced following fertilization of *Hordeum vulgare* with *Hordeum bulbosum*, as *H. bulbosum* chromosomes are preferentially eliminated. Recently the *Hordeum* system has been extended to produce haploids in closely related cereals, as additional species have been used as the female parent. In potato pollination of *Solanum tuberosum* with wild-type pollen, particularly *Solanum phureja*, results in parthenogenic development of *S. tuberosum*. Potato doubled haploids and haploids can be used to aid in the introduction of wild-species genes into the tetraploid cultivated potato. Haploid tobacco has been produced following pollination with *Nicotiana africana* (Burk et al., 1979). Each of these methods results in production of maternal haploids of the cultivated crop. On the other hand, the indeterminate gametophyte (ig) gene can be used in corn to produce haploids with unique mixtures of nuclear and cytoplasmic DNA. Both paternal and maternal haploids can be produced using the ig gene in heterozygous condition (Kermicle, 1969). This system may be modified in the future to aid in the transfer of cytoplasmic DNA between breeding lines without the transfer of nuclear genes.

Haploid tissue and plants can be produced in higher frequency in many species using anther culture. Haploid plants were first produced by this method in *Datura innoxia*. For each species examined the best developmental stage of cultured anthers must be ascertained to optimize the frequency of haploid production. First pollen grain mitosis is optimal for tobacco and *Datura*, while an earlier stage is required for tomato and a later stage is required for *Brassica* (Sunderland, 1974). In some species the culture medium does not appear to be as important as anther stage in determining the conditions for haploid production, as the nutrient requirements for cultured anthers may be quite simple. On the other hand, in some species the response of cultured anthers is medium dependent (e.g., rice varieties). Numerous other factors affect the degree of success in anther culture. The growth environment and age of the donor plant are important. Care should be taken to use the first floral buds that appear on the plant. Pretreatment of the anthers after removal from the plant but prior to culturing in vitro may be essential. Both cold shock (Nitsch, 1974) and heat treatment (Keller and Armstrong, 1979) have been proposed to increase the number of haploid plants produced per cultured anther.

Gametoclones have been recovered either via androgenesis or by plant regeneration from microspore-derived haploid cells following callus formation. From a recent review (Sharp et al., 1984) it is evident that most species capable of haploid production proceed via direct androgenesis. Taxonomic differences are apparent, though, between androgenesis and callus-mediated regeneration. The

Table 1. Commercial Food Crops for Which Haploid Plants Have Been Produced

Alfalfa	Cucumber	Rye
Asparagus	Grape	Strawberry
Barley	Kale	Sugarcane
Broccoli	Peanut	Sweet potato
Citrus	Pepper	Tomato
Clover	Potato	Triticale
Coffee	Rapeseed	Wheat
Corn	Rice	

Source: After Sharp et al. (1984).

majority of solanaceous species capable of producing haploid plants undergo direct androgenesis, while the majoirty of graminaceous species undergo callus-mediated haploid plant production. Commercially important crops for which haploid plants have been produced are listed in Table 1.

As anthers are a mixed population of diploid and haploid cells, all capable of cell reproduction, great effort has been directed toward isolated pollen culture. Pollen can be liberated by squashing anthers in a liquid culture medium and subsequently collected via filtration. Isolated pollen can be cultured on a complex medium or using nurse culture (reviewed by Nitsch, 1971). Glutamine and serine are important additives to pollen culture medium.

Haploids are integrated into a breeding program as homozygous diploid lines. Diploidized haploid lines can be produced using a colchicine treatment or, alternatively, using leaf midrib culture. Selection from a population of doubled haploids, particularly an F_1 population, can result in rapid fixation of desired characteristics. Griffing (1975) has statistically demonstrated that use of double haploids, when rapidly obtained, is more efficient than conventional selection.

Doubled haploids have been incorporated into breeding programs to produce new cultivated varieties of barley (Kasha and Reinbergs, 1980) and tobacco (Collins and Genovesi, 1982). Although not used as extensively in other crop species, doubled haploids have also been used in *Asparagus*, *Brassica*, rice, corn, barley, wheat, rye, and potato (see Nitzsche and Wenzel, 1977). In *Asparagus* anther culture of mature male (XY) plants can be used when chromosomes are doubled to produce supermales (YY). The supermales, when crossed with females (XX), have been very useful in the establishment of high-yielding, uniform all-male (XY) lines of *Asparagus*. Doubled haploid techniques are being utilized in *Brassica* to breed for lowered glucosinolate content. Varietal development in rice and peppers also currently involves double haploids. In corn doubled haploids are being utilized for analytical breeding. Because of the genetic uniformity of doubled haploids when compared to regular diploid lines, doubled haploids of inbred lines are used for the evaluation of the breeding lines for use as parents to produce F_1 hybrids. Following such analysis, F_1 hybrids are constructed with more confidence (Nitzsche and Wenzel, 1977).

Doubled haploids can also be used in genetic analysis to study the inheritance of qualitative and quantitative traits. Because haploids and doubled haploids exhibit the genotype of the gamete, ratios obtained are less complex if doubled haploids rather than diploids are used for genetic analysis (Collins and Legg, 1980). Doubled haploids have been utilized for the genetic analysis of several quantitative traits in tobacco. Haploids are also useful in cellular mutagenesis programs, as recessive alleles are expressed in haploids while they may be undetected in diploids. Anther culture can also be used to manipulate chromosome number in intraspecific (Schieder, 1978) and interspecific (Evans et al., 1983) somatic hybrids and to generate nullisomics useful for genetic analysis (Moore and Collins, 1982).

CELLULAR AND MOLECULAR GENETICS

Techniques developed for the plating of single cells for selection of desired genotypes at the cellular level suggest that cellular genetics can be used to produce genetically modified plants. With the use of cell suspension cultures, large numbers of cells can be screened for the isolation of agriculturally useful variants. The underlying requirement for successful agricultural application of cellular genetics is that variation identified in cultured cells continue to be expressed in regenerated plants. Variation can be introduced into cultured cells via mutagenesis, protoplast fusion, or uptake of exogenous DNA.

Mutant Isolation

Cultured plant cells have been used for the isolation of mutants in vitro with subsequent plant regeneration (Flick, 1983). Mutants may be regenerated directly for incorporation into conventional breeding programs or mutated cell lines could also be useful in the establishment of biochemically stable and genetically marked cell lines for protoplast fusion or DNA uptake experiments. Variant cell lines with direct potential agricultural application include lines selected for pathotoxin or herbicide resistance as well as lines selected for salt or cold tolerance. Mutant lines used as cell genetic markers would ideally have genetic lesions that are recessive to permit identification of genetically modified cells as corrected variants. It has been proposed that auxotrophic or temperature-sensitive mutants could be very useful in cell genetic studies. Dominant variants may nonetheless be useful to select for genetic modifications that confer resistance to toxic chemicals. For example, fusion products of two cell lines, in which each parental line was resistant to a different amino acid analog, expressed resistance to both amino acid analogs (White and Vasil, 1979). Cell lines resistant to amino acid analogs may be quite useful in protoplast fusion, as protoplasts are susceptible to very low concentrations of these chemicals, permitting discrimination between sensitive and resistant phenotypes and hence easy identification of heterokaryons. In lieu of induced recessive variants, most researchers have used genetically marked cell lines with lesions in photosynthesis. Albino mutants occur naturally or may be induced by chemical treatment. Most albinos are recessive and some albino mutants have been biochemically analyzed in great detail. While mutated and corrected cells following protoplast fusion or DNA uptake cannot normally be distinguished in vitro, corrected cells could subsequently be identified as green regenerating shoots. Isolation of more biochemically marked cell lines would permit the analysis of genetic modification experiments.

Protoplast Fusion

Protoplast fusion has often been suggested as a means to develop unique hybrid plants impossible to develop via conventional sexual hybridization. While any two plant cells can be fused using a modified PEG method, creation of unique somatic hybrid plants is limited by the ability to regenerate plants from isolated plant protoplasts (Evans, 1983). Interspecies somatic hybrid plants have been produced in the following genera: *Datura, Daucus, Nicotiana, Petunia, Brassica,* and *Solanum.* In most cases these hybrids have been between sexually compatible species and have not been incorporated into conventional breeding programs. Much of the emphasis of early fusion experiments was directed toward production of distant somatic hybrids not possible using conventional sexual hybridization.

Recently several intergeneric hybrid plants have been recovered. In each case only aneuploid plants were recovered, and gross morphological abnormalities were reported for each combination. These intergeneric combinations include *Solanum* + *Lycopersicon* (Melchers et al., 1978), *Atropa* + *Datura* (Krumbiegel and Schieder, 1979), *Daucus* + *Aegopodium* (Dudits et al., 1980), *Arabidopsis* + *Brassica* (Gleba and Hoffmann, 1980), and *Nicotiana* + *Atropa* (Gleba et al., 1982). Unfortunately, none of these fusion products has resulted in crop improvement, as the plants were morphologically and chromosomally abnormal. In most cases a wide range of aneuploid plants was recovered that resulted in a wide range of morphological phenotypes. In the *Daucus* + *Aegopodium* experiment, all the *Aegopodium* chromosomes were lost, resulting in plants with the same chromosome number as *Daucus carota*. However, evidence was presented that a small amount of genetic information was transferred from *Aegopodium* into *Daucus* (Dudits et al., 1980).

As it has now been demonstrated that distant hybrids can be produced by protoplast fusion, attention should be directed toward the use of fusion products in crop improvement. Somatic hybridization should be critically analyzed for its use as an aid to crop improvement. The primary limitation to the application of protoplast technology is certainly the inability to regenerate plants from protoplasts. Numerous hybrids could be proposed to complement cereal and legume breeding programs, but very little success has been reported in plant regeneration from these important crops. Hence the limitation of plant regeneration from protoplasts precludes the short-term application of this technology to cereals and legumes.

We have developed techniques for the production of unique somatic hybrids in the genus *Nicotiana* between species that cannot normally be hybridized (Evans et al., 1981). Production of these somatic hybrids has been directed toward the production of agriculturally useful hybrid germplasm. Protoplasts from leaves of *Nicotiana nesophila* and *Nicotiana stocktonii*, wild species that are resistant to numerous diseases to which cultivated tobacco is susceptible, were fused with cell suspension culture protoplasts from an albino mutant (Su/Su) of cultivated *Nicotiana tabacum*. Hybrid plants produced by protoplast fusion were distinguished as light-green shoots while *N. stocktonii* or *N. nesophila* shoots were dark green and *N. tabacum* shoots were albino. The light-green plants recovered following fusion were verified as somatic hybrids using morphological, chromosomal, isoenzymic, and genetic criteria. A number of clones have been identified with the amphiploid chromosome number (2n = 96). Stable incorporation of disease resistance into somatic hybrids was tested using resistance to tobacco mosaic virus. These somatic hybrids should be resistant to numerous diseases of cultivated tobacco. Ability to sexually propagate these hybrids was variable between clones. At least one clone capable of self-fertilization has been identified and nearly all clones could be backcrossed to *N. tabacum*. Seed from backcrosses (BC_1 and BC_2) is being evaluated for disease resistance. Useful material will be incorporated into a breeding program to develop resistant tobacco varieties.

Another use of protoplast fusion is the transfer of cytoplasmic genetic information. During fertilization the male cytoplasm is preferentially excluded from the developing embryo. Thus in most crops conventional sexual hybrids contain and express only maternally derived cytoplasmic genes. As protoplast fusion combines both parent cytoplasms into a single protoplast, fusion can be used to produce unique nuclear—cytoplasmic combinations not possible using conventional breeding (Gleba and Evans, 1983).

Evidence from a number of somatic hybrids suggests that although two types of cytoplasms are initially mixed during protoplast fusion, resulting in heteroplasmons, eventually one parent-type cytoplasm predominates, resulting in cytoplasmic segregation. Following segregation, which may not occur until after meiosis, genetic information from the second cytoplasm is irreversibly lost. This phenomenon was first reported by examination of the fate of a large subunit of fraction 1 protein (F-1-P) in *Nicotiana glauca* + *Nicotiana langsdorffii* somatic hybrids (Chen et al., 1977). Random chloroplast segregation resulted in fixed *langsdorffii*- or *glauca*-type F-1-P in each clone prior to meiosis (10 *langsdorffii* type and 7 *glauca* type), except for one clone, in which segregation followed self-fertilization. Cytoplasmic segregation has been observed for other cytoplasmically controlled traits. Segregation of male sterility versus male fertility has been reported in several cybrids (see Gleba and Evans, 1983). Cosegregation has been reported for several cytoplasmic traits (Aviv et al., 1980). We have found that F-1-P and tentoxin sensitivity cosegregated in *N. glauca* + *N. tabacum* somatic hybrids (Flick and Evans, 1982). Cosegregation implies that following cytoplasmic segregation the cytoplasm contains all characters from one parent or the other and therefore precludes widespread cytoplasmic recombination. Evidence has been presented though that mitochondria and chloroplasts sort independently in somatic hybrids (Galun, 1982).

Despite reports of the cosegregation of cytoplasmic genes, biochemical evidence using restriction analysis of mitochrondrial DNA of some cybrids has suggested that recombination occurs between parental mitochondrial DNAs prior to cytoplasmic segregation in somatic hybrids between different male sterile and fertile parent plants (Belliard et al., 1979). In these reports mitochrondrial recombination following protoplast fusion produced a wide range of morphological phenotypes controlling male sterility in the hybrid plants. Similarly, Nagy et al. (1981) detected recombination in the mitochondrial DNA of *N. tabacum* + *Nicotiana knightiana* somatic hybrids resulting in novel mitochrondrial DNA restriction enzyme patterns. Recombination of chloroplast DNA in higher plants has not yet been documented. Most likely these intriguing results of cytoplasmic segregation and recombination predate an era of extensive research on cytoplasmic genetics with higher plants. Newly established cytoplasmic markers for disease resistance (Gengenbach et al., 1977) and antibiotic resistance (Maliga, 1982) should facilitate research in this area. The production of unique nuclear–cytoplasmic combinations using protoplasts will aid in the development of novel germplasm not available using conventional methods.

Plant Molecular Biology

Numerous attempts have been made to use exogenous DNA to induce transformation in higher plants. While early reports were directed toward injection of exogenous radioactively labeled bacterial or plant DNA into seed or isolated pollen grains, difficulty in analyzing the fate of the exogenous DNA has hampered the widespread application of this method of DNA incorporation. The success of these whole-plant experiments has been critically reviewed (Kleinhofs and Behki, 1977). As recombinant DNA techniques have been developed that permit the routine transfer of genes between different prokaryotes and between eukaryotes and prokaryotes, more attention has recently been directed toward the genetic modification of higher plants using cultured plant cells and isolated plant protoplasts.

Purified DNA is susceptible to digestion by host cell nucleases; hence it is probably necessary to use a vector system to transfer DNA into a plant host. Gene vectors should facilitate the uptake, stabilization, and replication of foreign DNA inside the plant cell. While many potential vectors for plant transformation have been proposed, greatest attention has been directed to the use of the Ti plasmid of *Agrobacterium tumefaciens*, a bacterium involved in the formation of crown gall tumors in dicotyledonous plants. The genes that confer oncogenic properties, including auxin autotrophy, are harbored on the Ti plasmid, as well as DNA for the synthesis of other tumor-specific gene products (Montoya et al., 1977). The Ti plasmid DNA is degraded at a slower rate than bacterial chromosomal DNA following uptake by plant protoplasts. During crown gall infection part of the Ti plasmid integrates into the host cell nuclear DNA (Willmitzer et al., 1980), suggesting a natural method for the stable introduction of exogenous DNA into the plant cells. Methods have been developed that permit high-frequency delivery of Ti DNA into plant protoplasts (Marton et al., 1979). Despite these attractive features, there are some limitations that impede the routine use of the Ti plasmid as a vector for plant transformation:

1. Once protoplasts are transformed, they must be cloned, redifferentiated to nontumorous cells, and regenerated to complete plants. Protoplasts of *N. tabacum* transformed with Ti plasmid DNA have been regenerated to complete plants that retain nopaline synthesis derived from the Ti plasmid (Wullems et al., 1981). The

ability to synthesize nopaline, a plasmid trait, is sexually transmitted.

2. Genetically modified plants must be stably maintained through sexual reproduction or asexual propagation. It is encouraging that it has recently been shown that some Ti plasmid DNA sequences in certain *Agrobacterium* strains or mutants can be transmitted through meiosis to seeds of tobacco (Yang and Simpson, 1981; Otten et al., 1981).

3. Specific desired selectable genes must be identified and isolated and then integrated into the Ti plasmid. The Ti-mediated transfer and expression of prokaryotic genes into plant cells resulting in transformed plants has been recently reported (Horsch et al., 1984).

In addition to the Ti plasmid, other plasmids have been suggested as possible vectors for gene transfer. Plasmids are commonly found and can be easily transferred into a number of bacteria. Some of these plasmids have been found in bacteria commonly associated with plant diseases, for example, *Pseudomonas savastanoi* (Comai and Kosuge, 1980). In addition to pathological bacteria, plasmids were found in 14 strains of cyanobacteria (Lau et al., 1980), including both laboratory and natural strains. Plasmid-like DNA has recently been found to occur naturally in mitochondria of higher plants, as it has been associated with certain strains of male sterile corn (Levings et al., 1980). These higher-plant plasmids replicate within the mitochondria and are capable of integration into mitochondrial DNA in revertant male fertile lines of corn. The presence of naturally occurring plasmid DNA in plant mitochondria when combined with cybrid transfer methods mentioned above may offer a unique system of gene transfer in higher plants.

The DNA-containing plant viruses are also attractive as vectors, particularly since virus DNA replicates autonomously without integration into the host genome. Foreign DNA could therefore be introduced into plants by simply inoculating leaves (Howell et al., 1981). As there are a limited number of plant DNA viruses, greatest attention has been directed toward cauliflower mosaic virus (CaMV). Unfortunately, CaMV has a limited host range, as it infects only species of the *Cruciferae.* There is evidence, though, that foreign DNA can be inserted into CaMV without altering viral infectivity (Howell et al., 1981), thereby permitting gene transfer. As molecular genetic methods continue to advance, it is expected that useful host–vector systems will be developed that permit the routine incorporation of foreign DNA into higher plants.

SYNTHESIS OF SECONDARY PRODUCTS

Most proposed benefits of plant tissue culture require the regeneration of a genetically modified or cloned plant to achieve successful application of tissue culture methodology. It has been proposed, however, that cultured plant cells may produce useful chemicals. While plant cells cannot compete with bacterial or yeast batch cell culture for cost of production, certain unique compounds, synthesized exclusively by plant cells, may have commercial value.

While there are some similarities between the large-scale culture of microbes and plant cells, the striking number of physiological differences between these cell types precludes the use of microbial fermentation systems for plant cell culture (Prenosil and Pedersen, 1983). Plant cells are generally much larger than microbial cells and they possess rigid cell walls. These features render plant cells much more susceptible to the shear forces that develop in conventional microbial blade fermenters. Plant cells also grow much more slowly than microbial cells and therefore stringent aseptic conditions need to be observed. Owing to the tendency of plant cells to aggregate, settling becomes a problem in large-scale cultures in terms of oxygen transfer. Most importantly, plant cells generally do not excrete their secondary products but retain them inside the cell vacuole. Therefore a destructive harvest would be necessary to release intercellular secondary compounds. This would preclude long-term recyclable cell cultures and increase the overall cost of production. Studies on plant cell excretion have suggested that accumulation and excretion of secondary products may be conveniently modulated by strict control of external pH (Renaudin, 1981). Precise definition of specific excretion and accumulation parameters for individual cell lines would undoubtedly prove invaluable in designing cost-effective bioreactors for the scale-up of producing cell cultures. Recently nondestructive permeabilization of immobilized plant cells by treatment with organic chemicals has been reported (Brodelius and Nilsson, 1983).

Clearly the major hurdle to the cost-effective production of secondary compounds by plant cells is the isolation of high-producing cell lines. While cell cultures have been shown to produce a number of valuable secondary metabolites (Table 2), generally production levels are low and sometimes quite variable. The use of somaclonal variation technology in conjunction with cell aggregate cloning methods developed by Yamada and Fujita (1983) has already produced dramatic results in the induction and selection of high-yielding cell

Table 2. Secondary Metabolites with Commercial Value Produced in Cell Culture

Product	Use	Species
Anthraquinones	Laxative, dye	*Morinda citrifolia*
Ajmalicine	Tranquilizer	*Catharanthus roseus*
Camptothecin	Antileukemic, antitumor agent	*Camptotheca acuminata*
Cephalotaxine	Antitumor agent (esters of)	*Cephalotaxus harringtonia*
Diosgenin	Raw materials for hormone synthesis	*Dioscorea deltoides*
Rosmarinic acid	Spice, antioxidant	*Coleus blumei*
Shikonin	Dye, pharmaceutical	*Lithospermum erythrorhizon*
Stevioside	Nonnutritive sweetener	*Stevia rabaudiana*
Thebaine	Source of codeine	*Papaver bracteatum*
Ubiquinone-10	Cardiovascular agent	*Nicotiana tabacum*

Source: Zenk (1978) and Nickell (1980).

lines. Cell aggregate cloning has been used successfully to select for photoautotrophic cells (Yasuda et al., 1980), high-vitamin-producing cells (Watanabe and Yamada, 1982), high-pigment cells (Yamamoto et al., 1982), and high-alkaloid-containing cells (Zenk et al., 1977; Yamada and Hashimoto, 1982) in various plant species. In some instances cell cultures have been selected that produce significantly higher concentrations of a particular secondary metabolite than is found in the intact plant. An illustrative example of cell aggregate cloning is the selection of high-anthocyanin-producing cell lines from cultured cells of *Euphorbia millii* by Yamamoto et al. (1982). In these experiments cell aggregates were plated on solid medium and cultured. The resulting calli were then divided, one-half for continued growth and the other for analysis of anthocyanin content. The highest-pigmented calli were continually subcultured in this manner for 24 selections. The amount of pigment found in the highest-producing lines after this period of time was seven times greater than in the original cells.

The most economically successful example of the plant cell culture production of valuable chemicals is shikonin, a naphthoquinone used both as a dye and a pharmaceutical (Fujita et al., 1981a,b). The development of high-producing cell cultures was based on the selection of variant cell aggregates that produced shikonin followed by detailed investigations of proper nutritional and cultural techniques that further increased production 13-fold.

Cell aggregate cloning is simply a tissue culture method that permits the identification of cells with increased biosynthetic capacities for a particular secondary product. The genetic variation that is the basis of the observed chemical production is the result of spontaneous genetic variation already present in the original explant material or variation that was induced during the process of tissue culture initiation and subculture, that is, somaclonal variation. Therefore the same principle which has been successfully applied to agricultural crop plants to identify and select agronomically improved varieties is also widely applicable to the isolation of cell cultures that produce high levels of secondary metabolites. The only difference in the two applications is the material being evaluated for genetic alterations. Somaclonal variation technology, as it is applied to crop plants, relies on the regeneration of whole plants, their self-fertilization, and the analysis of the resulting F_1 progeny, whereas the application of somaclonal variation for secondary product synthesis relies on the generation of cell aggregates that can be individually selected and evaluated for specific chemical production.

A detailed cost analysis of secondary product synthesis is necessary for plants. It is important to consider the cost of the final product per kilogram. Unless the cost of the chemical is high, it will be impossible to use cell cultures to produce a commercially competitive product. Cost evaluation should also consider the demand of the product, opportunities and value of producing a product of improved purity, and government regulations on distribution. Finally, it should be emphasized that if there is any possibility that a microbe can make the product, plant cell biosynthesis will not be economical. At present only the production of expensive drug compounds and selected, valuable flavor and fragrance chemicals is commercially feasible (Zenk, 1978; Whitaker and Hashimoto, 1985).

CONCLUDING REMARKS

The potential agricultural application of plant cell culture to crop improvement is astonishing. Tissue culture represents a loose collection of techniques, that, when carefully integrated into an existing breeding program, should result in the development of unique germplasm. In addition, as techniques of cellular genetics continue to develop, there exists the possibility of altering the nature of future crop species. Even if only the less technical methods of meristem culture and plant regeneration for cloning and genetic variability are utilized, plant tissue culture should have a tremendous impact on crop improvement in the near future.

REFERENCES

Aviv, D., Fluhr, R., Edelman, M., and Galun, E. (1980). Progeny analysis of the interspecific somatic hybrids: *Nicotiana tabacum* (cms) + *Nicotiana sylvestris* with respect to nuclear and chloroplast markers. *Theor. Appl. Genet. 56*:145–150.

Belliard, G., Vedel, F., and Pelletier, G. (1979). Mitochondrial recombination in cytoplasmic hybrids of *Nicotiana tabacum* by protoplast fusion. *Nature 281*:401–403.

Brodelius, P., and Nilsson, K. (1983). Permeabilization of immobilized plant cells, resulting in release of intracellularly stored products with preserved cell viability. *Curr. J. Appl. Microbiol. Biotechnol. 17*:275–28.

Burk, L. G. (1970). Green and light-yellow haploid seedlings from anthers of sulfur tobacco. *J. Hered. 61*:279.

Burk, L. G., Gerstel, D. U., and Wernsman, E. A. (1979). Maternal haploids of *Nicotiana tabacum* L. from seed. *Science 206*:585.

Chaleff, R. S. (1981). *Genetics of Higher Plants—Applications of Cell Culture*, Cambridge University Press, Cambridge.

Chen, K., Wildman, S. G., and Smith, H. H. (1977). Chloroplast DNA distribution in parasexual hybrids as shown by polypeptide composition of fraction-1 protein. *Proc. Nat. Acad. Sci. U.S.A. 74*:5109–5112.

Collins, G. B. and Genovesi, A. D. (1982). Anther culture and its application to crop improvement. In *Application of Plant Cell and Tissue Culture to Agriculture and Industry* (D. T. Tomes, B. E. Ellis, P. M. Harney, K. J. Kasha, and R. J. Peterson, eds.). University of Guelph Press, Ontario, pp. 1–24.

Collins, G. B. and Legg, P. D. (1980). Recent advances in the genetic applications of haploidy in *Nicotiana*. In *The Plant Genome* (D. R. Davies and D. A. Hopwood, eds.), Johns Innes Charity, Norwich. pp. 197–213.

Comai, L. and Kosuge, T. (1980). Involvement of plasmid DNA in indoleacetic acid synthesis in *Pseudomonas savastanoi*. *J. Bacteriol. 143*:950–957.

D'Amato, F. (1977). Cytogenetics of differentiation in tissue cell cultures. In *Plant, Cell, Tissue and Organ Culture* (J. Reinert and Y. P. S. Bajaj, eds.), Springer-Verlag, Berlin, pp. 343–357.

Dudits, D., Fejer, O., Hadlaczky, G., Koncz, C., Lazar, G. B., and Horvath, G. (1980). Intergeneric gene transfer mediated by plant protoplast fusion. *Mol. Gen. Genet.* *179*:283–288.

Evans, D. A. (1983). Protoplast fusion. In *Handbook of Plant Cell Culture*, (D. A. Evans, W. R. Sharp, P. V. Ammirato, and Y. Yamada, eds.) Vol. 1, Macmillan, New York, pp. 291–321.

Evans, D. A. and Sharp, W. R. (1983). Single gene mutations in tomato plants regenerated from tissue culture. *Science 221*: 949–951.

Evans, D. A., Flick, C. E., and Jensen, R. A. (1981). Incorporation of disease resistance into sexually incompatible somatic hybrids of the genus *Nicotiana*. *Science 219*:907–909.

Evans, D. A., Flick, C. E., Bravo, J. E., and Kut, S. A. (1983). Genetic behavior of somatic hybrids in the genus *Nicotiana*: *N. otophora* + *N. tabacum* and *N. sylvestris* + *N. tabacum*. *Theor. Appl. Genet.* *65*:93–101.

Flick, C. E. (1983). Isolation of mutants from cell culture. In *Handbook of Plant Cell Culture* (D. A. Evans, W. R. Sharp, P. V. Ammirato, and Y. Yamada, eds.), Vol. 1, Macmillan, New York, pp. 393–441.

Flick, C. E. and Evans, D. A. (1982). Evaluation of cytoplasmic segregation in somatic hybrids in the genus *Nicotiana*: Tentoxin sensitivity. *J. Hered.* *73*:264–266.

Fujita, Y., Hera, Y., Ogino, Y., and Suga, L. (1981a). Production of shikonin derivatives cell suspension cultures of *Lithospermum erythrorhizon* I: Effects of nitrogen sources of production of shikonin derivatives. *Plant Cell Reports* *1*:59–60.

Fujita, Y., Hera, Y., Suga, L., and Moumoto, M. (1981b). Production of shikonin derivatives by cell suspension cultures of *Lithospermum erythrorhizon*. II. A new medium for the production of shikinon derivatives. *Plant Cell Reports* *1*:60–63.

Galun, E. (1982). Somatic cell fusion for inducing cytoplasmic exchange: A new biological system for cytoplasmic genetics in higher plants. In *Plant Improvement and Somatic Cell Genetics* (I. K. Vasil, W. R. Scowcroft, and K. J. Frey, eds.), Academic, New York, pp. 205–220.

Gengenbach, B. G., Green, C. E., and Donovan, C. M. (1977). Inheritance of selected pathotoxin resistance in maize plants regenerated from cell cultures. *Proc. Nat. Acad. Sci. U.S.A.* *74*:5113–5117.

Gleba, Y. Y. and D. A. Evans, (1983). Genetic analysis of somatic hybrid plants. In *Handbook of Plant Cell Culture* (D. A. Evans, W. R. Sharp, P. V. Ammirato, and Y. Yamada, eds.), Vol. 1, Macmillan, New York, pp. 322–357.

Gleba, Y. Y. and Hoffmann, F. (1980). "Arabidobrassica": A novel plant obtained by protoplast fusion. *Planta* *149*:112–117.

Gleba, Y. Y., Momot, V. P., Cherep, N. N., and Skarzynskaya, M. V. (1982). Intertribal hybrid lines of *Atropa belladonna* × *N. chinensis* obtained by cloning individual protoplast fusion products. *Theor. Appl. Genet. 62*:75–79.

Gregorini, G. and Lorenzi, R. (1974). Meristem-tip cultures of potato plants as a method of improving productivity. *Potato Res. 17*:24–33.

Griffing, B. (1975). Efficiency change due to use of doubled-haploids in recurrent selection methods. *Theor. Appl. Genet. 46*:367–385.

Heinz, D. J., Krishnamurathi, M., Nickell, L. G., and Maretzki, A. (1977). Cell, tissue, and organ culture in sugarcane. In *Plant Cell, Tissue, and Organ Culture* (J. Reinert and Y. P. S. Bajaj, eds.), Springer-Verlag, Berlin, pp. 3–17.

Hollings, M., Stone, O. M., and Dale, W. T. (1972). Tomato ringspot virus in *Pelargonium* in England. *Plant Pathol. 21*:46–47.

Horsch, R. B., Fraley, R. T., Rogers, S. G., Sanders, P. R., Lloyd, A., and Hoffmann, N. (1984). Inheritance of functional foreign genes in plants. *Science 223*:496–498.

Howell, S. H., Walker, L. L., and Walden, R. M. (1981). Rescue of in vitro generated mutants of cloned cauliflower mosaic virus genome in infected plants. *Nature 293*:483–486.

Hu, C. Y. and Wang, P. J. (1983). Meristem and shoot tip cultures. In *Handbook of Plant Cell Culture* (D. A. Evans, P. V. Ammirato, W. R. Sharp, and Y. Yamada, eds.), Vol. 1, Macmillan, New York, pp. 177–227.

Kasha, K. J. and Reinbergs, E. (1980). Achievements with haploids in barley research and breeding. In *The Plant Genome* (D. R. Davies and D. A. Hopwood, eds.), Johns Innes Charity, Norwhich, pp. 215–230.

Keller, W. A. and Armstrong, K. C. (1979). Stimulation of embryogenesis and haploid production in *Brassica campestris* anther cultures of elevated temperature treatments. *Theor. Appl. Genet. 55*:65–67.

Kermicle, J. L. (1969). Androgenesis conditioned by a mutation in maize. *Science 166*:1422–1424.

Kleinhofs, A. and Behki, R. (1977). Prospects for plant genome modification by non-conventional methods. *Annu. Rev. Genet. 11*:79–101.

Krumbiegel, G. and Schieder, O. (1979). Selection of somatic hybrids after fusion of protoplasts from *Datura innoxia* Mill. and *Atropa belladonna* L. *Planta 145*:371–375.

Larkin, P. J. and Scowcroft, W. R. (1981). Somaclonal variation—A novel source of variability from cell cultures for plant improvement. *Theor. Appl. Genet. 60*:197–214.

Lau, R. H., Sapienza, D., and Doolittle, W. F. (1980). Cyanobacterial plasmids: Their widespread occurrence and the existence of regions of homology between plasmids in the same and different species. *Mol. Gen. Genet. 178*:203–211.

Levings, C. S., Kim, B. D., Pring, D. R., Conde, M. F., Mans, R. J., Laughnan, R. J., and Gabay-Laughnan, S. J. (1980). Cytoplasmic reversion of cms-s in maize: Association with a transpositional event. *Science 209*:1021–1023.

Levy, L. W. (1981). A large-scale application of tissue culture: The mass propagation of pyrethrum clones in Ecuador. *Environ. Exp. Bot. 21*:389–395.

Maliga, P. (1982). Cell culture procedures for *Nicotiana plumbaginifolia. Plant Mol. Biol. Newslett. 3*:88–94.

Marton, L., Wullems, G. J., Molendijk, L., and Schilperoot, R. A. (1979). In vitro transformation of cultured cells from *Nicotiana tabacum* by *Agrobacterium tumefaciens. Nature 277*:129–131.

Melchers, G., Sacristan, M. D., and Holder, A. A. (1978). Somatic hybrid plants of potato and tomato regenerated from fused protoplasts. *Carlsburg Res. Commun. 43*:203–218.

Montoya, A. L., Chilton, M. D., Gordon, M. P., Sciaky, D., and Nester, E. W. (1977). Octopine and nopaline metabolism in Agrobacterium tumefaciens and crown galltumor cells: Role of plasmid genes. *J. Bacteriol. 129*:101–107.

Moore, G. A. and Collins, G. B. (1982). Identification of aneuploids in *Nicotiana tabacum* by isozyme banding patterns. *Biochem. Genet. 20*:555–568.

Mullin, R. H., Smith, S. H., Frazier, N. W., Schlegel, D. E. and McCall, S. R. (1974). Meristem culture frees strawberries of mild yellow edge, pallidosis and mottle diseases. *Phytopathology 64*:1425–1429.

Murakishi, H. H. and Carlson, P. S. (1976). Regeneration of virus-free plants from dark green islands of tobacco mosaic infected tobacco leaves. *Pythopathology 661*:931–932.

Murashige, T. (1974). Plant propagation through tissue culture. *Annu. Rev. Plant Physiol. 25*:135–166.

Murashige, T. (1978). The impact of tissue culture on agriculture. In *Frontiers in Plant Tissue Culture* (T. A. Thorpe, ed.), University of Calgary Press, Calgary, Alberta, pp. 15–26.

Nagy, F., Torok, I., and Maliga, P. (1981). Extensive rearrangements in the mitochondrial DNA in somatic hybrids of *Nicotiana tabacum* and *Nicotiana knightiana. Mol. Gen. Genet. 183*: 437–439.

Nakamura, A., Yamada, T., Kadotani, N., Itagaki, R., and Oka, M. (1974). Studies on the haploid method of breeding in tobacco. *Sabrao J. 6*:107–131.

Nakata, K. and Kurihara, T. (1972). Competition among pollen grains for haploid tobacco plant formation by anther culture. II. Analysis with resistance to tobacco virus (TMV) and wildfire diseases, leaf color, and leaf base shape characters. *Jpn. J. Breed. 22*:92–98.

Nickell, L. G. (1980). Products. In *Plant Tissue Culture as a Source of Biochemicals* (E. J. Staba, ed.), CRC Press, Boca Raton, Fla., pp. 236–256.

Nitsch, C. (1974). Pollen culture: A new technique for mass production of haploid and homozygous plants. In *Haploids in Higher Plants, Advances and Potential* (K. J. Kasha, ed.), University of Guelph Press, Ontario, pp. 123–135.

Nitsch, J. P. (1971). La Production in vitro d' embryons haploides: Resultats et perspectives. *Coll. Int. CNRS 193*:282–294.

Nitzsche, W. and Wenzel, G. (1977). *Haploids in Plant Breeding*, Verlag Paul Parey, Berlin.

Oglesby, R. P. (1978). Tissue cultures of ornamentals and flowers: Problems and perspectives. In *Propagation of Higher Plants Through Tissue Culture* (K. W. Hughes et al., eds.), U. S. Department of Energy, Washington, D. C., pp. 59–61.

Otten, L., DeGreve, H., Hernalsteens, J. P., VanMontagu, M., Schieder, O., Straub, J., and Schell, J. (1981). Mendelian transmission of genes introduced into plants by the Ti plasmids of *Agrobacterium tumefaciens*. *Mol. Gen. Genet. 183*:209.

Prenosil, J. E. and Pedersen, J. (1983). Immobilized plant cell reactors. *Enzyme Microb. Technol. 5*:323–331.

Quak, R. (1977). Meristem culture and virus-free plants. In *Plant, Cell, Tissue, and Organ Culture* (J. Reinert and Y. P. S. Bajaj, eds.), Springer-Verlag, Berlin, pp. 598–615.

Reisch, B. (1983). Genetic variability in regenerated plants. In *Handbook of Plant Cell Culture* (D. A. Evans, W. R. Sharp, P. V. Ammirato, and Y. Yamada, eds.), Macmillan, New York, pp. 748–769.

Renaudin, J. P. (1981). Tabernanthine by cell suspension cultures of *Catheranthus roseus* (L). G. Don and *Acer pseudoplatanus* L. *Plant Sci. Lett. 22*:59–69.

Schieder, O. (1978). Genetic evidence for the hybrid nature of somatic hybrids from *Datura innoxia* Mill. *Planta 141*:333–334.

Sharp, W. R., Reed, S. M., and Evans, D. A. (1984). Production and application of haploid plants. In *Contemporary Bases for Crop Breeding* (P. B. Vose and S. Blirt, eds.), Pergamon, Elmsford, N. Y., pp. 347–381.

Shepard, J. (1982). The regeneration of potato plants from leaf cell protoplasts. *Sci. Am. 246*:154–166.

Skirvin, R. M. and Janick, J. (1976). Tissue culture-induced variation in scented *Pelargonium* spp. *J. Am. Soc. Hort. Sci. 101*:281–290.

Sunderland, N. (1974). Anther culture as a means of haploid induction. In *Haploids in Higher Plants—Advances and Potential* (K. Kasha, ed.), University of Guelph, Ontario, pp. 91–122.

Walkey, D. G. A. and Cooper, V. C. (1975). Effect of temperature on virus eradication and growth of infected tissue cultures. *Ann. Appl. Biol. 80*:185–190.

Watanabe, K. and Yamada, Y. (1982). The selection of cultured plant cell lines producing high levels of biotin. *Phytochemistry 21*:513–516.

Whitaker, R. J. and Hashimoto, T. (1985). Plant tissue culture biotechnology and the production of secondary metabolites. In *Handbook of Plant Cell Culture,* Vol. 4 (D. A. Evans, P. V. Ammirato, W. R. Sharp, and Y. Yamada, eds.), Macmillan, New York (in press).

White, D. W. R. and Vasil, I. K. (1979). Use of amino acid analogue-resistant cell lines for selection of *Nicotiana sylvestris* somatic cell hybrids. *Theor. Appl. Genet. 55*:107–112.

Willmitzer, L., De Beucckeleer, M., Lemmers, M., Van Montagu, M., and Schell, J. (1980). DNA from Ti plasmid present in nucleus and absent from plastids of crown gall plant cells. *Nature 287*:359.

Wullems, G. J., Molendijk, L., Oooms, G., and Schilperoort, R. A. (1981). Differential expression of crown gall tumor markers in transformants obtained after in vitro *Agrobacterium tumefaciens* induced transformation of cell wall regenerating protoplasts derived from *Nicotiana tabacum. Proc. Nat. Acad. Sci. U.S.A. 78*:4344.

Yamada, Y. and Fujita, Y. (1983). Production of useful compounds in culture. In *Handbook of Plant Cell Culture* (D. A. Evans, P. V. Ammirato, W. R. Sharp, and Y. Yamada, eds.), Vol. 1, Macmillan, New York, pp. 717–728.

Yamada, Y. and Hashimoto, T. (1982). Production of tropane alkaloids in cultured cells of *Hyosyamus niger. Plant Cell Reports 1*:101–103.

Yamamoto, Y., Muzriquchi, R., and Yamada, Y. (1982). Selection of a high and stable pigment-producing strain in culture *Euphorbia millii* cells. *Theor. Appl. Genet. 61*:113–116.

Yang, F. and Simpson, R. B. (1981). Revertant seedlings from crown gall tumors retain a portion of the bacterial Ti plasmid DNA sequences. *Proc. Nat. Acad. Sci. U.S.A. 78*:4151.

Yasuda, T., Hashimoto, T., Sato, F., and Yamada, Y. (1980). An efficient method of selecting photoautotrophic cells from cultural heterogeneous cells. *Plant Cell Physiol. 21*:729–732.

Zenk, M. H. (1978). The impact of plant cell culture on industry. In *Frontiers of Plant Tissue Culture 1978* (T. A. Thorpe, ed.), University of Calgary Press, Calgary, Alberta, pp. 1–13.

Zenk, M., El-Shagri, H., and Ulrich, B. (1977). Production of rosmarinic acid by cell suspension cultures of *Coleus blumei. Naturwissenschaften 64*:585–586.

13

Single-Cell Protein: Production Modification and Utilization

CARL A. BATT* and ANTHONY J. SINSKEY / Massachusetts Institute of Technology, Cambridge, Massachusetts

INTRODUCTION

Single-cell protein (SCP) refers to any unicellular source of protein, including yeast, bacteria, fungi, and algae. The value of SCP is in its use as a nutritional supplement where conventional protein sources are not available or are uneconomical.

The production of SCP can be simply defined as the process of converting raw materials into cellular biomass. The production cost of SCP is dependent upon substrate cost, operating expenses, and capital investment for fermentation equipment. A significant reduction in the cost of SCP would be realized if cheaper substrates could be developed without loss of conversion efficiency.

Another important factor in SCP production is protein content and quality. The chemical composition of bacteria, yeast, fungi, and algae vary, depending upon the genera and growth conditions (Reed, 1981; Krug et al., 1979). The gross chemical composition of various microorganisms is presented in Table 1. Although the protein content can be varied by growth conditions, genetic manipulation can also be employed to alter the amino acid spectrum (see the section on nutrition).

The production of SCP is most amenable to manipulation as a biotechnological process. Improvements in SCP yields, productivity, and quality can be obtained by optimizing the various stages in the process. This review will highlight some of the recent developments in SCP production and strategies to improve SCP production via genetic engineering. Recently Litchfield (1983) has reviewed SCP

*Current affiliation: Cornell University, Ithaca, New York

Table 1. Protein Content of Various Microorganisms

Microorganisms	Protein (%)
Yeast	45–55
Algae	47–63
Bacteria	50–83
Fungi	31–55

production and described methods for producing SCP from various substrates using both photosynthetic and nonphotosynthetic microorganisms.

GENETIC ENGINEERING OF THE IDEAL SCP MICROORGANISM

Most SCP processes are designed to take advantage of an available substrate using a microorganism which can readily convert that substrate into microbial biomass. The choice of SCP microorganism is usually limited to that particular process, and a change in substrate often necessitates a change in the type of SCP microorganism used. Other considerations include the potential toxicity, functionality, and organoleptic performance of the SCP. In most SCP processes the selection of the SCP microorganism involves some compromise in each of these areas. It would be ideal if the best attributes of each SCP microorganism could be combined. Recent developments in genetic engineering have made the "construction" of SCP microorganisms possible. The required tools for the genetic engineering of a microorganism are a vector and a transformation system. A vector is a DNA sequence which functions to maintain the desired gene in the host. A vector is usually constructed from an extrachromosomal element, for example, a plasmid or an integrative virus. The only requirement is that it replicate whenever the host replicates to avoid its segregation and loss during mitosis.

The second tool for the genetic engineering of SCP microorganisms is a *transformation* system. Transformation is the uptake of naked DNA by a cell. Since most genetic engineering is performed in vitro, it is essential that introduction of the engineered gene into the host be possible. A cell can be transformed through a variety of techniques which make its competent (capable of DNA uptake).

Competence can be achieved either naturally or by treatment with divalent cations. Alternatively, the cell wall can be removed, rendering the protoplast capable of DNA uptake.

Few studies have been reported on improving SCP production using genetic engineering. This is directly attributable to two factors: (1) a lack of sophisticated genetic tools for manipulating SCP microorganisms and (2) the relatively low product cost of SCP. The low cost of SCP as compared to high-value pharmaceuticals (e.g., interferon) will limit any commercial research and development efforts for the next few years. As more and more recombinant DNA techniques become generic, they may be used to address the problems of SCP. Fortunately, several other current research problems are being pursued whose achievements are applicable to SCP production. Most notable are the efforts directed toward (biomass utilization for the production of low molecular weight fuels). These types of processes can be loosely categorized as SCP processes and frequently the resulting microbial biomass is used for animal feed. The technology developed for the treatment of agricultural biomass for fuel production is directly applicable, since the breakdown of polymer carbon substrates (e.g., starch, cellulose) into monosaccharides is frequently required in both cases.

SACCHAROMYCES CEREVISIAE AS A MODEL SOURCE OF SCP

Recent advances in biotechnology have facilitated the in vitro construction of recombinant genes and their transformation into a suitable host. A wide diversity of prokaryotic and eukaryotic organisms have been manipulated via genetic engineering resulting in new catabolic and anabolic functions. Although many yeast strains can serve as a source of SCP, the most sophisticated tools for the genetic manipulation of SCP organisms are available for the yeast *Saccharomyces cerevisiae*. *Saccharomyces cerevisiae* is therefore a suitable candidate for strain improvement via classical and recombinant DNA manipulation to yield a better SCP or improved SCP processes.

The present levels of recombinant DNA technology permits the in vitro construction of many genes and new methods are available to express foreign genes in *S. cerevisiae*. The only limitations are the scope of the biotechnologist's imagination and the cooperation of the host *S. cerevisiae*. The following sections describe the current status of genetic engineering of SCP microorganisms. Although this review emphasizes the potential for improving *S. cerevisiae*, the strategies could be generally applied to other microorganisms given the available genetic tools.

RAW MATERIALS

Substrate Utilization

A major factor in the cost of producing SCP is the raw materials and the efficiency of their conversion into SCP biomass. The choice of substrate is usually dependent upon local availability, since the transportation of substrates over long distances is not cost effective. It is usually advantageous to couple SCP production to another existing process whose waste by-products can be utilized as substrates for SCP.

The primary substrates for SCP production are petroleum-based hydrocarbons, carbohydrates, and methane (or methanol). Each substrate has its own benefits, depending upon their demand for other end uses, and several SCP processes have been developed to utilize them.

Agricultural Wastes as Substrates for SCP

Agricultural wastes represent an inexpensive source of substrates for the production of SCP. The types of carbon substrates available in these wastes include cellulose, hemicellulose, lactose, and starch. For the utilization of these waste substrates by SCP microorganisms, saccharification and metabolism are usually necessary. The utilization of these carbon sources by a given SCP microorganism is variable; for example, *Kluyveromyces fragilis* can metabolize lactose whereas *S. cerevisiae* cannot (Bernstein et al., 1977). *Saccharomyces cerevisiae* cannot utilize lactose because of the absence of both a lactose permease and β-galactosidase (Dickson, 1980). In other cases certain SCP microorganisms can utilize cellulose or xylose. The choice of SCP microorganism must take into account its ability to metabolize a substrate and the yield and quality of the protein obtained from growth on that substrate. The solution to the case of an SCP microorganism with high protein quality which cannot utilize the desired substrate is to either (1) treat the substrate to render it metabolizable by the SCP microorganism or (2) genetically engineer the SCP microorganism to metabolize the substrate.

The production of SCP from cellulose by hydrolysis with *Trichoderma reesei* and *Pellicularia filamentosa* has been reported (Kamikubo et al., 1981). The hydrolyzed cellulose supported the growth of both *Candida utilis* and *S. cerevisiae*. Alternatively, by genetically engineering an SCP microorganism to produce, for example, cellulase, the pretreatment enzymatic hydrolysis can be circumvented. The following describes the current status of cloning and the expression of various catabolic enzymes which could be used for improving the substrate range of SCP microorganisms.

Cellulose is a $\beta(1\rightarrow4)$ glucose polymer which must be hydrolyzed to glucose prior to glycolysis. There are a wide variety of cellulases and those derived from the filamentous fungus *Trichoderma* have been well characterized (Shoemaker et al., 1983a). At least three separate cellulase activities in *T. reesei* have been detected: cellobiohydrolase (CBHI), endoglucanase (EGI), and β-glucosidase (BGI).

The *T. reesei* cellulases are coordinately regulated to ensure the synergism required for breakdown of the cellulose matrix. Both EGI and CBHI are induced by cellulose and repressed by cellobiose. The synthesis of BGI is constitutive and its activity is feedback-repressed by glucose.

The gene coding for *T. reesei* CBHI has been cloned into *Escherichia coli* and its DNA sequence and translated amino acid sequence reported (Shoemaker et al., 1983b; Teeri et al., 1983). The CBHI gene was identified by differential hybridization using messenger RNA (mRNA) from induced as compared to uninduced *T. reesei* cultures.

Expression of CBHI in an SCP microorganism will require correct processing of the mRNA, including the removal of the two introns. Another potential problem is the secretion of the pro-CBHI and the efficacy of the native signal peptide. If the CBHI signal peptide is not properly exported, it may be necessary to use another signal, for example, invertase, the yeast signal peptide (Hitzman et al., 1983). Protein secretion in yeast has been investigated extensively for acid phosphatase and invertase (Schekman and Novick, 1982). The 5'-end of the invertase (Carlson and Bostein, 1983) and acid phosphatase (Haguenauer-Tsapis and Hinnen, 1984) have been identified and these signal peptides could be fused in vitro to the desired protein for secretion.

Lastly, CBHI, as well as the other *T. reesei* cellulases, is glycosylated. It is not known if glycosylation is required for biological activity or stability or if the SCP microorganism can properly glycosylate it.

The endocellulase gene from the bacterium *Thermomonospora* YX has been cloned and expressed in *E. coli* (Collmer and Wilson, 1983). This thermostable endocellulase has a molecular weight of 94,000 and cleaves $\beta(1\rightarrow4)$ linkages in carboxymethylcellulose (CMC). The endocellulase gene was identified by direct selection for CMC degradation in *E. coli* transformed with a *Thermomonospora* genomic bank constructed using pBR 322.

The *Clostridium thermocellum* endocellulase gene has also been cloned and expressed in *E. coli* using a strategy similar to that described for *Thermomonospora* (Cornet et al., 1983). A genomic cosmid bank (pHC 79) of *Cl. thermocellum* was constructed and transformed into *E. coli*. The *E. coli* clone carrying the *Cl. thermocellum* endocellulase gene was identified by CMCase activity in pools of transformants. The CMCase activity was cotransduced with the pHC 79 marker (ampicillin resistance). No further characterization of the gene has been reported.

Finally, the *Cellulomonas fimi* cellulase gene has been cloned and expressed in *E. coli* (Whittle et al., 1982). The gene was identified in a *C. fimi* genomic bank constructed in pBR 322 by screening with ^{125}I-labeled rabbit antibody against the extracellular supernatant of a *C. fimi* culture grown on CMC. An SCP process has been reported using *Cellulomonas* and bagasse as a substrate (Han et al., 1970).

No attempts to express either the *Thermomonospora*, *C. fimi*, or *Cl. thermocellum* cellulase genes in heterologous organisms have been reported. The potential problems with the expression of a bacterial cellulase gene are somewhat different from those encountered for *T. reesei* genes. Neither RNA splicing nor glycosylation is required for expression of any prokaryotic cellulase. The prokaryotic promoter would probably not function in a eukaryote and would therefore require its replacement with a yeast promoter (see next paragraph). Lastly, whether the bacterial procellulase protein would be secreted is not clear and, as mentioned previously, may require the introduction of a new signal peptide.

Hemicellulose is another fraction of agricultural biomass. It consists primarily of a pentose sugar, xylose in its polymeric form, xylan. Certain yeasts, including *S. cerevisiae*, cannot utilize xylose as sole carbon source, although the metabolic deficiency is not clear. There are, however, several yeasts that can catabolize xylose and which are used for SCP (e.g., *Candida*). Xylose can be transported (Cirillo, 1968) into the cell and *S. cerevisiae* can utilize the keto isomer of xylose, xylulose (Wang and Schneider, 1980). The missing catalytic function is the enzyme(s) to isomerize xylose to xylulose. A solution via genetic engineering is to introduce a gene(s) coding for an enzyme to isomerize xylose, xylose isomerase. Xylose isomerase has been detected in a wide variety of prokaryotic organisms, including *E. coli*, *Salmonella typhimurium*, *Lactobacillus*, and *Streptomyces*. The *E. coli* xylose isomerase gene has been cloned into *S. cerevisiae*; the *E. coli* xylose isomerase gene is stable in *S. cerevisiae* but is not expressed (Batt et al., 1983). Current efforts are focusing on expressing the xylose isomerase gene using a native yeast promoter.

The major sugar component of whey is lactose, which can be catabolized by several SCP microorganisms, for example, *Kluyveromyces lactis* (Giec and Kosikowski, 1982). On the other hand, *S. cerevisiae* cannot utilize lactose owing to an apparent lack of the enzyme(s) necessary for its metabolism.

The construction of a lactose-utilizing strain of *S. cerevisiae* would permit the growth of *S. cerevisiae* on whey. The inability of *S. cerevisiae* to utilize whey appears to be due to the absence of a lactose transport system and β-galactosidase, the enzyme which hydrolyzes lactose to galactose and glucose.

The gene coding for the β-galactosidase has been cloned from *K. lactis* into *S. cerevisiae* (Dickson, 1980). The *K. lactis* gene is expressed in *S. cerevisiae* and β-galactosidase activity is detectable, but the *S. cerevisiae* strain cannot grow on lactose as a sole carbon source. Although lactose can be hydrolyzed by the *S. cerevisiae* strain containing the cloned β-galactosidase gene, it cannot transport lactose into the cell.

Starch is another inexpensive substrate suitable for SCP production. It is a by-product of many food industries, such as rice and potato processing. The Symba process was developed to utilize starch as a substrate for the production of SCP. The Symba process employs two microorganisms: *Saccharomycopsis fibuligera* to hydrolyze the starch to glucose and maltose, which *Can. utilis* then metabolizes for growth (Skogman, 1976). The limiting step in the Symba process is the rate of starch hydrolysis by *Saccharomycopsis fibuligera* (Lemmel et al., 1979). A simplification of this coculture process would be to develop a SCP microorganism which could hydrolyze starch. This could be accomplished through genetic engineering by introducing an amylase gene into the desired SCP microorganism.

The glucoamylase gene from *Aspergillus awamori* has been cloned using a strategy similar to that used for cloning the CBH1 gene from *T. reesei* (Nunberg et al., 1984). The glucoamylase gene was identified by the differential mRNA levels in *A. awamori* grown on xylose and starch. Glucoamylase is only partially repressed by growth on glucose. This *A. awamori* gene contains four introns. As discussed previously, the expression of the glucoamylase gene in an SCP microorganism would depend upon proper mRNA processing, posttranscriptional modification, and secretion.

Other amylase genes have been cloned from *Bacillus* sp. (Palva, 1982; Cornelis et al., 1982). These amylase genes would not require mRNA splicing for expression, although the problems encountered in expressing its prokaryotic promoter in *S. cerevisiae* would exist.

Methanol

Several C_1 compounds (e.g., methanol) have been investigated as substrates for SCP production. The yeast strains which are suitable for growth on hydrocarbons are *Candida lipolytica* and *Candida tropicalis* (Reed, 1981). The feasibility of using higher molecular weight hydrocarbons has decreased drastically as petroleum prices have increased in the past decade. Methanol has the advantage of generating less heat from its oxidation as compared to higher molecular weight hydrocarbons (Krug et al., 1979). The heat generated during fermentation must be dissipated, resulting in additional operating expenses.

A process for SCP production using *Methylophilus methylotrophus* grown on methanol is an example of improving conversion by genetic engineering (Windass et al., 1980). The conversion of methanol by *M. methylotrophus* is limited by ammonia assimilation. Glutamate synthesis from ammonia and oxoglutarate in this organism involves two enzymes and requires adenosine triphosphate as a cofactor for the glutamine synthetase. Other microorganisms (e.g., *E. coli*) catalyze the same reactions using glutamate dehydrogenase (GDH), which is more efficient, since it does not consume adenosine triphosphate. The *gdh* gene from *E. coli* was cloned using a broad host range vector by complementation of a gdh^- mutant. The *gdh* gene was subcloned onto a conjugal vector and transferred from *E. coli* to *M. methylotrophus*. The *E. coli gdh* gene was expressed in *M. methylotrophus*, although GDH activity was 10- to 20-fold lower in the heterologous host (Windass et al., 1980). The engineered *M. methylotrophus* strain carrying the *E. coli gdh* gene gave 4–7% higher carbon conversion as compared to the parental strain.

Increasing the substrate range of SCP microorganisms will permit SCP production from many inexpensive substrates and therefore decrease the product cost. The problem is to integrate the new substrates and their metabolites into the normal biochemical pathways of the host. Not only must the host synthesize new enzymes but also the pool of substrates must be properly balanced with respect to the cofactors and other catabolic functions necessary for complete metabolism. New and novel control strategies based upon the physiology of the organism must be developed.

NUTRITIONAL CONTENT

The nutritional content of SCP depends on the metabolic state of the organism at the time of harvest and the effect of postharvest processing necessary to yield the final product. The balance of essential amino acids will determine the protein quality of the SCP, in addition to digestibility and bioavailability of the protein, as well as the presence of compounds detrimental to protein utilization (Young and Scrimshaw, 1975).

The protein content and quality of a given SCP are partially determined by the substrate on which the SCP is grown. The amino acid content of *S. cerevisiae* compared to that of other yeast strains is different both quantitatively and qualitatively. The amino acid spectrum of the different yeast strains has a pronounced effect on the protein efficiency ratio (Vaughan Martini et al., 1979). The differences in amino acid spectrum reflects the differences in the metabolism of the different organisms as regulated by the genes coding for the individual biochemical pathways.

Altering the balance of amino acid pools can be accomplished by deregulation of the biosynthetic pathways to overproduce the limiting amino acids. The concentration of the limiting amino acid may be increased by removing the biochemical feedback mechanisms which control the amino acid concentration. A similar strategy has been successfully employed with many gram-positive bacteria for the commercial production of amino acids (Soda et al., 1983). The regulation of amino acid biosynthesis has been recently reviewed and is controlled both transcriptionally and by the activity of the biosynthetic enzymes (Jones and Fink, 1982).

At present few attempts have been reported to develop an amino acid-overproducing strain of *S. cerevisiae*. Many of the same principles for isolating amino acid-overproducing bacteria apply to *S. cerevisiae*, although basic differences in amino acid biosynthesis regulation and accumulation will have to be accounted for (Hutter et al., 1983). The development of *S. cerevisiae* strains to overproduce limiting amino acids may reduce the need to add amino acid supplements to SCP products. The manipulation of amino acid biosynthesis can also benefit the flavor of SCP. Diacetyl and 2,3-pentanidione are components of beer flavor and result from side reactions of the isoleucine—valine pathway. Altering the activity of the isoleucine—valine pathway would have a direct effect on the production of diketones (Holmberg, 1984).

In addition, the composition of a protein may be enriched for a given amino acid by the insertion of a synthetic polynucleotide sequence through genetic engineering of the protein. This approach has been demonstrated by modifying the ampicillinase protein of pBR 322 by the insertion of a poly(G—C) sequences which increased the proline content of the ampicillinase protein in *E. coli* (Kangas et al., 1982). The addition of 41 G—C base pairs into the *Pst*I site of pBR 322 translated into a truncated 21,000-dalton protein with approximately 9 "new" proline residues added. Similarly, a synthetic DNA coding for a poly(l-aspartyl-L-phenylalanine) has been cloned and expressed into *E. coli* (Doel et al., 1980).

The nutritional availability of the protein upon consumption is at least partially determined by the degree of cellular lysis. This will be discussed below.

Toxic Components

Single-cell protein may be beneficial as a dietary supplement for animals or humans; however, certain toxic compounds may also be present (Reed, 1981). The nucleic acids present in SCP have been reported to cause high levels of uric acid in the blood, resulting in gout. The recommended maximum intake of nucleic acids by humans is 2 g/day. Several methods of reducing the nucleic acid of SCP have been developed, including alkali, acid, or enzymatic hydrolysis, as well as induction of the endogenous nucleases (Sinskey and Tannenbaum, 1975). Reducing the problem of nucleic acids in SCP can be addressed by genetic engineering. The solution would involve the engineering of a gene coding for a nuclease whose synthesis could be externally triggered during processing. The transcription of the structural gene for the nuclease could be placed under the control of a heat shock promoter and its synthesis induced by heat treatment (Lindquist, 1981).

CELLULAR LYSIS

The bioavailability of protein in SCP is limited by the degree of cellular lysis which releases the protein components of the cell. These are various methods to break yeast cells, including high-pressure, freeze–thaw, sonication, chemical, and enzymatic treatment (Sinskey and Tannenbaum, 1975; Knorr et al., 1979). Autolysis is an attractive method to disrupt yeast cells, especially if accomplished without additional chemical agents, such as salt or energy (i.e., heat), thereby reducing the cost of SCP production.

A temperature-sensitive lysis mutant of *S. cerevisiae* JD 109 has been isolated which will lyse at 37°C, the nonpermissive temperature. *Saccharomyces cerevisiae* JD 109 lysed more readily at pH 8 as compared to pH 5.6 and the protein content of the cell was reduced from 45 to 35% (Schaffeld et al., 1982). The genetic lesion responsible for cellular lysis in *S. cerevisiae* JD 109 is not known but must involve some perturbation of the cell wall. Maximal lysis of *S. cerevisiae* autolytic mutants occur at logarithmic phase and lysis begins within 1–3 hr of the temperature shift-up (Boudrant et al., 1979).

The development of *S. cerevisiae* strains which rapidly lyse have been obtained through chemical mutagenesis. The introduction of a gene coding for a lytic enzyme, for example, zymolase, under the control of a yeast promotor which could be externally triggered at the proper time is a possible method for obtaining an autolytic strain of *S. cerevisiae*. The restrictions in developing other autolytic *S. cerevisiae* strains relate to the viability of the mutant strain. The autolytic mutant must retain normal growth and protein content under permissive conditions in the absence of the agent to trigger cell lysis. This technology may be applied to the development of novel flavor-generating systems in addition to recovery of protein.

FUNCTIONAL PROPERTIES

Certain functional properties of SCP may be desirable, depending on the final food product. If used as a nutritional supplement, SCP could still provide certain functional properties, that is, as a gelling or emulsifying agent, or at least the SCP should not be detrimental to the food system (Rha, 1975). Various factors, including polysaccharides, amino acids, and proteins, can affect the functional properties of the SCP. Some of the functional properties of *S. cerevisiae* are dependent on the structure of the polymers in the cell wall. By modification of the structure of the cell wall, the functional attributes can be manipulated to yield the desired properties.

Several morphological mutants of *S. cerevisiae* have been isolated which exhibit mycelial forms under certain environmental conditions, including some involving temperature and medium composition. All the morphological mutants characterized have a defective cell division cycle (CDC). Over 150 CDC mutants have been isolated and grow as normal yeast cells at permissive temperatures but exhibit mycelial forms at nonpermissive temperatures (Hartwell et al., 1973).

A morphological mutant of *S. cerevisiae* designated JD7, which exhibits a normal yeastlike form when grown with 20% sorbitol but a mycelial form on complex medium without sorbitol, has been rheologically characterized (Miyasaka et al., 1980). *Saccharomyces cerevisiae* JD7 cells in the mycelial form settle out of solution faster as compared to the parent strain *S. cerevisiae* A364A. The viscosity of *S. cerevisiae* JD7 in the mycelial form increases very sharply as a function of cell concentration, whereas *S. cerevisiae* JD7 in the yeast form exhibits little increase in viscosity. The mycelial shape, which permits a larger surface interaction between cells, obviously contributes to the increased viscosity of the cell suspension.

The rheological properties of temperature-sensitive CDC mutants are similar to those reported for *S. cerevisiae* JD7. *Saccharomyces cerevisiae* 374 and 377 displayed a higher relative viscosity compared to wild-type *S. cerevisiae* A364A. The apparent viscosity is related to the structure of cell wall polymers, including the glucan component. The matrix of the isolated glucan fraction from the cell wall of *S. cerevisiae* 374 and 377 is denser than the glucan matrix of *S. cerevisiae* A 364A. The $\beta(1\rightarrow6)$ glucosidic crosslinking appears to be important in determining the functional properties of the yeast glucan (Jamas, 1983).

By controlling the glucan structure of *S. cerevisiae* strains, one could adjust the viscosity of the food product to meet the desired specifications. The key to controlling the structure–function relationship is in understanding the genetics of the polymer biosynthesis and developing methods to manipulate the structure–function relationship by classical genetics or recombinant DNA techniques. The genetic lesions in CDC mutants have been mapped at various positions on the yeast chromosome (Hartwell et al., 1973), although the CDC lesions are not specific for glucan biosynthesis and affect the general cell division process. The genes specifically controlling polymer structure have not been identified. Their elucidation is essential for manipulating the structure–function properties of SCP.

FUTURE PROSPECTS

Despite an incomplete understanding of the expression of eukaryotic protein syntehsis, strategies have been successfully developed and carried out to synthesize foreign proteins in *S. cerevisiae*. Once the genes responsible for the desired phenotype are identified, they can be manipulated in vitro to obtain the desired results. Clearly, novel and new functional proteins could be produced. As stated previously, the only limitations relate to the compatability of the recombinant gene in the host. It is obvious that any "cloned" product which is toxic to the host will not be stable.

The use of promoter sequences to turn on a desired gene function (e.g., cell lysis), when an external triggering agent is presented would be advantageous in developing *S. cerevisiae* strains for SCP production. Suitable triggering agents include temperature or a chemical inducer. This method of externally triggering a gene function would facilitate the design of two-stage processes for SCP production as a by-product of another fermentation process. For example, the primary fermentation may be the production of alcohol. After the primary fermentation is complete, the spent yeast could be utilized for SCP and the desired SCP properties "turned on" by the external triggering agent during the second fermentation. The external triggering agent would activate the gene(s) for cell lysis or morphological changes to suit the specification of the food product.

The development of strains of *S. cerevisiae* which possess new and novel catabolic and functional properties will have applications in areas other than SCP. The isolation of self-lysing mutants of *S. cerevisiae* may be used for the production of yeast autolysates as flavoring agents. Current methods of lysing yeast cells require the addition of heat, salt, or other lytic agents. Furthermore, the flavor profile of a yeast autolysate may be altered by manipulation of the amino acid content or peptide profile of the yeast strain. Many flavor compounds are derived from Maillard reactions between reducing sugars and amino acids. The Maillard reaction products will depend in part on the amino acid reactant. Yeast strains with the appropriate functional properties may be used as gelling agents in foods or chemical products, either as whole cells or using cell wall fractions.

Novel applications of yeast SCP are possible if the biotechnologist can elucidate the appropriate controlling genes and design methods to manipulate them via genetic engineering.

REFERENCES

Batt, C. A., Brown, A. J. P., Picataggio, S. K., and Sinskey, A. J. (1983). Molecular cloning of the *Escherichia coli* xylose isomerase in *Saccharomyces cerevisiae* (unpublished results).

Berstein, S., Tzeng, C. H., and Sisson, D. (1977). *Biotechnol. Bioeng. Symp.* 7:1.

Boudrant, J., DeAngelo, J., Sinskey, A. J., and Tannenbaum, S. R. (1979). Process characteristics of cell lysis mutants of *Saccharomyces cerevisiae*. *Biotechnol. Bioeng.* *21*:659–670.

Carlson, M. and Botstein, D. (1983). Organization of the *SUC* gene family in *Saccharomyces*. *Mol. Cell. Biol.* *3*:351–359.

Cirillo, V. P. (1968). Relationship between sugar structure and competition for the sugar transport system in baker's yeast. *J. Bacteriol.* *95*:603.

Cornelis, P., Digneffe, C., and Willemot, K. (1982). Cloning and expression of a *Bacillus coagulans* amylase gene in *Escherichia coli*. *Mol. Gen. Genet.* *186*:507–511.

Dickson, R. C. (1980). Expression of a foreign eukaryotic gene in *Saccharomyces cerevisiae*: β-Galactosidase from *Kluyveromyces lactis*. *Gene* *10*:347.

Doel, M. T., Eaton, M., Cook, E. A., Lewis, H., Patel, T., and Carey, N. J. (1980). The expression in *E. coli* of synthetic repeating genes for poly(L-aspartyl-L-phenylalanine). *Nucleic Acid Res.* *8*:4575–4502.

Giec, A. and Kosikowski, F. V. (1982). Activity of lactose fermenting yeasts in producing biomass from concentrated whey permeates. *J. Food Sci.* *47*:1892–1902.

Haguenauer-Tsapis, R. and Hinnen, A. (1984). A deletion that includes the signal peptidase cleavage site impairs processing. Glycolysation, and secretion of cell surface yeast acid phosphatase. *Mol. Cell. Biol.* *4*:2668–2675.

Han, Y. W., Dunlap, C. E., and Callihan, C. D. (1970). Single cell protein from cellulosic wastes. *Food Technol.* *25*:130–132.

Hartwell, L. H., Mortimer, R. K., Culotti, J., and Culotti, M. (1973). Genetic control of the cell division cycle in yeast. V. Genetic analysis of CDC mutants. *Genetics* *74*:267.

Holmberg, S. (1984). Genetic improvement of brewers' yeast. *Trends Biotechnol. 2*:98–102.

Hutter, R., Neiderberger, P., and Aebi, M. (1983). Regulation of amino acid biosynthesis in eucaryotic microorganisms. In *Genetics of Industrial Microorganisms* (Y. Ikeda and T. Beppu, eds.), Kodansha, Tokyo, p. 235.

Jamas, S. (1983). The effect of β-glucan structure on the rheological properties of yeast cell walls. M.Sc. thesis, Department of Nutrition and Food Science, Massachusetts Institute of Technology, Cambridge.

Jones, E. W. and Fink, G. R. (1982). Regulation of amino acid and nucleotide biosynthesis in yeast. In *The Molecular Biology of the Yeast Saccharomyces. Metabolism and Gene Expression* (J. N. Strathern, E. W. Jones, and J. R. Broach, eds.), Cold Spring Harbor Laboratory, Cold Spring Harbor, N. Y., pp. 181–299.

Kamikubo, T., Tanaka, M., Taniguchi, M., Morita, T., and Matsuno, R. (1981). Production of SCP from cellulose. In *Advances in Biotechnology*, Vol. 2 (M. Moo-Young and C. W. Robinson, eds), Pergamon, New York, pp. 311–318.

Kangas, T. T., Cooney, C. L., and Gomez, R. F. (1982). Expression of a proline enriched protein in *Escherichia coli*. *Appl. Environ. Microbiol. 43*:629.

Knorr, D., Shetty, K. J., and Kinsella, J. E. (1979). Enzymatic lysis of yeast cell walls. *Biotechnol. Bioeng. 21*:2011.

Krug, E. L., Lim, H. C., and Tsao, G. T. (1979). Single cell protein from C_1 compounds. In *Annual Reports on Fermentation Processes*, Vol. 3 (D. Perlman, ed.), Academic, New York, pp. 141–195.

Lemmel, S. A., Heimsch, R. C., and Edwards, L. L. (1979). Optimizing the continuous production of *Candida utilis* and *Saccharomyces fibuligera* on potato processing waste water. *Appl. Environ. Microbiol. 37*:227–232.

Lindwuist, S. (1981). Regulation of protein synthesis during heat shock. *Nature 293*:311–315.

Litchfield, J. H. (1983). Single-cell protein. *Science 219*:740.

Miyasaka, Y., Sinskey, A. J., DeAngelo, J., and Rha, C. K. (1980). Characterization of a morphological mutant of *Saccharomyces cerevisiae* for single-cell protein production. *J. Food Sci. 45*:588.

Nunberg, J. H., Meade, J. H., Cole, G., Lawyer, F. C. McCabe, P., Schweickart, V., Tal, R., Wittman, V. P., Flatgaard, J. E., and Innis, M. A. (1984). Molecular cloning and characterization of the glucoamylase gene of *Aspergillus awamori*. *Mol. Cell. Biol. 4*:2306–2315.

Palva, I. (1982). Molecular cloning of α-amylase gene from *Bacillus amyloliquefaciens* and its expression in *B. subtilis*. *Gene 19*:81–87.

Rha, C. K. (1975). Utilization of single-cell protein for human food. In *Single Cell Protein* (S. R. Tannenbaum and D. I. C. Wang, eds.), MIT Press, Cambridge, p. 587.

Rolf, M. J., Hennigan, P. J., Mohler, R. D., Weigand, W. A., and Lim, H. C. (1982). Development of a direct digital-controlled fermentor using a microminicomputer hierarchical system. *Biotechnol. Bioeng. 24*:1191.

Schaffeld, G., Sinskey, A. J., and Rha, C. K. (1982). Release of single-cell protein by induced cell lysis. *J. Food Sci. 47*:2072.

Schekman, R. and Novick, P. (1982). The secretory process and yeast cell surface assembly. In *The Molecular Biology of the Yeast Saccharomyces* (J. N. Strathen, E. W. Jones, and J. R. Broach, eds.), Cold Spring Harbor Laboratory, Cold Spring Harbor, N. Y., p. 351.

Shoemaker, S., Watt, K., Tristovsky, G., and Cox, R. V. (1983a). Characterization and properties of cellulases purified from *Trichoderma reesei* strain L27. *BioTechnol. 1*:687–690.

Shoemaker, S., Schweickart, V., Ladner, M., Gelfand, D., Kwok, S., Myambo, K., and Innes, M. (1983b). Molecular cloning of exo-cellobiohydralase I derived from *Trichoderma reesei* strain L27. *BioTechnol. 1*:691–696.

Sinskey, A. J. and Tannenbaum, S. R. (1975). Removal of nucleic acids in SCP. In *Single Cell Protein* (S. R. Tannenbaum and D. I. C. Wang, eds.), MIT Press, Cambridge, p. 158.

Skogman, H. (1976). The Symba process. *Starch 25*:278–282.

Soda, K., Tanaka, H., and Esaki, N. (1983). Amino acids. In *Biotechnology*, Vol. 3 (H. Dellweg, ed.), Verlag-Chemie, Wernheim, pp. 479–532.

Udaka, S., Tsukagashi, N., Yamada, N., and Miyashiro, S. (1981). Extracellular production of proteins by bacteria. In *Advances in Biotechnology*, Vol. 2 (M. Moo-Young and C. W. Robinson, eds.), Pergamon, New York, p. 381.

Vaughan Martini, A. E., Miller, M. W., and Martini, A. (1979). Amino acid composition of whole cells of different yeasts. *J. Agric. Food Chem. 27*:982.

Wang, P. Y. and Schneider, H. (1980). Growth of yeasts on D-xylulose. *Can. J. Microbiol. 26*:1165.

Windass, J. D., Worsey, M. J., Pioli, E. M., Pioli, D., Barth, P. T., Atherton, K. T., and Dart, E. C. (1980). Improved conversion of methanol to single-cell protein by *Methylophilus methylotrophus*. *Nature 287*:396–401.

Young, V. R. and Scrimshaw, N. S. (1975). Clinical studies on the nutritional value of single cell proteins. In *Single Cell Protein* (S. R. Tannenbaum and D. I. C. Wang, eds.), MIT Press, Cambridge, p. 564.

14

Functional Proteins from Yeast Nucleoprotein for Food Uses: Methods for Isolation

JOHN E. KINSELLA / Cornell University, Ithaca, New York

INTRODUCTION

Biotechnology and fermentation technology can become significant sources of nutrients for a burgeoning world population. Extensive starvation and protein/calorie malnutrition exists in most underdeveloped areas of the world (Milner et al., 1978). Because of the prevailing constraints on expanding productivity by conventional agriculture (arable land, climate, energy costs, etc.), it seems prudent to develop alternative sources of foods and nutrients that can supplement present agricultural sources. Fermentation technology for the production of microbes can provide a concentrated source of proteins that could help to meet the current 6% annual increase in protein required for an expanding world population, especially in the underdeveloped areas of the world.

The advantages of microbes as a possible protein source which can complement the conventional methods of food production have been documented (Tannenbaum, 1977; Cooney et al., 1980). The relative productivity of microbes is phenomenal; for example, it has been estimated that a fermentation plant making 10^4 tons/year produces as much protein as is obtained from 12×10^4 h of soybeans or 2×10^6 h used for beef. The productivity of bacteria exceeds that of yeast, and bacteria also have a higher protein content.

Microbe production can be continuous and is relatively independent of climate, geographical area, and so on. A multitude of different microbes can be grown on a wide range of substrates, many of which are unused by-products, and hence microbes may not compete with agricultural resources. Microbes have short generation times, which ensures a rapid biomass increase compared to conventional agriculture. The ability to grow yeast at very high cell densities (150 g/liter) compared to conventional methods (40 g/liter) should greatly expand their productivity (Krieger, 1983). Genetic flexibility via induced mutations and gene recombination and selection can be exploited to obtain desirable strains in terms of growth, substrate utilization, protein and essential amino acid composition, and so forth. Microbes are rich in protein (7–12% nitrogen) compared to other natural sources (Table 1). These attributes and the flexibility of production schedules warrant the continued research on microbes as sources of protein (Mateles and Tannenbaum, 1968; Litchfield, 1977, 1983).

The general status, technical aspects, and economics of biomass production have been reviewed (Kihlberg, 1972; Tannenbaum and Cooney, 1975; Tannenbaum, 1977; Cooney et al., 1980; Litchfield and Lipinsky, 1974; Litchfield, 1983). A wide range of microbes (bacteria, yeasts, fungi) can be grown on a wide range of substrates (hydrocarbons, cellulose, carbohydrates, waste by-products) (Cooney, 1975; Litchfield, 1977, 1983; Tannenbaum and Wang, 1975; Cooney et al., 1980); however, for food uses acceptable substrates may be limited to well-defined materials devoid of toxic materials.

The various fermentation methods have recently been described (Tannenbaum and Wang, 1975; Tuse, 1984). Microbial cells are usually harvested by centrifugation and/or filtration, and the cell mass is dried by spray- or drum-drying. This crude biomass, called single-cell protein (SCP), actually corresponds to a raw material

Table 1. Approximate Chemical Compositions of Microbes

	Chemical composition (%)		
Item	Fungi	Yeasts	Bacteria
Protein	31–50	47–56	72–83
Nucleic acids	9.2	6–15	8–16
Ash	9–14	5–9.5	3–7
Lipids	2–8	2–6	1.5–3

Source: From Reed (1981).

requiring further processing and refining to exploit the functional attributes of the protein in food processing.

YEASTS

Of all the microbes, yeast is the most widely accepted as a traditional food item and it has received much attention as a potential food protein source (Litchfield, 1977, 1983; Peppler, 1970, 1979; Reed, 1981). The yeasts *Saccharomyces cerevisiae* (baker's yeast), *Candida utilis* (torula yeast), and *Kluyveromyces fragilis* (whey yeast), when produced on suitable substrates (e.g., sugars, ethanol, lactose), are permitted in many foods in the United States, and the yeast market is currently valued around $130 million annually (Peppler, 1979). In addition, other microbes are being produced in quantity by fermentation on other substrates (e.g., *Methylophilus methylotropus* on methanol) and most are currently used in animal feeds (Litchfield, 1983). Yeasts are used as powders or tablets in the health food industry, as food additives in formulated foods (i.e., baby foods, soups, gravy, baked foods and comminuted meats); baker's yeast and torula yeasts are used as food flavorants (brothy and meaty flavors), as sources of enzymes and vitamins, and for the production of yeast extracts and autolysates (Chen and Peppler, 1978; Reed and Peppler 1973; Sinskey, 1978; Reed, 1981).

Composition

The protein and nucleic acid content of yeast ranges between 40–50 and 6–16% dry weight, or 8–25 g RNA/100 g of protein (Sinskey et al., 1975). Baker's yeast, *S. cerevisiae*, normally contains more protein and nucleic acid than *C. utilis*, that is, 48 and 16% versus 42 and 10%, respectively.

The content and composition of lipids are dependent on the nature of the growth medium. Food yeasts contain mostly straight-chain fatty acids, with approximately 20, 40, and 15% oleic, linoleic, and linolenic acids, respectively (Schnell and Akin, 1979). The high content of unsaturated fatty acids renders dried yeast cells susceptible to oxidative off-flavors and discoloration. The carbohydrate content of most food yeasts varies between 20 and 35% dry weight. Glucans and mannans and some chitin are the main structural carbohydrates in the cell wall (Phaff, 1977).

Generally the total proteins from microbes, including yeasts, are deficient in methionine and marginal in valine, isoleucine, and tryptophan. They are rich in other essential amino acids, including lysine and threonine, and are therefore excellent supplements for cereal foods. The total essential amino acid content of yeast

Table 2. Vitamin and Mineral Contents of Typical Yeast

Vitamin	Content (mg/100 g)	Mineral	Content (mg/100 g)
Thiamine	0.80	Phosphorus	2100
Riboflavin	4.50	Potassium	2000
Niacin	55.00	Magnesium	300
Folic acid (total)	0.40	Sulfur	200
Pyridoxine HCl	8.30	Sodium	100
Panthothenic acid	9.40	Calcium	15
Biotin	0.08	Iron	9.5
PABA	1.40	Zinc	9.3
Choline chloride	780.00	Fluoride	1.2
Inositol	460.00	Manganese	0.7
Vitamin B_{12}	0.0004		

Source: From Schnell and Akin (1979).

(*Saccharomyces fragilis*) protein was 44 compared to 52 g of essential amino acids per 100 g of egg protein (Vananuvat and Kinsella, 1975a). The vitamin and mineral contents of yeast are shown in Table 2.

The nutritional value of yeast protein per se is good, but it is not fully available from the intact yeast cells because of the tough yeast cell wall, which impairs digestion. The protein efficiency ratio (PER) of yeast cells, about 2.02, can be increased to 2.8 by adding 0.5% methionine. Isolated yeast protein has a PER of about 2.5, and supplementation with methionine enhances this to 3.0 (Bressani, 1968).

The nutritional value and safety of microbes for human food have been studied to a limited extent (Scrimshaw, 1975; Young and Scrimshaw, 1975). Feeding trials have shown that *C. utilis* cells are not as good as animal protein, partly because of cell wall materials and limiting methionine. Isolation of the protein improves digestibility by 50% over the homogenized cells (Kihlberg, 1972), and supplementation with methionine enhances nutritional value. Human tolerance tests are essential to determine whether microbial cells cause allergic reactions or digestive disturbances when ingested by humans (Young and Scrimshaw, 1975). Kapsiotis (1978) listed nutritional, safety, and regulatory concerns requiring careful study before microbial protein should be used in significant amounts in human foods.

PROBLEMS IN EXPLOITING YEAST PROTEINS FOR FOOD USES

Ideally, microbial biomass should be consumable directly as food or as food ingredients; however, several problems prevent this: The indigestible cell wall reduces the bioavailability of the proteins; in ruptured cells the presence of physiologically active substances and allergens are problematical; the high concentrations of nucleic acid (RNA) associated with protein is undesirable because it can cause uricacidemia and gout; and, finally, the appearance, quality attributes (flavor, color, taste, texture), and functional properties of intact dried cell biomass are limited.

Thus, despite its nutritional value and copious supply, microbial biomass, including yeast, is unlikely to be developed into a major food source without further processing. There are several important reasons for further processing: The cell wall must be removed, because it impairs digestion and nutrient bioavailability and may cause flatulence, allergic responses, and diarrhea; the component lipids contribute to off-flavors via oxidation and impair the functional properties of the proteins and the protein must be extracted from the cell biomass to obtain the biological value of the protein and realize the full range of functional properties; and, finally, where microbes may become a significant source of dietary protein the nucleic acid content must be reduced to avoid uricacidemia and gout (Young and Scrimshaw, 1975; Tannenbaum and Wang, 1975).

The nature of the cell wall and physical methods for its removal have been reviewed (Dunnill and Lilly, 1975; Phaff, 1977). Autolysis, thiol-stimulated autolysis, and enzyme-facilitated lysis have been studied (Kinsella and Shetty, 1978). Unfortunately, the latter methods are not suitable for the isolation of functional proteins, because extensive proteolysis occurs with greatly reduced protein yields. The selection of yeast strains with weaker cell walls (Batt and Sinskey, 1984) and low protease activity should facilitate cell disruption and enhance protein extraction and yield.

Effective disintegration of yeast cell walls has been achieved using homogenization, freeze—thawing, pressurization, and so on (Dunhill and Lilly, 1975; Vananuvat and Kinsella, 1975c; Newell et al., 1975). Treatment of yeast cells with alkali, pH > 10, weakens the cell wall and facilitates the recovery of yeast proteins; however, severe alkali treatment causes undesirable changes in proteins (Shetty and Kinsella, 1979).

FUNCTIONAL PROPERTIES AND PROTEIN RECOVERY

While nutritional and safety criteria are important in developing microbes as a food source, the successful adoption and acceptance of proteins from microbial sources by the food industry and consumer depend on their possession of the appropriate organoleptic and functional properties (Kinsella, 1982). The functional properties determine the usefulness of proteins in food formulation and fabrication. The functional properties of proteins are those physicochemical properties which govern the behavior of proteins in food systems during their preparation, processing, storage, and consumption, that is, those properties which, in the aggregate, affect the organoleptic and quality attributes of foods. Examples of the structural and functional roles of proteins are the myofibrillar proteins of meat, which impart structure, water-holding, and thermosetting properties to meats, collagen in gelatin gels, and glutenin in bread. Different foods and food applications require quite different functional properties (Table 3). For example, in a beverage, solubility, flavor compatibility, controlled viscosity, and turbidity may be required at different pH values. In comminuted meat systems good adhesive properties, water holding, emulsion stabilization, and gelatin during cooking are important properties of the constituent proteins. These are some examples of the important properties a functional protein ingredient should ideally possess. No food protein possesses all the possible requisite properties, and yeast biomass protein is no exception, though some effort has gone into attempts to commercialize it as a universal ingredient protein and many preparations have failed to perform as specified. Processors and technologists are now more realistic and recognize that cell biomass, that is, SCP, has limited properties and that the heterogeneous class of compounds called proteins do not possess identical properties and cannot be indiscriminately interchanged in the fabrication of food products.

The lack of information on the functional properties of proteins isolated from microbial biomass is a significant factor limiting their wider use. The use of unprocessed microbial biomass—so-called single-cell protein, or SCP, a misnomer, for at best it contains only 50% protein encapsulated in a cell wall envelope—is limited. The need for a better knowledge of the functional properties of microbial proteins has been largely overlooked, though this information is critical before they can be adopted and accepted by the food industry in both developed and developing countries. Numerous efforts to formulate protein-rich foods based on novel proteins have met

Table 3. Functional Requirements of Ingredient Proteins in Selected Food Systems[a]

Generic food	Example	Some typical functional requirements
Beverage	Breakfast drink, pH 6.5	Solubility, colloidal stability, flavor release
	Soft drink, pH 3.0	Acid solubility, color, flavor, stability
	Milk system	Colloidal stability, flavor, mouth-feel
Gel system	Yogurt	Viscosity, limited protein–protein interaction, water holding, smooth mouth-feel
	Meat/sausage	Strong protein–protein association, emulsion stability, gelation, water holding, moisture release
	Cheese	Strong protein–protein association, matrix formation, elastic/friable texture, mixability
Emulsion	Spreads	Interfacial spreading, film formation, cohesiveness, water retention
Foam	Frappe	Viscoelastic film formation, rapid air entrapment, lamellar moisture retention, heat stability
Dough	Breads	Compatible with dough formation, limited water binding, browning
	Cake batters	Surface activity for foam stabilization, heat setting, moisture retention

[a] Protein should lack color and off-flavor, be soluble and/or dispersible, not bind flavors or pigments, and not impair the functional behavior of other food components.

with limited success because the principal concern was the delivery of balanced nutrients and insufficient attention was given to organoleptic and functional attributes, which are critical in determining food acceptability (Kinsella, 1981).

In considering the development of new or formulated foods or a functional ingredient for specific applications, it is critically important to become familiar with the food habits and preferences of the target population. For the successful simulation of a traditional food using new raw materials, it is necessary to understand the physicochemical properties of both. Thus, in developing new foods or food ingredients for developed and developing economies, acceptability, nutritional value (organoleptic and functional), and cost are critical criteria in determining consumer acceptance, and more research emphasis on these is essential for expanding the food uses of microbial proteins.

The determination of the physical and functional properties should be an integral part of research concerned with the isolation of food proteins from microbes. Only when the relationships between the structure and the physical basis of function is understood can we truly manipulate and design proteins appropriate to specific functional applications. At present the food technologist tries to use proteins from various sources, each with different properties, for a specific functionality, for a specific functionality, for which in many cases the proteins are unsuitable. The need for a greater knowledge of the functional properties of microbial proteins has been largely overlooked, although this information is critical for determining their application in foods (Kinsella and Shetty, 1978; Cooney et al., 1980; Batt and Sinskey, 1984). Systematic exploration of the physical and functional properties of yeast proteins should be an essential part of programs concerned with food applications of microbial proteins. Furthermore, elucidation of the relationships between protein structure and functional properties should greatly facilitate the exploitation of recombinant DNA techniques for the production of proteins possessing specific functional properties for food uses.

However, for the study and practical exploitation of the functional properties of yeast proteins, it is desirable to extract the proteins, preferably using mild conditions to recover a maximum amount of undenatured proteins. Alkaline conditions are usually employed because of improved extractability, and at high temperatures (i.e., 90°C, pH > 10) the isolation of proteins low in nucleic acid is achieved (Hedenskog and Mogren, 1973). However, this causes denaturation of proteins and destruction of some functional properties. For food uses it is extremely important to obtain undenatured protein preparations, because this ensures a superior range of functional properties and a greater range of applications in foods (Kinsella, 1976). Proteins obtained by conventional cell disruption and extraction methods tend to be denatured, possess poor solubility, and have limited use in foods (Vananuvat and Kinsella, 1975b). Improved methods for the isolation of highly functional protein from microbes are needed to validly assess functional properties.

NUCLEIC ACIDS AND NUCLEOPROTEIN COMPLEXES

A significant problem associated with the preparation, utilization, and consumption of microbial protein is the high content of nucleic acids, mostly RNA, which ranges from 8 to 25 g/100 g of protein. Humans lack uricase and consequently consumption of microbial proteins rich in RNA may result in uricacidemia, kidney stones, and arthritic gout. If microbes are to be used as a protein source for humans, the nucleic acid content should be reduced to levels which would allow a maximum intake of protein providing less than 2 g/day of nucleic acids (Kapsiotis, 1978; Scrimshaw, 1975).

Because of the undesirability of ingesting nucleic acids, several approaches for reducing RNA content of yeast proteins have been tested. The nucleic acid content of yeast cells may be reduced by controlling their growth rate (Sinskey and Tannenbaum, 1975); however, this also decreases productivity. Alkali treatments of the crude disrupted yeast biomass (e.g., at pH 10.5, 80°C, for 1–4 hr or pH 12, 55°C, for 1–2 hr) can reduce the RNA content to approximately 2% in the final isoelectrically precipitated product (Lindblom, 1974; Vananuvat and Kinsella, 1975b; Hedenskog and Mogren, 1973). However, alkali treatment reduces cysteine, cystine, and serine via β-elimination, causes crosslinking and polymerization via ε-NH_2 of lysine, and denaturation. These alterations impair functional properties and reduce nutritional value, thereby rendering the sodium hydroxide method unsuitable for preparing functional proteins for food uses from yeast biomass (Shetty and Kinsella, 1979). The use of ammonium hydroxide may circumvent these problems (Schlingman and Vertesy, 1980).

Nucleic acids can be reduced enzymatically using high-temperature (55°C) activation of endogenous ribonuclease (heat shock process) and/or exogenous ribonuclease (Newell et al., 1975; Sinskey and Tannenbaum, 1975; Robbins et al., 1975; Lindblom, 1977). Unfortunately, these treatments concomitantly activate proteases, which cause extensive proteolysis and decrease protein yields. Hence these methods have limited value in preparing functional proteins.

Because these methods and conventional biochemical procedures are unsuitable, innovative approaches for isolating functional proteins low in nucleic acid for food uses are needed. Therefore an understanding of the structure and interactions stabilizing the nucleoprotein complex should indicate useful approaches for dissociating this complex and recovering native protein with little contaminating nucleic acid.

Nucleoprotein Structure

In the intact yeast cell soluble cytoplasmic proteins (mostly enzymes), ribosomal proteins, and cell wall- and/or membrane-bound proteins account for approximately 40, 40, and 20%, respectively, of the total protein. During cellular disruption some of the cytoplasmic proteins become complexed with nucleic acids, and this, together with ribosomal protein, means that 50–60% of the protein isolated from yeast cells by isoelectric precipitation may exist as a nucleoprotein complex containing 10–15% nucleic acid.

The eukaryotic 80S ribosome is composed of two subunits, 40S and 60S. The 40S subunit contains 45% RNA and 30 discrete proteins; the 60S subunit contains 59% RNA and approximately 44 proteins (Weinberg and Penman, 1970; Otaka and Osawa, 1981). The ribosomal subunit is apparently organized as a core of RNA molecules enveloped by associated ribosomal proteins (Kuhlbrandt and Unwin, 1982; Helene and Lancelot, 1982). Neutron-scattering studies reveal that the radii of gyration of proteins and RNA in the 80S yeast ribosome are 105 and 70A, respectively, indicating that the ribosomal RNA exists as a compact mass in the interior of the ribosomes surrounded by the associated proteins (Kuhlbrandt and Unwin, 1982). This is supported by nuclear magnetic resonance data, which indicate that 80% of the RNA in ribosomes has restricted motion (Bolton et al., 1982). The molecular weights of the ribosomal proteins range from 10×10^3 to 60×10^3 and their amino acid composition reveals a consistent high content of lysine, arginine, and histidine (Otaka and Osawa, 1981); hence these proteins are quite basic and positively charged around pH 6.8. In addition, these proteins have a high concentration (40–50%) of apolar amino acids, which makes them quite hydrophobic (Table 4).

Hydrophobic, van der Waals, stacking and electrostatic interactions and hydrogen bonding are apparently involved in the formation and stabilization of the RNA–protein complexes. Extensive electrostatic interactions between the negatively charged phosphate groups on the RNA and positively charged arginyl and lysyl (and possibly protonated histidyl) side chains are possible (Helene and Lancelot, 1982). However, if electrostatic interactions are the sole forces involved, then it should be possible to neutralize these interactions and destabilize RNA–protein complexes by increasing the ionic strength of the medium to 1 M. However, this is not possible,

Table 4. Molecular Weights and Amino Acid Compositions (g/100 g) of Some Proteins Isolated from Yeast Ribosomal Subunits

	Protein molecular weight of subunit ($\times 10^3$)								
Amino acid	60.0	48.0	31.5	24.0	24.0	22.5	21.5	21.5	20.5
Aspartic acid	6.7	6.8	8.1	7.8	9.2	12.6	8.6	8.4	7.3
Threonine	6.5	7.2	4.0	3.7	4.9	5.9	3.1	3.1	5.2
Serine	4.8	6.5	5.5	4.0	2.8	4.1	4.7	4.4	4.2
Glutamic acid	8.0	8.9	7.1	11.9	9.8	9.5	8.9	10.9	11.7
Proline	3.4	5.1	4.0	4.5	3.3	2.5	4.5	1.1	4.9
Glycine	8.8	9.0	14.3	7.0	7.3	6.5	6.5	5.5	4.6
Alanine	8.9	13.3	10.7	10.4	7.3	4.1	10.7	14.3	10.4
Valine	9.0	9.3	7.1	6.1	7.2	13.4	7.7	7.0	10.7
Methionine	1.3	0.2	0.5	0.4	0.0	1.5	1.3	0.0	0.1
Isoleucine	4.7	3.9	5.8	7.6	2.6	8.3	4.0	3.3	2.8
Leucine	6.0	8.4	6.6	8.6	6.9	6.1	5.8	7.1	6.5
Tyrosine	3.2	0.7	2.2	4.1	5.8	2.7	4.2	1.9	2.9
Phenylalanine	4.2	2.4	2.2	4.1	2.4	4.2	4.0	0.6	4.0
Histidine	4.2	2.7	3.7	1.7	2.7	2.5	2.5	3.7	1.3
Lysine	11.6	9.0	8.0	12.1	11.6	10.5	11.1	12.1	14.1
Arginine	9.0	6.9	10.4	6.2	16.5	6.2	10.6	14.9	5.6

Source: From Otaka and Osawa (1981).

indicating that other forces are involved in maintaining the structural stability of these complexes. Furthermore, in an aqueous medium hydration of polar groups and the high dielectric environment should weaken electrostatic interactions. However, if localized apolar domains with low dielectric constants exist, then electrostatic interactions become very effective. Such low dielectric regions may occur within the ribosomal complexes and facilitate the formation of strong protein–protein and protein–RNA electrostatic bonds (5–7 kcal/mol).

In addition, numerous functional groups (i.e., —OH, —SH, $—NH_2$, and —COOH) can potentially form one to two hydrogen bonds with functional groups (NH, N, OH^-, CO^-) on nucleotide bases (Helene and Lancelot, 1982). However, hydrogen bonding with water is thermodynamically favored in aqueous environments; nevertheless, in apolar environments hydrogen bonds between protein and RNA are considerably enhanced.

Thus an apolar, relatively anhydrous environment is necessary to create regions of low dielectric for effective electrostatic and hydrogen-bonding-type interactions to occur. This is provided by the hydrophobically induced association of the ribosomal proteins to form nonpolar interior regions of low dielectric constant where electrostatic and hydrogen bonding are considerably strenghthened and van der Waals interactions are facilitated. The aromatic amino acids in the proteins can engage in stacking interactions with bases of the RNA (Hogan et al., 1979), and these are stabilized by van der Waals interactions. Although individually weak, in the aggregate these contribute significantly to stabilization of the nucleoprotein complexes (Helene and Lancelot, 1982).

Hydrophobic interactions reflect the negative entropy effects of apolar compounds on water structure. Apolar compounds, for example, apolar proteins, induce the formation of hydration shells around their periphery via dipole–dipole interactions. This decreases the entropy of the involved water by loss of rotational and translational motion (Hatefi and Hanstein, 1969). In order to minimize this thermodynamically unfavorable effect, the apolar compounds associate to the maximum extent possible to reduce the surface area exposed to the water and form a single sphere of hydration, thereby releasing much of the structured hydration water and increasing the entropy of the system.

Thermodynamic data are consistent with the involvement of hydrophobic, electrostatic, and van der Waals interactions and hydrogen bonding in protein–nucleic acid complexes (Ohlendorf and Matthews, 1983; Helene and Lancelot, 1982). The thermodynamic indices are complex, reflecting a number of sequential cooperative interactions. The association of 5S RNA with individual ribosomal proteins showed K, ΔH, and ΔS values of $2.25 \times 10^8\ M^{-1}$; −2.7

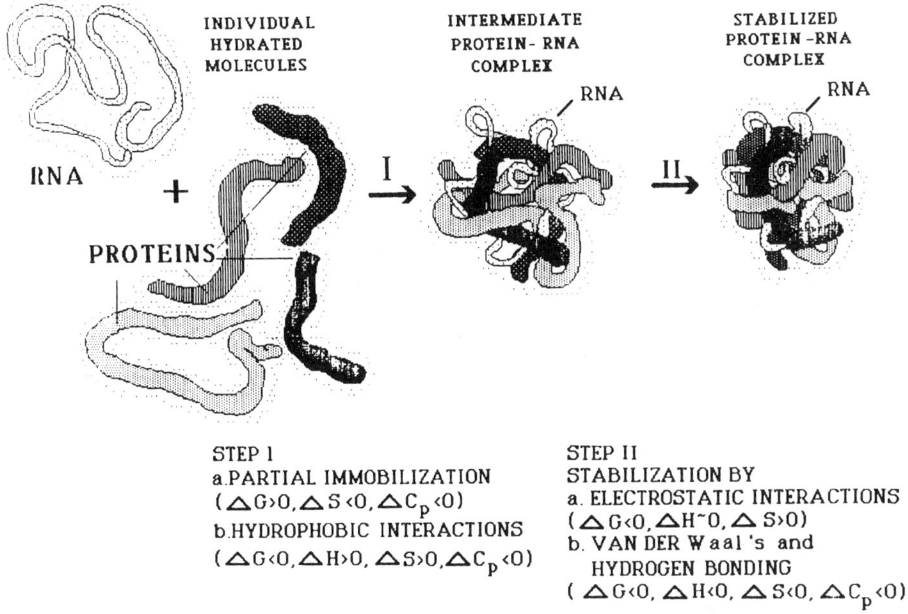

Fig. 1. Schematic of the (step I) association (hydrophobically driven) and (step II) stabilization (via electrostatic and van der Waals interactions and hydrogen bonding) of protein and ribonucleic acid (RNA) in nucleoprotein complexes.

kcal/mol, and 29 e.u., respectively, reflecting mostly entropy-driven reactions (Spierer et al., 1978). The entropy change may result from association of the apolar moieties of the molecules; the disruption of hydration shells around the phosphate groups on RNA and the charged groups of the proteins when these form electrostatic bonds in anhydrous domains, and the release of bound counterions into solution (Flogel et al., 1975; Helene and Lancelot, 1982). The association of RNA with protein is characterized by a negative enthalpy, a large positive entropy, and a decrease in heat capacity and is entropy driven at low temperatures (Fig. 1).

Conceivably protein–nucleic acid complex formation may occur in two sequential steps. Initially the hydrated protein associates hydrophobically in an entropy-driven process. Based on structural studies, most of the RNA becomes located in the interior, being largely surrounded by associated ribosomal proteins, though extensive interdigitation and interaction of the molecules may occur. This facilitates stacking and van der Waals interactions between apolar aromatic amino acids and nucleotide bases and concomitantly creates anhydrous domains, or pockets, by squeezing out water. These pockets of low dielectric constant then facilitate the formation of hydrogen bonds and electrostatic interactions in the RNA–protein complex to minimize free energy to attain a stable conformation. Hydrogen bonding and electrostatic interactions are paramount in stabilizing this structure (Record et al., 1978; Helene and Lancelot, 1982). The physical properties and unique structure of water are critical phenomena responsible for the integrity this structure. Based on this model and a knowledge of the stabilizing forces involved, we explored a number of approaches for destabilizing this complex in order to separate yeast proteins from contaminating RNA.

DISSOCIATION OF NUCLEOPROTEINS AND ISOLATION OF PROTEINS

Chaotropic Anions

Based on the rationale that hydrophobic interactions are critical in stabilizing the nucleoprotein complex and that hydrophobic forces result from the structural and physical properties of water, we speculated that agents which perturb water structure might be useful in dissociating nucleoprotein complexes by weakening hydrophobic interactions (Kinsella and Damodaran, 1984). Chaotropic anions, especially the larger anions thiocyanate and trichloroacetate, by weakening the normal hydrogen-bonded structure of water and altering interfacial properties, alter the thermodynamics of water stabilized structures (Von Hippel and Schleich, 1969; Hatefi and Hanstein, 1969; Damodaran and Kinsella, 1982). Chaotropic anions, in concentrations ranging from 0.5 to 1.0 M, were effective in dissociating yeast RNA–protein complexes and reducing the RNA content of the isolated proteins (Table 5). Thus anions like perchlorate (ClO_4^-), trichloroacetate ($Cl_3C_2OO^-$), and thiocyanate (SCN^-) at 0.5 M reduced the RNA content of nucleoproteins by over 80%, whereas chloride reduced it by less than 10% (Table 5). Repeated washings with $NaClO_4$ or Cl_3C_2OONa (1.0 M) reduced the RNA content by 98% (Fig. 2); see Damodaran and Kinsella, 1983a,b, 1984b). The effectiveness of the anions is directly related to their capacity to destructure water and thereby reduce the negative entropy effects accompanying the resultant solution and dissolution of apolar ribosomal protein molecules in water. The larger anions alter water structure and concurrently weaken the hydrophobic associations between the proteins on the periphery of the nucleoprotein complex. They may also cause conformational changes in the nucleic acids. The dissociation of the protein matrix permits water molecules into

Table 5. Effectiveness of Various Anions in Reducing the RNA Content of Isoelectrically Precipitated Microbial Proteins

Anion treatment (0.5 M)	Nucleic acid in yeast nucleic protein (%)	Reduction in Nucleic acid (%)
No salt added	20.7±1.3	0
NaF	21.0±1.5	0
NaCl	19.7±1.1	6
NaBr	18.0±1.3	13
$NaNO_3$	15.6±1.2	25
NaI	5.1±0.9	75
$NaClO_4$	2.7±0.7	87
NaSCN	2.2±0.6	90

[a]Mean ± SD.

the interior of the complex, increasing the dielectric constant in these regions. This greatly weakens hydrogen bonding between the component molecules and the concomitant influx of ions progressively weakens electrostatic interactions. Overall, this cascade of events, initiated by the alteration of water structure, facilitates the dissociation of the proteins and RNA and the subsequent preparation of isoelectrically precipitated proteins with 2% nucleic acid from yeast biomass (Damodaran and Kinsella, 1983b). This method is practical because, by manipulating the salt concentration and number of extractions, one can obtain the desired RNA level in the isolated protein, and the salt is easily removed for reuse by ultrafiltration or reverse osmosis. Proteins are recovered in good yields and have a good amino acid composition.

A considerable proportion of the isolated protein (50%), particularly the apolar ribosomal protein components, are poorly soluble at pH 6–7 because of spontaneous aggregation to macromolecular complexes (> 100,000 daltons), presumably via hydrophobic interactions, reflecting their high content of apolar amino acids. These proteins may be useful in food applications requiring network formation, surface activity, viscosity, and gel formation.

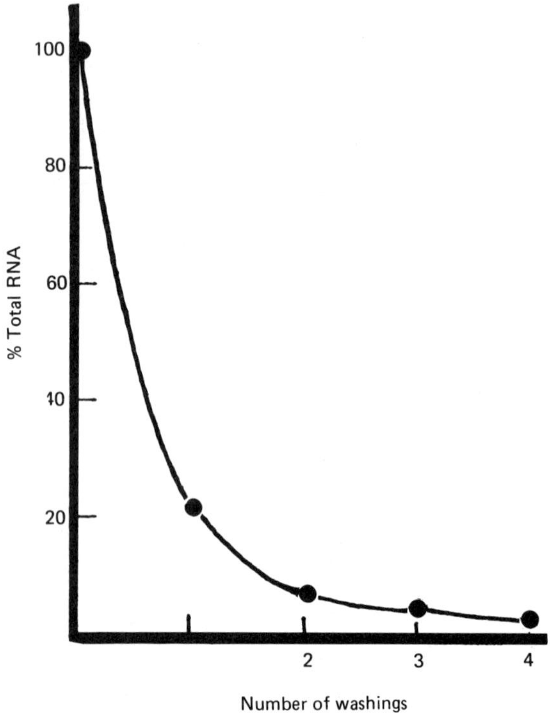

Fig. 2. The progressive reduction in the RNA content of protein isolated from yeast nucleoprotein by successive washings (or dialysis) with chaotropic anions (trichloroacetate or thiocyanate, 1.0 M).

Succinylation

Perturbation of electrostatic interactions also affords methods for isolating proteins low in nucleic acid from yeast biomass and in addition yields soluble proteins. Chemical modification of free amino groups using acid anhydrides at pH 9.0, by enhancing the net negative charge (following acylation of cationic amino groups with anionic carboxyl acid groups), destabilizes the nucleoprotein complex via electrostatic repulsion between the anionic proteins and RNA (Kinsella and Shetty, 1978; Shetty and Kinsella, 1979):

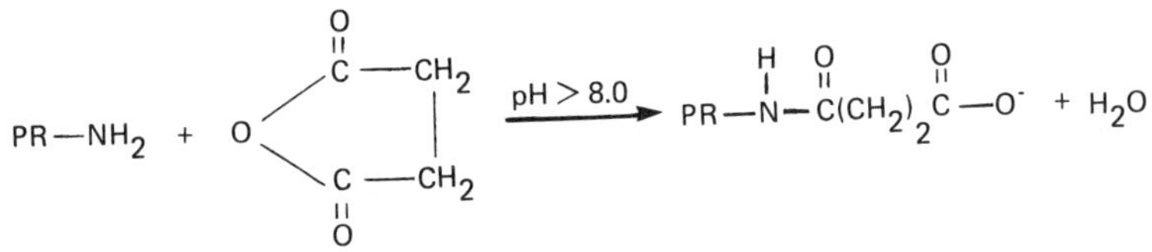

—NH_2 of protein (PR) + succinic anhydride ⟶ succinylated protein

Succinylation of homogenized yeast biomass using succinic anhydride at pH 9.0 enhanced the yield of protein precipitated at pH 4.2 from 60 to 85% and reduced RNA contamination to under 2% (Table 6). This procedure inactivated endogenous proteases and ribonuclease and gave a protein isolate (> 90% protein) that was fully soluble at pH 7.0 and which possessed an excellent amino acid profile (Table 7), including more than 2% methionine (Shetty and Kinsella, 1979).

As the degree of succinylation was increased, the rate of precipitation of the derivatized protein increased in the isoelectric region and larger protein flocs were obtained, facilitating recovery.

Table 6. Chemical Compositions of Yeast, Yeast Nucleoprotein, and Yeast Proteins Prepared by Different Methods

Sample	Protein (%)	Nucleic acid (%)	Carbohydrate (%)	Lipid (%)
Whole yeast cell	42.4	11.4	28.8	4.0
Nucleoprotein complex	64.0	20.0	6.0	5.1
Protein isolate ($NaClO_4$)	76.9	2.5	3.6	6.3
Succinylation	90.0	1.8	3.0	3.5
Citraconylation	84.0	2.2	3.7	5.1
Phosphorylated protein	82.0	2.7	5.1	5.7

Table 7. Amino Acid Compositions (g/100 g) of Yeast, Yeast Nucleoprotein, and Proteins Isolated by Different Methods

Amino acid	Whole yeast	Nucleoprotein	$NaClO_4^-$ isolated protein	Succinylated protein	Phosphorylated protein	Alkali-treated protein
Aspartic acid	8.0	10.9	10.2	11.2	10.6	9.5
Threonine	3.8	5.6	5.4	4.7	5.2	5.0
Serine	3.7	4.7	4.5	4.3	4.1	3.7
Glutamic acid	10.8	10.7	10.6	10.7	10.7	13.5
Proline	6.5	4.2	4.4	4.6	4.3	4.4
Glycine	3.1	5.0	4.3	3.8	4.5	4.0
Alanine	6.6	6.4	6.5	5.6	6.8	5.6

Cystine (half)	1.5	1.0	1.9	1.6	1.0	—
Valine	5.0	6.3	7.2	6.7	7.8	7.0
Methionine	1.8	1.9	1.0	2.3	1.3	2.5
Isoleucine	6.4	5.6	6.0	6.0	6.3	6.4
Leucine	6.6	8.2	9.8	8.8	9.7	9.4
Tyrosine	3.2	4.3	4.4	4.5	4.2	4.7
Phenylalanine	4.0	5.0	5.5	5.4	5.6	5.8
Lysine	8.5	9.1	9.5	8.4	10.0	7.7
Histidine	2.0	2.2	2.7	2.7	2.0	2.8
Arginine	4.7	5.0	5.5	5.8	6.4	2.1
Ammonia	—	—	2.0	2.3	1.1	5.8

The pH solubility profile of succinylated proteins revealed the typical increased solubility between pH 4 and 6. Succinylated yeast proteins were very stable to heat precipitation above pH 5. The emulsifying capacity of the yeast proteins was significantly and progressively improved with the extent of succinylation (Pearce and Kinsella, 1978). Succinylation improved the foaming capacity of yeast protein, which was almost equivalent to that of ovalbumin, whereas the unmodified yeast failed to stabilize foams. The modified proteins were susceptible to hydrolysis by both α-chymotrypsin and trypsin, though the α-chymotrypsin was the more effective of the two (Kinsella and Shetty, 1978).

The succinylation procedure has significant practical benefits. The succinylated protein is white, bland, and highly soluble and possesses good functional properties. The disadvantage is that the final product is a succinylated protein. While the succinic residue is a normal metabolite, succinylated protein should have no deleterious effects when consumed in limited amounts as a functional protein. However, there is concern that it reduces the bioavailability of the lysine, and this could be a problem if succinylated yeast protein were a major source of dietary protein.

Citraconylation

Because of the problem of lysine bioavailability, the feasibility of using reversible modifying reagents (citraconic or maleic anhydride) to disrupt electrostatic interactions and separate proteins from nucleic acids and subsequently removing the modifying groups under mildly acidic conditions was explored (Shetty and Kinsella, 1980, 1982). As with succinylation, the addition of negative charges to the lysine ε-NH_2 group destabilizes the supramolecular nucleoprotein complex by disrupting the noncovalent interactions. This facilitates the separation of anionic derivatized proteins from the RNA by isoelectric precipitation at pH 4.2. Citraconylation is as effective as succinylation in preparing yeast protein isolates with low levels of contaminating RNA. The isopeptide bond formed between acid anhydrides containing a cis double bond and the ε-amino group of lysine is acid labile; thus complete removal of the citraconic residue was achieved by incubation at pH 4.0 (30°C) to yield a protein isolate with less than 2% RNA (Shetty and Kinsella, 1979; see Tables 6 and 7):

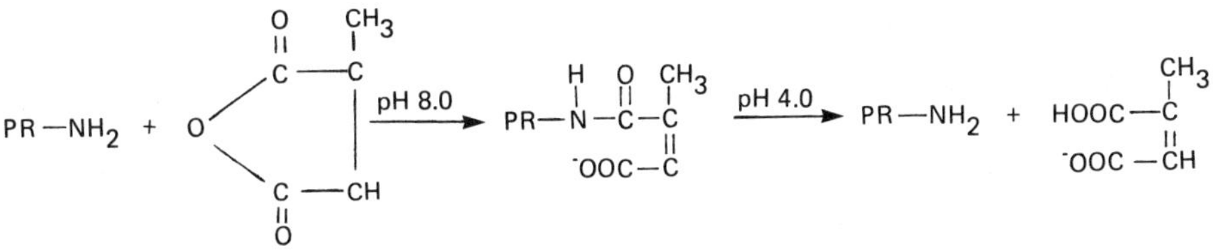

$—NH_2$ of protein (PR) + citraconic anhydride ⟶ citraconylated protein ⟶ protein

Citraconylation and removal of RNA improved the solubility of yeast protein from 50 to 100% at pH 7.0. Decitraconylation reduced solubility to about 70%, presumably because of loss of hydrated carboxylic acid groups and some aggregation of the protein components. The emulsifying and foaming properties of decitraconylated protein were comparable to those of other functional proteins; for example, soy protein (Shetty and Kinsella, 1979). The decitraconylated yeast proteins were readily digested by pepsin, but pancreatin digestion in vitro was somewhat reduced.

Phosphorylation

Because of concerns about the safety and cost of reversible acylation, the feasibility of phosphorylation as a method for separating RNA from microbial nucleoproteins was studied:

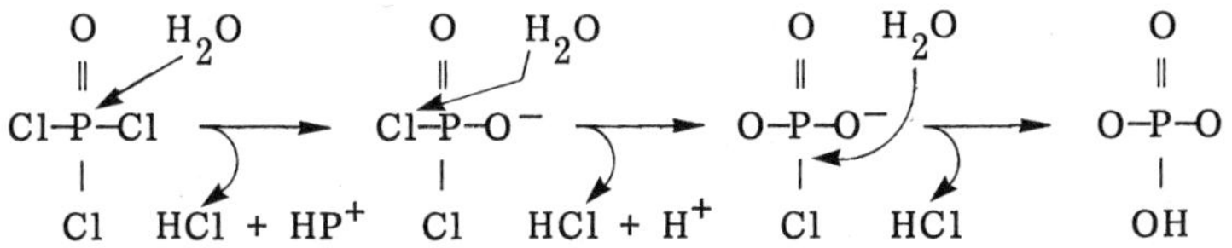

Phosphorous oxychloride | intermediate (I) | intermediate (II) | phosphoric ion

Because Cl^- is a good leaving group, $POCl_3$ and the two intermediates I and II are very reactive and phosphorylation of the $—NH_2$ and —OH groups of proteins can be easily achieved by the following mechanisms:

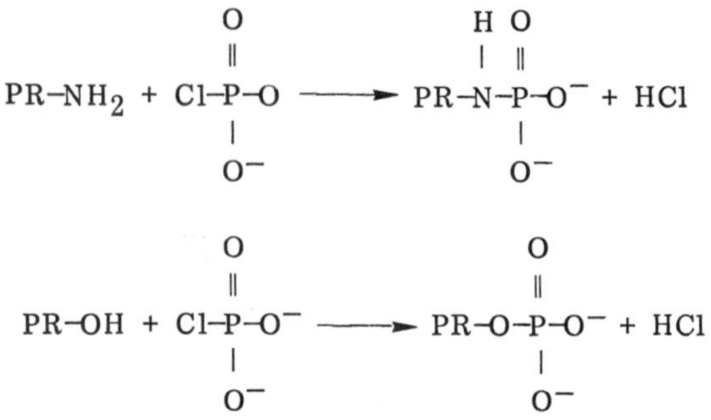

Phosphorylation has been used to alter the properties of several food proteins (Matheis et al., 1983; Huang and Kinsella, 1985). Phosphorylation of yeast nucleoproteins via ε-NH_2 groups of lysine using phosphorous oxychloride ($POCl_3$) at pH 9.0 progressively reduced nucleic acid, and a 90% reduction in the RNA content of isoelectrically precipitated protein was obtained when 30% of the available ε-NH_2 groups were phosphorylated (Damodaran and Kinsella, 1984a; Huang and Kinsella, 1985, 1986). The precipitated phosphorylated protein contained 72% protein and had an excellent amino acid spectrum (see Tables 6 and 7).

The phosphorylated yeast protein possessed some unique and useful functional properties. It showed a remarkable water binding capacity (i.e., 18 g H_2O/100 g protein at pH 7.0) and formed viscous dispersions at concentrations from 3 to 10%. This may reflect hydration of the phosphate groups and/or some network formation by phosphate crosslinking. Dispersions of phosphorylated yeast proteins showed shear thinning ($n = 0.67$), and all concentrations showed very high consistency coefficients k compared to those of other functional proteins. Phosphorylated yeast proteins possessed good emulsifying and foaming properties. Both dispersions and emulsions made from the phosphorylated proteins were heat stable. Phosphorylation did not affect the in vitro digestibility of the yeast proteins (Huang and Kinsella, 1986).

An outline of these various procedures is presented in Figure 3.

CONCLUSIONS

The successful development of a market for functional proteins from yeast and other microbial sources depends on their possession of the appropriate functional properties that are equivalent or superior to those of existing functional ingredient proteins. With the rapid developments in genetic engineering, it seems possible that microbes can become a significant source of functional proteins, in addition to

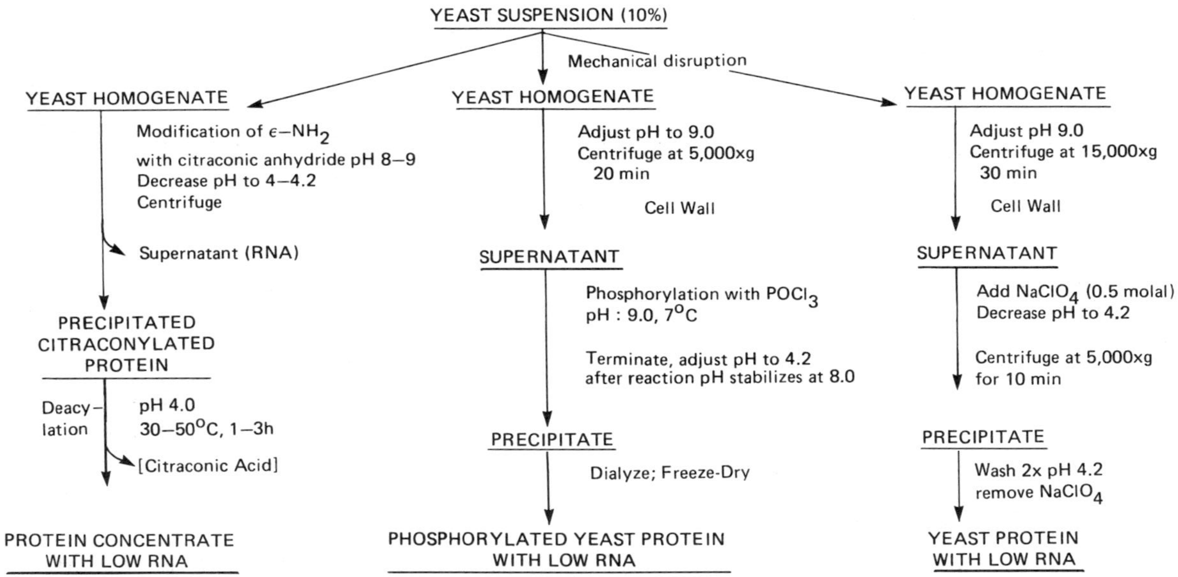

Fig. 3. Outline of chemical methods for separating protein from yeast ribonucleoproteins.

Table 8. Summary of Research Methods for the Reduction of RNA in Isolated Yeast Protein

Methods	Advantages	Disadvantages
Control cell growth by substrate limitation	Proper design of fermenter	Limited reduction of RNA, low protein production
Alkaline hydrolysis pH 10–10.5, 90°C, 1–4 hr pH 11.5, 60°C, 1–2 hr	Simple, rapid	Protein loss (30%), destruction of amino acids, formation of lysinoalanine, denaturation of protein
Exogenous ribonuclease, 56°C, pH 6.7–8.0	Simple, rapid	Cost of enzyme, proteolysis reduces protein yield
Endogeneous RNase, heat shock at 68°C, incubation at 52.5°C for 2 hr	Simple, economic	Slow process, proteolysis reduces protein yield
Succinylation	High yield, good functional properties	Succinyl group, safety, cost
Citraconylation, –decitraconylation	High yield, no chemical residue	Complicated chemical reaction, cost, safety
Chaotropic salt	Simple extraction	Denaturation of some proteins
Phosphorylation	Simple reaction, nutritionally acceptable, good functional properties	Corrosive chemicals, cost
Sulfitolysis	Simple, effective	Regulatory

other food-grade materials, and thereby supplement agricultural sources in time. Such developments will require the concurrent development of practical procedures for isolating yeast proteins with low nucleic acid contents and good functional properties. Most of the current methods have technical disadvantages, as summarized in Table 8, and most add to production costs. Thus continuing systematic studies of practical methods for isolating and fractionating functional proteins from yeast and microbial biomass are warranted.

ACKNOWLEDGMENT

This work was supported by National Science Foundation Grant CBT 8506243.

REFERENCES

Batt, C. A. and Sinskey, A. J. (1984). Use of biotechnology in production of single cell protein. *Food Technol. 38*:108.

Bolton, P. H., Clowson, G., Basis, V. J., and James, T. L. (1982). Comparison of ribonucleic acid–protein interactions in messenger ribonucleoproteins, robosomes, MS2 virus, and QB virus examined via phosphorus-31 nuclear magnetic reasonance relaxation. *Biochemistry 24*:6073.

Bressani, R. (1968). The use of yeast in human foods. In *Single-Cell Protein* (R. I. Mateles and S. R. Tannenbaum, eds.), MIT Press, Cambridge, p. 90.

Chen, S. L. and Peppler, H. J. (1978). Single cell proteins in food applications. *Dev. Ind. Microbiol. 19*:79.

Cooney, C. (1975). SCP production from methand by yeast. In *Single-Cell Protein II* (S. R. Tannenbaum and D. I. C. Wang, eds.), MIT Press, Cambridge, p. 402.

Cooney, C. L., Rha, C. K., and Tannenbaum, S. R. (1980). Single cell protein: Engineering economics and utilization in food. *Adv. Food Res. 26*:1.

Damodaran, S. and Kinsella, J. E. (1982). Effect of ions on protein conformation and functionality. *Am. Chem. Soc. Symp. Ser. 206*:327.

Damodaran, S. and Kinsella, J. E. (1983a). Dissociation of nucleoproteins by chaotropic salts. *FEBS Lett. 158*:53.

Damodaran, S. and Kinsella, J. E. (1983b). Use of chaotropic salts for separation of RNA and proteins from yeast nucleoprotein. *Biotechnol. Bioeng. 25*:761.

Damodaran, S. (1986). Removal of nucleic acids from yeast nucleoprotein complexes by sulfitolysis. *J. Agric. Food Chem. 34*:100.

Damodaran, S. and Kinsella, J. E. (1984a). Dissociation of yeast nucleoproteins by chemical phosphorylation. *J. Agric. Food Chem. 32*:1030.
Damodaran, S. and Kinsella, J. E. (1984b). Dissociation of yeast 80S ribosomes by chaotropic salts. *Biochim. Biophys. Acta. 801*:416.
Dunnill, P. and Lilly, M. D. (1975). Protein extraction and recovery from microbial cells. In *Single-Cell Protein II* (S. R. Tannenbaum and D. I. C. Wang, eds.), MIT Press, Cambridge, p. 179.
Flogel, M., Albert, A., and Biltonen, R. (1975). The magnitude of electrostatic interactions in inhibitor binding and during catalysis by ribonuclease A. *Biochemistry 14*:2616.
Hatefi, W. and Hanstein, W. G. (1969). Solubilization of particulate proteins and nonelectrolytes by chaotropic agents. *Proc. Nat. Acad. Sci. U.S.A. 62*:1129.
Hedenskog, G. and Mogren, H. (1973). Some methods for processing of single-cell protein. *Biotechnol. Bioeng. 15*:129.
Helene, C. and Lancelot, G. (1982). Interactions between functional groups in protein–nucleic acid associations. *Prog. Biophys. Mol. Biol. 39*:1.
Hogan, M., Dattagupta, N., and Crothers, D. M. (1979). Transient electric dichroism studies of the structure of the DNA complex with intercalated drugs. *Biochemistry 18*:280.
Huang, Y. T. and Kinsella, J. E. (1985). Chemistry and functional properties of phosphorylated proteins. Thesis, Cornell Univer-
Huang, Y. T. and Kinsella, J. E. (1986). Functional properties of phosphorylated yeast proteins. *J. Agric. Food Chem. 34*:400.
Huang, Y. T. and Kinsella, J. E. (1986). Phosphorylation of yeast protein: Reduction of nucleic acid. *Biotechnol. Bioeng. 28*:800.
Kapsiotis, G. D. (1978). Single cell protein: Review and assessment. *Food Nutr. 4*:2.
Kihlberg, R. (1972). The microbe as a source of food. *Annu. Rev. Microbiol.*, p. 427.
Kinsella, J. E. (1976). Functional properties of proteins in foods: A survey. *CRC Crit. Rev. Food Sci. Nutr. 7*:219.
Kinsella, J. E. (1981). Nutritional, chemical and physical criteria affecting the use and acceptability of proteins in foods. In *Criteria of Food Acceptance* (J. Solms and R. Hall, eds.), Forster-Verlag, Zurich, p. 296.
Kinsella, J. E. (1982). Relationship between structure and functional properties of food proteins. In *Food Proteins* (P. F. Fox and J. J. Condon, eds.), Applied Science, London, pp. 51–103.
Kinsella, J. E. and Damodaran, S. (1984). Method for separation and recovery of proteins and nucleic acids from nucleoproteins

using water destructuring salts. U.S. Patent No. #4,427,580.

Kinsella, J. E. and Shetty, K. J. (1978). Yeast proteins: Recovery, nutritional and functional properties. In *Nutritional Improvements in Food and Feed Proteins* (M. Friedman, ed.), Plenum, New York, pp. 797–825.

Kinsella, J. E. and Shetty, K. J. (1979). Chemical modification for improving functional properties of plant and yeast proteins. *Am. Chem. Symp. 92*:3–50.

Krieger, J. (1983). Single cell protein process targeted for licensing. *Chem. Eng. News 61*:21.

Kuhlbrandt, W. and Unwin, P. (1982). The structure of the Ribosome. *J. Mol. Biol. 156*:431.

Lindblom, M. (1974). The influence of alkali and heat treatment on yeast protein. *Biotechnol. Bioeng. 16*:1495.

Lindblom, M. (1977). Properties of intracellular ribonuclease utilized for RNA reduction in disintegrated cells of *Saccharomyces cerevisiae*. *Biotechnol. Bioeng. 19*:199.

Litchfield, J. (1977). Single-cell proteins. *Food Technol. 31*:175.

Litchfield, J. H. (1983). Single-cell proteins. *Science 219*:740.

Litchfield, J. and Lipinsky, E. C. (1974). Single-cell protein in perspective. *Food Technol. 28*:16.

Mateles, R. I. and Tannenbaum, S. R. (1968). *Single Cell Protein I*, MIT Press, Cambridge.

Matheis, G., Penner, M. H., Feeney, R. E., and Whitaker, J. R. (1983). Phosphorylation of casein and lysozyme by phosphorous oxychloride. *J. Agric. Food Chem. 31*:379.

Milner, M., Scrimshaw, N., and Wang, D. (1978). *Protein resources and Technology*, AVI, Westport, Conn.

Newell, J. A., Robbins, A. E., and Seeley, R. D. (1975). Manufacture of yeast protein isolate having a reduced nucleic acid content by an alkali process. U.S. Patent No. 3,867,555.

Ohlendorf, D. H. and Matthews, B. W. (1983). Structural studies of protein: Nucleic acid interactions. *Annu. Rev. Biophys. Bioeng. 12*:409.

Otaka, E. and Osawa, S. (1981). Yeast ribosomal proteins: V. Correlation of several nomenclatures and proposal of a standard nomenclature. *Mol. Gen. Genet. 181*:176.

Pearce, K. N. and Kinsella, P. E. (1978). Emulsifying properties of proteins: Evaluation of a turbidimetric technique. *J. Agric. Food Chem. 26*:176.

Peppler, H. J. (1970). *The Yeasts*, Vol. 3, p. 421.

Peppler, H. J. (1979). Production of yeasts and yeast products. In *Microbial Technology*, Vol. 1 (H. J. Peppler and D. Perlman, eds.), Academic, New York, p. 157.

Phaff, H. J. (1977). Enzymatic yeast cell wall degradation. *Adv. Chem. Ser. 160*:244.

Record, Jr., M. T., Anderson, C. F., and Lohman, T. M. (1978). Thermodynamic analysis of ion effects on binding and conformational equilibria of proteins and nucleic acid: The role of ion association of release, screening, and ion effects on water activity. *Q. Rev. Biophys. 11*:103.

Reed. G. (1981). Use of microbial cultures: Yeast products. *Food Technol. 35*:89.

Reed, G. and Peppler, H. J. (1973). *Yeast Technology.* AVI, Westport, Conn.

Robbins, E. A. and Sucher, R. W., Seeley, R. D., and Newell, J. A. (1975). Yeast protein isolate with reduced nucleic acid content. U.S. Patent No. #3,887,431.

Schlingman, M. and Vertesy, L. (1980). Ammonium hydroxide to reduce nucleic acid in single cell protein. U.S. Patent No. #4.206,243.

Schnell, P. and Akin, C. (1979). Functional properties of yeast grown on ethanol. *J. Am. Oil Chem. Soc. 56*:82A.

Scrimshaw, N. S. (1975). Single-cell protein for human consumption—An overview. In *Single-Cell Protein II* (S. R. Tannenbaum and D. I. C. Wang, eds.), MIT Press, Cambridge, p. 24.

Shetty, J. K. and Kinsella, J. E. (1979). Preparation of yeast protein isolate with low nucleic acid by succinylation. *J. Food Sci. 44*:663.

Shetty, J. K. and Kinsella, J. E. (1980). Ready separation of proteins from nucleoproteins by reversible modification of lysine residues. *Biochem. J. 191*:269.

Shetty, J. K. and Kinsella, J. E. (1982). Isolation of yeast protein with reduced nucleic acids using reversible acylating agents. *J. Agric. Food Chem. 30*:1166.

Sinskey, A. J. (1978). Yeast. In *Food and Beverage Mycology.* (L. Beuchat, ed.), AVI, Westport, Conn., p. 334.

Sinskey, A. J. and Tannenbaum, S. R. (1975). Removal of nucleic acids in SCP. In *Single-Cell Protein II* (S. R. Tannenbaum and D. I. C. Wang, eds.), MIT Press, Cambridge, p. 158.

Spierer, P., Bogdonov, A. A., and Zimmerman, R. A. (1978). Parameters for the interaction of ribosomal proteins L5, L18, and L25 with 5S RNA from *Escherichia coli. Biochemistry 17*:5 394.

Tannenbaum, S. R. (1977). Single-cell protein. In *Food Proteins* (J. R. Whitaker and S. R. Tannenbaum, eds.), AVI, Westport, Conn., p. 315.

Tannenbaum, S. R. and Cooney, C. (1975). Removal of nucleic acid in SCP. In *Single Cell Proteins II* (S. R. Tannenbaum and D. I. C. Wang, eds.), MIT Press, Cambridge, p. 170.

Tannenbaum, S. R. and Wang, D. I. C. (1975). *Single Cell Proteins II*, MIT Press, Cambridge.

Tuse, D. (1984). Single cell protein current status and future prospects. *CRC Crit. Rev. Food Sci. Nutr. 19*:273.

Vananuvat, P. and Kinsella, J. E. (1975a). Amino acid composition of protein isolates from *Saccharomyces fragilis*. *J. Agric. Food Chem. 23*:3, 595–597.

Vananuvat, P. and Kinsella, J. E. (1975b). Extraction of protein, low in nucleic acid, from *Saccharomyces fragilis* grown continuously on crude lactose. *J. Agric. Food Chem. 23*:216.

Vananuvat, P. and Kinsella, J. E. (1975c). Some functional properties of protein isolates from yeast. *Saccharomyces fragilis*. *J. Agric. Food Chem. 23*:613.

Von Hippel, P. H. and Schleich, T. (1969). In *Structure and Stability of Biological Macromolecules* (S. N. Timasheff and G. D. Fasman, eds.), Marcel Dekker, New York, p. 417.

Weinberg, R. A. and Penman, S. (1970). Processing of 45S nucleolar RNA. *J. Mol. Biol. 47*:169.

Young, V. and Scrimshaw, N. S. (1975). Clinical studies on the nutritional value of SCP. In *Single Cell Proteins II* (S. Tannenbaum and D. Wang, eds.), MIT Press, Cambridge, p. 564.

15

Molecular Cloning of Carbohydrases for the Food Industry

JAMES H. MEADE, THOMAS J. WHITE, SHARON P. SHOEMAKER,* DAVID H. GELFAND, SHING CHANG, and MICHAEL A. INNIS / Cetus Corporation, Emeryville, California

INTRODUCTION

Enzymes are widely used in the food industry. The major factor limiting greater utilization of enzymes in food processes is the inability to cheaply produce sufficient quantities of stable, highly active enzymes that have acceptable safety for food use. The application of recombinant DNA technology to the production of food enzymes can potentially reduce the cost and create new uses. Generally, the yield and purity of an enzyme can be increased through molecular cloning of the gene and subsequent modification for higher levels of expression. Enzyme properties such as turnover number, enzyme substrate affinity and specificity, pH and temperature optima and stability, and resistance to proteases and chemical agents can increasingly be altered using techniques such as site-specific mutagenesis to make the enzymes more suitable for the processes in which they are utilized. Finally, the metabolic capabilities of microorganisms used in the food industry can be altered to provide microorganisms better adapted to food or beverage application.

Genetic engineering can have an immediate impact on the food industry by improving the utilization and/or modification of complex carbohydrates. Polymeric carbohydrates, such as starch and cellulose, are present in most agricultural raw materials. In the processing of these materials to food products, cellulose and starch are either removed as waste, converted to other products such as glucose, or included in the product as dietary fiber or as an essential component for the desired consistency or texture of the product.

**Current affiliation*: Genencor, Inc., South San Francisco, California

Specific carbohydrases can be used to impart specific structural changes or to convert these polysaccharides to glucose. This can result in improvements in the functional properties of these materials in foods and increases in product yield. This review will focus on the status of the molecular cloning and expression of enzymes which degrade starch and cellulose.

Starch and cellulose are both homopolymers of glucose. Starch consists of α-linked glucose, including both amylose (linear 1,4-α-D-glucan) and amylopectin (linear 1,4-α-D-glucan with 1,6-α-D-glucan branches), whereas cellulose consists solely of linear chains of 1,4-β-D-linked glucose. In aqueous suspensions these polysaccharides exhibit polymorphism; however, in general, starch is a hydrated polymer and cellulose is a crystalline polymer. This difference contributes to the approximately 100 times higher rates of hydrolysis by amylases as compared to cellulases.

The enzymes involved in the degradation of starch and cellulose comprise multicomponent enzyme systems. The amylolytic and cellulotytic enzymes can be grouped into four general categories (Table 1). Multiple forms of each of these enzymes exist within each category. Differences in amino acid composition, extent of glycosylation, substrate specificity, and activity have been found among the various forms of these enzymes (Fogarty and Kelley, 1979; Mandels, 1981; Brown and Gritzali, 1984; Woodward and Wiseman, 1982).

Some of the properties of these enzymes are summarized in Table 1. In general, α-amylases and endoglucanases act on internal bonds to significantly decrease the chain length of the polymers and the viscosity of modified, soluble polymers. These enzymes typically have broad substrate specificity and high temperature stability. Furthermore, these endoacting enzymes participate in transglycosylation reactions under conditions where the oligosaccharide acceptor is in excess.

β-Amylases and cellobiohydrolases are exoacting enzymes that cleave disaccharide units from the nonreducing end of the polymer. β-Amylases hydrolyze α-1,4 bonds but not α-1,6 bonds in starch and thus produce maltose and limit dextrin. Cellobiohydrolases hydrolyze β-1,4 bonds of cellulose to produce cellobiose as the principal product. Small amounts of glucose (< 10%) have also been detected under certain conditions using purified cellobiohydrolase. In contrast to the endoacting enzymes, these enzymes generally do not participate in transglycosylation reactions and have lower temperature stability and a narrower substrate specificity.

α-Glucosidases and β-glucosidases have no activity on starch or cellulose but hydrolyze oligosaccharides (G_2-G_6) to glucose. Because of their relatively high activity on the shorter-chain oligosaccharides, especially disaccharides, these enzymes have been

Table 1. Starch- and Cellulose-Degrading Enzymes

Starch (1,4-α-D-glucan)	Cellulose (1,4-β-D-glucan)	Characteristics
α-Amylases	Endoglucanases	Hydrolyze internal linkages of starch or cellulose
		Decrease chain length and viscosity
		Broad substrate specificity
		High temperature stability
		Some transglycosylation activity
β-Amylases	Cellobiohydrolases	Hydrolyze starch or cellulose to dissaccharides
		Narrow substrate specificity
		No transglycosylation activity
α-Glucosidases	β-Glucosidases	Hydrolyze malto- or cello-oligosaccharides to glucose
		Generally high arylglucosidase and transglycosylation activity
Glucoamylases		Hydrolyze starch to glucose
		Hydrolyze both α-1-6 and α-1-4 bonds
		Low arylglucosidase activity
		No transglycosylation activity

called maltases and cellobiases, respectively. In addition, many, but not all, of the glucosidases are active on arylglucosides. These enzymes readily participate in transglycosylation reactions.

Exoglucanases, such as glucoamylase, produce glucose from the nonreducing end of starch chains. Some glucoamylases acts on both α-1-4 and α-1-6 bonds. They have low arylglucosidase activity and do not participate in transglycosylation reactions. There does not appear to be a cellulase with an activity analagous to that of glucoamylase.

These enzymes act synergistically to degrade cellulose or starch to glucose. Complete and efficient degradation of crystalline cellulose to glucose requires the action of endoglucanase, cellobiohydrolase, and β-glucosidase. In contrast, starch can be degraded completely to glucose using only two of the four amylolytic enzymes, the α-amylase and the glucoamylase.

AMYLASES

α-Amylase (1,4-α-D-Glucan Glucanohydrolase, EC 3.2.1.1)

The α-amylases of principal commercial interest are produced by *Bacillus stearothermophilus*, *Bacillus licheniformis*, and *Bacillus amyloliquefaciens*. The genes for these three α-amylases and two other *Bacillus* α-amylases (*Bacillus subtilis* and *Bacillus coagulans*) have been isolated by molecular cloning of DNA fragments into phage or plasmids and subsequent screening for α-amylase activity in the transformed bacteria (Mielenz, 1983; Palva, 1982; Cornelis et al., 1982; Yamazaki et al., 1983; Ortlepp et al., 1983). For example, Mielenz (1983) isolated DNA from *B. stearothermophilus*, cleaved it and the bacterial plasmid pBR 322 with the restriction endonuclease *Hind*III, ligated the mixture with T4 ligase, and transformed the ligated mixture into *Escherichia coli*. Large-scale screening for α-amylase production among the transformants relied on detection of a zone of starch hydrolysis around lysed colonies on starch plates. Tsukagoshi et al. (1984) have shown that when the *B. stearothermophilus* α-amylase gene is expressed in *E. coli*, the level of expression is at least threefold higher than that of the same gene expressed in *B. stearothermophilus*. The majority of α-amylase produced in *E. coli* is secreted to the periplasmic space. Aiba et al. (1983) have expressed the *B. stearothermophilus* gene in *B. subtilis* and *B. stearothermophilus*. In both organisms the α-amylase is secreted to the extracellular culture medium. Reintroduction of the cloned α-amylase gene on a multicopy plasmid into *B. stearothermophilus* increased the level of production in that organism fivefold. This is an example of how recombinant DNA technology can significantly increase enzyme yield within the original production organism.

The complete nucleotide sequence of the *B. stearothermophilus* α-amylase has been determined (S. Chang, unpublished data); the deduced amino acid sequence codes for a polypeptide of 549 amino acids. The complete nucleotide sequences of the α-amylases of *B. amyloliquefaciens* (Takkinen et al., 1983) and *B. subtilis* (Yang et al., 1983) and the NH_2 terminal 75 residues of the *B. licheniformis* α-amylase (Stephens et al., 1984) have also been reported. Comparison of the deduced amino acid sequences of the mature proteins shows substantial homology between the sequences of the thermophilic α-amylases from *B. amyloliquefaciens*, *B. stearothermophilus*, and *B. licheniformis*. For example, the mature protein sequences of *B. amyloliquefaciens* and *B. stearothermophilus* share a total of 325 conserved amino acid residues; this represents 67% homology at the amino acid level. In contrast, the sequence of the *B. subtilis* α-amylase, a mesophilic α-amylase, is significantly different from that of the other *Bacillus* α-amylases; there is, for example, no more than 30% homology with the enzyme from *B. amyloliquefaciens*.

The cDNA clones of two plant α-amylase genes, barley (Rogers and Milliman, 1983; Chandler et al., 1984) and wheat (Baulcombe and Buffard, 1983), have been isolated. In germinating wheat and barley embryos, the prevalent mRNA of the aleurone cells encodes α-amylase. Messenger RNA was isolated from these cells, converted to cDNA with reverse transcriptase, and molecularly cloned into the plasmid pBR 322. The cDNA clones were screened by hybridization to aleurone cDNA probes under conditions favoring hybridization to prevalent cDNAs, and the selected clones were confirmed to encode α-amylase by hybridization selection of α-amylase mRNA. The DNA sequences of the two barley α-amylase clones are not identical; they share approximately 77% homology between the two inferred amino acid sequences in the region corresponding to the mature polypeptide. An earlier study (Jacobsen and Higgins, 1982) had shown that at least four distinct isozymes of α-amylase appeared in gibberellic acid-treated barley aleurone cells; two of the isozymes now appear to have been cloned. Chandler et al. (1984) have purified one of the secreted barley α-amylases and sequenced the amino terminal 11 amino acids. This sequence is identical with amino acids 25–35 of the sequence from the clone isolated by Rogers and Milliman (1983) and differs by only one amino acid from the clone isolated by Chandler et al. (1984). These sequence data and the α-amylase amino acid composition data published by Chandler et al. (1984) provide confirmation that the clones do indeed code for α-amylase. Only a 36-amino acid sequence of the wheat pre-α-amylase has been published (Rothstein et al., 1984). With this limited sequence, it is not possible to determine the extent of possible homology between the wheat and barley α-amylases.

The wheat α-amylase has been expressed in *Saccharomyces cerevisiae* (Rothstein et al., 1984). A protein corresponding in size to the native protein (42,000 daltons) is produced by the transformed yeast, and some of this protein is found in the extracellular culture medium. Preliminary data indicate that the wheat α-amylase signal sequence may have been recognized and cleaved during the secretion of the α-amylase from *S. cerevisiae*.

In summary, several mesophilic and thermophilic α-amylase genes have been cloned from bacterial and plant sources. The use of recombinant DNA technology has increased the yield of some of these enzymes.

β-Amylases (1,4-α-D-Glucan Maltohydrolase, EC 3.2.1.2)

At present there are no reports of β-amylases being cloned either from a plant (Robyt and Whelan, 1968) or from one of the *Bacillus* species that have also been reported to produce β-amylase (Robyt and French, 1964; Higashihara and Okada, 1974; Takasaki, 1976; Napier, 1977).

Glucoamylases (1,4-α-D-Glucan Glucohydrolase, EC 3.2.1.3)

Aspergilli secrete high levels of glucoamylase into the culture medium when grown on starch. As a result, they are the primary microbial producers of glucoamylase for commercial applications. The first *Aspergillus* glucoamylase gene to be cloned was isolated from *Aspergillus awamori* (Nunberg et al., 1984; White et al., 1984). The glucoamylase mRNA is the predominant mRNA produced by *A. awamori* when it is grown on starch as the sole carbon source. Using cDNA complementary to the glucoamylase mRNA as a hybridization probe, the glucoamylase gene was identified in a λ-phage library containing *A. awamori* genomic DNA. The glucoamylase gene was characterized by DNA sequence analysis and confirmed to encode glucoamylase by comparison of the deduced amino acid sequence with a partial amino acid sequence of the glucoamylase protein. There was no evidence by DNA hybridization for the presence of a second gene. An initial evaluation of the glucoamylase genomic DNA sequence indicated the presence of several introns. Therefore cDNA clones were also isolated and sequenced. By comparison of the genomic and cDNA sequences, it was established that there are four intervening sequences which are spliced from the *A. awamori* glucoamylase mRNA. There are two forms of glucoamylase produced by *A. awamori* that differ by approximately 10,000 daltons. The cDNA cloned by Nunberg et al. (1984) coded for the high molecular weight form.

Boel et al. (1984a,b) have isolated cDNA and genomic clones for the *Aspergillus niger* glucoamylase. Two different-sized cDNA clones were isolated. By comparing the nucleotide sequences of the two cDNA clones and the genomic clone, the authors concluded that the larger mRNA was formed by removing four intervening sequences from the original mRNA transcript and that the smaller mRNA was formed by removing the same four intervening sequences and an additional intervening sequence. In *A. niger* there are also two different molecular weight forms of the glucoamylase. Boel et al. (1984a) concluded that this differential splicing of the original mRNA transcript into two smaller transcripts explained why there is a single gene coding for two glucoamylase proteins differing by 10,000 in molecular weight. Interestingly, the glucoamylases from *A. awamori* and *A. niger* have the same amino acid sequence and differ only slightly in their nucleotide sequence; therefore it is likely that the lower molecular weight form in *A. awamori* is also generated by differential splicing of the glucoamylase mRNA.

The *A. awamori* glucoamylase gene was not expressed when cloned directly in yeast (Innis et al., 1985). Subsequent analysis indicated that, despite similarities to yeast control sequences, neither the transcription initiation nor the termination sequences are recognized by yeast and that proper splicing of the intervening sequences does not occur. An intron-free glucoamylase gene is expressed in yeast, however, using yeast promoter and terminator sequences derived from a yeast enolase gene (*ENO1*). More than 95% of the glucoamylase produced is secreted into the extracellular culture medium, the natural leader sequence of preproglucoamylase is correctly processed by yeast, and the secreted enzyme is glycosylated at both N- and O-linked glycosylation sites at a level comparable to that of the native *Aspergillus* enzyme.

The expression of the *A. awamori* glucoamylase gene in yeast produces a strain capable of simultaneous saccharification and fermentation of starch substrates. Such yeast can be used to shorten or eliminate separate saccharification steps in current industrial ethanol production processes and may also be useful in the production of light beer by converting nonfermentable malto-oligosaccharides to fermentable glucose.

The *A. awamori* glucoamylase cDNA has also been expressed in *E. coli* (M. A. Innis, unpublished data) using bacterial control sequences. In *E. coli* the glucoamylase is not glycosylated but does retain some activity. There is no evidence of extracellular secretion of the glucoamylase.

A glucoamylase from *Saccharomyces diastaticus* (*STA3*) has also been cloned and expressed in *S. cerevisiae* (Yamashita and Fukui, 1983). This glucoamylase can only hydrolyze α-1,4 bonds, in contrast to the *Aspergillus* enzyme, which also cleaves α-1,6 glycosidic bonds. Fragments of *S. diastaticus* DNA were cloned into a yeast–*E. coli* bifunctional plasmid. DNA from the library was transformed into *S. cerevisiae*, and the transformants were screened for glucoamylase activity. The level of expression of the *S. diastaticus* glucoamylase in *S. cerevisiae* is 5 to 10 times higher than that from the original *S. diastaticus* strain, and the glucoamylase is secreted into the extracellular culture medium.

Other interesting glucoamylases are currently being cloned. For example, Sills et al. (1983) are attempting to clone and express the glucoamylase of *Schwanniomyces castellii* in *S. cerevisiae*. Not only can this yeast glucoamylase hydrolyze both α-1,4 and α-1,6 glycosidic bonds, but it is also reported to have a higher specific activity on maltose and isomaltose than it does on starch. The glucoamylases from *Aspergillus* species and *S. diastaticus* have very low levels of activity on these low molecular weight glucose polymers. The *Schw. castellii* enzyme is thermolabile (Stewart et al., 1984); this property is desirable in the production of light beers because the ability to inactivate the glucoamylase during pasteurization is essential in order to produce a stable, consistent product. Continued activity of glucoamylase would change the glucose concentration in the beverage during storage.

α-Glucosidases (α-D-Glucoside Glucohydrolase, EC 3.2.1.20)

An intracellular α-glucosidase (Maltase) gene from the yeast *Saccharomyces carlsbergensis* has been isolated by Federoff et al. (1982). Sheared fragments of yeast DNA from a maltase-producing yeast strain were inserted into a yeast—*E. coli* bifunctional plasmid and transformed into *E. coli*. DNA from this yeast genomic library was subsequently transformed into a maltase-deficient yeast strain, and maltose-utilizing transformants were selected. Subsequent analysis has shown that an 11.4-kb DNA fragment that contains the α-glucosidase gene also contains a maltose permease gene and a regulatory gene for the permease and maltase (Needleman et al., 1984).

Other α-glucosidases are likely to be molecularly cloned in the near future, including secreted, extracellular maltases such as that produced by *Bacillus brevis* (McWethy and Hartman, 1979).

CELLULASES

Endoglucanases [1,4-(1,3;1,4)-β-D-Glucan 4-Glucanohydrolase, EC 3.2.1.4]

Endoglucanases have been molecularly cloned from both bacterial and fungal sources. A highly active, thermostable endoglucanase gene was isolated from *Clostridium thermocellum*, a gram-positive thermophile (Cornet et al., 1983). A genomic library of *Cl. thermocellum* DNA was prepared in a cosmid vector and transformed into *E. coli*.

The 1200 *E. coli* transformants that were isolated were distributed into pools of 10 and then grown, lysed, and assayed for carboxymethylcellulase activity. One of the cosmid clones was shown, by activity and immunological assays, to contain the endoglucanase structural gene. The reported level of expression of this endoglucanase in *E. coli* was about 30% the level observed in *Cl. thermocellum*. The endoglucanase produced by *Cl. thermocellum* is secreted to the extracellular culture medium; when produced by *E. coli*, the endoglucanase is intracellular.

An endoglucanase gene has also been isolated from another gram-positive bacterium, *Cellulomonas fimi* (Whittle et al., 1982; Gilkes et al., 1984a,b). Fragments of *C. fimi* DNA were inserted into the plasmid pBR 322 and transformed into *E. coli*. The initial screen for cellulase production was by immunoassay of lysed *E. coli* colonies. This assay for gene expression was used initially because it is more sensitive than enzyme activity assays; that is, it could detect 1 ng of anitgen. However, sufficient endoglucanase was produced by *E. coli* to be detectable in a colony activity assay. *Escherichia coli* containing the endoglucanase plasmid secreted 70% of the endoglucanase to the periplasmic space, but very little activity was found in the extracellular culture medium. The *C. fimi* endoglucanase may be glycosylated, since on SDS–polyacrylamide gels the protein bands corresponding to the endoglucanase can also be stained with a carbohydrate stain (periodic acid–Schiff base; see Gilkes et al., 1984b). It is unusual for a bacterial protein to be glycosylated, and it is unlikely that the recombinant endoglucanase produced by *E. coli* is glycosylated. Thus glycosylation of this endoglucanase is probably not essential for activity.

Another thermostable endoglucanase has been isolated from the thermophilic, gram-variable bacterium *Thermomonospora* YX (Collmer and Wilson, 1983). Purified *Thermomonospora* DNA was partially digested with *Sau*3A, ligated into *Bam*HI-cleaved pBR 322 DNA, and transformed into *E. coli*. The transformants were screened for carboxymethylcellulase activity, and several cellulase-producing clones were identified. The enzyme produced by the transformed *E. coli* strains has been shown to be homologous to the *Thermomonospora* YX endoglucanase by immunological criteria. Interestingly, while most if not all of the proteins secreted by *E. coli* are restricted to the cell membranes or the periplasmic space, about 30% of the *Thermomonospora* YX endoglucanase produced by *E. coli* is found in the extracellular culture medium. Collmer and Wilson (1983) believe that this is due to active secretion into the medium, and not due to lysis, because less than 5% of a periplasmic enzyme, alkaline phosphatase, is found in the culture medium, compared to 30% of the endoglucanase. Also, SDS gels of periplasmic and supernatant proteins show completely different protein patterns.

A cellulase with activity at high pH has been isolated from a alkalophilic *Bacillus* species (Sashihara et al., 1984). The native and cloned enzymes have a broad pH optimum ranging from pH 8 to 10. The alkalophilic enzyme was isolated by molecular cloning of *Hind*III restriction endonuclease-generated fragments of DNA into the plasmid pBR 322, transformation of *E. coli*, and subsequent screening of the transformants for carboxymethylcellulase activity. A significant amount of the carboxymethylcellulase activity was found in the periplasmic space, while only a little of the activity was found in the extracellular culture medium. While the enzyme activity has not been characterized in detail and the enzyme has been referred to only as a carboxymethylcellulase, it is likely to be an endoglucanase, since only endoglucanases have been reported to efficiently hydrolyze carboxymethylcellulose.

One of the *Trichoderma reesei* endoglucanases (EGI) has also been cloned (M. A. Innis et al., unpublished data). In contrast to the cellulases described above, this enzyme was cloned by hybridization to an enriched cDNA probe. The mRNA from induced and uninduced cultures of *T. reesei* was fractionated, and specific fractions containing the EGI mRNA were identified by in vitro translation and immunoprecipitation with endoglucanase antiserum. Comparably sized fractions from the induced and uninduced mRNA preparations were used to make cDNA probes. The probes were used to screen λ-phage banks of *T. reesei* genomic DNA. Putative endoglucanase clones were defined as those which hybridized to probes from the induced but not the uninduced cultures. Hybrid selection translation using specific antiserum to identify in vitro translation products subsequently confirmed that these clones encoded endoglucanase. Finally, comparison of the DNA sequence with the amino acid sequence (K. W. K. Watt, personal communication; Bhikhabhai and Pettersson, 1984) confirmed molecular cloning of the EGI gene. (Note: The same endoglucanase is referred to as EGI in the United States and as EGII in Europe.) The sequenced DNA fragment included 66 nucleotides for a 22-amino acid leader sequence preceding the coding sequence for the 437 amino acid residues of the mature protein (as deduced from the known amino terminal sequence of the purified secreted EGI). The gene also contained two small introns of approximately 60 nucleotides. The introns were removed, and an intron-free EGI gene was inserted into a yeast expression vector under the control of the yeast *ENO*1 promoter and termination sequences (M. A. Innis, unpublished data). The EGI expression vector was transformed into yeast and initial confirmation of endoglucanase expression was obtained by a plate assay for hydrolysis of carboxymethylcellulose (Teather and Wood, 1982). Subsequently immunological analysis confirmed that the *T. reesei* EGI gene had been cloned. More than 70% of the endoglucanase has been shown to be secreted by the transformed yeast, and the enzyme is glycosylated. Interestingly, while the native EGI enzyme from *T. reesei* contains carbohydrate attached solely through O-linked glycosidic bonds, the recombinant EGI produced by yeast has a similar amount of O-linked carbohydrate but also a significant amount of N-linked glycosylation.

In summary, in the last 2 years endoglucanases have been cloned from a variety of sources and expressed in several different hosts. These enzymes clearly have different physical properties in terms of catalytic efficiency and temperature and pH optimum and stability. These enzymes might be used separately to modify cellulosic fibers in order to provide new textures and functionality as noncaloric fillers in various food preparations. In conjunction with other components of the cellulase system (e.g., cellobiohydrolase or β-glucosidase), their use could be expanded.

Cellobiohydrolases (β-1,4-Glucan Cellobiohydrolase, EC 3.2.1.91)

At present the molecular cloning of only two cellobiohydrolase genes has been reported. The first was isolated from *C. fimi* (Gilkes et al., 1984a,b) by the same immunological screening technique used for isolating endoglucanase. The cellobiohydrolase gene was expressed in *E. coli*, and the majority of the cellobiohydrolase activity was found in the periplasmic space. Like the *C. fimi* endoglucanase described above, the cellobiohydrolase is also reported to be glycosylated; the active enzyme produced by *E. coli* presumably is not.

One of the cellobiohydrolase genes (CBHI) of the cellulolytic fungus *T. reesei* has been isolated in two different laboratories (Shoemaker et al., 1983; Teeri et al., 1983). In both laboratories essentially the same approach was used to isolate the gene; the gene was identified in *T. reesei* genomic DNA libraries using a cDNA probe and was subsequently confirmed by hybrid selection of mRNA. Shoemaker et al. (1983) have sequenced the entire CBHI gene and compared the nucleotide sequence with the published amino acid sequence (Fagerstam, 1981). The CBHI gene codes for a 17-amino acid hydrophobic signal peptide sequence and 497 amino acids of mature protein. Within the region coding for the mature protein, two small introns of approximately 65 bp were found. The endoglucanase and cellobiohydrolase genes of *T. reesei* do not hybridize with each other and hybridize poorly, if at all, to other cellulase genes. This indicates that considerable variation exists at the DNA level among the many genes comprising the cellulase gene family of *T. reesei*. In contrast, there is extensive homology between EGI and CBHI of *T. reesei* at the amino acid level. The homologies occur in discrete clusters within the protein sequences and are interrupted by polymorphic regions. Introduction of gaps into the sequence allows an alignment which shows 47% homology using only identical matches. The most striking homologies correspond to regions postulated to include the active site (Yaguchi et al., 1983; Paice et al., 1984). Chou–Fasman analysis (1978) indicates substantial conservation of secondary structural elements between the two enzymes. These results suggest that the *T. reesei* EGI and CBHI enzymes share a common evolutionary origin and appear to have retained similar structural conformations throughout their evolutionary development. An intron-free construct of the CBHI gene has been expressed in yeast using a yeast *ENO1* expression vector (D. H. Gelfand, unpublished data). Like glucoamylase and endoglucanase produced by yeast, the cellobiohydrolase produced by yeast is active, and the majority is secreted to the extracellular culture medium. The CBHI enzyme is glycosylated by yeast and, similar to the *T. reesei* endoglucanase described above, contains N-linked glycosylation not found in the native enzyme.

β-Glucosidase (β-D-Glucoside Glucohydrolase, EC 3.2.1.21)

In the preceding two sections we have described the cloning and expression of enzymes which hydrolyze cellulose. The additional enzyme required in order to produce high levels of glucose is β-glucosidase. The β-glucosidase of *A. niger* has been cloned (Penttila et al., 1984). A genomic bank of *A. niger* DNA was made in *E. coli* using a yeast cosmid shuttle vector. Yeast transformed with DNA from this bank were subsequently screened for expression of five *Aspergillus* genes; only one, β-glucosidase, was expressed in yeast. The *Aspergillus* β-glucosidase is normally secreted to the extracellular culture medium, but no information is currently available as to whether or not the cloned enzyme is secreted by yeast. It is unlikely that many fungal genes will be cloned by direct expression in yeast or *E. coli*. Many fungal genes have been shown to contain introns (Dons et al., 1984), and yeasts do not appear to recognize and process heterologous introns (Reggs et al., 1980; Langford et al., 1983; Innis et al., 1985).

In contrast to the *Aspergillus* enzyme, the β-glucosidase of *Kluyveromyces fragilis* is an intracellular enzyme. To isolate the β-glucosidase gene, high molecular weight fragments of *K. fragilis* DNA were ligated into a yeast cosmid vector and transformed into *E. coli* (Raynal and Guerineau, 1984). The *E. coli* transformants were lysed and screened for β-glucosidase activity (hydrolysis of p-nitrophenyl-β-D-glucoside). The β-glucosidase gene was also transformed into *S. cerevisiae* and shown to be expressed at a level at least 300-fold higher than that of the original *K. fragilis* strain. In *S. cerevisiae* β-glucosidase remains intracellular, as it does in

K. fragilis. In spite of the high level of expression, *S. cerevisiae* containing the *K. fragilis* β-glucosidase grows only poorly on cellobiose. This appears to result from lack of transport of cellobiose into the yeast cell. Therefore construction of a strain of *S. cerevisiae* that is able to efficiently grow on cellobiose will require either a secreted β-glucosidase or an intracellular β-glucosidase and a cellobiose permease.

An enzyme involved in cellobiose hydrolysis has been molecularly cloned from *Escherichia adecarboxylata* and expressed in *E. coli* (Armentrout and Brown, 1981). This enabled the *E. coli* to grow on cellobiose. The enzyme is not found in the extracellular culture medium or in the periplasmic space but, rather, appears to be an intracellular enzyme. The enzyme requires phosphate ions for activity. It is possible that the enzyme is not a β-glucosidase but, instead, a cellobiose phosphorylase (Alexander, 1972) which cleaves cellobiose to produce glucose and glucose-1-phosphate.

SUMMARY

Between 1981 and 1984 at least 19 amylase or cellulase genes have been molecularly cloned, and many have been expressed in heterologous microorganisms. The genes isolated from prokaryotic microorganisms were isolated from genomic DNA libraries, while those isolated from eukaryotes were isolated from either genomic DNA or cDNA libraries. The use of cDNA libraries for cloning and expression was necessary owing to the presence of introns in many eukaryotic genes. The genes have been identified by several different techniques. In some cases transformants were screened or selected on the basis of functional expression of the gene in the host. In other cases a more sensitive immunological screen for expression was used. Finally, in some cases where functional expression could not be used, cDNA probes were used for the initial screening.

The capability now exists to molecularly clone and express any desired carbohydrase. Food technologists are no longer limited to using only enzymes that are produced in high yield, since genetic engineering can usually increase enzyme production. Enzymes can be "genetically purified" by cloning and expression of an enzyme in an alternate host organism. For example, cloning and expression of the cellulases of *T. reesei* result in the production of only endoglucanase or cellobiohydrolase by the transformed host. Endoglucanase may therefore be more economically purified and used by itself to modify cellulosic substrates such as in the preparation of crystalline cellulose for tablet formation in the pharmaceutical industry (Zabriskie, 1984). The natural source of the enzyme does not have to be an acceptable food microorganism, since it can be cloned and then expressed in an organism generally recognized as safe by the food industry (e.g., the yeast *S. cerevisiae*). In principle, an enzyme can be chosen for use solely on the basis of its suitability for a specific process. The capability also exists to modify enzymes to improve their characteristics. While at present no specific modifications of amylases or cellulases have been reported, modifications of other enzymes for use in the food industry, for example, proteases (Perry and Wetzel, 1984), have been described. The ability to express enzymes in alternate hosts also provides the opportunity to produce microorganisms with improved performance in a food or beverage process. For example, Windass and co-workers (1980) modified the nitrogen assimilation pathway of *Methylophilus methylotrophus*, a bacterium grown for single-cell protein production, to increase the cell yield. Additionally, the expression of amylases in yeast may result in a more economical production of low-carbohydrate beer.

Finally, while no cloned enzymes are currently being used in commercial applications in the food industry, the economic potential and the availability of the appropriate technology virtually guarantee that commercial applications of cloned carbohydrases and other food enzymes will begin within the next few years.

ACKNOWLEDGMENTS

We would like to thank Vaughan Wittman, Judy Davis, Edna McCallan, and Kay Pharis for their assistance in the preparation of this manuscript.

REFERENCES

Aiba, S., Kitai, K., and Imanaka, T. (1983). Cloning and expression of thermostable α-amylase from *Bacillus stearothermophilus* in *Bacillus stearothermophilus* and *Bacillus subtilis*. *Appl. Environ. Microbiol.* *46*:1059–1065.

Alexander, J. K. (1972). Cellobiose phosphorylase from *Clostridium thermocellum*. *Methods Enzymol.* *28*:944–948.

Armentrout, R. W. and Brown, R. D. (1981). Molecular cloning of genes for cellobiose utilization and their expression in *Escherichia coli*. *Appl. Environ. Microbiol.* *41*:1355–1362.

Baulcombe, D. C. and Buffard, D. (1983). Gibberellic-acid-regulated expression of α-amylase and six other genes in wheat aleurone layers. *Planta* *157*:493–501.

Beggs, J. D., van der Berg, J., van Ooyen, A., and Weissmann, C. (1980). Abnormal expression of chromosomal rabbit β-globin gene in *Saccharomyces cerevisiae*. *Nature* *283*:835–840.

Bhikhabhai, R. and Pettersson, L. G. (1984). The cellulolytic enzymes of *Trichoderma reesei* as a system of homologous proteins: Cyanogen bromide peptides and partial sequence of endoglucanase II. *FEBS Lett.* *167*:301–308.

Boel, E., Hjort, I., Svensson, B., Norris, F., Norris, K. E., and Fiil, N. P. (1984a). Glucoamylases G1 and G2 from *Aspergillus niger* are synthesized from two different but closely related mRNA's. *EMBO J.* *3*:1097–1102.

Boel, E., Hansen, M. T., Hjort, I., Hoegh, I., and Fiil, N. P. (1984b). Two different types of intervening sequences in the glucoamylase gene from *Aspergillus niger*. *EMBO J.* *3*:1581–1585.

Brown, Jr., R. D. and Gritzali, M. (1984). Microbial enzymes and lignocellulose utilization. In *Genetic Control of Environmental Pollutants* (G. S. Omenn and A. Hollaender, eds.), Plenum, New York, pp. 239–265.

Chandler, P. M., Zwar, J. A., Jacobsen, J. V., Higgins, T. J. V., and Inglis, A. S. (1984). The effects of gibberellic acid and abscisic acid on α-amylase mRNA levels in barley aleurone layers studies using an α-amylase cDNA clone. *Plant Mol. Biol.* *3*:407–418.

Chou, P. Y. and Fasman, G. D. (1978). Prediction of the secondary structure of proteins from their amino acid sequence. *Adv. Enzymol.* *47*:45–148.

Collmer, A. and Wilson, D. B. (1983). Cloning and expression of a *Thermomonospora* YX endocellulase gene in *E. coli*. *Biotechnology* *1*:594–601.

Cornelis, P., Digneffe, C., and Willemot, K. (1982). Cloning and expression of a *Bacillus coagulans* amylase gene in *Escherichia coli*. *Mol. Gen. Genet.* *186*:507–511.

Cornet, P., Tronik, D., Millet, J., and Aubert, J. (1983). Cloning and expression in *Escherichia coli* of *Clostridium thermocellum* genes coding for amino acid synthesis and cellulose hydrolysis. *FEMS Microbiol. Lett.* *16*:137–141.

Dons, J. J. M., Mulder, G. H., Rouwendal, G. J. A., Springer, J., Bremer, W., and Wessels, J. G. H. (1984). Sequence analysis of a split gene involved in fruiting from the fungus *Schizophyllum commune*. *EMBO J.* *3*:2101–2106.

Fagerstam, L. G. (1981). Cellulases from *Trichoderma reesei* QM9414: Enzymatic and structural properties. Doctoral thesis, University of Uppsala, Uppsala, Sweden.

Federoff, H. J., Cohen, J. D., Eccleshall, T. R., Needleman, R. B., Buchferer, B. A., Giacalone, J., and Marmur, J. (1982). Isolation of a maltase structural gene from *Saccharomyces carlsbergensis*. *J. Bacteriol.* *149*:1064–1070.

Fogarty, W. M. and Kelley, C. T. (1979). Starch-degrading enzymes of microbial origin. *Prog. Ind. Microbiol.* *15*:87–150.

Gilkes, N. R., Kilburn, D. G., Langsford, M. L., Miller, R. C., Jr., Wakarchuk, W. W., Warren, R. A. J., Whittle, D. J., and Wong, W. K. R. (1984a). Isolation and characterization of *Escherichia coli* clones expressing cellulase genes from *Cellulomonas fimi*. *J. Gen. Microbiol.* *130*:1377–1384.

Gilkes, N. R., Langsford, M. L., Kilburn, D. G., Miller, Jr., R. C., and Warren, R. A. J. (1984b). Mode of action and substrate specificities of cellulases from cloned bacterial genes. *J. Biol. Chem.* *2259*:10455–10459.

Higashihara, M. and Okada, S. (1974). Studies on β-amylase of *Bacillus megaterium* strain No. 32. *Agric. Biol. Chem.* *38*: 1023–1029.

Innis, M. A., Holland, M. J., McCabe, P. C., Cole, G. E., Wittman, V. P., Tal, R., Watt, K. W. K., Gelfand, D. H., Holland, J. P., and Meade, J. H. (1985). Expression, glycosylation, and secretion of an *Aspergillus* glucoamylase from *Saccharomyces cerevisiae*. *Science* *228*:21–26.

Jacobsen, J. V. and Higgins, T. J. V. (1982). Characterization of the α-amylase synthesized by aleurone layers of Himalya barley in response to GA_3. *Plant Physiol.* *70*:1647–1653.

Langford, C., Nellen, W., Niessing, J., and Gallwitz, D. (1983). Yeast is unable to excise foreign intervening sequences from hybrid gene transcripts. *Proc. Nat. Acad. Sci. U.S.A.* *80*: 1496–1500.

McWethy, S. J. and Hartman, P. A. (1979). Extracellular maltase of *Bacillus brevis*. *Appl. Environ. Microbiol.* *37*:1096–1102.

Mandels, M. (1981). Cellulases. *Annu. Rep. Ferment. Processes* 5:35–78.

Mielenz, J. (1983). *Bacillus stearothermophilus* contains a plasmid-borne gene for α-amylase. *Proc. Nat. Acad. Sci. U.S.A.* *80*:5975–5979.

Mapier, E. J. (1977). Biochemical process. U.S. Patent No. 4,011,136.

Needleman, R. B., Kaback, D. B., Dubin, R. A., Perkins, E. L., Rosenberg, N. G., Sutherland, K. A., Forrest, D. B., and Michaels, C. A. (1984). *MAL6* of *Saccharomyces*: A complex genetic locus containing three genes required for maltose fermentation. *Proc. Nat. Acad. Sci. U.S.A.* *81*:2811–2815.

Nunberg, J. H., Meade, J. H., Cole, G., Lawyer, F. C., McCabe, P., Schweickart, V., Tal, R., Wittman, V. P., Flatgaard, J. E., and Innis, M. A. (1984). Molecular cloning and characterization of the glucoamylase gene of *Aspergillus awamori*. *Mol. Cell. Biol.* *4*:2306–2315.

Ortlepp, S. A., Ollington, J. F., and McConnell, D. J. (1983) Molecular cloning in *Bacillus subtilis* of a *Bacillus licheniformis* gene encoding a thermostable α-amylase. *Gene* *23*:267–276.

Paice, M. G., Desrochers, M., Rho, D., Jurasek, L., Roy, C., Rollin, C. F., DeMiquel, E., and Yaguchi, M. (1984). Two forms of endoglucanase from the Basidiomycete *Schizophyllum commune* and their relationship to their β-1,4-glycoside hydrolases. *Biotechnology* *2*:535–539.

Palva, I. (1982). Molecular cloning of α-amylase gene from *amyloliquefaciens* and its expression in *B. subtilis*. *Gene* *19*:81–87.

Penttila, M. E., Nevalainen, K. M. H., Raynal, A., and Knowles, J. K. C. (1984). Cloning of *Aspergillus niger* genes in yeast. Expression of the gene coding *Aspergillus* β-glucosidase. *Mol. Gen. Genet.* *194*:494–499.

Perry, L. J. and Wetzel, R. (1984). Disulfide bond engineered into T4 lysozyme: Stabilization of the protein towards thermal inactivation. *Science* *226*:555–557.

Raynal, A. and Guerineau, M. (1984). Cloning and expression of the structural gene for β-glucosidase of *Kluyveromyces fragilis* in *Escherichia coli* and *Saccharomyces cerevisiae*. *Mol. Gen. Genet.* *195*:108–115.

Robyt, J. F. and French, D. (1964). Purification and action pattern of an amylase from *Bacillus polymyxa*. *Arch. Biochem. Biophys.* *104*:338–345.

Robyt, J. F. and Whelan, W. J. (1968). The β-amylases. In *Starch and Its Derivatives*, 4th ed. (J. A. Radley, ed.), Chapman and Hall, London, pp. 477–497.

Rogers, J. C. and Milliman, C. (1983). Isolation and sequence analysis of a barley α-amylase cDNA clone. *J. Biol. Chem.* *258*:8169–8174.

Rothsetin, S. J., Lazarus, C. M., Smith, W. E., Baulcombe, D. C., and Gatenby, A. A. (1984). Secretion of a wheat α-amylase expressed in yeast. *Nature* *308*:662–665.

Sashihara, N., Kudo, T., and Horikoshi, K. (1984). Molecular cloning and expression of cellulase genes of alkalophilic *Bacillus* sp. strain N-4 in *Escherichia coli*. *J. Bacteriol.* *158*:503–506.

Shoemaker, S., Schweickart, V., Ladner, M., Gelfand, D., Kwok, S., Myambo, K., and Innis, M. (1983). Molecular cloning of exocellobiohydrolase I derived from *Trichoderma reesei* strain L27. *Biotechnology* *1*:691–696.

Sills, A. M., Sauder, M. E., and Stewart, G. G. (1983). Amylase activity in certain yeasts and a fungal species. *Dev. Ind. Microbiol.* *24*:295–303.

Stephens, M. A., Ortlepp, S. A., Ollington, J. F., and McConnell, D. J. (1984). Nucleotide sequence of the 5' region of the *Bacillus licheniformis* α-amylase gene: Comparison with the *B. amyloliquefaciens* gene. *J. Bacteriol.* *158*:369–372.

Stewart, G. G., Panchal, C. J., Russell, I., and Sills, A. M. (1984). Biology of ethanol-producing microorganisms. *Crit. Rev. Biotechnol.* *1*:161–188.

Takasaki, Y. (1976). Purifications and enzymatic properties of β-amylase and pullulanase from *Bacillus cereus* var. *mycoides*. *Agric. Biol. Chem.* *40*:1523–1530.

Takkinen, K., Pettersson, R. F., Kalkkinen, N., Palva, I., Soderlund, H., and Kaariainen, L. (1983). Amino acid sequence of α-amylase from *Bacillus amyloliquefaciens* deduced from the nucleotide sequence of the cloned gene. *J. Biol. Chem.* *258*:1007–1013.

Teather, R. M. and Wood, P. J. (1982). Use of Congo Red–polysaccharide interactions in enumeration and characterization of cellulolytic bacteria from the bovine rumen. *Appl. Environ. Microbiol.* *43*:777–780.

Teeri, T., Salovuori, I., and Knowles, J. (1983). The molecular cloning of the major cellulase gene from *Trichoderma reesei*. *Biotechnology* *1*:696–699.

Tsukagoshi, N., Ihara, H., Yamagata, H., and Udaka, S. (1984). Cloning and expression of a thermophilic α-amylase gene from *Bacillus stearothermophilus* in *Escherichia coli*. *Mol. Gen. Genet.* *193*:58–63.

White, T. J., Meade, J. H., Shoemaker, S. P., Koths, K. E., and Innis, M. A. (1984). Enzyme cloning for the food fermentation industry. *Food Technol.* *38*:92–98.

Whittle, D. J., Kilburn, D. G., Warren, R. A. J., and Miller, Jr., R. C. (1982). Molecular cloning of a *Cellulomonas fimi* cellulase gene in *Escherichia coli*. *Gene* *17*:139–145.

Windass, J. D., Worsey, M. J., Pioli, E. M., Pioli, D., Barth, P. T., Atherton, K. T., Dart, E. C., Byrom, D., Powell, K., and Senior, P. J. (1980). Improved conversion of methanol to single-cell protein by *Methylophilus methylotrophus*. *Nature* *287*:396–401.

Woodward, J. and Wiseman, A. (1982). *Enzyme Microb. Technol.* *4*:73–79.

Yaguchi, M., Roy, C., Rollin, C. F., Paice, M. G., and Jurasek, L. (1983). A fungal cellulase shows sequence homology with the active site of hen egg-white lysozyme. *Biochem. Biophys. Res. Commun.* *116*:408–411.

Yamashita, I. and Fukui, S. (1983). Molecular cloning of a glucoamylase-producing gene in the yeast *Saccharomyces*. *Agric. Biol. Chem.* *47*:2689–2692.

Yamazaki, H., Ohmura, K., Nakayama, A., Takeichi, Y., Otozai, K., Yamasaki, M., Tamura, G., and Yamane, K. (1983). α-Amylase genes (amyR2 and amyE+) from an α-amylase-hyperproducing *Bacillus subtilis* strain: Molecular cloning and nucleotide sequences. *J. Bacteriol.* *156*:327–337.

Yang, M., Galizzi, A., and Henner, D. (1983). Nucleotide sequence of the amylase gene from *Bacillus subtilis*. *Nucleic Acids Res.* *11*:237–249.

Zabriskie, D. W. (1984). Enzymatic preparation of particulate cellulose for tablet making. U.S. Patent No. 4,427,778.

16

Bioconversions: Enzyme Technology

DON SCOTT, FRANK E. HAMMER, and THOMAS J. SZALKUCKI* /
Fermco Development Inc., Subsidiary of Finnsugar LTD, Elk Grove Village, Illinois

INTRODUCTION

The traditional uses of enzymes in food processing and future potential uses have been very adequately treated in the publications of Reed (1975), Godfrey and Reichelt (1983), and Schwimmer (1981); between them, these authors "cover the field" up until the last few years. In this chapter we have chosen to deal with new and novel kinds of applications, commercially important ones used now or virtually certain to be used in the very near future. The changes in the past few years make for interesting and important reading. Because of the brevity of this chapter, necessitated by the scope of the book, neither all new uses nor all references to the uses discussed are listed. Nevertheless, the impact of biotechnology and the revolution taking place to improve the quality, quantity, economics of production, and types of foods available for human and animal use through the application of enzymes, old and new, in ways heretofore not considered possible, becomes clearly evident.

ENZYMES AS PRESERVATIVES

Lysozyme for Cheese

One of the recurring problems in the manufacture of hard cheeses is "late blowing" (hole formation, especially multiple small or unusually large and irregular holes formed slowly during cheese ripening). This is usually attributed to the "contamination" of milk with

**Current affiliation*: Finnsugar Biochemicals Inc., Subsidiary of Finnsugar LTD, Elk Grove Village, Illinois

organisms from the farm and animal environment, including the feed. Silage is often blamed as the source of the heat-resistant and gas-forming organism *Clostridium tyrobutyricum* contaminating the milk and then causing late blowing in the cheese (see the section on enzymes for ensiling forage and other crops as clostridial growth in silage results in butyric acid production and lowered acceptability to the diary animal).

The traditional way in which late blowing has been overcome in areas famed for their quality cheeses is by the use of nitrates. (Nitrates cannot be used in cheeses made in the United States, but imported cheeses containing nitrates are permitted, at least on a de facto basis!). The growing concern over nitrites and nitrates in foods (related to the formation of carcinogenic nitrosamines) is fueling the use of lysozyme in place of nitrates.

One of nature's antimicrobial agents, lysozyme (muramidase) (EC 3.2.1.17), has been shown to be effective in preventing the growth of *C. tyrobutyricum* and preventing late blowing when added to cheese or milk destined for cheese production. The spore germinates in the normal manner, but the growth of the emerging vegetative cell is stopped by the lysozyme (Carminati et al., 1984). In 1984 an estimated 100 metric tons of lysozyme, isolated from hen egg whites, were used in Europe alone for this purpose.

Lysozyme (muramidase) cleaves the β-1,4-glycosidic bond between N-acetyl-D-glucosamine and N-acetylmuramic acid in certain bacterial cell walls; it has been used to make "naked protoplasts" for decades in the laboratory. Commercial hen egg lysozyme has a known structure, consisting of 129 amino acids, with four disulfide bonds that tend to stabilize the molecule by crosslinking. It has a molecular weight of about 14,400. Its high isoelectric point (about 10.5) makes it easy to selectively separate. The older method of salting out the lysozyme at pH 10 with 5% NaCl has been replaced with processes involving acidic ion exchange resins (Ghielmetti and Trinchera, 1968), deaminated squid chitin (Weaver and Kroger, 1977), or other adsorptive materials. When the salting-out process was used, the residual salt in the remaining egg whites made these whites unsuitable for normal use in the food industry. Egg white contains about 0.35% lysozyme, and about 80% is readily separated, usually with minimal effect on the functional properties of the egg white. This may be done by batch or column processes, with columns being generally preferred. A process described in a 1968 patent (Ghielmetti and Trinchera, 1968) to make lysozyme for per os medical use (largely in Japan and Germany at that time) is still employed to make substantial amounts of the lysozyme used. In this process the egg white is passed over a column of weakly acidic resin such as Amberlite IRC-50 previosly equilibrated to pH 6.5; the lysozyme is picked up on the column. The column is washed with an aqueous buffer at pH 6.5 to remove other materials physically present but not strongly adsorbed. Then the lysozyme is eluted with a weak salt (NaCl or other salt) solution, and the crude lysozyme precipitated by increasing the salt content. If further purification is necessary, the crude product can be resuspended and, using more modern membrane technology, desalted by diafiltration. Commercial lysozyme preparations are generally about 85–95% protein (based on the specific absorbance of lysozyme) and contain as much as 5% moisture and some salt. Activity is expressed in "Shugar" units (Shugar, 1952), an assay method based on the lysis of a suspension of *Micrococcus lysodeikticus* (*Micrococcus luteus*). Most people now employ various modifications of the original method that used a standard curve to measure activity. Kinetic methods are now more popular, but method variations result in reported activities that can differ by a factor of 2. A good commercial lysozyme will assay about 22,500 Shugar units by most commercial suppliers, while some modifications of the Shugar method report 45,000 units for the same materials (L. Ray, personal communication, 1985).

Lysozyme appears to be particularly useful in the manufacture of Provolone, Grana, Emmenthal, Asiago, and Montasio cheeses. Usage levels are 25 mg/liter milk to be made into cheese, or 300 mg/kg cheese. The enzyme is added to the milk intended for cheese at the appropriate rate (e.g., if ultrafiltration concentrated milk is used, the dosage is calculated at 25 mg/liter milk prior to concentration). Addition is made prior to rennet addition.

The proper use of lysozyme normally does not interfere with the subsequent growth of lactic inoculum in commercial use, but in some instances strains of suitable culture resistant to lysozyme must be selected.

T4 Lysozyme

While the usual biological source of lysozyme is hen egg white, recently a T4 lysozyme was cloned into *Escherichia coli* (Perry and Wetzel, 1984). The expressed lysozyme was, however, thermally unstable, which may have been due to the lack of disulfide bonds. In globular proteins disulfide bonds provide conformational stability. The detailed mechanisms by which this takes place have yet to be defined. Theoretical calculations indicate that the extent of conformational stability due to crosslinking increases with the number of amino acid residues it spans.

The crystal structure of the T4 lysozyme was studied for appropriate residues that had a large span of amino acids with some close enough so that they could be joined by a disulfide bond. Here Cys^{97} occurs naturally and Ile^{3} was changed to Cys by site-directed mutagenesis. The formation of the disulfide bond between Cys^3 and Cys^{97} was then accomplished with the mild oxidizing agent sodium tetrathionate or glutathione redox buffer. The oxidized lysozyme derivative (Ile^3 to Cys) was fully stable for 180 min at 67°C, whereas the natural T4 lysozyme was almost wholly inactivated. When the oxidized lysozyme derivative was reduced by β-mercaptoethanol, its thermal stability was comparable to the poor stability exhibited by the expressed T4 lysozyme.

This work is an elegant example of the expression of a cloned enzyme and its subsequent specific alteration to a more stable form by site-directed mutagenesis. The T4 lysozyme is not likely to be readily approved for food use because of its source. It is more likely that the lysozyme from the hen will also be produced by cloning and, being identical to that made in the hen, will be more readily approved by regulatory authorities.

Lactoperoxidase: Nature's Preservative System

Mammalian secretions such as saliva, milk, tears, and mucus contain a peroxidase that, coupled with the thiocyanate ion (SCN^-) and H_2O_2, forms a powerful biocide believed to be the hypothiocyanate ion ($OSCN^-$). The hydrogen peroxide could be added per se or arise from the action of oxidases in the body. The instability and high reactivity of the hypothiocyanate prevent its accumulation. The only (current) practical commercial source for this type of peroxidase is nonpasteurized milk or sweet whey, and the enzyme preparation produced therefrom is referred to as lactoperoxidase. Our discussion will deal with lactoperoxidase and associated coproduced milk proteins, their application to the preservation of foods, and their use against "scours" (diarrhea) in young animals. Defeating scours has practical implications for feed efficiency by increasing the intestinal residence time of the food for more complete digestion and absorption, thereby increasing the yield of animal products for our food supply. (Lactoperoxidase is also involved in biological iodinations, but this will not be discussed here.)

The preserving action of lactoperoxidase requires hydrogen peroxide. In some systems the hydrogen peroxide can be produced in situ using an enzyme system such as glucose oxidase (from *Aspergillus niger*), in the presence of glucose and oxygen, to produce the peroxide. This is the basis for a toothpaste sold under the name Zendium that utilizes the lactoperoxidase and SCN^- in saliva with amyloglucosidase (to produce glucose) and glucose oxidase in the toothpaste (Hoogendoorn, 1974).

The lactoperoxidase system has been investigated for the preservation (extension of shelf-life without refrigeration) of unpasteurized (raw) milk. While hydrogen peroxide has been used in some countries for 30 years, the level of peroxide used (300–500 ppm) is sufficient to destroy the lactoperoxidase naturally present in the milk. The preservative action at these levels of H_2O_2 is the direct action of the hydrogen peroxide on the organisms present. At lower peroxide levels the lactoperoxidase thiocyanate system comes into play (Bjorck et al., 1979).

Bjorck et al. (1979) found that augmenting the thiocyanate level in milk increased the preserving action of the lactoperoxidase and hydrogen peroxide, greatly reducing the microbial count (as measured by the resazurin decolorization method). In colostrum, the milk from the cow in the first days following parturition, the concentrations of lactoperoxidase and thiocyanate are very high; the lactoperoxidase may be present at 10 times the levels found in milk at other times (J. Perraudin and J. Preel, private communication, 1984). Bjorck et al. (1979) attribute the success of the system in milk to the relative absence of available SH^- groups, as they attribute the antibacterial action of the $OSCN^-$ ion to its reactivity with the sulfhydryl enzymes. The inhibitory action can be reversed by reducing agents containing free sulfhydryl groups, such as cysteine or glutathione. Reiter (1979) states that the enzyme system is active against "pathogenic Gram-negative organisms such as *Escherichia coli*, *Salmonella typhimurium*, and *Pseudomonas aeruginosa*" and that the system "damages the inner membrane causing leakage and cessation of uptake of nutrient, leading to death of the organism and lysis."

Lactoferrin–Lactoperoxidase in Calf Milk Replacers

Calf milk replacers compounded from dry skim milk, whey, vegetable fat, emulsifiers, and other nutrients, wherein the lactoperoxidase indigenous to the whey or milk is largely destroyed in the processing, has advantages that are beginning to be used by at least two European firms. The approach of EWOS AB (Sodertal ja, Sweden) is described by Gudmundsson (1984). Oleofina is now marketing a lactoperoxidase–lactoferrin preparation for use with calf milk replacement formulations. Oleofina (no date) reported on two groups of 10 calves fed twice daily, one group receiving 10 g of "lactoferrin–lactoperoxidase system" per meal (Table 2) for 4 weeks and the other group acting as a control. Both groups of animals were followed for 19 weeks. The results (Table 1) clearly favor the group fed the enzymatic diet. In addition, the enzymatic group showed almost no weight loss in the first few days, whereas the control group showed a definite weight loss. The enzymatic group started gaining weight after the first week, while the control group lost weight for 2 weeks before gaining.

Table 1. 19-Week Comparison of Calves on Milk Replacer with and Without Enzymatic Addition

Parameter	Control group	Enzyme group	Change (%)
Average initial weight (kg)	48.0	48.5	
Weight increase (kg)	140	154	+10
Feed efficiency (kg feed/ kg gain)	1.66	1.48	−11
Diarrhea (days/ calf)	3.3	1. 3	−60
Feed refusal (kg/calf)	3.3	0.49	−85

Table 2. Composition of Base Feed Used with Enzymatic Diet Improver Evaluation

Ingredient	Percent
Milk powder	60
Fat	17.65
Whey powder	14.15
Glucose	5
Mineral–vitamin premix	2.5
Ethoxyquin	0.125
Choline chloride	0.025
Radiamuls LR2 emulsifier	0.55

STARCH-PROCESSING ENZYMES

Glucoamylase

Glucoamylase produced by *A. niger* has dropped dramatically in price over the last 5 years, owing primarily to lowered production costs resulting from yield improvement. In at least one case this yield and processing improvement resulted from a strain in which the organism was mutated by "conventional" biotechnological means (mutation by chemical and physical agents) so that 75% of the excreted protein is glucoamylase (Carbonell, 1982). Finnsugar Co. coupled this improved strain with ultrafiltration to eliminate the low molecular weight materials in the medium, creating a light-colored, stabilized, more concentrated glucoamylase that is now the "standard."

Regenerable Glucose Isomerase

Finnsugar Co. is now producing crystalline glucose isomerase (at least 80% pure enzyme) literally by the ton (K. Visuri, personal communication, 1985). Figure 1 shows typical glucose isomerase crystals under the microscope. This high enzyme purity has made possible the use of a reusable carrier based on DEAE-cellulose in a granular base containing food-grade polystyrene for rigidity and TiO_2 for weighting. The preparation of this immobilized glucose isomerase is shown in Figures 2 and 3 (Antrim and Auterinen, 1985). The actual immobilized glucose isomerase is shown at approximately 80×, 500×, and 5000× in the scanning electron micrograms of Figures 4–6. Because it is electrostatically bound, the exhausted enzyme can be stripped from the carrier, by high pH or high ionic strength solutions, and the carrier "reloaded" with fresh enzyme without removal from the column (Fig. 7). Reloads are reported to be at least 95% as active as the original column, so that in practice the column can be reloaded a number of times. Use of crystalline enzyme and reusable carrier in place of whole-cell preparations immobilized by crosslinking or chemical bonding of glucose isomerase to a support appears to offer a significant saving in materials cost and labor, further reducing the cost of processing starch into high-fructose corn syrup (HFCS).

Barley β-Amylase

Barley β-amylase, produced from ungerminated barley, was introduced during the past few years for the production of high-maltose syrups. The absence of α-amylase, an enzyme associated with germination, is claimed to make a high-maltose syrup with less glucose

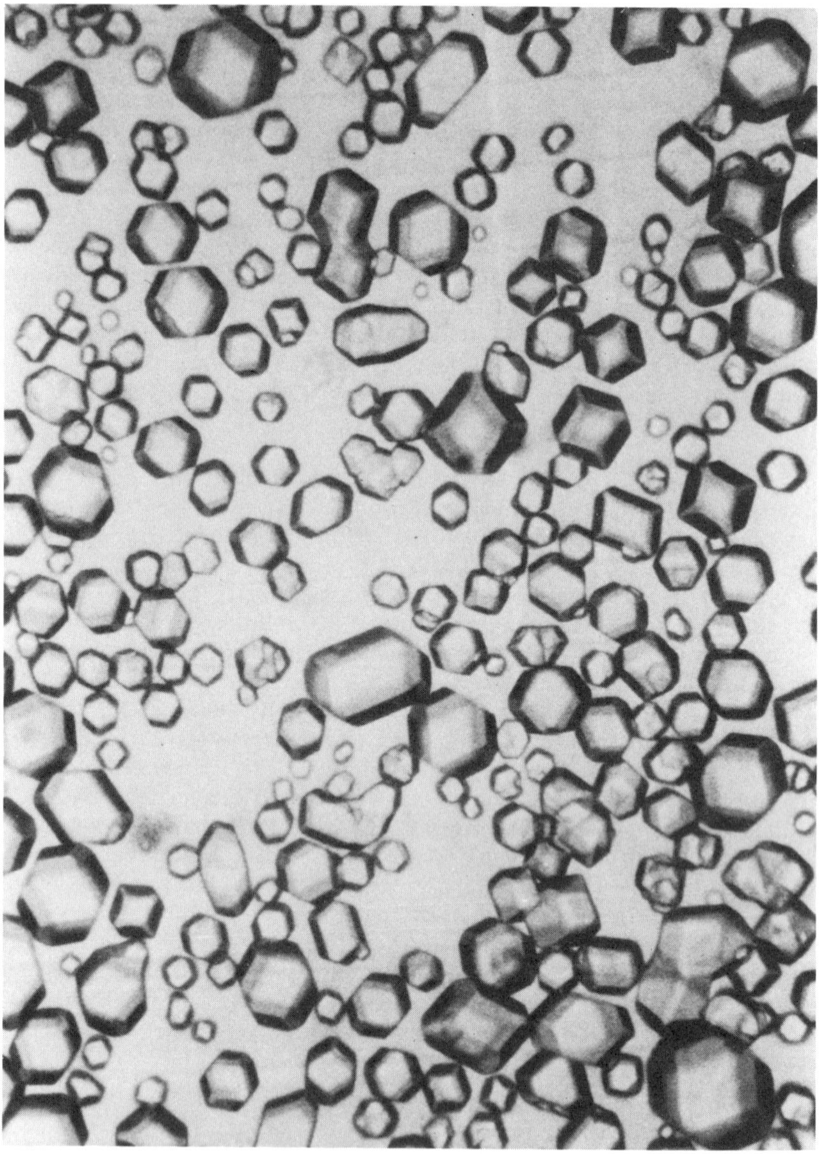

Fig. 1. Glucose isomerase crystals (approx. 200×).

PREPARATION OF IMMOBILIZED G.I.

FERMENTATION
|
EXTRACTION
|
FILTRATION
|
ULTRAFILTRATION
|
CRYSTALLIZATION
|
DISSOLUTION
| ← CARRIER
ADSORPTION
|
WASHING
|
DRYING

Fig. 2. Preparation of immobilized glucose isomerase.

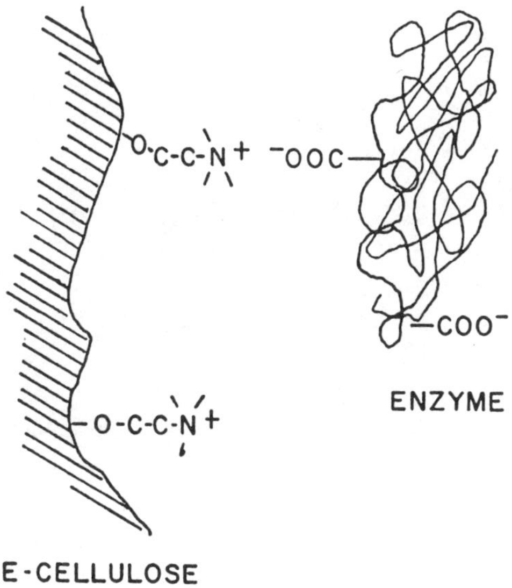

Fig. 3. Schematic of immobilized glucose isomerase.

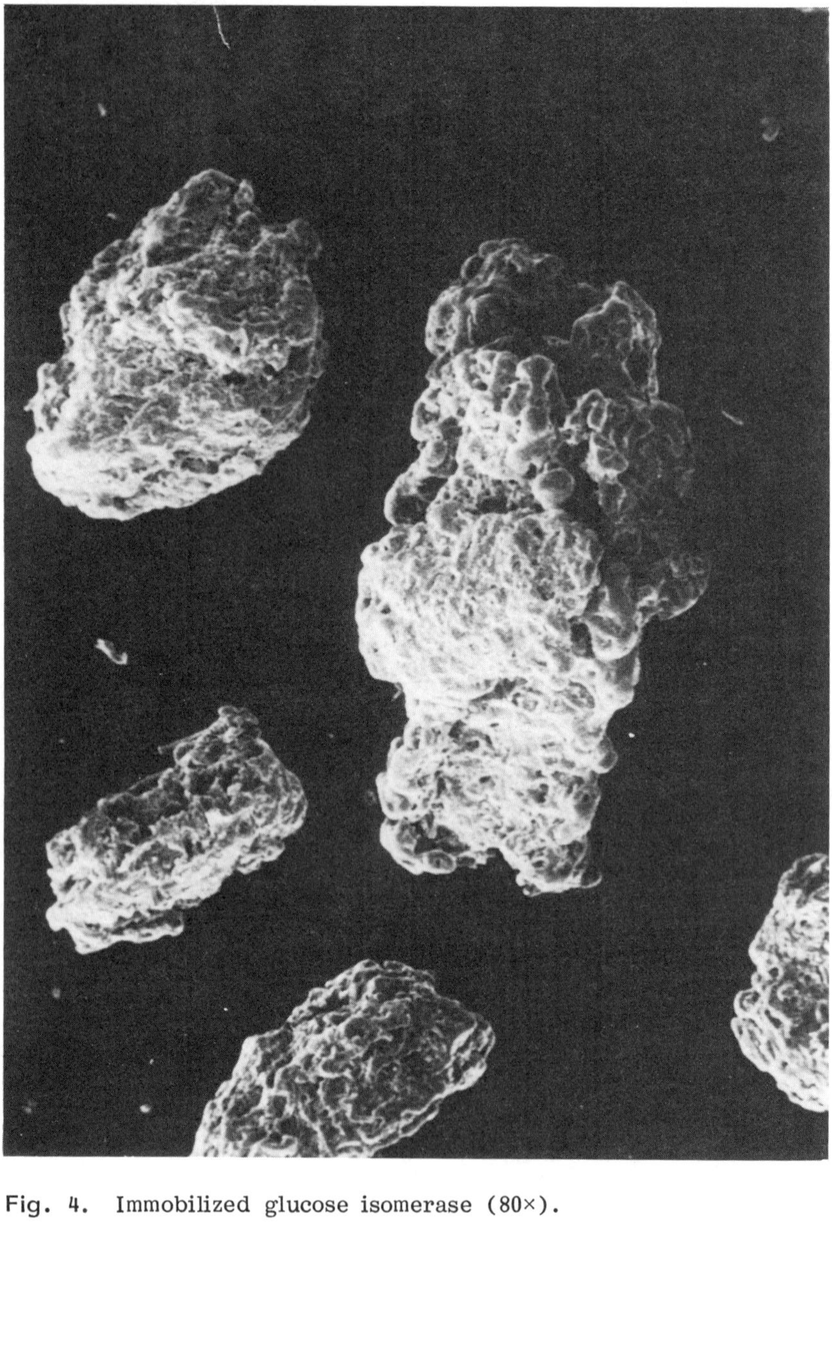

Fig. 4. Immobilized glucose isomerase (80×).

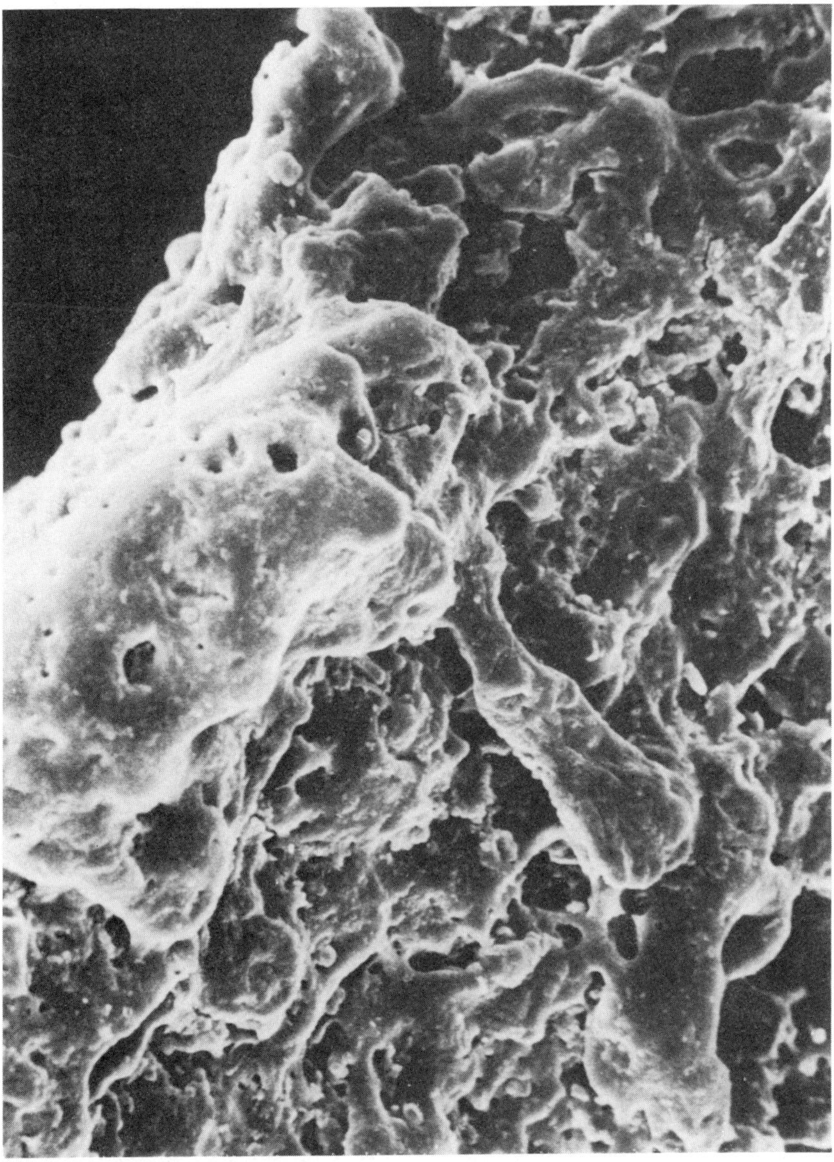

Fig. 5. Immobilized glucose isomerase (500×).

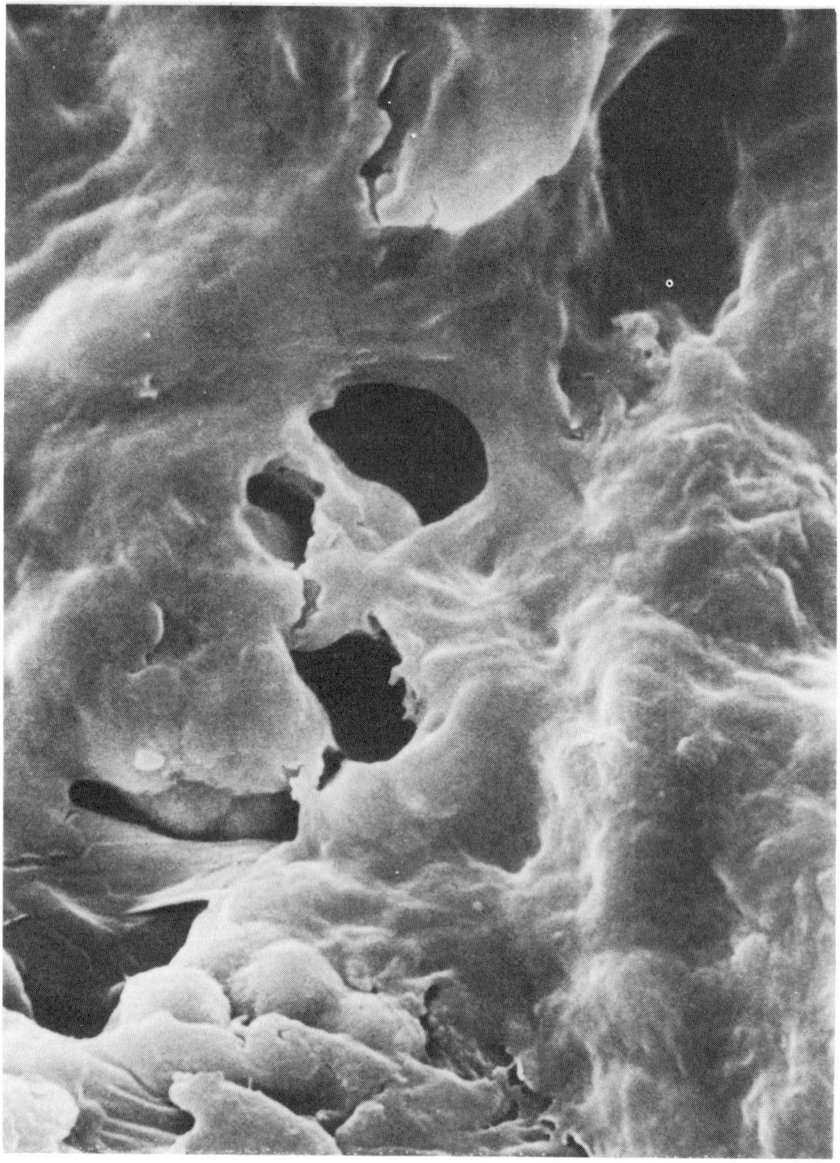

Fig. 6. Immobilized glucose isomerase (5000×).

REGENERATION

SWEETEN-OFF WITH WATER

2% SODIUM HYDROXIDE WASH

WATER WASH

BUFFER WASH

WATER RINSE

ENZYME LOADING

Fig. 7. Regeneration of immobilized glucose isomerase.

formation (Finnsugar, 1984). Barley β-amylase cleaves successive maltose units from the nonreducing end of amylose and amylopectin molecules. It hydrolyzes only the α-1,4-glucosidic bonds, so that the principal reaction products are maltose, maltotriose, and β-limit dextrins. The use of barley β-amylase on enzyme-liquefied starch (DE 10–16) gives 50–60% maltose and less than 2% glucose, while the use of acid-liquefied starch (DE 17–25) yields only 45–55% maltose and between 3 and 8% glucose. The production of syrups above 70% maltose requires the use of debranching enzymes (e.g., pullulanase) in conjunction with the barley β-amylase.

"REVERSE REACTIONS": SYNTHESIS BY HYDROLYTIC ENZYMES

Aspartame Synthesis

Enzymes are acknowledged to reversibly catalyze a reaction, and the conditions of commercial use are generally arranged to favor the so-called "forward" reaction (i.e., proteases catalyze the hydrolysis of proteins). Yet it is known that pepsin at a pH of 4.5 will synthesize the protein plastein from the hydrolysis products formed by pepsin at pH 2. In a similar manner other proteases can also synthesize under the proper conditions (Isowa et al., 1977, 1978, 1979; Isowa and Ichikawa, 1979).

The advantages of using selected proteases as synthetic catalysts in place of conventional chemical means, particularly the use of thermolysin in the synthesis of aspartame, are that it permits the use of ambient conditions instead of highly energy-intensive refrigerated systems; it allows the use of racemic reactants to selectively produce only the L-L "natural" α-aspartame, which is sweet, and not the β-aspartame, which is bitter; and it increases the yield of desirable product and eliminates the need to block the side-chain carboxylic group, as in chemical synthesis.

The process originally used soluble thermolysin, but now an immobilized version is used. While other proteases can be used, thermolysin, EC 3.4.24, a metalloproteinase produced by *Bacillus thermolyticus*, does not exhibit the esterase activity shown by some other endopeptidases, such as the serine proteases, EC 3.4.21 (trypsin, subtilisin, etc.) or thiol proteinase, EC 3.4.22 (papain).

The preferred aspartame synthesis process involves aspartic acid and phenylalanine as starting materials; these are "standard articles of commerce." The aspartic acid is carbobenzoxylated to produce the benzyloxycarbonyl-L-aspartate. The phenylalanine is esterified to produce the phenylalanine methyl ester. The *enzymatic* coupling of these two substances then takes place under near-neutral pH in an aqueous or biphasic system to produce benzyloxycarbonyl-L-aspartyl-L-phenylalanine-methyl ester, which precipitates as the addition compound with D-phenylalanine-methyl ester. The addition compound is easily separated and racemized before being recycled. Simple hydrogenation of the separated benzyloxycarbonyl-L-aspartyl-L-phenylalanine-methyl ester then splits off the benzyloxycarbonyl group, leaving the sweet product, aspartame (Oyama and Kihara, 1984). Figure 8 presents a schematic of aspartame synthesis.

Lipases for Synthetic Reactions: Transesterification

Since water is an essential reactant in the hydrolysis of triglycerides, it is not unexpected that, in low-water situations, lipases can and do catalyze the reverse or synthetic reaction. Pursuing "unnatural reactions" (i.e., different substrates or modifying conditions to reverse the "usual" reaction) has been spearheaded by the landmark work of A. M. Klibanov. A real application of this is in transesterification. Let us suppose we start with a triglyceride in abundant supply and of limited value. If we put this into a reactive environment (very low water, less than perhaps 0.2%) with a supply of a fatty acid or alcohol (primary or secondary alcohol) and a suitable catalyst (e.g., a lipase), then an interchange between the fatty acids in the fat and the externally supplied fatty acid or alcohol will take place. This is transesterification. This process

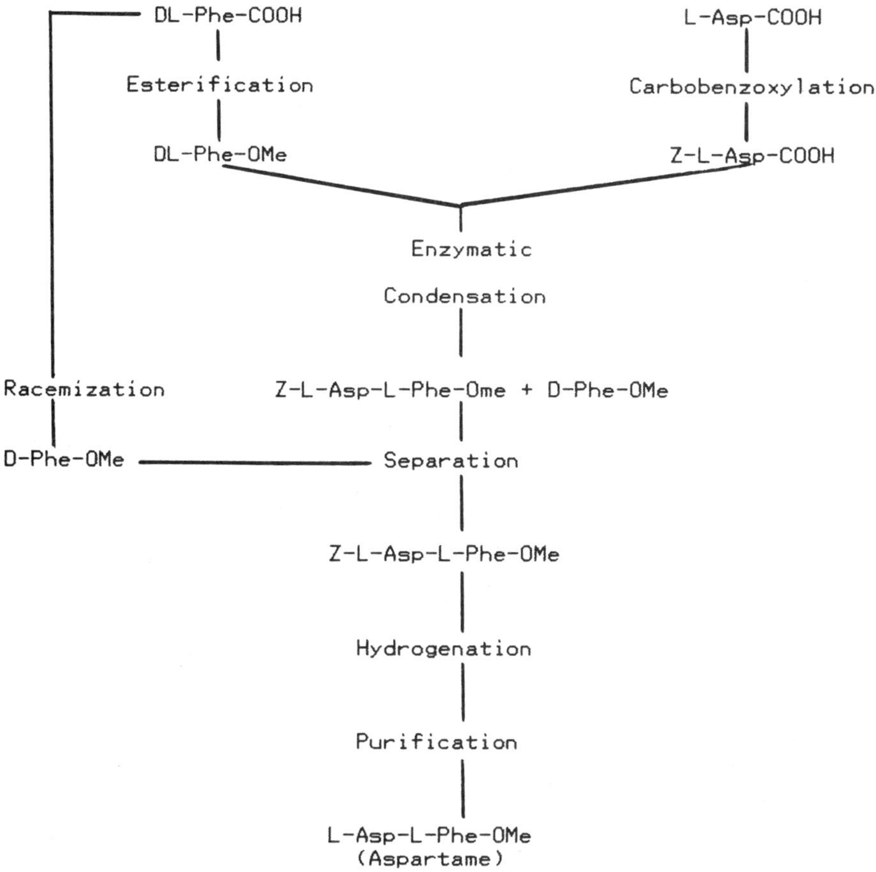

Fig. 8. Schematic of aspartame synthesis.

can be accomplished with a suspension of dry enzyme in a nonaqueous organic medium such as heptanol, benzene, or the triglyceride itself (at a temperature at which it is liquid, even at 100°C) (Matsuo et al., 1984; Zaks and Klibanov, 1984).

The Fuji Oil Petition (1984) pending before the Food and Drug Administration for the safe use of cocoa butter substitute from palm oil prepared by the direct esterification of partially saturated 1,2-triglycerides from palm oil and ethyl stearate in the presence of *A. niger* lipase shows one facet of the commercial utility of enzymes in synthetic reactions.

Triglyceride Synthesis in Nonaqueous Media

The modification of lipoprotein lipase (true lipases as compared to esterases) by polyethylene glycol to make it soluble in the organic phase (as compared to a suspension of a lipase powder preparation) has now been successfully applied to the synthesis of triglycerides from mono- and diglycerides with added fatty acids, as well as esters from fatty acids and alcohols (Takahashi et al., 1984a,b).

MODIFIED PHOSPHOLIPIDS: APPLICATIONS IN BAKING

A very new application of enzymes to improve the performance of gluten in the baking process has resulted in the commercial use of an *activated gluten* in Japan under the trade name Provian (T. Uno, private communication, 1985). Activated gluten is a gluten complexed with phospholipids modified by the action of a phospholipase; the actions of the different phospholipases give very different products with, consequently, different applications.

Phospholipase A acts on lecithin to split the fatty acid from C-2, which results in lysophospholipids that are ionic, mostly neutral, and hydrophilic. Phospholipase C splits the phosphatide from the lecithin, leaving a nonionic 1,2-diglyceride. Phospholipase D splits the "other side" of the phosphate, leaving the phosphate attached to C-3, which results in a phosphatidic acid (anionic) (Ohta et al., 1983). Figure 9 is a schematic of the action of phospholipases A, C, and D.

Ohta et al. (1983) reported several different possibilities: If soy lecithin is modified and added to wheat flour or to vital gluten, then the sequential use of phospholipase D and then phospholipase A gives the best results. To modify the phospholipids that are an integral part of the wheat flour, treatment with phospholipase A alone is sufficient. Ohta et al. (1983) report that phospholipids, even though a minor constituent of wheat flour, are "essential to the full development of baking potential of wheat flour." A third alternative, and the one now used in Japan, is to add soy lecithin modified with phospholipase A to wheat flour and then separate from this flour the enzyme-modified phospholipid–gluten complex (EMPL–gluten complex). The addition of this EMPL–gluten complex in place of vital gluten in bread formulations has resulted in increased dough stability, vastly increased dough breakpoint times, reduced development time, improvement in the mechanical tolerance of the bread dough, and a somewhat improved loaf volume (Kyowa Hakko Kogyo Co., no date). The phospholipase A used by Kyowa Hakko is separated from hog pancreas and is prepared essentially devoid of protease to avoid degradation of the gluten. Phospholipase A is

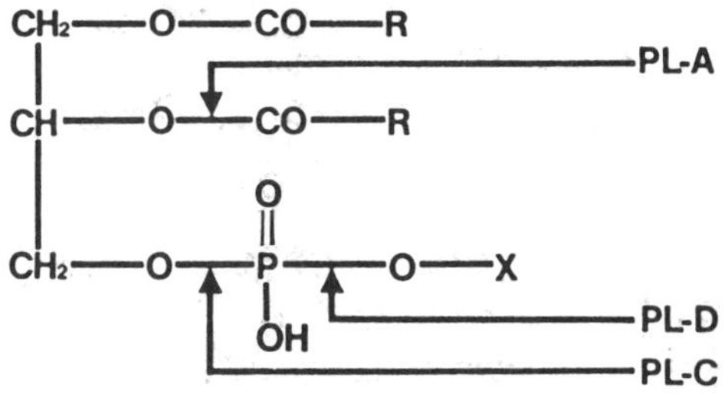

Fig. 9. Schematic of the action of phospholipases A, C, and D. R = Fatty Acid Residue; X = Choline, Ethanolamine, Inositol, Glycerol, etc.

also produced by microorganisms; one can expect that large-scale use will come about after the development of suitable microbiological sources and associated sales price reductions.

ENZYMES FOR CHEESE

Cloned Chymosin from *E. coli*

The conversion of fluid milk into a solid called cheese and a liquid whey historically involves use of the enzyme complex rennet. Fluid milk is a colloidal suspension of protein, fat, and other constituents. The initial phase of the cheese-making process, the K-casein which protects the casein micelle and keeps the casein in solution, is broken down by rennet. With the breakdown of K-casein, the unprotected casein forms a semisolid matrix interacting with itself, as well as fat- and water-soluble milk constituents such as vitamins and minerals.

Rennet is composed of chymosin (rennin, EC 3.4.4.3) and pepsin (EC 3.4.4.1). Veal or calf rennet is composed of 75–95% chymosin while the remainder is bovine pepsin. Chymosin is specific for the K-casein bond, which means that chymosin will destabilize the micelle without unduly hydrolyzing the rest of the protein. This specificity results in cheese of better texture and flavor. The most preferred rennet is the one with the highest concentration of chymosin, to obtain maximum milk-clotting action with minimal proteolysis.

Worldwide, there is an insufficient supply of calf vells (fourth stomach of the calf) for the production of veal rennet. As cheese production increases and calf slaughter decreases, this shortage will become more severe. Because of this continuing shortage of veal rennet, microbial rennet is being used for most of the cheese made in the United States. These microbial rennets are produced by the pure culture fermentation of microorganisms such as *Endothia parasitica*, *Mucor pusillus*, and *Mucor miehei*. Microbial rennet is not as satisfactory as veal rennet because of its higher proteolytic action; thus a microbial source for a rennet more similar to veal rennet has long been sought. The recent advances in genetic engineering have made it possible to clone the chymosin gene into a suitable microorganism.

Chymosin has a molecular weight of about 35,600 and contains 257 amino acid residues. Disulfide bonds link residues 116–121, 123–136, and 141–156. The immediate translation protein product contains a pre, pro, and structural (active) component. The pre portion, also called the signal sequence, containing 16 residues, which presumably directs the cell to excrete the protein, is removed during the excretion process. Chymosin is secreted as the inactive zymogen called prochymosin. The inactive prochymosin is activated in the stomach of the ruminant. Presumably the production of the zymogen protects the enzyme from self-proteolysis. If the gene for chymosin could be isolated and cloned, the protein expressed would probably contain the pre, pro, structural, and intervening sequences and may be nonfunctional.

The intervening sequences are not found in the ribosomal mRNA or in the protein produced. The intervening sequences are probably present on the RNA gene transcript but are removed during mRNA processing. Therefore the mRNA contains the pre, pro, and structured components only. The mRNA, because it contains a poly-A tail, preferentially binds to an oligo-dT-cellulose column while the other RNAs pass through. A single-stranded DNA (ssDNA) is then produced from the purified mRNA using reverse transcriptase. This ssDNA serves as the template to produce the double-stranded complementary DNA (cDNA).

Plasmid pBR 322 was chosen as the cloning vector. The plasmid was treated with the restriction endonuclease Pst I, a poly dC tail was introduced, and the cDNA was annealed to produce the fused gene product containing the gene for chymosin. The loop was closed with a ligase and the chimeric plasmid was used to transform *E. coli*. Immunodiffusion and electrophoresis techniques were designed to detect proteolytic activity at a low pH. The transformed *E. coli* was grown in various media and cell-free extracts were then prepared. These extracts were assayed for chymosin using anti-chymosin in an immunodiffusion technique. Chymosin expression was not detected.

An electrophoretic technique was also tried using salt-free casein in the gel. After electrophoresis and incubation a clear zone was detected ahead of the clear zones produced by authentic chymosin. It seemed, therefore, that chymosin was being expressed in

E. coli as an altered protein or in a configuration that migrated more rapidly owing to folding or fusing of the protein (Moskowitz et al., 1984). It was later determined that the protein was produced in an inactive, improperly folded form (G. Moskowitz, private communication, 1985). The work of Moskowitz et al. (1984) demonstrates the progress of genetic engineering efforts in this area. Thus in the near future "calf rennet" will likely be available from the fermenter.

Destabilized Microbial Rennet

There are some instances when it is not desirable for an enzyme to be too stable. For example, when a microbial rennet has been used to coagulate milk while making cheese, there should be little or no residual proteolytic activity in the cheese or in the pasteurized whey. Significant proteolysis can occur in cheeses with even minimal remnant proteolytic activity because of the long storage time for cheeses. In conventional cheese processing a portion of the coagulating enzyme preparation remains with the cheese, the remainder going with the whey. For cheeses produced by first ultrafiltration concentration of the milk there is no whey separation and *all* the enzyme activity remains in the cheese. (the "whey proteins" remain with the concentrated milk in ultrafiltration cheeses and the milk permeate is not whey). In conventional whey, if undue proteolysis occurs, the whey loses its economic and nutritional value as a source of protein. To prevent this proteolysis, collected whey is pasteurized at about 60–70°C. This temperature is usually high enough to inactivate at least 80–90% of the residual rennet coagulant. Residual levels of much more than 20% after pasteurization cause whey protein proteolysis and a bitter taste due to the presence of lower molecular weight peptides and amino acids. This same phenomenon occurs in cheeses with excess residual protease activity. Several microbiological and chemical approaches have been tried to decrease the thermal stability of microbial rennet.

Cornelius (1982) oxidized the methionine residues of microbial rennet from *M. miehei* and *M. pusillus* by treating with 3% vol/vol hydrogen peroxide for 24 hr at 4°C (the residual peroxide was removed with beef liver catalase). The milk clotting activity of the altered rennet was then determined on 10% wt/vol solutions of milk solids containing 0.01% $CaCl_2$. The altered enzymes had essentially the same milk clotting activity but their thermal stabilities were reduced. The thermal stability of a rennet from *M. pusillus* was reduced by a factor of about 10, and in the case of *M. miehei* it was reduced to essentially zero.

Activation of Milk-Clotting Activity of Microbial Rennet

Instead of destabilizing the microbial rennet, as described above, Higashi et al. (1983) altered the relative "proteolytic–chymosin-like" activity ratios. Higashi et al. (1983) found that acylating rennet from *M. pusillus* increases its milk coagulating activity (MCA). The proteolytic activity (PA) MCA index (i.e., PA/MCA) was reduced from 100 to 50–90 when the rennet was acylated. It is important that the PA/MCA ratio be as low as possible, because if the rennet contains too high a PA, the resulting cheese may be bitter owing to the increased quantity of lower molecular weight peptides or amino acids formed by the proteolytic activity. The acylation procedure involved treatment of the microbial rennet with succinic anhydride. It is well known that when a protein is treated with succinic anhydride, the amino groups are mainly acylated. Succinates occur widely in plants and animals and have long been known as seasonings. The Food Chemicals Codex (1981) describes succinic acid as a food additive.

The acylated microbial rennet contains at least 4 mol of the succinyl group per mole of rennet. This quantity may vary between 4 and 20 mol, depending on acylation conditions.

Accelerating Ripening and Flavor Development

The role of lipases, esterases, and peptidases in cheese ripening and flavor development have been under extensive study. The traditional sources for these enzymes have been the milk itself and the microorganisms associated with the development of the characteristic attributes of a particular cheese. Often this enzyme development and activity manifestation take many months of storage. If the same flavor and texture could be obtained in a shorter time by the addition of selected enzymes, the advantages would be substantial at even modest interest rates. In addition, the opportunity to increase the proportion of high-quality cheese increases with each measure of control, and addition of enzymes per se does provide significant control as compared to, say, leaving everything to "Mother Nature."

The opportunity to intensify cheese flavors also has strong economic consequences. For example, a flavor-intensified cheddar cheese could permit the use of 20% enzyme-modified cheddar in a cheese snack food coating as compared to 50% for the natural-intensity product. The use of enzymes for cheese flavor development and the acceleration of ripening is still more of an art than a science. Enzyme preparations sold for these purposes are "black boxes" because of the great research investment of the company selling the product and also, in some instances, the enzyme activities in the preparation have not yet been fully characterized or the relative importance of their interactions established. For example, one such product, described as being able to double the rate of formation of cheddarlike flavor, is comprised of "selected strains of lactic acid-producing bacteria, enzymes and polysorbate 80" (Miles Laboratories, no date). Although the subject is of considerable interest (virtually every issue of the *Journal of Dairy Science* has at least one article dealing with cheese cultures or flavor), even a meaningful introduction to it is really beyond the scope of this chapter.

ENZYMES FOR ANIMAL FEED

Enzymes for Ensiling Forage and Other Crops

One of the key elements in the economic production of milk and meat from ruminants is on-the-farm production of most or at least part of the feed. Farm crops for this purpose vary according to what grows best in each locale; in the north it may be orchard grass or other grasses whereas further south it would be alfalfa and corn, as well as other whole-grain crops, such as wheat, triticale, and sorghum. What is grown depends on climate and water supply; silage practices also vary based on these same factors. Traditional farming methods provide for the storage of farm-produced animal feed for supplemental use during winter feeding. As farmers have become more cognizant of the factors involved in efficient production, basic practices have changed. For example, instead of field-drying grasses to make hay (with the heavy loss of nutrients, especially protein), farmers with small herds cut and briefly wilt the grasses in the field and then store them in tower silos. When the stored product has enough fermentable carbohydrate (marginal in grass and alfalfa, plentiful in corn plants with stalk and fully developed seed heads) and the right organisms are present, and if it is packed well to eliminate air, natural fermentation preserves all but the top portion, which, being exposed to air, molds. As herd sizes increase, tower silos become an expensive and inefficient way to store silage. A more efficient method involves the use of bunkers. Bunker silos are large concrete chambers, perhaps 40 ft by 120 ft, with walls 8–12 ft high on three sides. The fourth side is used to load in the cut crop and pack it down. The entire bunker is then covered with a heavy plastic sheet that is suitably weighted down (tires are frequently used). Where there is sufficient fermentable carbohydrate, the organisms normally present (*Lactobacillus plantarium*, *Leuconostoc* sp., and others) convert a portion of it to lactic acid. This lowers the pH and the redox potential to the point where *Clostridium* cannot grow. *Clostridium tyrobutyricum* growth in silage produces butyric acid, which reduces the palatability of the silage and therefore the feed intake of the ruminant.

The use of cellulases from *Trichoderma reesii* is briefly described by Godfrey (1983) as a means of increasing fermentable sugars in such crops as grass, alfalfa, and red clover. Where fruit wastes are involved, he suggests the use of pectinase as well, and for cereal husks or straw, hemicellulase and pentosanases.

More recently a patented product/process has been introduced which results in in situ acid generation along with the production of fermentable sugars and the simultaneous consumption of free oxygen in the silo. This involves using a balanced mixture of cellulases, hemicellulases, miscellaneous glucanases, pentosanases, catalase, and glucose oxidase but negligible protease on partly wilted forage crops with limited fermentable carbohydrate. There is evidence that the system promotes a drop in pH through initial gluconic acid production along with the release of fermentable sugars for conversion to lactic acid by the organisms normally present or by added inocula (M. Virkki, personal communications, 1984, 1985). A product designed for use on the surface of bunker silos before covering and closing, to avoid the approximately 5% "normal" loss of materials to mold (estimated at 40—50 tons for a typical bunker), was introduced in 1985 as Topzyme (Forum Chemical, Surrey, England). Both of the above-mentioned products have been shown effective in preventing the clostridial growth that results in butyric acid production and loss of palatability. There is also evidence of a possible increase in roughage utilization by ruminants, increasing the energy value of treated silage.

Cultures are also used in conjunction with enzymes for silage. In general, the cost of using a suitable blend is lower than the cost of the direct addition of molasses or other fermentable carbohydrates, a past practice of small farmers.

In general, whatever grows well in a particular area is ensiled for winter feeding. It is particularly important that these crops be prepared so as to conserve their nutritional value. Only in this way can the modern farmer meet the competitive standards and survive in a situation that is moving steadily in the direction of larger herds and more efficient operators.

Poultry Feed

Enzyme supplements to aid digestion have been used in animal feed for many years; however, there have been few controlled experiments with a sufficiently large number of animals, so that feed lot operators and others interested in the use of enzymes have often had to rely on subjective judgments. Results published by Finnsugar (1985) show that, for poultry, feeds with a suitable β-glucanase-containing enzyme preparation permit the substitution of barley for wheat and dehulled oats, even where the barley constitutes almost 70% of the feed. This is of particular importance in Finland, where barley is locally grown and is cheaper than wheat; such feeds have been in use there since June 1984. Results are shown in Table 3.

Table 3. Broiler Performance from Three Trials on a Barley + Enzyme[a] Diet Compared to a Wheat–Dehulled Oat Control Diet at Days 21–42

	Control	Barley + Enzyme
Diet composition (%)		
Barley	8.6–8.8	67.4–67.4
Dehulled oats	25	—
Wheat	37.0–40.0	—
Soybean meal	13.4–15.7	14.5
Fat	2.3–2.4	6.1–6.3
Crude protein	20.0	18.0
Lysine	1.04–1.12	1.04–1.13
Methionine + cysteine	0.70–0.72	0.70
Ca	1.05–1.06	1.05
P	0.68–0.70	0.70
Metabolizable energy (MJ/kg)	12.35–12.40	12.20–13.35
Results		
Number of broilers	18,300	18,342
Mortality (%)	5.0	4.5
Meat total (kg)	16,846	17,070
Empty weight (g)	970	976
Feed conversion (kg/kg empty weight)	3.40	3.29

[a] β-Glucanase-containing enzyme preparation.
Source: Finnsugar (1985).

FATTY ACID PRODUCTION BY LIPASE

With energy costs and pressurized vessel capital costs generally rising, it seems only natural to consider the use of lipase instead of high-temperature, high-pressure fat splitters to hydrolyze fats into the constituent fatty acids and glycerol, for subsequent resynthesis into desired surfactants and emulsifiers.

The positional specificity of the animal lipases (e.g., pancreatic) and their low rate of activity on di- and monoglycerides rule them out as enzymes of choice. The microbial enzymes seem much less specific for fatty acid position and chain length and hence seem more suitable. In recent years a lipase from *Candida cylindracea* has been used for this purpose, since this enzyme results in over 90% hydrolysis of vegetable fats at moderate temperatures such as 30–50°C. However, the hydrolysis of animal fats is generally not as good as, for example, that of soybean or olive oil (Meito Sangyo, Tokyo, no date). Other microbial enzymes, especially those from *Pseudomonas* and *Geotrichium*, are also being investigated for this purpose, but at this time only the *Candida* lipase appears to be in commercial use. Fungal lipases now available from *Aspergillus* and *Rhizopus* species seem to be more like pancreatic lipase in their positional preference and lowered activity on di- and monoglycerides.

POTATO VIRUS TEST

In an analytical sense, enzymes are quite important in determining various parameters before, during, and after food processing. In a more esoteric sense, enzymes are used as sensing agents for many enzyme immunoassays. One of these is an enzyme immunoassay to determine potato viruses in vitro. The principle involved is the detection of the formation of an antigen–antibody complex; the antigen is one of a variety of potato viruses and the antibody is specific for this potato virus. Microtiter wells are coated with the anti-potato virus antibody and the sample allowed to react with this bound antibody. In the third step antibody labeled with alkaline phosphatase is added. If virus is present, the labeled antibody will bind specifically to it. The amount of bound antibody is directly related to the amount of virus. The alkaline phosphatase level is then determined by measuring the rate of conversion of p-nitrophenylphosphate to p-nitrophenol, which absorbs strongly at 405 nm (Boehringer Mannheim, Mannheim, 1977).

HYPERPRODUCING CELLULASE ORGANISM

Cellulose comprises a major storage form of photosynthesized glucose and is the major component of biomass energy. It has been estimated that cellulose makes up more than 50% of the total organic carbon in the biosphere (Lehninger, 1970). It is the simplest structural and cell-wall polysaccharide in the plant world. Wood is comprised of about 50% cellulose, while cotton is almost pure cellulose.

The polysaccharide cellulose is made up of glucoses linked by 1,4-bonds. The minimum molecular weight of cellulose is estimated to vary from 50,000 to 500,000, equivalent to 300–3000 glucose residues.

Because of the recent energy crisis and the search for renewable resources, work on utilizing this vast store of cellulose as energy has been greatly accelerated. The use of cellulose as a combustible fuel is not widespread, because the form of resulting energy, that is, heat, cannot be easily converted for use in internal combustion engines.

If cellulose could be hydrolyzed to glucose in a cost-effective manner, the resulting glucose could be converted to alcohol using ordinary yeast fermentation. The alcohol could then be added to or used as a substitute for gasoline, as is done in Brazil. The glucose could also be used as a carbon source to produce protein. Cellulose can be completely hydrolyzed by strong acids and heat, but this is not cost effective. It can also be hydrolyzed with cellulase, which may be cost effective, depending on the price of the enzyme. Various methods of increasing the production of cellulase by microorganisms have been tried. One method that has been used successfully is to mutate the microorganisms so that they hyperproduce the enzyme. A number of fungal species are known to produce cellulase; among these are the *Ascomycetes*, such as *Neurospora* and *Trichoderma*. One fungus that was mutated into a hyperproducing form was *T. reesei* (Gallo, 1984). The synthesis of cellulase by wild-type *T. reesei* involves stringent metabolic controls of induction and repression. If the ratio of these two processes could be altered, more cellulase could be produced.

The presence of a repressor prevents the expression of the gene coding for that enzyme and in some cases an inducer is also necessary for gene expression. For wild-type *T. reesei* cellulose is an inducer and glucose and glycerol are repressors. The necessary conditions for cellulase production are the presence of cellulose or other inducers, such as lactose, and the almost complete absence of glucose. However, in a fermentation, as cellulase is produced, glucose is also produced, which results in the repression of cellulase production. Consequently, wild-type *T. reesei* never produced much cellulase.

The mutagenesis of *T. reesei* was brought on by ultraviolet light and the mutated spores were transferred to Kabacidin agar plates for incubation and growth. The colonies obtained were isolated and tested for cellulase production in liquid culture. Typical results obtained from one of the mutated strains, designated MCG 80, showed that about 200 filter paper units could be produced per hour. This mutant represents a significant improvement in cellulase production compared to wild-type *T. reesei*. The high economic incentive for success in this area will continue to generate interest and further improvements. We feel that cellulase is likely to become a significant commercial reality in the near future.

REFERENCES

Antrim, R. and Auterinen, A. L. (1985). A new regenerable immobilized glucose isomerase. Presented at the Association of Cereal Research Starch Conference, Detmold, Germany, April 25, 1985.

Bjorck, L., Claesson, O., and Schulthess, W. (1979). The lactoperoxidase–thiocyanate–hydrogen peroxide system as temporary preservative for raw milk in developing countries. *Milchwissenschaft 4*:726–729.

Boehringer Mannheim (1977). Enzyme Immunoassay for the In Vitro Determination of Potato Virus, Boehringer Mannheim, Mannheim 31, West Germany.

Carbonell, R. J. (1982). In-house commercialization by a major corporation: laboratory and marketplace. Presented at The Energy Bureau's Genetic Engineering in Food and Agriculture Conference, Arlington, Va.

Carminati, D., Mucchetti, G., Neviani, E., and Emaldi, G. C. (1984). La germinazione di *Clostridium tyrobutyricum* in presenza di lisozima. *Latte 9*:897–904.

Cornelius, D. A. (1982). Process for decreasing the thermal stability of microbial rennet. U.S. Patent No. 4,348,482.

Finnsugar (1984). *Spezyme BBA 1500*, Bulletin BBA 102, April 1984; *Spezyme BBA 1500—Production of High Maltose Syrups*, Bulletin 203, April 1984; *Spezyme BBA 1500—Production of Very High Maltose Syrups*, Bulletin 204, April 1984, Finnsugar, Helsinki.

Finnsugar (1985). *Food, Feed, Pharmaceuticals Research and Special Know-how*, Finnsugar Group, Espoo, Finland.

Food Chemicals Codex, Third Edition (1981). National Academy Press, Washington, D.C.

Fuji Oil Petition (1984). *Fed. Reg.* 50477.

Gallo, B. E. (1984). Hyperproducing cellulase microorganism. U.S. Patent No. 4,472,504.

Ghielmetti, G. and Trinchera, C. (1968). Process for the production of lysozyme. British Patent No. 1,110,446.

Godfrey, T. and Reichelt, J. (1983). *Industrial Enzymology*, Nature Press, New York.

Gudmundsson, B. (1984). EWOS publication *The Lactoperoxidase System; a Defense System of Nature With Importance for Animal Health*, EWOS, Sodertalja, Sweden.

Higashi, T., Kobayashi, Y., and Iwasaki, S. (1983). Microbial rennet having increased milk coagulating activity and method for products thereof. European Patent Application 83103406.1.

Hoogendoorn, H. (1974). The effect of lactoperoxidase-thiocyanate-hydrogen peroxide on the metabolism of cariogenic microorganisms in vitro and in the oral cavity. In *Industrial Enzymology* (T. Godfrey and J. Reichelt, eds.), Nature Press, New York, p. 433.

Isowa, Y. and Ichikawa, T. (1979). Syntheses of N-acyl dipeptide derivatives by metalloproteinases. *Bull. Chem. Soc. Jpn.* *52*:796–800.

Isowa, Y., Ohmori, M., Ichikawa, T., Kurita, H., Masanari, S., and Mori, K. (1977). The synthesis of peptides by means of proteolytic enzymes. *Bull. Chem. Soc. Jpn.* *50*:2762–2765.

Isowa, Y., Ichikawa, T., and Ohmori, M. (1978). Peptide synthesis with proteinases. Fragment condensation of ZLeuGlnGlyOH or ZGlnGlyOH with $HLeuValNH_2$ using metalloproteinases. *Bull. Chem. Soc. Jpn.* *51*:271–278.

Isowa, Y., Ohmori, M., Mori, K., Ichikawa, T., Nonaka, Y., Kihara, K., Oyama, K., Satoh, H., and Nishimura, S. (1979). Addition compound of dipeptide derivative and amino acid derivative. U.S. Patent No. 4,165,311.

Kyowa Hakko Kogyo Co., Ltd. (no date). *Activated Gluten*, Kyowa Hakko Kogyo, Tokyo.

Lehninger, A. L. (1970). *Biochemistry*, Worth, New York.

Matsuo, T., Sawamura, N., Hashimoto, Y., and Hashida, W. (1984). Method for enzymatic transesterification of lipid and enzyme used therein. U.S. Patent No. 4,472,503.

Meito Sangyo Co. (no date). *Lipase OF for Enzymatic Fat Splitting* and *Fat Splitting by Lipase MY*, Meito Sangyo, Tokyo.

Miles Laboratories (no date). *Naturage*, technical information bulletin.

Moskowitz, G. J., Stout, J. T., and Howard, R. (1984). The production of bovine chymosin by genetic engineering and fermentation. Paper presented at the R&D Associates for Military Food and Packaging Systems.

Ohta, S., Torigoe, T., and Inoue, S. (1983). Application of enzymatic modification of phospholipids on breadmaking. Paper presented at the 68th Annual Meeting of the American Association of Cereal Chemists, Kansas City, MO., October 30–November 3, 1983.

Oleofina (no date). *Enzymatic Diet Improver for Calves, Lactoperoxidase,* and *Lactoferrin,* Oleofina, Brussels.

Oyama, K. and Kihara, K. (1984). A new horizon for enzyme technology. *Chemtech 14*:100–105.

Perry, J. L. and Wetzel, R. (1984). Disulfide bond engineered into T4 lysozyme: Stabilization of the protein toward thermal inactivation. *Science 226*:555–557.

Reed, G. (1975). *Enzymes in Food Processing,* Academic, New York.

Reiter, B. (1979). The lactoperoxidase–thiocyanate–hydrogen peroxide antibacterium system. *Ciba Found. Symp. 1979*:285–294.

Schwimmer, S. (1981). *Source Book of Food Enzymology,* AVI, Westport, Conn.

Shugar, D. (1952). The measurement of lysozyme activity and the ultraviolet inactivation of lysozyme. *Biochim. Biophys. Acta 8*:302–309.

Takahasi, K., Nishimura, H., Yoshimoto, T., Okada, M., Ajima, A., Matsushima, A., Tamaura, Y., Saito, Y., and Inada, Y. (1984a). Polyethylene glycol-modified enzymes trap water on their surface and exert enzymic activity in organic solvents. *Biotechnol. Lett. 6*:765–770.

Takahashi, K., Yoshimoto, T., Ajima, A., Tamaura, Y., and Inada, Y. (1984b). Modified lipoprotein lipase catalyzes ester synthesis in benzene. *Enzymes 32*:235–240.

Weaver, G. L. and Kroger, M. (1977). Deaminated chitin affinity chromatography: a method for the isolation, purification, and concentration of lysozyme. *Journal of Food Science 42*:1084–1087.

Zaks, A. and Klibanov, A. M. (1984). Enzymatic catalysis in organic media at 100°C. *Science 224*:1249–1251.

FOUR

Food Ingredients and Processing Aids from Biotechnological Processes

17

Corn Sweeteners

LOWELL E. COKER / The Hubinger Company, Subsidiary of H. J. Heinz Company, Keokuk, Iowa

K. VENKATASUBRAMANIAN / H. J. Heinz Company, Pittsburgh, Pennsylvania, and Rutgers University, New Brunswick, New Jersey

INTRODUCTION

The conversion of starch to sugars has undergone a very impressive increase in importance in this century. Current production of all starch-based products by the U.S. corn wet milling industry approaches nearly 20 billion lb. The sweetener consumption pattern in the United States is being reshaped by new and sweeter corn syrups, particularly high-fructose corn syrup. In 1984 sales of high-fructose corn syrup exceeded 10 billion lb, or about 34% of the U.S. sweetener market.

This chapter reviews the major technological developments of the corn sweetener industry from conventional acid-converted corn syrup to the modern, totally enzymatic manufacturing processes for high-fructose corn syrup. Products of virtually any combination of viscosity and sweetness, as well as other functional properties, can be made from corn starch. Economic and marketing aspects of corn sweeteners are also briefly discussed. A more detailed account of many of these aspects, including a historical perspective, can be found in Coker and Venkatasubramanian (1985).

DEVELOPMENT OF CORN SWEETENERS

The development of corn sweeteners can be traced back to the early nineteenth century, when the Russian chemist Kirchoff (1811) discovered that starch yielded a sweet substance when heated with acid. In 1815 de Saussure identified acid hydrolysis as the underlying reaction of Kirchoff's observation. He found that the end-product of the hydrolytic reaction was dextrose.

Early experiments established the basis for the commercial production of syrups and crude sugars from starch. As the demand for starch-derived syrups increased, corn emerged as the preferred source of starch—especially in the United States—because it was low in cost, plentiful, and easily stored. The result was the beginning of the present-day corn wet milling industry. This development paved the way for the corn-growing temperate agricultural zones of the world for the production of raw materials for sweeteners, with a profound and continued impact on national and international economics and politics.

In 1935 only one type of corn syrup was available. This product was the 42 DE (dextrose equivalent) acid-converted corn syrup. Although this product was useful in many applications, it lacked the sweetness of sucrose and could not compete as a sweetener. When corn syrup was acid-converted to higher degrees of hydrolysis, the resulting products were often highly discolored and contained bitter by-products from the acid-mediated reaction.

The first major technological breakthrough since Kirchoff was made in 1940, when Langlois and Dale patented the use of commercially available enzymes and hydrolyze starch. Although the new enzyme syrups found many commercial applications, their new technology was not used to produce large quantities of corn syrup until the 1950s.

The discovery, isolation, and application of various carbohydrase enzymes resulted in the development of many new corn syrups. These enzymes could be used singly, in sequence, or in combination on starch to produce a variety of saccharide components and a broad range of syrup compositions. This, in turn, resulted in a wide variety of different syrup properties.

In the early 1960s the first commercially significant quantities of crystalline dextrose were being marketed. It was produced from corn starch by an all-enzyme process using bacterial α-amylase for starch liquefaction and dextrinization and fungal glucoamylase for saccharification of the hydrolysate to produce approximately 95% dextrose levels. The significant features of this new technology were patented (Wallerstein, 1950; Rentshler et al., 1962).

The commercial development of glucose isomerase, which converts glucose to its sweeter isomer fructose, was a major milestone in the corn sweetener industry. A historical perspective of this exciting development is presented by Casey (1977).

The enzymatic transformation of glucose to fructose was first introduced to corn sweetener production in 1967. The first high-fructose corn syrup, commonly referred to as HFCS, contained 15% fructose. The manufacturing process, known as isomerization, originally involved the direct addition of an isomerase enzyme to a dextrose substrate in a batch reactor. Further process improvements resulted in HFCS products containing 42 and 55% fructose.

In 1972 batch production was replaced by a continuous process utilizing isomerase enzyme immobilized in an insoluble carrier. This continuous process for the production of high-fructose corn syrup involved the world's first large-scale use of an immobilized enzyme system. The continuous process resulted in a significant reduction in production costs. The design and operation of continuous immobilized isomerase reaction for HFCS have been discussed extensively (Oestergaard and Knudson, 1976; Hupkes and Van Telburg, 1976; Venkatasubramanian, 1978; Venkatasubramanian and Harrow, 1979).

FUNCTIONAL PROPERTIES OF CORN SYRUP

The term *corn sweetener* has been the generic term for a wide variety of nutritive carbohydrates prepared by the hydrolysis of corn starch. These products are differentiated principally by the degree of hydrolysis. The functional properties of a corn sweetener are a consequence of the particular type and mixture of hydrolysis products.

The hydrolysis products of starch can be classified conveniently on the basis of the "reducing sugars" they contain. Since starch is a homopolymer of anhydroglucose, its depolymerization through hydrolysis results in a mixture of glucose oligomers, ranging typically from the monomer glucose to glucose multiples containing many units of glucose linked together. The reducing sugars contained in these mixtures can be assayed and expressed as they relate to the reducing power of dextrose, in terms of a dextrose equivalent (DE). The greater the degree of hydrolysis, the higher the DE value.

Corn sweeteners are conveniently classified according to their DE values (Table 1). High-fructose corn syrups (HFCSs) do not fall under this classification, since they contain substantial amounts of fructose. Indeed, different HFCS syrups are differentiated on the basis of their fructose content.

Table 1. Types of Corn Sweeteners

Product	DE value
Maltodextrins	<20
Corn syrups	
Type I	20–37
Type II	38–57
Type III	58–73
Type IV	>73
Dextrose	>99.5

Table 2. Compositional Data

Sample	Dextrose equivalent	Percentage of saccharides on a carbohydrate basis						
		DP_1	DP_2	DP_3	DP_4	DP_5	DP_6	DP_7
Maltodextrin	12	1	3	4	3	3	6	80
Corn syrup AC[a]	27	9	9	8	7	7	6	54
Corn syrup AC	36	14	12	10	9	8	7	40
Corn syrup AC	42	20	12	12	9	8	7	30
Corn syrup AC	55	31	18	12	10	7	5	17
Corn syrup HM, DC[b]	43	8	40	15	7	2	2	26
Corn syrup HM, DC	49	9	52	15	1	2	2	19
Corn syrup DC	65	39	31	7	5	4	3	11
Corn syrup DC	70	47	27	5	5	4	3	9
Corn syrup DC	95	92	4	1	1	Sum of DP_{5-7+}		2
High-fructose corn syrup	—	94[c]	4	Sum of DP_{3-7+}				2

[a]AC = acid-converted syrup; DP = degree of polymerization.
[b]HM = high maltose; DC = acid plus enzyme-converted syrup.
[c]Dextrose plus fructose.
Source: Nutritive Sweeteners from Corn, *Corn Refiner's Association Handbook*, Second Edition, Corn Refiner's Association, Washington, D.C., 1979.

Table 3. Physical Properties of Corn Sweeteners

Properties	Significance
Solubility	Control of fermentation rates in baking
Hygroscopicity	Moisture conditioning; food, plasticizing, crystallization inhibition
Textural properties	Body; chewiness
Osmotic pressure	Inhibition of microbial spoilage
Freezing point depression	Ice cream and frozen deserts
Viscosity	Handling characteristics

The carbohydrate compositions of different hydrolysis products determine their functional properties. Typical compositions of different products are shown in Table 2. Maltodextrins and type I corn syrups contain little glucose, while type II and type IV corn syrups are characterized by a high content of mono- and disaccharides. The important physical and chemical properties of different starch-derived products and their significance in various applications are outlined in Tables 3 and 4. A more detailed analysis of the composition—properties—applications matrix can be found in Horn (1981).

Maltodextrin and various corn syrups are versatile ingredients which find numerous applications in the food processing and related industries. In fact, there is hardly any sector of the food industry in which some starch-derived product is not used. These applications are based on a wide variety of functional properties. An

Table 4. Chemical Properties of Corn Sweeteners

Property	Significance
Sweetness	Determine application; cost
Fermentability	Baking and brewing industries
Browning reactions	Nonenzymatic browning
Reducing properties	Decreases oxidative degradation in foods; color

extensive range of applications can be found in many manufacturers' catalogs and a convenient handbook by the Corn Refiners Association (1979).

HIGH-FRUCTOSE CORN SYRUP PRODUCTS

Three high-fructose corn syrup products are commercially available; they contain 42, 55, and 90% fructose. The typical carbohydrate composition of these products is shown in Table 5.

In most applications HFCS syrups replace sucrose as the sweetener. High-fructose corn syrups containing 42% fructose are used in most food products that make use of a liquid sweetener. The development of "second-generation" syrups with higher fructose levels greatly extended the use of HFCs in many applications. This is particularly true with respect to the use of HFCs with 55% fructose as a replacement for sucrose in soft drinks.

Fructose corn syrup containing 90% fructose has found limited applications in many new and specialty food products, especially as a sweetener for reduced-calorie foods such as jams and jellies.

Today there are several companies in the United States and abroad manufacturing high-fructose corn syrup. The U.S. companies, together with their location, plant size, and HFCS production capacities, are listed in Table 6.

Table 5. Carbohydrate Composition of High-Fructose Corn Syrups

	Typical analysis[a]		
Carbohydrate	42 HFCS	55 EFCS[b]	90 VEFCS[c]
Fructose	42	55	90
Dextrose	52	42	7
Monosaccharides	94	97	97
Higher saccharides	6	3	3

[a] Percent dry basis.
[b] Enriched fructose corn syrup.
[c] Very enriched fructose corn syrup.

Table 6. U.S. HFCS Producers

Producer	Plant location	Plant size (bu/day)	HFCS capacity[a] (lb C.B./year)
Archer Daniels Midland	Cedar Rapids, Iowa	220,000	1,264,000
	Decatur, Ill.	200,000	1,714,000
American Maize Products	Decatur, Ala.	35,000	500,000
Amstar	Dimmitt, Tex.	30,000	336,000
Cargill	Dayton, Ohio	150,000	696,000
	Memphis, Tenn.	90,000	696,000
Corn Products Company	Argo, Ill.	145,000	551,000
	Stockton, Calif.	32,000	352,000
	Winston-Salem, N.C.	32,000	351,000
Clinton Corn Processing	Clinton, Iowa	110,000	948,000
	Montezuma, N.Y.	35,000	423,000
Hubinger	Keokuk, Iowa	83,000	623,000
A. E. Staley	Decatur, Ill.	150,000	600,000
	Morrisville, Pa.	85,000	700,000
	Lafayette, Ind.	155,000	1,300,000
	Loudon, Tenn.	70,000	600,000
		Total =	11,553,000

[a] 42 HFCS and 55 EFCS (55% enriched fructose corn syrup).
C. B. = commercial basis.

MODERN PROCESS TECHNOLOGY

A simplified flow diagram for the manufacture of 42% high-fructose corn syrup from starch is shown in Figure 1. This diagram also outlines the production of 55 and 90% fructose syrups from 42% HFCS. The manufacturing process may be divided into about 18 separate steps in 5 principal areas of operation. These areas include dextrose production, primary refining and chemical treatment to produce dextrose feedstock, isomerization of dextrose feedstock to produce 42% fructose, secondary refining of 42% fructose, and fractionation of 42% fructose for the production of 55% fructose.

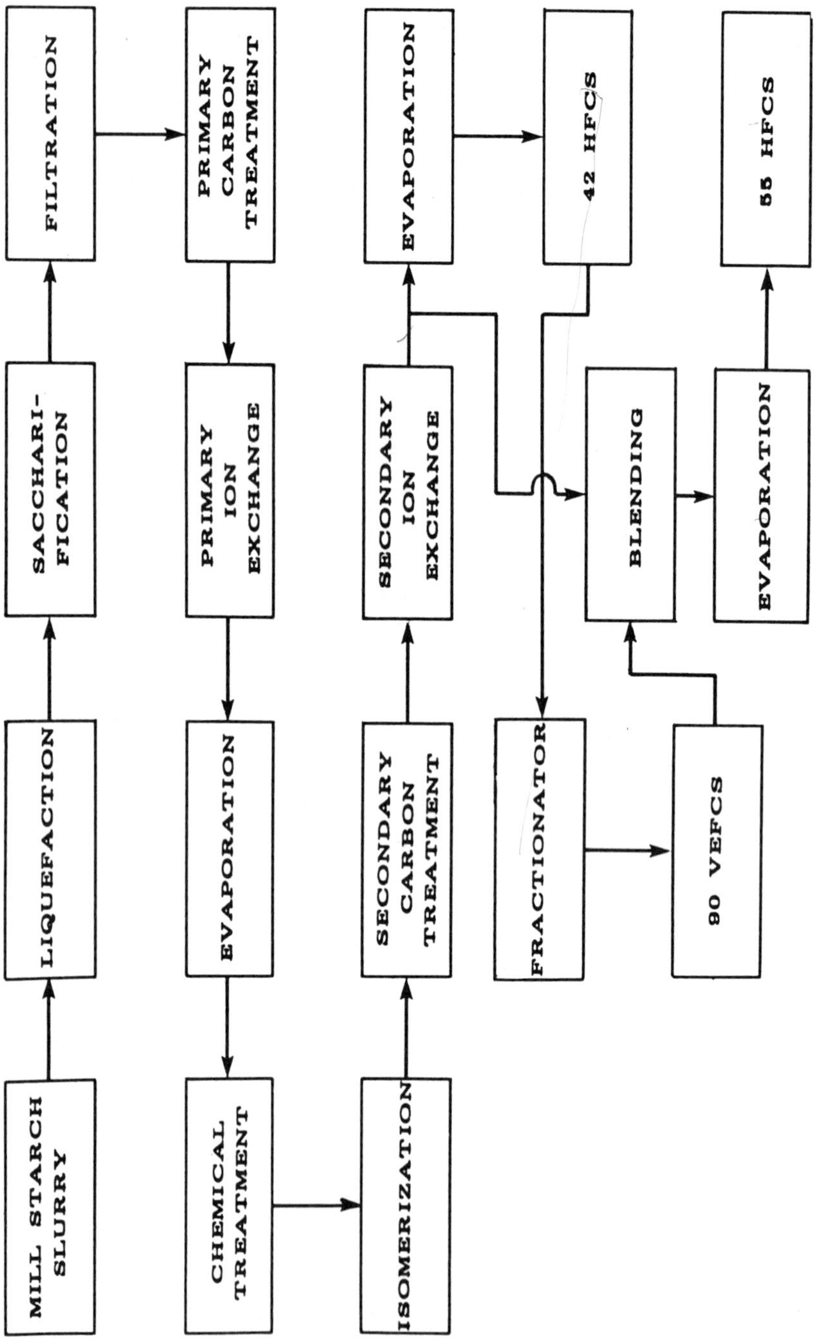

Fig. 1. Flow chart for the manufacture of 42% HFCS from starch, as well as the production of 55 and 90% fructose syrups from 42% HFCS.

The heart of the entire process is the enzymatic isomerization step utilizing immobilized glucose isomerase.

The economic and technical success of the isomerization reaction depends upon the production and delivery of high-quality dextrose feedstock to the isomerization reactors.

MANUFACTURE OF DEXTROSE FROM STARCH

The manufacture of dextrose feedstock from starch is a multistage process involving thermostable α-amylase and glucoamylase in successive enzymatic steps. These enzymes catalyze the ultimate conversion of the starch polymer to dextrose monomer.

In the first step starch slurry is gelatinized by cooking at high temperature. The gelatinized starch is then liquefied and dextrinized by thermostable α-amylase in a continuous two-stage reaction. The product of this reaction is a soluble dextrin hydrolysate with a DE of 10–15, suitable for the subsequent saccharification step. Typical conditions for the liquefaction–dextrinization reaction are summarized in Table 7.

During the liquefaction–dextrinization reaction certain key process variables (starch quality and concentration, α-amylase

Table 7. Liquefaction–Dextrinization Reaction Conditions

Starch slurry	30–35% wt/wt d.b.
Total protein	⩽ 0.3%
Soluble protein	⩽ 0.03%
pH	6.0–6.5
Thermostable α-amylase	0.05–0.10% d.b. starch
First-stage liquefaction	
Temperature	104–107°C
Hold	5–8 min
DE	0.5–1.5
Second-stage liquefaction	
Temperature	94–97°C
Hold	90–120 min
DE	10–15

dosage, temperature, pH, starch flow rate, and contact time) must be maintained within relatively narrow limits to ensure that the starch is properly cooked and dextrinized. If any one of these variables deviates significantly from process specifications, the finished liquor may contain undercooked and unconverted starch. This, in turn, leads to poor conversion and filtration problems or the production of undesirable saccharides such as maltulose, which can result in flavor problems in the finished high-fructose corn syrup.

The total soluble protein levels in the starch slurry should be maintained below about 0.3% total protein and 0.03% soluble protein. This is essential to minimize color formation as a result of the Maillard reaction between amino acids and sugars under conditions of high temperature and pH. If the starch slurry is high in protein, the syrup produced has a greater potential to develop color bodies exceeding the capacity of the carbon and ion exchange refining systems.

Following liquefaction–dextrinization, the pH and temperature of the 10–15 DE hydrolysate is adjusted for the saccharification step. During saccharification the hydrolysate is further hydrolyzed to dextrose by the action of glucoamylase enzyme. Although saccharification can be carried out as a batch reaction, a continuous saccharification is practiced in most modern plants. In the continuous saccharification reaction glucoamylase is added to 10–15 DE hydrolysate following pH and temperature adjustment. The saccharifying liquor is then pumped through a number of large stirred tank reactors in series. Typical saccharification reaction conditions are summarized in Table 8.

The total time for saccharification is dictated by the amount of glucoamylase. Normally a reaction time of 48–72 hr is used to obtain a hydrolysate containing 94–96% dextrose.

During saccharification, the important variables to be controlled are the initial DE, pH, temperature, dry substance, glucoamylase dose, the time course of conversion, and the presence of unconverted starch in the liquor during this reaction. These variables

Table 8. Saccharification Reaction Conditions

Dry substance	30–35%
pH	4.0–4.4
Temperature	60–62°C
Glucoamylase	1 liter/ton d.s. starch[a]
Reaction time	65–75 hr

[a] d.s. = dry substance.

Table 9. Dextrose Saccharification Product: Typical Analysis

Component	Percent, dry basis
Dextrose	94–96
Maltose	2–3
Maltotriose	0.3–0.5
Higher saccharides	1–2
Dry substance	35–37

must again be controlled within relatively narrow limits to ensure that a minimum 94% dextrose level is reached at the end of the reaction. This minimum level is necessary to meet the specifications for the carbohydrate composition of 42% HFCS in which the higher-saccharides level cannot exceed 6%. The carbohydrate composition of typical high-dextrose saccharification liquor is summarized in Table 9. The high-dextrose hydrolysate is then refined to produce dextrose feedstock for the isomerization reaction.

PREPARATION OF DEXTROSE FEEDSTOCK FOR ISOMERIZATION

Preparation of very high-quality dextrose feedstock for isomerization is first necessary because of the very low color and ash specifications for the finished high-fructose corn syrup. A high-purity feedstock is also required for efficient utilization of the immobilized isomerase enzyme column.

Immobilized isomerase enzyme columns are used continuously over a period of several months. During this period very large volumes of dextrose feedstock pass through the columns. Extremely low levels of impurities such as ash, metal ions, or protein in the feedstock can accumulate and lead to decreased productivity of the enzyme. For these reasons dextrose feedstock is refined to a color of 0.1 (CRA × 100) and a conductivity of 5–10 μmho.

In the refining process the high-dextrose conversion liquor is filtered on rotary precoat filters to remove "mud" or coagulated protein and oil. This filtered liquor is then passed through a series of check filters and polish filters to remove traces of particulate matter.

Color in the hydrolysate is first removed in a series of granulated carbon columns. These columns are renewed by the removal of spent carbon and the addition of regenerated carbon on a regular basis.

Carbon-treated liquor is filtered again and passed through an ion exchange system, where it is deionized by ion exchange resin. This resin is usually arranged in a dual-pass cation–anion/cation–anion system. Ion exchange is designed to remove all heavy metals and ash that might be detrimental to the immobilized isomerase enzyme. Ion exchange resin also removes significant amounts of color bodies that are not removed by the carbon columns.

The carbon-treated and deionized high-dextrose liquor is evaporated to the proper solids level for isomerization. In addition, the feedstock is chemically treated by the addition of magnesium ions, which not only activate the immobilized isomerase but also competitively inhibit the action of any residual calcium ions, which are potent inhibitors of isomerase.

ISOMERIZATION PROCESS

The isomerization reaction is carried out under the conditions summarized in Table 10. The conversion of glucose to fructose is a reversible reaction with an equilibrium constant of about 1.0 at 60°C. Thus one would expect to obtain a fructose level of about 47–48% at equilibrium, starting from a feedstock containing 94–96% dextrose. However, the reaction rate near the equilibrium value is so slow that it is prudent to terminate the reaction at a conversion level of 42% fructose to achieve practical reactor residence times.

Table 10. Isomerization Feedstock and Reaction Conditions

Dry substance	40–45%
Dextrose	94–96%
Higher saccharides	4–6%
pH	7.5–8.2 at 25°C
pH drop	0.2–0.4
Temperature	55–65°C
Activator	0.004 M Mg^{2+}
Residence time	0.5–4 hr

In a given isocolumn (immobilized isomerase column) the rate of conversion of dextrose to fructose is proportional to the enzyme activity of the immobilized isomerase. This activity decays in a nearly exponential manner as a function of time. When the column is new and the activity is high, the flow of feedstock through the column is relatively high, since a shorter residence time is required to achieve the 42% fructose level. The flow through the column must be reduced proportionately to provide a longer residence time, compensating for the lowered activity in order to achieve a constant conversion level as the usage life of the column increases.

Since the activity of the immobilized enzyme decreases continuously, it is necessary to have a number of isocolumns to minimize production fluctuations with respect to capacity and conversion level. Both series and parallel operation of the isocolumn is possible. In practice, the parallel operation of at least six isocolumns offers the greatest operational flexibility. In this arrangement each isocolumn can be operated essentially independently of the others. Each isocolumn can very readily be brought into and taken out of service.

It is necessary to operate the isocolumn battery to obtain a finished product of uniform quality and a constant average fructose content of 42%. The variation in total flow of the isocolumns must be maintained within relatively narrow limits because of the requirements of evaporation and other finishing operations. In practice, flow cannot be precisely controlled at all times to obtain 42% fructose, but this can easily be achieved on an average basis.

A number of important process control strategies can be used to achieve an approximately steady-state operation. These include modest variations in operating temperature, conversion level, and feedstock pH control. Final uniformity of product quality and fructose level is usually accomplished by automatic back-blending operations controlled by an in-line polarimeter, which measures the relative levels of glucose and fructose.

The effect of temperature on overall productivity can be dramatic. An operating temperature of 60°C is considered as an optimum. Higher temperatures result in faster flow rates but also give rise to accelerated enzyme decay rates. Feed temperatures as low as 55°C can be used to extend enzyme life at the expense of slower flow rates. Some risk of microbial contamination exists at the lower operation temperature.

One of the most critical operating variables is the internal isocolumn pH. The operating pH is usually a compromise between the pH of maximum activity, typically around pH 8, and the pH of maximum stability, typically pH 7.0–7.5. This complicated by the fact that the dextrose feedstock is not pH stable at temperatures around 60°C. Some decomposition to produce acidic by-products results in a pH drop across the isocolumn during operation.

Table 11. Principal Producers of Immobilized Isomerase

Company	Trade name of product
Gist-Brocades	Maxazyme GI Immob.
Miles Laboratories, Inc.	Takasweet
Novo Industries	Sweetzyme Q
UOP Process Division	Ketomax GI-100

Since it is difficult to control pH directly in the column, the pH of the feedstock is adjusted externally to maintain a constant pH in the column effluent.

The operational stability of the immobilized isomerase system can be characterized by its half-life, or the time span during which the enzyme activity is reduced by one-half. Typically, a single isocolumn is operated for a period of at least two half-lives, after which the enzyme is discarded and replaced with a fresh batch. The operating life of a column is determined by such considerations as the number of isocolumns in the battery, the average decay rate of the individual columns, the maximum allowable variance in individual isocolumn flow, minimum total flow, and total required production capacity. Enzyme half-lives of 70–120 days are common, resulting in a column replacement frequency of 1.5–2 times per year.

Isomerization enzyme accounts for a significant fraction of the total operating cost. The enzyme can be purchased commercially or manufactured by the user. In the former case most enzyme is supplied on a performance guarantee with a minimum stated activity. The quality of immobilized isomerase has improved, with a longer half-life and higher initial activity with a net higher productivity. In general, isomerization costs have decreased significantly from the original cost of 50–70¢ per centiweight HFCS dry basis.

The principal producers of immobilized glucose isomerase are listed in Table 11. Most of these preparations consist of fixed whole cells containing glucose isomerase activity. The products of NOVO and UOP are manufactured from isolated and purified glucose isomerase.

Following isomerization, the manufacturing process involves the secondary refining or polishing of the 42% HFCS product. Some additional color is picked up during the chemical treatment and isomerization when the feedstock is held at a higher pH and temperature for a period of time. The product also contains some additional ash from the chemicals added for isomerization. This color and ash are removed by the secondary carbon and ion exchange systems. The refined 42% HFCS is then evaporated to 71% solids for shipment.

MANUFACTURE OF ENRICHED FRUCTOSE PRODUCTS

The HFCS product from the isomerization reaction typically contains 42% fructose, 52% unconverted dextrose, and about 6% oligosaccharides. For reasons previously discussed, this product represents the practical maximum level of fructose attainable. In order to obtain products with higher levels of fructose, it is necessary to selectively concentrate the fructose. Many common separation techniques are not applicable for this purpose, since they do not readily discriminate between the two isomers of essentially the same molecular size. However, fructose preferentially forms a complex with different cations, such as calcium. This difference has been exploited to develop commercial separation processes.

There are basically two different commercial processes currently available for the large-scale purification of fructose. In both instances resins in the preferred cationic form are used in packed bed systems. One process employs an inorganic resin leading to a selective molecular absorption of fructose (Jensen, 1978).

Chromatographic fractionation using organic resins is the basis for the second commercial separation process (Venkatasubramanian, 1982). When an aqueous solution of dextrose and fructose such as 42% HFCS is fed to a fractionating column, fructose is selectively held by the resin to a greater degree than dextrose. Deionized and deoxygenated water is used as the eluant. Typically, the separation is achieved in a column packed with a bed of low-crosslinked fine-mesh polystyrene sulfonate cation exchange resin using calcium as the preferred salt form. The enriched product containing approximately 90% fructose is referred to as very enriched fructose corn syrup (VEFCS). This VEFCS fraction can be blended back with the 42% HFCS feed material to obtain products having a fructose content between 42 and 90%. The most typical of these products is 55% enriched fructose corn syrup called 55 EFCS. The fractionation and blending process is schematically outlined in Figure 1.

The treatment of other raffinate streams in the fractionation process is an important consideration. In general, the dextrose-rich raffinate stream is recycled to the dextrose feed of the isocolumn system for further conversion to 42 HFCS. The raffinate stream containing dextrose with fructose levels higher than the feed level is generally recycled through the fractionator to maintain a high solids level and reduce water usage. The raffinate stream rich in oligosaccharides is recycled back to the saccharification system.

Since water is used as the elution medium, it has a great impact on the overall evaporation load on the system. Very low solids concentrations contribute to the risk of microbiological problems within the system. Thus the most important design parameter dictating overall process economics is the maximization of solids yield at acceptable purity while minimizing the dilution effect of the eluant rinse. The efficiency of feed and water usage must be maximized for optimal yield. The yield is important to reduce the cost of reisomerization.

Procedures available for achieving these goals include recycling techniques, higher equalization of the resin phase with proper redistribution in a packed column, and the addition of multiple entry/exit points in the column. These approaches to increase the purity and the yield are sometimes referred to as feed enrichment. A small apparent increase in the purity of feed to the column, that is, higher fructose levels, results in a much larger gain in production through increased yield at a given product purity. In practice, this translates into maximization of the ratio of the sugar volume fed per volume of resin per cycle, minimization of the ratio of the water volume required per volume of resin per cycle, and careful fluid distribution to the columns.

MARKETING AND ECONOMIC CONSIDERATIONS

Sucrose has long been the dominant caloric sweetener in the United States; however, since 1972 it has been losing ground to HFCS. The remarkable growth of the HFCS industry in the last 15 years was dramatically triggered by high sugar prices in the early 1970s. In 1971 the wholesale price of sugar (Northeast) was 11.5¢ per pound. By 1976 the price rose to 19.2¢ per pound and in 1980 a record price of 41.0¢ per pound was reached. In comparison, in 1976 high-fructose corn syrup (Illinois) sold for 14.0¢ per pound, or 73% of the cost of sugar. In 1980, during the record rise in sugar prices, HFCS was selling for 23.6¢ per pound, or only 58% of the sugar cost. In 1981 sugar prices dropped about 25%, to 30.6¢ per pound; HFCS prices dropped by only about 9%, to 21.5¢ per pound, or 70% of the sugar cost (Anonymous, 1982).

The price differential between HFCS and sugar offered strong incentive for the substitution of HFCS for sugar in soft drinks, canned fruits, ice cream, and certain bakery products. As a result, sugar usage by industrial users has been declining relative to total sugar usage and particularly relative to total sweeteners because of the inroads of high-fructose corn syrup. This decline in sugar usage is dramatically illustrated by the beverage industry, the largest industrial users of sugar. In 1978 annual sugar usage peaked at 5.12 billion lb. By 1981 this usage had declined by 28.5%, to 3.66 billion lb. The total industrial sugar usage declined about 18% from 13.9 billion pounds in 1978 to 11.4 billion pounds in 1981. In late 1984 all major soft drink companies approved the total substitution of sucrose by HFCS. The trend of HFCS substitution for sugar in canned fruits, ice cream, and certain bakery items is expected to slow down as HFCS saturates these markets by 1985.

Caloric sweetener consumption in the United States reached a peak of 129.3 lb per capita in 1977, after growing at a rate of about 1 lb per person per year since 1960. By 1982 this had declined to about 122.4 lb per person. An annual consumption of about 130 lb per capita has been considered a safe plateau. Future growth in total caloric sweetener consumption is expected to occur only in direct proportion to population growth.

It is expected that sugar will continue to be replaced by HFCS, particularly in the processed foods sector. Consequently, the sale of HFCS is projected to grow, but at a decreasing rate.

ACKNOWLEDGMENT

The authors are grateful to Ms. Mary K. Higgins for her impeccable assistance in the preparation of this chapter.

REFERENCES

Anonymous (1982). The Future of Fructose, *Beverage World*, August, pp. 26–28.

Casey, S. P. (1977). High Fructose Corn Syrup: A Case History of Innovation, *Stärke 29*(6):196–204.

Coker, L. E. and Venkatasubramanian, K. (1985). Starch Conversion Process, In *Comprehensive Biotechnology*, M. Moo-Young, C. L. Cooney, and A. E. Humphrey (Eds.), Pergamon Press, Oxford, England, pp. 777–787.

Corn Refiners Association (1979). *Nutritive Sweeteners from Corn*, Second Edition, Corn Refiners Association, Inc., Washington, D.C.

Dale, J. K. and Langlois, D. P. (1940). U.S. Patent 2,201,609. Syrup and Method of Making the Same, May 21, 1940, assigned to A. E. Staley Mfg. Co.

de Saussure, T. (1967). in J. N. Bemiller, Acid Hydrolysis and Other Lytic Reactions of Starch, in *Starch Chemistry and Technology*, Vol. I., R. L. Whistler and E. F. Paschall (Eds.), Academic Press, New York.

Horn, H. E. (1981). Corn Sweeteners: Functional Properties, *Cereal Foods World 26*(5):219–223.

Hupkes, J. V. and van Tillburg, R. (1976). Production and Properties of an Immobilized Glucose Isomerase, *Stärke 28*(10): 356–360.

Jensen, R. J. (1978). The Sarex Process for the Fractionation of High Fructose Corn Syrup, Abstracts of the Institute Chemical Engineers, 85th National Meeting, Philadelphia, Pa., 1978.

Kirchoff, G. S. C. (1967). In J. N. Bemiller, Acid Hydrolysis and Other Lytic Reactions of Starch, in *Starch Chemistry and Technology*, Vol. I, R. L. Whistler and E. F. Paschall (Eds.). Academic Press, New York.

Oestergaard, J. and Knudson, S. L. (1976). Use of Sweetzyme in Industrial Continuous Isomerization. Various Process Alternatives and Corresponding Product Types, *Stärke 28*(100):350–356.

Rentschler, D. F., Langlois, D. P., Larson, R. F., Alverson, L. H., and Liggett, R. W. (1962). U.S. Patent 3,039,935. Production of Crystalline Glucose, June 19, 1962, assigned to A. E. Staley Mfg. Co.

Venkatasubramanian, K. (1978). High Fructose Corn Syrup: Plant Design and Process Economics. In *Enzymes: The Interface Between Technology and Economics*, J. P. Dansky and B. Wolnak (Eds.), Marcel Dekker, New York, pp. 35–48.

Venkatasubramanian, K. (1982). Integration of Large Scale Production and Purification of Biomolecules, *Enzyme Engineering 6*:37–43.

Venkatasubramanian, K. and Harrow, L. S. (1979). Design and Operation of a Commercial Immobilized Enzyme Reactor System, *Ann. N. Y. Acad. Sci. 326*:141–155.

Wallenstein, L. (1950). U.S. Patent 2,531,999. Manufacture of Crystalline Dextrose, Nov. 28, 1950, assigned to Wallenstein Co.

18

Plant Tissue Culture for Lipid Production

MING C. WEN and JOHN E. KINSELLA / Cornell University, Ithaca, New York

INTRODUCTION

Plant tissue culture offers great potential in the agricultural and life sciences. Following routine subculturing, the tissues can be maintained over a period of years. Growing these tissues in a liquid medium is analogous to growing industrial microorganisms using submerged fermentation techniques and in certain respects offers advantages over conventional field cropping (Zenk, 1978; Crocomo, 1981). Tissue culture can provide a steady, year-round supply of products without climatic or geographical limitations, production can be free of contamination by pests or microorganisms, and the genetics and metabolism of cultured tissues can be modified or regulated to obtain maximum yield.

Cultured tissues may produce useful products, that is, pigments, enzymes, and alkaloids used for the food or pharmaceutical industry (Nickell, 1980). The possibility that plant tissues may be exploited to produce special edible fat products has received limited attention. Jones (1974) was the first to mention that plant tissue culture might be a possible way for improving vegetable oil production. Radwan and Mangold (1976, 1980) discussed the possibility of the industrial production of lipids using plant tissue culture. This chapter will focus on the synthesis of lipids by plant tissue culture, with an emphasis on cocoa bean tissue cultures.

PLANT TISSUE CULTURE

History

White (1934) was the first to successfully grow excised tomato root tips in culture media. The first true plant tissue cultures were achieved almost simultaneously by Gautheret (1939), Nobecourt (1939), and White (1939). They cultured the cambial tissues of tobacco and carrot in an agar medium and observed the formation of undifferentiated callus which grew freely after repeated subculturing. By dispersing fragments of callus of *Tagetes erecta* and *Nicotiana tabacum* in liquid media agitated on a reciprocal shaker, Muir (1953) and Muir et al. (1954) started suspension cell cultures. The advantages of a suspension culture are that it can be used to develop plating techniques later to obtain single-cell clones (Bergmann, 1960), to study many facets of cell biology (Nickell, 1956), and to develop a chemostat (Street, 1977a) for the mass production of cells or cell products.

Initiation

Plant calli can be initiated from seedlings, young shoots or buds, root tips or developing embryos, fruits, floral parts, tubes, and bulbs (Gamborg and Shyluk, 1981). Generally the more juvenile the explant, the easier it is to produce a viable callus. However, various qualities of the explant, such as ontogenetic age, preculture treatment, and size, influence the successful initiation, proliferation, and differentiation of callus (Seabrook, 1980). Juvenile plant tissue produces calli which are more likely to regenerate tissues or organs than older tissue from the same plant.

Media

Being heterotrophic, plant tissues need complex media. Gautheret (1939) described the medium formula for the initiation of carrot callus culture. This consists of Knop's solution (Gautheret, 1937, 1938) supplemented with Berthelot's salt mixture (Berthelot, 1934), glucose, gelatin, thiamine, cysteine HCl, and indoacetic acid. Later Steward and co-workers found that a combination of 2,4-dichloroacetic acid (2,4-D) and coconut milk enhanced the growth of cultured carrot and potato callus (Caplin and Steward, 1948; Steward and Caplin, 1951; 1952). More complete formulations were developed by Murashige and Skoog (1962) and Gamborg et al. (1968). These formulations consist basically of inorganic salts, carbon source, vitamins, plant growth hormones, amino acids, casein hydrolysate, or natural extracts such as coconut water, and yeast extract, which may be added in the media to enhance the initiation and growth of the culture.

Environmental Factors

Environmental conditions affect the growth, metabolism, and differentiation of tissues in culture. Different types of culture have different optimum growth temperatures in the range of 25–30°C. In *Ipomoea* tissue culture maximum utilization of sucrose and amino nitrogen occurs between 30 and 32°C (Rose and Martin, 1975). During the growth cycle the pH of the medium may change, depending on the release of organic acid and utilization of ammonium and nitrate. The pH of the medium is usually adjusted to 5.5–5.8 before autoclaving. This initial pH influences the uptake of magnesium (Veliky et al., 1977) and the production of tryptophol, an indole metabolite of tryptophan (Veliky, 1977). Plant tissues in culture are aerobic and need shaking to maintain oxygen supply. Shaking enhances oxygen supply and nutrient uptake and prevents the accumulation of volatile toxic factors in the media (Rajasekhar et al., 1971). Light is not essential for heterotrophic plant tissue culture; however, it may be necessary for morphogenesis and the growth of some autotrophic tissue cultures. In general, heterotrophic culture is maintained in darkness.

Differentiation

The primary objective of tissue culture in agriculture is crop improvement. This can be achieved if some cellular genetic techniques are applied to the cultured tissues and then the latter are induced to differentiate and finally generate new plants (Evans et al., 1981). Basically there are two types of plant regeneration, namely, organogenesis and embryogenesis.

Skoog and Miller (1957) were the first to observe that by adjusting the ratio of auxin to cytokinin in the media, one can induce organogenesis in tobacco tissue culture. A high auxin-to-cytokinin ratio induced root formation, while a low auxin-to-cytokinin ratio favored shoot formation. Although the relative concentrations of auxin and cytokinin influence the initiation of organogenesis, other factors are also involved. For example, carbohydrate, illumination, and photoperiod control are required for root formation (Gautheret, 1966), and other hormones, such as gibberelic acid, also induce shoot formation in chrysanthemum callus (Street, 1977b).

Since most seed oils are produced in the mature embryos, somatic embryogenesis may be very important in the production of oilseeds without requiring field cropping. Embryogenesis, that is, somatic embryogenesis, implies the development of asexual embryos ("embryoids") directly from callus or suspension cells. Somatic embryogenesis was observed by Steward et al. (1958) in carrot tissue culture and later by Reinert (1959) in carrot callus culture. Since then it has been reported for tissues from more than 40 species

(Evans et al., 1981). Induction of somatic embryogenesis consists of two steps. Specific concentrations of growth regulators and/or particular cultural conditions (primary medium) are required to initiate the callus and to epigenetically reprogram the cells to the embryogenic stage (Evans et al., 1981). Then different types of culture media (secondary medium) are used to induce embryo development and growth. Usually the primary medium contains higher levels of growth regulators than the secondary medium; for example, for the somatic embryogenesis of carrot the primary medium contains 4.5 μM 2,4-D, which was omitted from the secondary medium (Halperin and Wetherell, 1964).

Cocoa Bean Tissue Culture

Because of the unique physical properties of cocoa butter reflected by the specific structure of the component triacylglycerols, attempts to produce this product by tissue or embryo culture from cocoa bean embryos are the focus of current research. Cocoa bean callus culture was first initiated by Archibald (1954) from cambial tissue. A systematic study of the initiation and growth of cacao callus was done by Hall and Collin (1975). In our laboratory cacao callus was initiated from embryos harvested 120–130 days after pollination, that is, 50–60 days prior to maturity (Tsai and Kinsella, 1981). The calli were maintained actively growing by subculturing every 4 weeks. By dispersing calli in a liquid medium of the same composition, a liquid suspension culture was obtained. The suspension culture exhibited an approximate doubling time of 3 days, with fresh weight increasing 20-fold from 300 mg to 6 g in 2 weeks (Tsai and Kinsella, 1981). The suspension culture has been maintained for many years for the study of lipid biosynthesis in the cultured tissues.

Somatic Embryogenesis of Cacao

Because cocoa butter is actually produced by cacao embryos, attempts have been made to induce embryos in vitro (somatic embryogenesis) and to determine whether they can produce cocoa butter. Embryogenesis of cacao tissues was first reported by Esan (1977), who observed the budding of adventive embryos from parts of immature cacao zygotic embryos cultured in vitro. These adventive embryos seemed to be epidermal in origin. Later Pence et al. (1980, 1981) repeated the same phenomenon using zygotic embryos of cocoa bean cultured in Murashige–Skoog (1962) medium containing 0.1% casein hydrolysate, 10% coconut water, and 1.5 mg/liter naphthalene acetic acid (NAA). Somatic embryos are obtained in many ways (Pence et al., 1979, 1980). In the budding process the somatic embryos develop from specific epidermal cells of cotyledon and hypocotyl origin. In the nonbudding process portions of the cotyledon swell, fold, and form somatic embryos with axes and cotyledons. Esan (1980) reported the initiation of somatic embryos from embryogenic callus. Pence et al. (1980) observed that embryogenesis in vitro occurs more frequently in liquid media than in agar media. Tissue explants initiating embryos can be transferred to basal Murashige–Skoog medium without auxin and coconut water and will continue to initiate somatic embryos during a full year reculturing in this medium.

In our laboratory somatic embryos are initiated from immature zygotic embryos cultured in medium with 8 μM 2,4-D or NAA. In some reports somatic embryos can be grown to sizes equivalent to 100- to 120-day-old zygotic embryos (Pence et al., 1979).

LIPID CONTENT AND COMPOSITION OF CULTURED PLANT TISSUES

Total Lipids

The lipid contents of various plant tissues are summarized in Table 1. It is important to note that seed tissues contain much larger amounts of lipid compared with the callus or suspension culture of the same species. The lipid content of seed tissues is quite variable among species. Generally speaking, the total lipid content of seed tissues falls in the range of 8.5–44.7% on a fresh weight basis, or 9.2–65.0% on a dry weight basis. The lipid content is usually low for immature seeds; for example, the lipid of cocoa beans increased from 10.5–11.5 to 53.0–55.0% during 60 days of maturation (Tsai et al., 1982). The lipid content of somatic cocoa embryos covers the range of that of callus, suspension, and immature seeds (Pence et al., 1981; Wright et al., 1983); thus it is conceivable that these somatic embryos are comparable to the early stages of embryo development. In contrast, lipid contents of callus or suspension cultures are only a fraction of that of seed lipid. The values lie between 5.3 and 7.7% on a dry weight basis (Tsai et al., 1982).

Lipid Classes

The lipid classes of different plant tissues are summarized in Table 2. The major lipids of seeds are neutral lipids, most of which are triacylglycerols, accounting for 80–97% of total lipids. However, the predominant lipids in callus or suspension cultures are polar lipids. They account for more than half of the total lipids. Polar lipids increase during the conversion of heterotrophic (nongreen) to photoautotrophic (green) cultures. However, when photoautotrophic cultures were changed to heterotrophic cultures, the content of polar

Table 1. Total Lipid Contents of Different Plant Tissues

Plant species	Tissue	Lipid (%) Fresh weight	Lipid (%) Dry weight	References
Acer pseudoplatanus	Suspension	—	6.5–7.9	Bligny et al. (1979)
Arachis hypogaea	Seed	47.7	—	Shin et al. (1971)
	Callus	0.20–0.30	—	Shin et al. (1971)
Artemisia absinthium	Seed	34.8	—	Shin et al. (1971)
	Callus	0.20–0.40	—	Shin et al. (1971)
Brassica campestris	Seed	44.7	—	Shin et al. (1971)
	Callus	0.30	—	Shin et al. (1971)
Brassica juncea	Seed	23.2	—	Shin et al. (1971)
	Callus	0.20	—	Shin et al. (1971)
Brassica napus	Seed	39.9	—	Shin et al. (1971)
	Callus	0.30	—	Shin et al. (1971)
	Callus	—	4.2	Radwan et al. (1978)
Cicer arietinum	Suspension	—	3.3	Radwan et al. (1974)
Citrullus vulgaris	Cotyledon	—	25.9	Halder and Gadgil (1983)
	Callus	—	2.3	Halder and Gadgil (1983)
Cucumis melo	Cotyledon	—	21.9	Halder and Gadgil (1983)
	Callus	—	3.7–4.3	Halder and Gadgil (1983), Pandey and Gadgil (1984)
Cucumis melo var. *utilissimus*	Cotyledon	—	28.0	Halder and Gadgil (1983)
	Callus	—	3.7	Halder and Gadgil (1983)

Cucumis sativus	Callus	—	2.8–3.5	Halder and Gadgil (1983), Pandey and Gadgil (1984)
	Cotyledon	—	30.3	Halder and Gadgil (1974)
Caucus carota	Callus	—	2.1–2.3	Radwan et al. (1974)
	Suspension	0.05	—	Gregor (1977)
Glycine maxima	Suspension	0.33	—	Tattrie and Veliky (1973)
Glycine max	Suspension	0.06–0.12	—	Stearns and Morton (1975b)
	Suspension	0.50	—	Tattrie and Veliky (1973)
	Suspension	—	6.0	Wilson et al. (1978)
Glycine soja PI-153	Seed	21.0	—	Shin et al. (1971)
	Suspension	0.17–0.24	—	Shin et al. (1971)
	Callus	0.14–0.16	—	Shin et al. (1971)
Glycine soja PI-194	Seed	18.1	—	Shin et al. (1971)
	Suspension	0.20–0.40	—	Shin et al. (1971)
	Callus	0.10–0.20	—	Shin et al. (1971)
Glycine soja	Suspension	—	6.0–8.1	Radwan and Mangold (1976)
Hydnocarpus anthelminthica	Callus	0.35–0.45	—	Spencer et al. (1974)
Ipomoea sp.	Suspension	—	3.5–7.0	Song and Tattrie (1973)
	Suspension	0.33	—	Tattrie and Veliky (1973)
Linum usitatissimum	Seed	38.6	—	Shin et al. (1971)
	Callus	0.20	—	Shin et al. (1971)
Luffa acutangula	Cotyledon	—	21.6	Halder and Gadgil (1983)
	Callus	—	2.6	Halder and Gadgil (1983)
Momordica charantia	Cotyledon	—	24.7	Halder and Gadgil (1983)
	Callus	—	3.2	Halder and Gadgil (1983)

Table 1. (Continued)

Plant species	Tissue	Lipid (%) Fresh weight	Lipid (%) Dry weight	References
Nicotiana tabacum				
Nongreen	Suspension	—	1.7	Siebertz et al. (1978)
Green	Suspension	—	6.1–6.3	Siebertz et al. (1978)
Petroselinum crispum	Seed	8.51	—	Ellenbracht et al. (1980)
	Callus	0.08	—	Ellenbracht et al. (1980)
	Suspension	0.14	—	Ellenbracht et al. (1980)
	Photomixotrophic callus	0.51	—	Ellenbracht et al. (1980)
Petroselinum hortense	Suspension	—	5.0	Ellenbracht et al. (1980)
Phaseolus aureus	Suspension	—	2.6	Radwan et al. (1974)
Pinus elliotti	Seed	—	65.02	Laseter et al. (1973)
	Callus	—	4.01	Laseter et al. (1973)
Theobroma cacao	Immature seed[a]	—	10.5–11.5	Tsai et al. (1982)
	Mature seed[b]	—	53.0–55.0	Tsai et al. (1982)
	Callus	—	5.1–5.5	Tsai et al. (1982)
	Suspension	—	5.3–7.7	Tsai et al. (1982)
	Somatic embryos	—	3.5–14.7	Pence et al. (1981), Wright et al. (1983)
Tropaeolum majus	Callus	—	8.1–8.3	Radwan et al. (1978)

[a] 110 days after pollination.
[b] 170 days after pollination.

lipids reverted to the original amount (Barz et al., 1980). There are no obvious differences in composition between lipid classes of various callus and suspension cultures. Triacylglycerols occur in small amounts in callus and suspension cultures of different species, the only exception being in one variety of carrot, which contained 30.3% triacylglycerols (Kleinig and Kopp, 1978).

Fatty Acid Composition

The fatty acid pattern of total lipids varies with different species of plants (Table 3). The content of palmitic acid is usually lower in seeds than in callus or suspension cultures. Stearic acid is low in most species; however, it is high in mature cacao seeds (Tsai, 1981). Oleic acid content is extremely high in seeds of parsley (*Petroselinum crispum*) (Ellenbracht, 1980) and also high in some seeds or tissue culture. When compared with oleic acid, linoleic acid seems to be the predominant unsaturated fatty acid. Linoleic acid comprises more than 50% of the total fatty acids in soybean (*Glycine max*) (Ezzat and Pearce, 1980) and pine oil (*Pinus elliottii*) (Laseter et al., 1973) and in lipids of suspension cultures of *Chenopodium rubrum* (Radwan et al., 1979), *P. crispum* (Ellenbracht et al., 1980), and *Solanum* species (Tattrie and Veliky, 1973). Considerable amounts of linolenic acid are found in suspension cultures of soybean (Stearns and Morton, 1975a; Wilson et al., 1978), morning glory (*Ipomonea* sp.) (Tattrie and Veliky, 1973), and some other species. It is interesting to observe that when heterotrophic suspension cultures turned autotrophic, the relative percentage of linoleic acid decreased while that of linolenic acid increased (Radwan et al., 1979; Barz et al., 1980; Ellenbracht et al., 1980). The fatty acid patterns of total lipids in tissue or cell cultures are quite different from those of the seed lipids of the same species. However, two exceptions were reported. The first exception was found in two varieties of rapeseed (*Brassica napus*) (Ezzat and Pearce, 1980). The fatty acid patterns of seeds and suspension culture are very similar and appreciable amounts of erucic acid unique to this seed were detected in the tissue culture lipids. Yano et al. (1972a) showed cyclic acids, such as malvalic acid, sterulic acid, and dihydrosterculic acid, in substantial amounts in callus lipids of *Malva parviflora*.

Because of the interest in triglyceride production, the fatty acid composition of triacylglycerols in different plants is summarized in Table 4. The data show that the fatty acid composition of triacylglycerols varies among different species.

In conclusion, it seems that the lipid contents and compositions of tissue or cell cultures are very different from the seeds of the same species. There is also a wide variation among lipids of the

Table 2. Lipid Classes of Different Tissues (Percent of Total Lipids)

	Neutral lipids				Polar lipids			
Plant species	Triacyl-glycerols	Sterols + steryl esters	Others	Total	Phospho-lipids	Glyco-lipids	Total	Reference
Artemisia absinthium[a]	3.2–3.9	23.7–24.4	12.1–14.9	39.4–42.9	—	—	49.2–52.8	Radwan et al. (1975)
Brassica napus								
var. *Maris Haplona*								
Seeds	—	—	—	98.9	0.9	0.2	1.1	Ezzat and Pearce (1980)
Suspension cells	—	—	—	57.3	32.0	10.7	42.7	Ezzat and Pearce (1980)
var. *Rapora*								
Seeds	—	—	—	98.5	1.3	0.2	1.5	Ezzat and Pearce (1980)
Suspension cells	—	—	—	44.7	42.6	12.6	55.2	Ezzat and Pearce (1980)
Chenopodium rubrum								
Hetrotrophic[b]	—	—	—	—	20.9 (1.65)[c]	79.1 (6.25)	100.0	Radwan et al. (1979)
Phototrophic[b]	—	—	—	—	28.2 (13.4)	71.8 (34.1)	100.0	Radwan et al. (1979)
Phototrophic–heterotrophic[b]	—	—	—	—	30.8 (3.3)	69.2 (7.4)	100.0	Radwan et al. (1979)
Daucus carota[b]	30.3	4.3	tr	34.6	59.1	6.4	65.5	Kleinig and Kopp (1978)
Daucus carota[b]	16.3	—	19.7	36.0	64.0	—	64.0	Gregor (1977)

Kalanchoe crenata[a]								
Nongreen	—	—	—	—	79.0 (2.07)	21.0 (0.55)	100.0 (2.62)	Tomas and Stobart (1970)
Green	—	—	—	—	20.6 (2.24)	79.4 (8.61)	100.0 (10.85)	Tomas and Stobart (1970)
Glycine max[b]	13.1	7.1	2.1	22.3	58.9	18.8	77.7	Wilson et al. (1978)
Glycine max								
var. *Bravalla*								
Seeds	—	—	—	96.5	3.1	0.4	3.5	Ezzat and Pearce (1980)
Suspension cells	—	—	—	26.4	18.2	5.4	23.6	Ezzat and Pearce (1980)
var. *Fiskeby V*								
Seeds	—	—	—	96.0	3.6	0.4	4.0	Ezzat and Pearce (1980)
Suspension cells	—	—	—	55.4	35.7	8.9	44.6	Ezzat and Pearce (1980)
Nicotiana tabacum[b]	8.0	—	—	8.0	73.0	19.0	92.0	Gawer et al. (1983)
Nicotiana tabacum[b]								
Nongreen	—	—	—	—	59.7 (6.9)	40.7 (10.1)	100.0 (17.0)	Siebertz et al. (1978)
Green	—	—	—	—	48.5–54.6 (27.7–32.5)	45.4–53.2 (29.6–33.3)	100.0 (57.3–65.8)	Siebertz et al. (1978)
Peganum harmala								
Heterotrophic[b]	11.3 (1.6)[c]	32.3 (4.55)	— —	43.6 (6.15)	46.1 (6.50)	10.3 (1.45)	56.4 (7.95)	Barz et al. (1980)
Photomixotrophic[b]	12.2 (2.90)	34.0 (8.10)	— —	46.2 (11.00)	33.5 (8.00)	20.3 (4.85)	53.8 (12.85)	Barz et al. (1980)
Photoautotrophic[b]	5.7 (1.90)	18.0 (6.00)	— —	23.7 (7.90)	46.9 (15.65)	29.4 (9.80)	76.3 (25.45)	Barz et al. (1980)

Table 2. (Continued)

Plant species	Neutral lipids: Triacyl-glycerols	Sterols + steryl esters	Others	Total	Polar lipids: PL	GL	Total	References
Petroselinum crispum								
Heterotrophic[b]	13.4	2.6	—	16.0	54.0	29.8	83.8	Ellenbracht et al.
	(18.8)[d]	(3.6)	—	(22.4)	(75.6)	(41.7)	(117.3)	(1980)
Heterotrophic[a]	7.8	1.3	—	9.1	57.9	33.0	90.9	Ellenbracht et al.
	(6.2)	(1.0)	—	(7.3)	(46.3)	(26.4)	(72.7)	(1980)
Photomixotrophic[a]	10.2	2.1	—	12.3	58.8	28.9	87.7	Ellenbracht et al.
	(52.0)	(10.7)	—	(62.7)	(299.9)	(147.4)	(447.3)	(1980)
Seeds	79.2	1.5	—	80.7	—	—	19.3	Ellenbracht et al. (1980)
Theobroma cacao								
Immature seeds (125 days post-pollination)	82.9–87.1	1.6–2.0	5.5–7.1	90.1–96.2	3.6–4.4	1.1–1.3	4.7–5.7	Tsai et al. (1982)
Ripe seeds (170 days post-pollination)	96.4–97.2	0.2	0.9–1.3	97.5–98.7	0.3–0.7	0.4–0.6	0.7–1.3	Tsai et al. (1982)
Callus	12.6 13.8	7.9–9.3	0.7–1.5	21.2–24.6	26.3–27.1	44.4–48.8	70.7–75.9	Tsai et al. (1982)
Suspension cultures	11.6–13.6	8.2–10.2	0.6–1.0	20.4–23.8	19.5–24.5	53.8–58.2	73.3–82.7	Tsai et al. (1982)

[a] Callus.
[b] Suspension culture.
[c] Absolute value (mg/g dry cells).
[d] Absolute value (mg/g fresh cells).

Table 3. Fatty Acid Compositions of Total Lipids in Different Plant Tissues (Weight Percent)

Plant species	<16:0	16:0	16:1	18:0	18:1	18:2	18:3	>18:0	Reference
Acer pseudoplatanus[a]	tr[b]	24.0	—	4.0	38.0	24.0	10.0	—	Bligny et al. (1979)
Atropa belladonna[a]	—	26.1	—	10.8	8.7	41.8	12.6	—	Tattrie and Veliky (1973)
Brassica napus									
Seeds	tr	2.5	tr	tr	23.3	14.2	1.7	58.3	Radwan et al. (1978)
Callus	tr	27.6	tr	7.2	19.0	22.6	17.6	6.0	Radwan et al. (1978)
Brassica napus									
var. *Maris Haplona*									
Seeds	—	7.0	—	—	58.0	18.0	6.0	11.0	Ezzat and Pearce (1980)
Suspension culture	—	17.0	—	—	41.0	18.0	12.0	13.0	Ezzat and Pearce (1980)
var. *Rapora*									
Seeds	—	4.0	—	—	41.0	13.0	6.0	37.0	Ezzat and Pearce (1980)
Suspension culture	—	21.0	—	—	28.0	21.0	16.0	14.0	Ezzat and Pearce (1980)
Cannabis sativa[a]									
95-C	—	30.0	—	6.1	9.2	42.2	12.5	—	Tattrie and Veliky (1973)
95-D	—	30.8	—	3.9	7.2	40.6	17.5	—	Tattrie and Veliky (1973)
Catharanthus roseus[a]	—	18.2–20.0	—	0.9–1.8	26.8 32.7	39.4–43.1	7.6–11.0	—	MacCarthy and Stumpf (1980)

Table 3. (Continued)

Plant species	<16:0	16:0	16:1	18:0	18:1	18:2	18:3	>18:0	Reference
Cicer arietinum[a]	1.7	25.4	—	10.8	8.4	20.2	17.8	11.4	Radwan et al. (1974)
Chenopodium rubrum[a]									
Heterotrophic	NA[c]	20.5	NA	3.6	11.3	50.4	6.6	NA	Radwan et al. (1979)
Phototrophic	NA	21.5	NA	1.2	4.3	34.6	33.8	NA	Radwan et al. (1979)
Heterotrophic–phototrophic	NA	22.5	NA	1.2	7.0	58.6	6.9	NA	Radwan et al. (1979)
Citrullus vulgaris	5.6	50.8	—	9.9	8.6	5.3	19.8	—	Halder and Gadgil (1983)
Cucumis melo									
Cotyledons	—	12.2	—	1.0	14.1	72.7	—	—	Halder and Gadgil (1983)
Callus	4.8	50.1	—	5.6	4.1	9.5	22.0	1.0	Halder and Gadgil (1983)
Cucumis melo var. *utilissimus*									
Cotyledons	—	13.3	—	6.1	19.5	61.1	—	—	Halder and Gadgil (1983)
Callus	3.2	53.2	—	5.5	6.9	5.6	20.1	5.5	Halder and Gadgil (1983)
Cucumis sativus									
Cotyledons	—	21.3	—	5.9	24.1	48.7	—	—	Halder and Gadgil (1983)

Callus	6.4	50.5	—	2.9	5.5	3.5	31.2	—	Halder and Gadgil (1983)
Daucus carota[a]	—	19.1	—	6.2	8.3	55.9	10.5	—	Gregor (1977)
Daucus carota[d]									
C1411	1.7	60.0	—	7.5	0.6	3.9	4.0	20.9	Radwan et al. (1974)
E1721	0.2	60.6	—	4.6	6.1	11.6	3.2	13.4	Radwan et al. (1974)
Glycine max[a]	—	21.9	—	4.0	6.6	16.3	51.2	—	Tattrie and Veliky (1973)
Glycine max[a]	—	22.0	—	3.1	5.5	18.9	50.9	—	Wilson et al. (1978)
Glycine max									
var. *Bravalla*									
Seeds	—	11.0	—	—	18.0	58.0	13.0	—	Ezzat and Pearce (1980)
Suspension culture	—	22.0	—	—	18.0	13.0	30.0	17.0	Ezzat and Pearce (1980)
var. *Fiskeby V*									
Seeds	—	12.0	—	—	16.0	58.0	13.0	—	Ezzat and Pearce (1980)
Suspension culture	—	22.0	—	—	28.0	17.0	24.0	9.0	Ezzat and Pearce (1980)
Glycine max									
Seeds	—	10.0	1.0	4.0	23.0	51.0	10.0	—	Stearns and Morton (1975a)
Suspension culture	—	37.0	1.0	8.0	7.0	4.0	44.0	—	Stearns and Morton (1975a)

Table 3. (Continued)

Plant species	<16:0	16:0	16:1	18:0	18:1	18:2	18:3	>18:0	Reference
Hydnocarpus anthelminthica[b]	—	34.5	—	10.8	15.0	26.3	4.4	8.4	Radwan et al. (1974)
Ipomonea ap[a]	—	23.0	—	6.7	3.0	29.5	37.7	—	Tattrie and Veliky (1973)
Ipomonea sp. var. *Heavenly Blue*	—	26.2	—	11.5	9.9	38.5	13.9	—	Tattrie and Veliky (1973)
Lactuca sativa[a]	—	54.8	—	14.6	10.2	16.8	3.6	—	Tattrie and Veliky (1973)
Luffa acutangual									
Cotyledons	—	21.3	—	10.1	28.4	40.2	—	—	Halder and Gadgil (1983)
Callus	11.5	53.6	—	6.1	3.3	8.4	17.0	—	Halder and Gadgil (1983)
Momordica charantia									
Cotyledons	—	2.7	—	24.2	—	7.2	65.9	—	Halder and Gadgil (1983)
Callus	—	52.0	—	12.1	15.6	10.4	10.0	—	Halder and Gadgil (1983)
Nicotiana tabacum[a]	—	19.0	—	4.0	2.0	52.0	23.0	—	Gawer et al. (1983)
Nicotiana tabacum[a]	—	19.1–23.4	—	1.4–2.5	1.9–4.2	57.2–63.2	11.4–15.8	—	MacCarthy and Stumpf (1980)

Nicotiana tabucum[a]									
Nongreen	—	26.1	0.3	4.6	3.5	53.1	11.3	1.2	Siebertz et al. (1978)
Green	—	20.3	0.7	4.3	5.9	34.6	32.9	0.9	Siebertz et al. (1978)
Peganum harmala									
Suspension culture	0.7	24.0	0.1	2.5	13.9	43.0	11.0	4.2	Barz et al. (1980)
Photomixotrophic suspension culture	0.7	24.0	0.1	2.1	14.3	34.9	17.5	5.6	Barz et al. (1980)
Photoautotrophic suspension culture	2.2	27.3	0.7	2.4	14.1	25.4	21.9	5.3	Barz et al. (1980)
Petroselinum hortense[a]	0.2	24.1	—	0.6	8.1	58.2	6.9	1.9	Radwan et al. (1974)
Petroselinum arietinum[a]	1.7	25.4	—	10.8	8.4	20.2	17.8	11.4	Radwan et al. (1974)
Petroselinum crispum									
Callus	0.3	34.6	—	1.2	4.0	44.2	6.8	8.9	Ellenbracht et al. (1980)
Suspension culture	0.2	19.0	—	0.5	4.7	62.2	7.8	5.6	Ellenbracht et al. (1980)
Photomixotrophic callus	0.3	25.8	—	1.0	3.2	51.2	13.0	5.3	Ellenbracht et al. (1980)
Phaseolus aureus[a]	0.3	32.8	tr	7.3	2.8	18.3	34.0	3.9	Radwan et al. (1974)
Phaseolus vulgaris[a]	—	34.0	—	5.7	6.6	33.8	19.9	—	Tattrie and Veliky (1973)
Pinus elliottii									
Callus	4.5	22.1	1.2	3.9	26.1	30.6	7.9	3.2	Laseter et al. (1973)
Seed	0.1	6.2	0.1	2.3	21.6	50.8	18.0	1.0	Laseter et al. (1973)
Solanum dulcamara[a]	—	20.0	—	5.1	3.6	60.9	10.4	—	Tattrie and Veliky (1973)

Table 3. (Continued)

Plant species	<16:0	16:0	16:1	18:0	18:1	18:2	18:3	>18:0	Reference
Solanum pseudocapsicum[a]	—	25.0	—	7.0	5.4	55.0	7.6	—	Tattrie and Veliky (1973)
Theobroma cacao	—	27.9–	0.7–	4.9–	21.1–	32.8–	4.8–	—	Tsai et al. (1982)
Callus from cotyledon		30.7	0.9	5.5	23.5	36.0	5.6		
Callus from flower bud	—	40.6	—	14.4	17.7	21.9	3.5	3.7	Janick et al. (1982)
Suspension culture	—	27.5–	0.8–	2.2–	10.8–	47.0–	6.9–	—	Tsai et al. (1982)
		30.1	1.4	2.6	12.2	50.2	8.5		
Somatic embryo	—	30.4–	—	8.3–	2.9–	37.2–	9.1–	2.2–	Janick et al. (1982)
		37.8		9.9	4.4	39.6	9.9	8.3	
Somatic embryo	—	23.6–	1.1–	9.9–	6.2–	37.6–	8.0–	—	Wen et al. (1984)
		31.4	2.7	14.9	12.0	39.8	13.0		
Immature seeds (125 days postpollination)	—	29.8–	—	5.4–	7.3–	42.8–	3.4–	—	Tsai et al. (1982)
		32.4		6.2	7.9	48.0	3.8		
Mature seeds (170 days postpollination)	—	22.6–	—	37.0–	21.6–	3.0–	—	—	Tsai et al. (1982)
		25.2		39.4	35.2	3.4			
Tropaeolum majus									
Seeds	tr	2.4	tr	tr	10.3	tr	tr	87.3	Radwan et al. (1978)
Callus	tr	27.1	tr	tr	35.2	14.6	23.0	tr	Radwan et al. (1978)

[a] Suspension culture.
[b] tr, trace.
[c] NA, not available.
[d] Callus.

Table 4. Fatty Acid Compositions of Triglycerides of Different Plant Tissues (Weight Percent)

Plant species	<16:0	16:0	16:1	17:0+ 17:1	18:0	18:1	18:2	18:3	>18:0	Reference
Arachis hypogaea										
Seed	tr[a]	12.4	—	—	0.2	48.3	34.5	1.0	1.9	Shin et al. (1971)
Callus	1.5–5.2	24.6–24.7	tr–2.0	0.0–tr	1.8–1.9	6.0–7.8	15.5–19.2	41.5–47.7	tr	Shin et al. (1971)
Artemisia absinthium										
Seed	tr	8.9	—	tr	0.7	6.5	83.2	tr	tr	Shin et al. (1971)
Callus	0.8–1.6	12.4–14.6	0.0–1.0	0.0–tr	tr–1.1	4.5–5.1	56.6–66.0	12.6–23.8	0.0–tr	Shin et al. (1971)
Brassica campestris var. *Echo*										
Seed	tr	2.9	0.4	—	0.8	35.9	17.1	15.9	25.4	Staba et al. (1971)
Callus	2.4–6.2	13.3–17.2	1.2–2.6	tr–0.4	3.7–11.0	13.8–17.8	3.2–14.9	27.8–62.2	tr–0.4	Staba et al. (1971)
Brassica juncea	3.9	21.1	3.5	tr	19.0	30.3	10.3	11.8	tr	Shin et al. (1971)
Brassica napus										
Seed	0.2	4.1	1.2	1.2	1.0	20.9	16.7	14.2	41.0	Shin et al. (1971)
Callus	1.0	16.1	1.0	tr	3.7	14.5	6.7	53.8	2.0	Shin et al. (1971)
Brassica napus var. *Target*										
Seed	0.2	4.1	4.2	—	1.0	20.9	16.7	14.2	41.3	Staba et al. (1971)
Callus	1.0	16.1	1.0	0.0	3.7	14.5	6.7	53.8	2.0	Staba et al. (1971)

Table 4. (Continued)

Plant species	<16:0	16:0	16:1	17:0+ 17:1	18:0	18:1	18:2	18:3	>18:0	Reference
Brassica napus										
30°C	0.6–1.6	16.4–20.9	2.3–2.6	—	4.0–5.6	27.7–30.9	28.0–30.9	9.6–14.2	1.1–3.2	Radwan et al. (1978)
5°C	1.0	1.2	4.4	—	4.6	29.5	25.7	10.3	3.3	Radwan et al. (1978)
Brassica napus										
var. *Maris Haplona*										
Seed NL[b]	—	7.0	—	—	—	58.0	18.0	6.0	12.0	Ezzat and Pearce (1980)
Suspension cell NL	—	17.0	tr	—	—	41.0	18.0	12.0	13.0	Ezzat and Pearce (1980)
var. *Rapora*										
Seed NL	—	4.0	—	—	—	41.0	12.0	6.0	38.0	Ezzat and Pearce (1980)
Daucus carota	tr	14.2	—	—	0.6	6.3	68.9	10.0	—	Gregor (1977)
Glycine max										
var. *Bravalla*										
Seed NL	—	11.0	—	—	—	19.0	57.0	13.0	—	Ezzat and Pearce (1980)
Suspension cell NL	—	22.0	tr	—	—	18.0	13.0	30.0	17.0	Ezzat and Pearce (1980)
var. *Fiskeby V*										
Seed NL	—	12.0	—	—	—	17.0	58.0	13.0	—	Ezzat and Pearce (1980)
Suspension cell NL	—	22.0	—	—	—	28.0	17.0	24.0	9.0	Ezzat and Pearce (1980)

Glycine soja PI-194										
Seed	tr	13.7	—	tr	2.7	33.1	44.2	6.3	tr	Shin et al. (1971)
Callus	2.1–26.8	18.8–43.8	2.1–6.8	0.0–1.4	8.0–9.3	8.8–15.2	3.9–7.5	tr–43.7	tr	Shin et al. (1971)
Suspension cell	4.6–4.9	21.9–29.5	1.7–4.0	0.7–2.4	5.2–17.3	7.3–24.4	4.2–16.5	11.1–41.9	0.0–2.1	Shin et al. (1971)
Linum usitatissimum										
Seed	tr	6.1	—	tr	4.5	17.2	15.1	57.2	tr	Shin et al. (1971)
Callus	1.9–3.7	20.2–21.2	1.1–1.7	0.4–0.7	2.0–2.3	4.8–7.8	37.7–38.2	30.0–30.6	0.0–tr	Shin et al. (1971)
Peganum harmala[c]	0.3	23.2	0.6	—	4.8	17.5	36.3	11.1	6.2	Barz et al. (1980)
P. harmala[d]	0.5	27.0	0.4	—	2.8	13.3	32.2	17.7	5.9	Barz et al. (1980)
P. harmala[e]	18.8	22.9	0.7	—	4.6	17.8	15.1	12.2	7.8	Barz et al. (1980)
Theobroma cacao										
Immature seeds (125 days post-pollination)	—	22.7–24.7	tr	—	36.6–38.2	31.8–32.4	4.2–5.0	tr	0.7–1.3	Tsai et al. (1982)
Ripe seeds (170 days post-pollination)	—	23.1–23.4	tr	—	36.0–39.6	31.8–33.0	4.2–4.8	tr	tr	Tsai et al. (1982)
Callus	tr	25.4–26.0	1.1–1.7	—	16.8–17.6	23.4–25.4	22.6–24.2	6.8–7.2	0.6–0.8	Tsai et al. (1982)
Suspension cell	tr	23.8–24.6	1.0–1.2	—	16.4–16.8	17.2–18.8	29.5–30.3	8.5–9.1	1.1–1.7	Tsai et al. (1982)

[a] tr, trace.
[b] NL, neutral lipids.
[c] Suspension cells.
[d] Photomixotrophic suspension cells.
[e] Photoauxotrophic suspension cells.

different species. Radwan and Mangold (1976) indicated that culture conditions such as media composition, aeration, and temperature can drastically alter lipid content and composition. It is thus very important to understand the effects of various environment conditions on the lipid production by tissue or cell cultures before exploring the possibility of producing seed lipid using tissue culture methods.

BIOSYNTHESIS OF LIPIDS IN PLANT TISSUE CULTURE

Plant tissue cultures are a useful model system for studying plant lipid biosynthesis (Stearns and Morton, 1975a; Stumpf and Weber, 1977; Bligny et al., 1979; Kates et al., 1979; MacCarthy and Stumpf, 1980). Cell growth is fast, uniform, and reproducible. The lipid composition of plant tissue cultures is sometimes similar to that of the organs of the plant from which they were derived (Ezzat and Pearce, 1980). Another advantage is that their metabolism is very easy to manipulate for biochemical studies. Previous reviews (Kates et al., 1979; Radwan and Mangold, 1980) will be updated in this section, with an emphasis on fatty and triacylglycerol biosynthesis.

Fatty acid biosynthesis in cell culture has been studied using radioactive acetate or fatty acid precursors. The species studied include *Malva* sp. (Yano et al., 1972b), soybean (Stearns and Morton, 1975a; Stumpf and Weber, 1977; Nothelfer et al., 1977; Wilson et al., 1978; Weber et al., 1979; MacCarthy and Stumpf, 1980), *Acer pseudoplatanus* (Bligny et al., 1979), and cacao (Tsai and Kinsella, 1982a;b).

Acetate is rapidly incorporated into a range of fatty acids, such as palmitic, stearic, oleic, linoleic, and linolenic acids. Data for soybean (Stearns and Morton, 1975a; Wilson et al., 1978; MacCarthy and Stumpf, 1980), tobacco (MacCarthy and Stumpf, 1980), and cacao (Tsai and Kinsella, 1982a) showed rapid desaturation of stearic to oleic, linoleic, and linolenic acids similar to the desaturation system in the intact plant. The desaturation pattern was not very clear in the cell culture of *Catharanthus roseus* (MacCarthy and Stumpf, 1980). The desaturation system was further demonstrated using oleic and linoleic acids in soybean (Stumpf and Weber, 1977) and cacao (Tsai and Kinsella, 1982b) cell culture.

The incorporation of exogenous fatty acids or fatty acids synthesized from exogenous acetate has also been studied. Fatty acids were rapidly incorporated into phospholipids of soybean (Stearns and Morton, 1975a; Stumpf and Weber, 1977; Wilson et al., 1978) and cacao cell cultures (Tsai and Kinsella, 1982b; Tsai et al., 1982). It seems that the synthesis of polar lipids is the major event in the cell culture and only small amounts of triacylglycerols are produced. This clearly indicates that suspension cultures actively synthesize membrane lipid instead of storage lipid. Thus cell suspension cultures seem a good system for the study of membrane rather than storage lipid biosynthesis.

An embryo culture system is needed to study the storage lipid metabolism. Currently there is one system which has been developed: oil palm (Jones, 1974; Turnham and Northcote, 1984). In Jones' study higher amounts, that is, 17% of acetate, was incorporated into triacylglycerols of oil palm somatic embryos, when compared with 12% into those of undifferentiated cell culture. In a later study Turnham and Northcote (1984) also found that as the somatic embryos developed to larger size in culture, the proportions of triacylglycerols in the total lipids increased drastically, possibly indicating a gradual deposition of storage lipid in the somatic embryo cells.

FACTORS AFFECTING LIPID PRODUCTION IN PLANT TISSUE AND CELL CULTURE

Growth Stage

Song and Tattrie (1973) found that the total lipid content of morning glory (*Ipomoea* sp.) cell culture peaked after 4 days of growth and then leveled off at 5% until 8 days after growth. However, triacylglycerol content increased from 2 μM (first day) to 12 μM (second day), decreased to 7 μM (third and fourth day), again increased to 11.5 μM (fifth day), and then rapidly decreased to the original value. Significant changes in fatty acids were also observed; oleic acids content remained constant (less than 5%) for 2 days and then increased to 40% in the next 4 days. In contrast, the total linolenic acids content gradually decreased from 47% (third day) to 28% (sixth day).

Significant changes in the triacylglycerols-to-phospholipid ratio in cultured rapecells (*B. napus*) were observed by Radwan et al. (1978). They found that this ratio remained constant (2:1) for the first 2 weeks in culture and then decreased to 1:2 during the third week. However, no change was observed in the fatty acid composition of triacylglycerols during this period. MacCarthy and Stumpf (1980) studied the change of fatty acid composition of *G. max*, *C. roseus*, and *N. tabacum* during growth at room temperature. They reported that the linoleic acid content of *C. roseus* and *G. max* decreased with time and that of *N. tabacum* increased with time. Nevertheless, the total fatty acid contents of tobacco and soybean decreased and that of *C. roseus* increased during culturing.

In cacao cell cultures no change was observed in the total lipid content and fatty acid composition during growth of callus and suspension culture (Tsai, 1981; Tsai et al., 1982). However, Tsai (1981) found that the triacylglycerol content decreased from 26.7% (fifth week) to 13.9% of total lipid (seventh week). From the above studies it seems that metabolic changes during growth among different species are variable and might be determined by the specific genotype of the cell (MacCarthy and Stumpf, 1980).

Nutrients

Addition of coconut water into the culture medium increased the total lipid content of soybean callus and cell suspension cultures and decreased that of wormwood callus cultures (Shin et al., 1971). Coconut water treatment also changed the fatty acid composition of triacylglycerols of soybean callus cultures (Shin et al., 1971). The palmitic acid content increased about threefold and linolenic acid content decreased from 51% to trace amounts under the same treatment. A total of 10% of coconut water increased the triacylglycerol content from 11 to 19% for cacao cell culture (Tsai et al., 1982). A concurrent decrease in the linoleic acid content from 37 to 19% and an increase in the oleic acid content from 10 to 33% were also observed. Radwan and Mangold (1976) found 35 mg of lipid in 100 ml of coconut water, but it did not contribute a significant amount of fatty acid (only 33.4 μg fatty acids/100 ml of coconut water) to the cultures (Wen et al., 1984). Organic nitrogen such as casein hydrolysate decreased the total lipid contents of callus and suspension culture (Radwan et al., 1974).

Sucrose is the major carbon source in cell culture media. A combination of coconut water and sucrose added 8 days after culture enhanced the lipid content of cocoa bean cells (Tsai et al., 1982). Increasing sucrose in the culture media from 3 to 27% increased the proportions of stearic acid and oleic acid and decreased those of linoleic and linolenic acids in somatic cacao embryos, which were thus similar to those of the zygotic embryos (Pence et al., 1981). Oleopalmitostearin, the major triacylglycerol in cocoa butter, was also identified in the somatic embryos (Janick et al., 1982). Sucrose treatment did not increase the total lipid content significantly but increased the total fatty acid content of somatic embryos from 1.2% (3% sucrose) to 3.1% (27% sucrose) on a dry weight basis (Pence et al., 1981).

Plant Growth Hormones

Stearns and Morton (1975b) first investigated the effect of 1 ppm levels of indole-3-butyric acid, kinetin, and gibberellin (GA) individually or in several possible combinations on the fatty acid composition of soybean suspension cultures. Cells from indole-3-butyric acid

(IBA) or IBA and GA treatment exhibited a higher palmitic acid content and a lower linolenic acid content than cells from other treatment groups. Combinations of kinetin and GA induced the highest amount of linolenic acid among all treatments. Pandey and Gadgil (1984) tested the effects of four combinations of growth factors on the fatty acid compositions of total lipids in *Cucumis melo* and *Cucumis sativus* callus cultures: naphthalene acetic acid (NAA) plus coconut water (CW), NAA plus kinetin, NAA plus 6-benzylaminopurine (BAP), and BAP plus IBA. A combination of IBA and BAP induced the highest myristic acid content and lowest linolenic acid content in these two species.

Different combinations of 2,4-D and kinetin were tested with cacao cell culture (Tsai, 1981). Although the response of total lipids or triacylglycerols to 2,4-D or kinetin at a level of $p=.05$ was not significant, there was a significant interaction between 2,4-D and kinetin. The optimum concentrations of 2,4-D and kinetin were found to be 2.26 and 0.465 μM, respectively. A combination of 2.26 μM 2,4-D, 5.0 μM gibberellic acid (GA_3), and 5.0 μM zeatin further reduced the linoleic acid and palmitic acid contents and increased the oleic acid content in the suspension culture (Wen et al., 1984). Although the oleic acid level was increased, the stearic acid level remained low. However, complete elimination of all hormones normally used in the cell culture systems had an apparently beneficial effect on the fatty acid pattern. More studies are needed to elucidate the effects of hormones.

Temperature

Radwan et al. (1978) first studied the effect of low temperature on the lipids of rape (*B. napus*) and nasturtium (*Tropaeolum majus*) callus cultures. Their results showed that low temperature increased the lipid content of rapeseed cells. Similar results were also observed from sycamore cell cultures (Gawer et al., 1980), which showed a threefold increase of total lipid content by 12°C treatment when compared with the 25°C control. Similar observations were reported by Wright et al. (1983) for somatic embryos cultured under different temperatures ranging from 10 to 35°C. In the latter system embryos cultured at 17°C showed the highest total lipid content. The total fatty acid content was also influenced by temperature: It was highest at 20°C for tobacco cell culture (Gawer et al., 1983) and at 26°C for cacao embryo cultures (Wright et al., 1983).

At low temperature oleic acid content was higher in *C. roseus* culture (MacCarthy and Stumpf, 1980) and lower in rape and nasturtium cultures (Radwan et al., 1978). In cacao embryo cultures, however, oleic acid content was highest at 26°C (Wright et al., 1983). Linoleic acid content was enhanced by low temperature for

G. max (MacCarthy and Stumpf, 1980), tobacco (Gawer et al., 1983), and nasturtium (Radwan et al., 1978) cell cultures. It is also interesting to note that the proportion of linoleic acid peaked at 17°C and was lowest at 26°C for cacao embryo cultures (Wright et al., 1983). Higher proportions of linolenic acid was found at low-temperature treatment for rape (Radwan et al., 1978) and tobacco (MacCarthy and Stumpf, 1980; Gawer et al., 1983). The relative portion of linolenic acid was highest at 10°C and lowest at 26°C for cacao embryo culture (Wright et al., 1983).

POTENTIAL OF PLANT CELL CULTURE FOR SEED OIL PRODUCTION

Breeding of Seed Oil Plants

Plant tissue culture offers the advantage of producing large quantities of plantlets in a shorter time when compared with other conventional propagational methods. This is very helpful for those plants for which the success of a breeding program takes a long time to determine because the propagation is very slow. These plant tissue techniques used for propagation include somatic organogenesis and embryogenesis. Each of these processes can be either direct or calus-mediated plant regeneration (Evans et al., 1981). The advantage of the direct process is that the plantlets regenerated are uniform in their characteristics (clones). However, callus-mediated regeneration often contributes variability to the regenerated plantlets. This variation results from somaclonal variation and is very helpful in generating variability in the breeding program. The best example using plant tissue culture for plant breeding is the oil palm (*Elaeis guineensis*), which is the second largest edible oil crop in the world (Jones, 1984). This crop cannot be propagated in large quantities because each tree has only a single terminal meristem (Turnham and Northcote, 1982). Successful cloning of this crop is now possible (Jones, 1974). Selection of crop with high oil yield and quality followed by clonal propagation is currently actively pursued by the industry (Jones, 1984).

Direct Production of Seed Oils

Jones (1974) was the first to discuss the possibility of producing seed oils using plant tissue culture. His conclusion was not optimistic owing to the fact that cultured cells or somatic embryos are low in fat, especially the types of triacylglycerols occurring in the seed oils. Radwan and Mangold (1976) suggested that plant tissue culture is expected to be a source of valuable specialty fats such as steryl glycosides and steryl glycolipids instead of lower-priced triacylglycerols. However, in view of the very high price of cocoa butter (the 1984 U.S. import price was $4.52 per kilogram), which is 3.3 times higher than the second most expensive edible oil, olive oil, and 6.2 times higher than soybean oil (Food and Agriculture Organization, 1985), there is potential for the development of cell culture technology for the production of cocoa butter. Much research has been done on the culture of cacao cells (Tsai and Kinsella, 1981; 1982a,b; Tsai et al., 1982; Wen et al., 1984) and somatic embryos (Esan, 1977; 1980; Pence et al., 1979; 1980; 1981; Janick et al., 1982; Wen et al., 1984). The cultured cells are totipotent (Schwann, 1839) and contain all the genes for the expression of any anabolism occurring in the parent plant. However, to date, lipid metabolism in the cultured cells or embryos can be manipulated to a very limited degree. Perhaps if the cells or embryos could be transformed to produce mature zygotic cells or embryos, it may become possible to produce cocoa butter using tissue culture techniques.

Economics

The economic potential of producing seed lipids using plant tissue and cell cultures was first discussed by Jones (1974). From his calculations, it is estimated that in order to produce 52.5 kg of extracted product (35 batch cultures per year) 2000 kg of sucrose are needed as the carbon source. Goldstein et al. (1980) carried out an extensive product cost analysis on plant tissue culture as a source of biochemicals. They found that the manufacturing cost was approximately $17/kg and the capital cost was $25/kg for a production scale of 10^6 kg/year. Thus it seems it is still too early for the commercialization of plant cell culture for seed oil production, even for the most expensive edible oil, cocoa butter. Since approximately 80% of the raw material cost comes from the carbon source (sucrose), it might be possible to lower this cost by switching to some other carbon source, such as molasses, whose price is about one-ninth that of sucrose (Sahai and Knuth, 1985). Another way to reduce the cost is to scale up production, which is more practical for oils of higher market volume and value (Goldstein et al., 1980; Sahai and Knuth, 1985).

REFERENCES

Archibald, J. F. (1954). Culture *in vitro* of cambial tissue of cocoa. *Nature 173*:351–352.

Barz, W., Herzbeck, H., Husemann, W., Schneiders, G., and Mangold, H. K. (1980). Alkaloids and lipids of heterotrophic, photomixotrophic and photoautotrophic cell suspension cultures of *Peganum harmala*. *Planta Med. 40*:137–148.

Bergmann, L. (1960). Growth and division of single cells of higher plants *in vitro*. *J. Gen. Physiol. 43*:841–851.

Berthelot, A. (1934). Nouvelles remarques d'ordre chimique sur le choix des milieux de culture naturels et sur la manière de formuler les milieux synthétiques. *Bull. Soc. Chim. Biol. 16*:1553–1557.

Bligny, R., Rebeille-Borgella, F., and Douce, R. (1979). Incorporation of [^{14}C]-acetate and [^{33}P]-phosphate into phospholipids of sycamore cell suspensions. In *Advances in the Biochemistry and Physiology of Plant Lipids* (L. A. Appelqvist and C. Liljenberg, eds.), Elsevier/North-Holland, Amsterdam, pp. 387–392.

Caplin, S. M. and Steward, F. C. (1948). Effect of coconut milk on the growth of explants from carrot root. *Science 108*:655–657.

Crocomo, O. J. (1981). Biosynthesis of secondary products. In *Plant Tissue Culture Methods and Applications in Agriculture* (T. A. Thorpe, ed.), Academic, New York, pp. 359–372.

Ellenbracht, F., Barz, W., and Mangold, H. K. (1980). Unusual fatty acids in the lipids from organs and cell cultures of *Petroselinum crispum*. *Planta 150*:114–119.

Esan, E. B. (1977). Tissue culture studies of cacao (*Theobroma cacao* L.)—A supplementation of current research. In *Proceedings of the Fifth International Cocoa Research Conference*, Cocoa Research Institute of Nigeria, Ibadan, Nigeria, pp. 116–125.

Esan, E. B. (1982). *In vitro* studies on morphogenesis and plant regeneration in tissue cultures of cacao and *Herrania* species—A progress report. In *Proceedings of the Eighth International Cocoa Research Conference*, Cocoa Producers' Alliance, Lagos, Nigeria, pp. 245–252.

Evans, D. A., Shapr, W. R., and Flick, C. E. (1981). Growth and behavior of cell cultures: Embryogenesis and organogenesis. In *Plant Tissue Culture Methods and Applications in Agriculture* (T. A. Thorpe, ed.), Academic, New York, pp. 45–113.

Ezzat, K. S. and Pearce, R. S. (1980). Fatty acids of lipids from cultured soybean and rape cells. *Phytochemistry 19*:1375–1378.

Food and Agriculture Organization (1985). *FAO Trade Yearbook*, Food and Agriculture Organization, Rome, pp. 193, 269, and 275.

Gamborg, O. L. and Shyluk, J. P. (1981). Nutrition, media and characteristics of plant cell and tissue cultures. In *Plant Tissue Culture Methods and Applications in Agriculture* (T. A. Thorpe, ed.), Academic, New York, pp. 21–44.

Gamborg, O. L., Miller, R. A., and Ojima, K. (1968). Nutrient requirements of suspension cultures of soybean root cells. *Exp. Cell Res. 50*:151–158.

Gautheret, R. J. (1937). Nouvelles recherches sur la culture du tissu cambial. *C.R. Acad. Sci. Paris 205*:572–573.

Gautheret, R. J. (1938). Sur le repiquage des cultures de tissu cambial de *Salix caprea*. *C.R. Acad. Sci. Paris 206*:125–127.

Gautheret, R. J. (1939). Sur la possibilité de réaliser la culture indéfinie des tissue de tubercules de carotte. *C.R. Acad. Sci. Paris 208*:118–121.

Gautheret, R. J. (1966). Factors affecting differentiation of plant tissues *in vitro*. In *Cell Differentiation and Morphologenesis* (W. Beerman, ed.), North-Holland, Amsterdam, pp. 55–95.

Gawer, M., Trapy, F., Guern, J., and Mazliak, P. (1980). Lipid composition of sycamore cells cultivated at various temperatures. In *Biogenesis and Function of Plant Lipids* (P. Mazliak, P. Benveniste, C. Costes, and R. Douce, eds.), Elsevier/North-Holland, Amsterdam, p. 199–202.

Gawer, M., Sansonetti, A., and Mazliak, P. (1983). Lipid composition of tobacco cells cultivated at various temperatures. *Phytochemistry 22*:855–859.

Goldstein, W. E., Lasure, L. L., and Ingle, M. B. (1980). Product cost analysis. In *Plant Tissue Culture as a Source of Biochemicals* (E. J. Staba, ed.), CRC Press, Boca Raton, Fla., pp. 191–209.

Gregor, H. D. (1977). Lipids of *Daucus carota* cell suspension cultures. *Chem. Phys. Lipids 20*:77–85.

Halder, T. and Gadgil, V. N. (1983). Fatty acids of callus tissues of six species of *Cucurbitaceae*. *Phytochemistry 22*:1965–1967.

Hall, T. R. H. and Collin, H. A. (1975). Initiation and growth of tissue cultures of *Theobroma cacao*. *Ann. Bot. 39*:555–570.

Halperin, W. and Wetherell, D. F. (1964). Adventive embryony in tissue cultures of the wild carrot, *Daucus carota*. *Am. J. Bot. 51*:274–283.

Janick, J., Wright, D. C., and Hasegawa, P. M. (1982). *In vitro* production of cacao seed lipids. *J. Am. Soc. Horticult. Sci. 107*:919–922.

Jones, L. H. (1974). Plant cell culture and biochemistry: Studies for improved vegetable oil production. In *Industrial Aspects of Biochemistry* (B. Spencer, ed.), North-Holland Publ., Amsterdam, pp. 813–833.

Jones, L. H. (1984). Novel palm oils from cloned palms. *J. Am. Oil Chemists' Soc. 61*:1717–1719.

Kates, M., Wilson, A. C., and de la Roche, A. I. (1979). Lipid biosynthesis in plant cell cultures. In *Advances in the Biochemistry and Physiology of Plant Lipids* (L.-Å. Appelqvist and C. Liljenberg, eds.), Elsevier/North-Holland, Amsterdam, pp. 329–342.

Kleinig, H. and Kopp, C. (1978). Lipids, lipid turnover, and phospholipase D in plant suspension culture cells (*Daucus carota*). *Planta 139*: 61–65.

Laseter, J. L., Lawler, G. C., Walkinshaw, C. H., and Weete, J. D. (1973). Fatty acid of *Pinus elliottii* tissues. *Phytochemistry 12*: 817–821.

MacCarthy, J. J. and Stumpf, P. K. (1980). Fatty acid composition and biosynthesis in cell suspension cultures of *Glycine max* (L.) Merr., *Catharanthus roseus* G. Don and *Nicotiana tabacum* L. *Planta 147*: 384–388.

Muir, W. H. (1953). *Culture conditions favoring the isolation and growth of single cells from higher plants in vitro.* Ph.D. thesis, University of Wisconsin, Madison.

Muir, W. H., Hildebrandt, A. C., and Riker, A. J. (1954). Plant tissue cultures produced from single isolated plant cells. *Science 119*: 877–887.

Murashige, T. and Skoog, F. A. (1962). A revised medium for rapid growth and bioassays with tobacco tissue cultures. *Physiol. Plant. 15*: 473–497.

Nickell, L. G. (1956). The continuous submerged cultivation of plant tissues as single cells. *Proc. Nat. Acad. Sci. U.S.A. 42*: 848–850.

Nickell, L. G. (1980). Products. In *Plant Tissue Culture as a Source of Biochemicals* (E. J. Staba, ed.), CRC Press, Boca Raton, Fla., pp. 236–269.

Nobecourt, P. (1939). Sur la perennité et l'augmentation de volume des cultures de tissus végétaux. *C.R. Soc. Biol. Paris 130*: 1270–1271.

Nothelfer, H. G., Barckhaus, R. H., and Spener, F. (1977). Localization and characterization of the fatty acid synthesizing system in cells of *Glycine max* (soybean) suspension cultures. *Biochim. Biophys. Acta 489*: 370–380.

Pandey, B. and Gadgil, V. (1984). Fatty acids in callus cultures: Influence of growth factors on fatty acid composition of total lipids in callus cells. *Phytochemistry 23*: 51–53.

Pence, V. C., Hasegawa, P. M., and Janick, J. (1979). Asexual embryogenesis in *Theobroma cacao*. *J. Am. Soc. Horticult. Sci. 104*: 145–148.

Pence, V. C., Hasegawa, P. M., and Janick, J. (1980). Initiation and development of asexual embryos of *Theobroma cacao* L. *in vitro*. *Z. Pflanzenphysiol. 98*: 1–14.

Pence, V. C., Hasegawa, P. M., and Janick, J. (1981). Sucrose-mediated regulation of fatty acid composition in asexual embryos of *Theobroma cacao*. *Physiol. Plant.* *53*:378–384.

Radwan, S. S. and H. K. Mangold (1976). The lipids of plant cell cultures. *Adv. Lipid Res.* *14*:171–211.

Radwan, S. S. and Mangold, H. K. (1980). Biochemistry of lipids in plant cell cultures. *Adv. Biochem. Eng.* *16*:109–133.

Radwan, S. S., Mangold, H. K., and Spener, F. (1974). Lipids in plant tissue cultures III. Very long-chain fatty acids in the lipids of callus cultures and suspension cultures. *Chem. Phys. Lipids* *13*:103–107.

Radwan, S. S., Spener, F., and Mangold, H. K. (1975). Lipids in plant tissue cultures IV. The characteristic patterns of lipid classes in callus cultures and suspension cultures. *Chem. Phys. Lipids* *14*:72–80.

Radwan, S. S., Grosse-Oetringhaus, S., and Mangold, H. K. (1978). Lipids in plant tissue cultures. VI. Effect of temperature on the lipids of *Brassica napus* and *Tropaeolum majus* cultures. *Chem. Phys. Lipids* *22*:177–184.

Radwan, S. S., Mangold, H. K., Barz, W., and Husemann, W. (1979). Lipids in plant tissue cultures. VII: Reversible changes in the composition of lipids and their constituent fatty acids in response to alternate shifts in the mode of carbon supply. *Chem. Phys. Lipids* *25*:101–109.

Rajasekhar, E. W., Edwards, M., Wilson, S. B., and Steet, H. E. (1971). Studies on the growth in culture of plant cells. XI. The influence of shaking rate on the growth of suspension cultures. *J. Exp. Bot.* *22*:107.

Reinert, J. (1959). Über die Kontrolle der Morphogenese und die Induktion von Adventivembryonen an Gewebekulturen aus Karotten. *Planta* *53*:318–333.

Rose, D. and Martin, S. M. (1975). Growth of suspension cultures of plant cells (*Ipomoea* sp.) at various temperatures. *Can. J. Bot.* *53*:315–320.

Sahai, O. and Knuth, M. (1985). Commercializing plant tissue culture processes: Economics, problems and prospects. The technology of phytoproduction in plant tissue culture and process economics. *Biotechnol. Prog.* *1*:1–9.

Schwann, T. (1839). Mikroskopische Untersuchungen über die Übereinstimmung in der Struktur und dem Wachsthume der Thiere und Pflanzen. Berlin. Prilim. statement: Froriep's Notizen No. 91:103, 112. 1838.

Seabrook, J. E. A. (1980). Laboratory culture. In *Plant Tissue Culture as a Source of Biochemicals* (E. J. Staba, ed.), CRC Press, Boca Raton, Fla., pp. 1–20.

Shin, B. S., Mangold, H. K., and Staba, E. J. (1971). Lipids of selected plant tissue cultures. In *Les cultures de Tissues de Plantes*, Colloq. No. 193, Centre National de Recherches Scientifiques, Paris, pp. 51–69.

Siebertz, H. P., Heinz, E., and Bergmann, L. (1978). Acyl lipids in photosynthetically active tissue cultures of tobacco. *Plant Sci. Lett.* *12*:119–126.

Skoog, F. and Miller, C. O. (1957). Chemical regulation of growth and organ formation in plant tissues cultured *in vitro*. *Symp. Soc. Exp. Biol.* *11*:118–130.

Song, M. and Tattrie, N. (1973). Lipid composition of morning glory (*Ipomoea* sp.) cells grown in suspension cultures. *Can. J. Bot.* *51*:1893–1897.

Spener, F., Staba, E. J., and Mangold, H. K. (1974). Lipids in plant tissue cultures II. Unusual fatty acids in lipids of *Hydnocarpus anthelminthica* cultures. *Chem. Phys. Lipids* *12*:344–350.

Staba, E. J., Shin, E. J., and Mangold, H. J. (1971). Lipids in plant tissue cultures I. The fatty acid composition of triglycerides in rape and turnip rape cultures. *Chem. Phys. Lipids* *6*:291–295.

Stearns, Jr., E. M. and Morton, W. T. (1975a). Biosynthesis of fatty acids from acetate in soybean suspension cultures. *Lipids* *10*:597–601.

Stearns, Jr., E. M. and Morton, W. T. (1975b). Effects of growth regulators on fatty acids of soybeans suspension cultures. *Phytochemistry* *14*:619–622.

Steward, F. C. and Caplin, S. M. (1951). A tissue culture from potato tubers. The synergistic action of 2,4-D and coconut milk. *Science* *113*:518–520.

Steward, F. C. and Caplin, S. M. (1952). Investigations on growth and metabolism of plant cells. IV. Evidence on the role of the coconut-milk factor in development. *Ann. Bot.* *16*:491–504.

Steward, F. C., Mapes, M. O., and Mears, K. (1958). Growth and organized development of cultured cells. II. Organization in cultures grown from freely suspended cells. *Am. J. Bot.* *45*:705–708.

Street, H. E. (ed.), (1977a). In *Plant Tissue and Cell Culture*, University of California Press, Berkeley and Los Angeles, pp. 1–10.

Street, H. E. (1977b). The anatomy and physiology of morphogenesis. Studies involving tissue and cell cultures. In *La Culture des Tissus des Végétaux. Resultats Généaux et Realisations Pratiques* (R. J. Gautheret, ed.), Masson, Paris, pp. 20–33.

Stumpf, P. K. and Weber, N. (1977). Uptake and metabolism of fatty acids by soybean suspension cells. *Lipids 12*:120–124.

Tattrie, N. H. and Veliky, I. A. (1973). Fatty acid composition of lipids in various plant cell cultures. *Can. J. Bot. 51*:513–516.

Tomas, D. R. and Stobart, A. K. (1970). Lipids of tissue cultures of *Kalanchoe crenata. J. Exp. Bot. 21*:274–285.

Tsai, C. H. (1981). Composition and metabolism of lipids in callus and suspension cultures of cocoa beans (Theobroma cacao), Ph.D. thesis, Cornell University, Ithaca, N.Y.

Tsai, C. H. and Kisella, J. E. (1981). Initiation and growth of callus and cell suspension of *Theobroma cacao* L. *Ann. Bot. 48*:549–557.

Tsai, C. H. and Kinsella, J. E. (1982a). Tissue culture of cocoa beans (*Theobroma cacao* L.): Incorporation of acetate and laurate into lipids of cultured cells. *Lipids 17*:367–371.

Tsai, C. H. and Kinsella, J. E. (1982b). Tissue culture of cocoa bean (*Theobroma cacao* L.): Incorporation of fatty acids into lipids of cultured cells. *Lipids 17*:848–852.

Tsai, C. H., Wen, M. C., and Kinsella, J. E. (1982). Cocoabean tissue culture: Lipid composition and fatty acid metabolism. *J. Food Sci. 43*:768–773.

Turnham, E. and Northcote, D. H. (1982). The use of acetyl-CoA carboxylase activity and changes in wall composition as measures of embryogenesis in tissue cultures of oil palm (*Elaeis guineensis*). *Biochem. J. 208*:323–332.

Turnham, E. and Northcote, D. H. (1984). The incorporation of [1-^{14}C]acetate into lipids during embryogenesis in oil palm tissue cultures. *Phytochemistry 23*:35–39.

Veliky, I. A. (1977). Effect of pH on tryptophol formation by cultured *Ipomoea* sp. plant cells. *Lloydia 40*:482–486.

Veliky, I. A., Rose, D., and Zink, M. W. (1977). Uptake of magnesium by suspension cultures of plant cells (*Ipomoea* sp.). *Can. J. Bot. 55*:1143–1147.

Weber, N., Richter, I., Mangold, H. K., and Mukherjee, K. D. (1979). Positional specificity in the incorporation of isomeric cis- and transoctadecenoic acids into glycerolipids of cultured soya cells. *Planta 145*:479–485.

Wen, M. C., German, B., and Kinsella, J. E. (1984). Cocoa bean cell and embryo culture. *J. Am. Oil Chemists' Soc. 61*:1720–1724.

White, P. R. (1934). Potentially unlimited growth of excised tomato root tips in a liquid medium. *Plant Physiol. 9*:585–600.

White, P. R. (1939). Potentially unlimited growth of excised plant callus in an artificial medium. *Am. J. Bot. 26*:59–64.

Wilson, A. C., Kates, M., and de la Roche A. I. (1978). Incorporation of [1-^{14}C]acetate into lipids of soybean cell suspensions. *Lipids 13*:504–510.

Wright, D. C., Janick, J., and Hasegawa, P. M. (1983). Temperature effects on *in vitro* lipid accumulation in asexual embryos of *Theobroma cacao* L. *Lipids 18*:863–867.

Yano, I., Nichols, B. W., Morris, L. J., and James, A. T. (1972a). The distribution of cyclopropane and cyclopropene fatty acids in higher plants (Malvaceae). *Lipids* 7:30–34.

Yano, I., Morris, L. J., Nichols, B. W., and James, A. T. (1972b). The biosynthesis of cyclopropane and cyclopropene fatty acids in higher plants (Malvaceae). *Lipids* 7:35–45.

Zenk, M. H. (1978). The impact of plant cell culture on industry. In *Frontiers of Plant Tissue Culture* (T. A. Thorpe, ed.), University of Calgary Press, Calgary, pp. 1–13.

19

Cold-Adapted Enzymes from Fish

BENJAMIN K. SIMPSON and NORMAN F. HAARD* / Memorial University of Newfoundland, St. John's, Newfoundland, Canada

INTRODUCTION

Industrial Enzymes

The present-day use of enzymes as food processing aids is a continuing application of ancient technology. It is on record that the ancient Egyptians used yeast to bake bread some 4500 years ago, that the lactic acid bacteria have been used since time immemorial in making fermented milks and cheeses, and that molds have been used to make a variety of oriental fermented foods (Demain, 1981; Litchfield, 1983). Other examples include the utilization of papaw leaves to tenderize meat and the fermentation of fish by the action of endogenous proteases. Some of these traditional practices have been refined to the present-day uses of chymosin, α-amylase, and papain in the food industry. Proteases are the most extensively used enzymes in the food industry, where they act to improve the quality, stability, and solubility of foods as in baking, brewing, cheese making, and meat processing. Some of the attributes of enzymes which make them useful in industrial operations include the following: (1) They are derived from plant, animal, and microbial sources and are invariably nontoxic substances that are able to catalyze specific reactions; (2) they are active at very low concentrations under mild conditions of temperature and pH where undesirable side reactions are minimized; and (3) they can be inactivated after a desired effect has been achieved. Presently proteases from plant, animal, and microbial sources find extensive use as food

**Current affiliation*: University of California-Davis, Davis, California

Table 1. Applications of Proteolytic Enzymes in the Food Industry

Food	Purpose
Baked foods	Softening action in doughs, reduce mixing time, increase extensibility, improve texture and grain loaf volume, liberate β-amylase
Brewing	Body, flavor, and nutrient development during fermentation, aid in filtraton and clarification, chill proofing
Cereals	Increase drying rate of proteins, improve product handling characteristics, production of miso and tofu
Cheese	Coagulate casein, flavor development during aging
Chocolate, cocoa	Facilitate fermentation
Egg, egg products	Improve drying products
Feeds	Waste product conversion to feed, digestive aid
Fish	Solubilization of fish protein concentrates, recover oil or meat scraps from inedible parts
Legumes	Hydrolyzed protein products, remove flavor, plastein formation
Meats	Tenderization, recover proteins from bones
Milk	Coagulate rennet puddings, prepare soybean milk
Protein hydrolysates	Soy sauce, fish sauce, bouillon, dehydrated soups, gravy powders, processed meats, special diets
Antinutrients	Remove phytate, gossypol, nucleic acids, and enzyme inhibitors
Wine	Clarification, decrease foaming, promote malolactic fermentation

processing aids. Some of the applications of proteases in the food industry are summarized in Table 1.

Proteases from various sources differ in their catalytic and physical properties, and whether or not a particular enzyme would be suitable to use for a particular industrial application depends on several factors. For many uses, the specificity of the protease is of paramount importance. For example, even though many proteases have the capacity to clot milk, most of them are not suitable for cheese making because their broad hydrolytic specificity culminates in lower yields, loss of fat from the curd, and development of undesirable changes in texture and flavor during aging of the cheese. The relatively narrower specificity of chymosin for the hydrolysis of the phenylalanine–methionine bond of K-casein makes it the enzyme of choice for cheese making. Other applications, such as the production of plant protein hydrolysates, are best achieved by the use of proteases with a broad specificity. Some other factors of considerable importance in the selection of an enzyme for an industrial process include pH, temperature, response to inhibitors and activators, cost and availability of the enzyme and technical service support.

The greatest variety of industrial enzymes are presently derived from microbial sources, with a lesser diversity coming from plant and animal sources (Godfrey and Reichelt, 1983). Enzymes derived from plant sources and which are used extensively in the food industry include papain, bromelin, ficin, and amylases. Animal enzymes of economic importance include trypsins, lipases, and gastric proteases. In spite of the potential diversity that can be achieved by the use of microbial enzymes, very few species of microorganism are used to produce industrial enzymes. The cost of getting a microorganism approved by regulatory authorities is substantial, and few of these organisms have been stringently evaluated and accepted as safe. Proteolytic enzymes obtained from livestock offal currently do not adequately meet the demand on a world basis and the future availability of traditional enzyme sources is dependent on the political and agricultural policies that control the production of livestock for slaughter (Godfrey and Reichelt, 1983). Moreover, traditional animal enzyme sources have been restricted to relatively few species, namely, bovine and porcine offal.

Fishery

The problem of providing adequate protein for an ever-increasing world population is second only to the overall food problem (Altschul, 1962). The primary nutritional importance of protein is as a source of amino acids. The aquatic habitat offers tremendous potential in supplying the world's protein requirements. The management of the fishery industry and new product development using underutilized fish is a major concern of the world's leading fish-producing and fish-exporting countries. One of the natural accompaniments of the expanding fishing industry is the increased production of fish offal.

In Canada alone, today about half of the fish offal generated is used as fish meal, while the remainder represents a disposal and pollution problem. The utilization of such materials as sources of industrial enzymes would not curtail the availability of food material for human consumption. At the same time it would serve as a means of minimizing the waste disposal problem of the fishing industry, as well as recover valuable biochemicals, such as proteases, that could be used as food processing aids. There have been relatively few attempts to use fish proteases as industrial processing aids. Fish are poikilothermic and vary considerably in their feeding habits and temperature preferences, and it is to be expected that their digestive enzymes will also exhibit diversity.

The position taken in this chapter is that digestive enzymes from fish have sufficiently unique properties to justify their use over conventional sources of proteases in certain food processing operations. In particular, enzymes from cold-adapted fish exhibit two salient properties that make them attractive choices for certain applications: thermal instability and high molecular activity at low process temperatures. This discussion is restricted to the influence of temperature on the activity and stability of proteolytic enzymes. Advantage can be taken of thermostable enzymes in reactions that proceed at elevated temperatures, such as the use of papain in barbecue sauce for the tenderization of meat (Metz et al., 1975).

However, there may be hindrances associated with the use of heat-stable enzymes: (1) high energy costs associated with elevated process temperatures, (2) destruction of heat-labile essential components in food materials, (3) proliferation of undesirable microorganisms, (4) alteration of the physical integrity of the products, (5) enhancement of undesirable side reactions, and (6) inability to stop the reaction when the process desired is complete (Haard et al., 1982; Hultin, 1978). For example, the use of papain to tenderize ham can result in continued proteolysis in the canned product and undesirable texture softening and even soupy products. Excessive proteolysis can also result in flavor deterioration, giving rise to bitterness in cheese, plant protein extracts, or biological fish protein concentrates.

On account of the foregoing, thermal instability may be regarded as a desirable property of enzymes in certain food processing applications. Moreover, other temperature-related characteristics of proteolytic enzymes may be beneficial. For example, if the desired proteolytic reaction has a temperature coefficient Q_{10} of 1.5 and an associated undesirable side reaction (e.g., enzymatic browning or lipid oxidation) has a Q_{10} of 2.0, then by lowering the reaction temperature by 10°C the desired reaction rate would be reduced by only 1.5-fold while the undesirable reaction rate would be reduced by 2-fold. In this way the desired reaction rate can be accomplished under conditions that slow down undesirable reactions.

ENZYMIC COLD ADAPTION IN FISH

General Considerations

Several poikilothermic organisms are known to subsist at extremely low temperatures. For instance, certain fish like the Greenland cod (*Gadus ogac*) remain active and grow at temperatures as low as −2−2°C (Bobbitt and Akenhead, 1982), while fish from temperate waters undergo general anesthesia at such low temperatures. Studies aimed at (1) elucidating the biochemical properties of gastric proteases of fish acclimated to low-temperature habitats,—for example, the Arctic cod (*Boreogadus saida*), Greenland cod (*G. agac*), Atlantic cod (*Gadus morhua*), and American smelt (*Osmerus mordax*)—(2) exploiting some of these properties in certain food processing operations have been carried out. These fish were obtained from Newfoundland and Labrador and represent stocks having a temperature preference near 0°C. The body temperature of poikilothermic organisms is normally within 1°C of the ambient water temperature (Linthicum and Carey, 1972), which implies that the digestive enzymes of fish are fashioned such that they can effectively utilize food at the habitat temperature of the fish. Many factors are involved in the adaptation of organisms to low temperature (Conrad, 1983). Among these factors are subtle changes in the structure of enzyme proteins which lead to specialized functional capabilities. Nature has endowed cold-adapted poikilotherms with enzymes that are, in one way or another, more effective catalysts at lower temperatures than their homologs from organisms adapted to the warm environment. Findings on the differences in the catalytic and thermodynamic properties of enzymes from poikilotherms adapted to the cold environment versus their homologs from warm-temperature-adapted organisms have been made using intracellular enzymes of intermediary metabolism, and more recently with extracellular enzymes like digestive proteases. Poikilotherms adapted to cold temperatures exhibit enzymic adaptability in a variety of ways: (1) by increasing the levels or concentrations of enzymes present in the system, (2) by changing the type of enzyme present in the system, and (3) by evolutionary adaptability of preexisting enzymes (Somero, 1969; Hochacka and Somero, 1971). It is beyond the scope of this chapter to deal with the nature of all facets of enzymic adaption to the cold environment, nor is it our intent to explore the mechanism

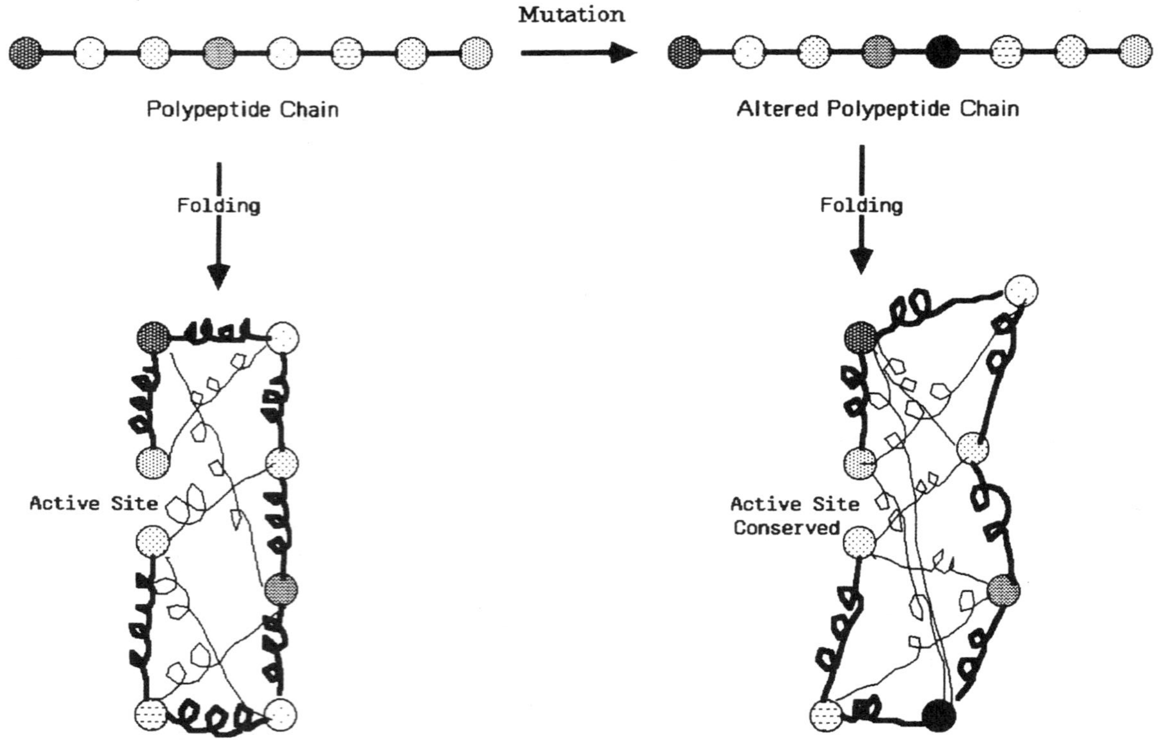

Fig. 1. Mutation–absorption paradigm. (Based on Conrad, 1983.)

of genotype transformation as relates to any given aspect of cold adaptability; rather, we will restrict this treatment to a discussion of the apparent outcome of the evolutionary adaptability of preexisting enzymes.

Molecular Adaptation: Genetic Basis

The essence of this mode of adaptability is that two versions of enzymes, E and E', may have the same physiological function; nevertheless, one may be more amenable to carrying out that function in a cold environment than the other. The conservation of a basic physiological function (e.g., specificity of trypsin for the hydrolysis of peptide bonds on the carboxyl side of arginine or lysine) together with the achievement of cold amenability would appear to be the result of appropriate alterations in the primary structure of the protein. Primary structure determines the distribution of possible tertiary structures in a given environment. It is apparent that subtle alterations in tertiary structure can allow for modification of certain aspects of function (e.g., binding constants or rate constants at a low reaction temperature) without loss of catalytic specificity. The ability of the molecule to buffer such change has been referred to as the mutation–absorption paradigm (Conrad, 1979). This model is represented simplistically with a ball and spring analogy in Figure 1. The balls represent amino acids, the springs on solid lines represent peptide bonds, and the springs on thin lines represent weak noncovalent bonds. The principle of graduated transformation of shape and function with stepwise changes in primary structure has been verified experimentally with a few enzymes, for example, alcohol dehydrogenases, where it has been demonstrated that point mutations give rise to slight changes in rate constants. While it is premature to relate the essence of how the detailed tertiary structure of an enzyme is related to cold adaptability, there is now considerable evidence pertaining to the phenotypic expression of enzymic cold adaptability.

Molecular Cold Adaptation: Enzymes

Enzymic properties affected include substrate binding affinity, thermodynamic properties, molecular activity at low temperatures, specificity, sensitivity to inhibitors and/or activators, and cold stability.

Substrate Binding Affinity

It has been the habit of various researchers to interprete K_m' as the dissociation constant (K_{diss}) for the enzyme–substrate complex. While this interpretation is only strictly valid when the reaction in question can be sufficiently described by the assumptions made under Michaelis–Menten kinetics, K_m' is nonetheless a valid index of

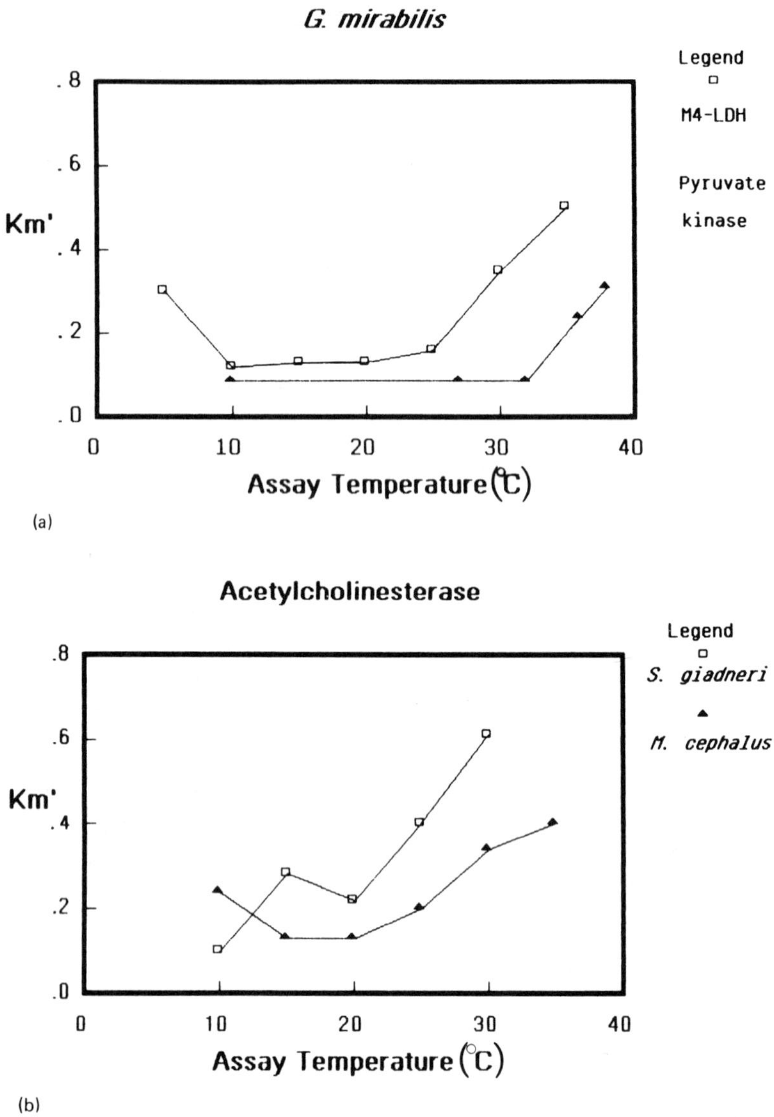

Fig. 2. Intracellular enzymes with temperature-dependent K_m' values. (a) Data from Somero (1973); (b) data from Baldwin (1971).

the sensitivity of a reaction to substrate concentration. This is because K'_m does represent the concentration of substrate required to attain half the maximum velocity, irrespective of whether K'_m represents a true K_{diss} or is merely a complex ratio of individual rate constants that have nothing to do with K_{diss}. In this discussion K'_m is used to represent substrate binding affinity.

The substrate binding affinity (K'_m) of enzymes is temperature dependent, (Cowey, 1967; Hazel and Prosser, 1974) and five types of relationships have been observed (Hultin, 1978). Examples of intracellular enzymes which exhibit temperature-dependent K'_m values are shown in Figure 2. For instance, the K'_m–temperature response curve for certain enzymes, such as phosphofructokinase from *Salmo gairdneri*, is U shaped, implying that such enzymes have definite minimum K'_m values (Somero and Hochacka, 1971). The temperature range at which the minimum K'_m occurs usually coincides quite closely with the natural habitat temperature of the organism. We shall refer to this type of K'_m–temperature response as the "type 1" response. Examples of other enzymes that show type 1 response include acetylcholinesterases from *S. gairdneri* (Baldwin and Hochacka, 1970) and *Mugil cephalus* and *Elops hawaiensis* (Baldwin, 1971). Other enzymes show "type 2, 3, 4, or 5" response where there is no defined minimum K'_m value. In the type 2 response K'_m does not increase or decrease with temperature and remains essentially constant. Examples of enzymes with the type 2 response include trypsins from *Salmo trutta, Rana amarus*, and *Tinca tinca* (Hofer et al., 1975). In the type 3 response K'_m continually increases with temperature at higher assay temperatures but is temperature insensitive at lower temperatures. This class of enzymes is exemplified by trypsins from *Salmo atra* and *Triturus alpestris* (Hofer et al., 1975), choline acetyltransferase from *Carassius auratus* (Hebb et al., 1972), and malate dehydrogenase from the garter snake, *Thamnophis sirtalis parietalis* (Hoskins and Aleksiuk, 1973). The type 4 response is where K'_m continually decreases with temperature at low assay temperatures but is insensitive at higher temperatures. This class is typified by trypsins from *Rana esculenta* and *Natrix tessellata* (Hofer et al., 1975) and acetylcholinesterase from tuna *Euthymus yaito* (Baldwin, 1971). The type 5 response is where the K'_m decreases at both high and low temperatures. Such enzymes appear to have a maximum K'_m where substrate binding would be expected to be lowest. The type 5 response has been observed with pyruvate kinase from rat (Somero, 1969). The type 1 and type 3 responses are perhaps the most commonly observed K'_m–temperature relationships.

The different binding of substrate to enzyme has been explained as follows: Enzyme–substrate interactions are stabilized by a set of weak bonds which exhibit opposing stability characteristics as a function of temperature. The formation of hydrogen bonds and

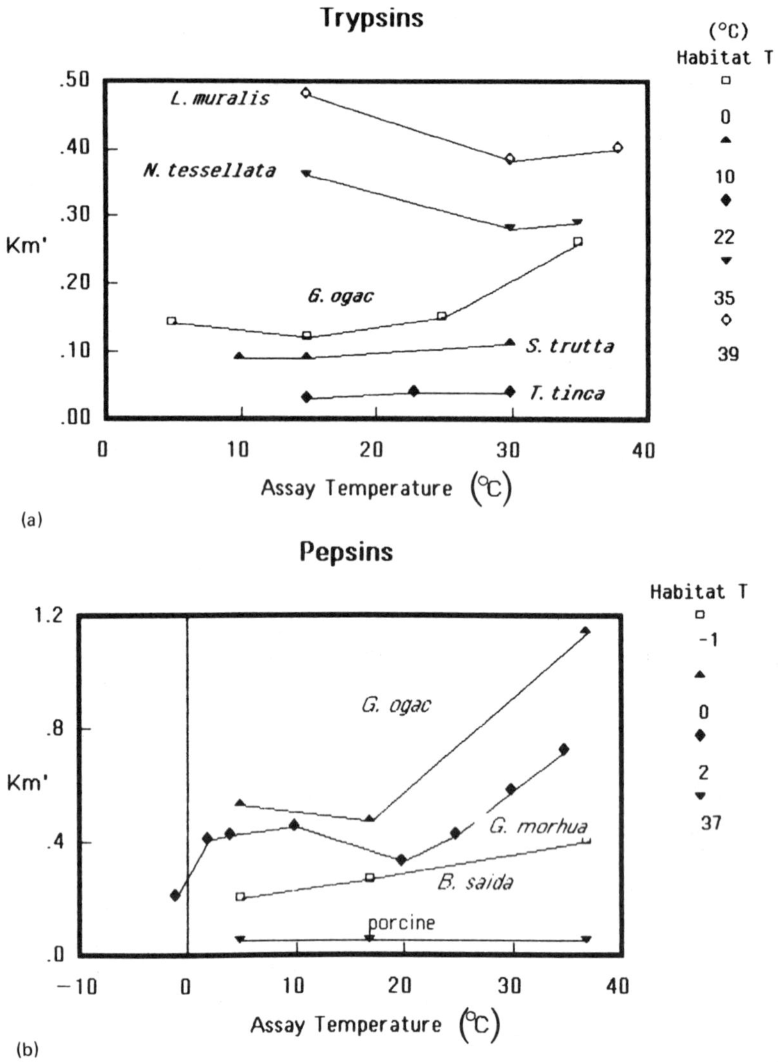

Fig. 3. Digestive enzymes with temperature-dependent K'_m values. (a) Data from Hofer et al. (1975), Simpson and Haard (1984); (b) data from Haard et al. (1982), Brewer et al. (1984), Arunchalam and Haard (1985).

electrostatic interactions proceed exothermically and will therefore be more important at low temperatures. However, hydrophobic bonds form endothermically and prevail at elevated temperatures. This is because, in order to achieve interaction of hydrophobic groups in an aqueous environment, the high order of structure of water molecules must be disrupted, a process which leads to an increase in the entropic factor in the free-energy change:

$$\Delta G^* = \Delta H^* - T \Delta S^*$$

As temperature is increased, the degree of disorderliness correspondingly increases and makes the entropic factor more important in lowering the free energy of formation to promote the reaction (Hochacka et al., 1975, 1976; Low and Somero, 1974, 1976; Somero, 1973). The positive correlation between K_m' and temperature in the case of poikilotherms is of adaptive value insofar as it ensures enhanced substrate binding at lower reaction temperatures, which leads to an increase in reaction rates and thereby nullifies the constraint that would have been imposed by the reduced thermal energy availability in the environment. Such an adaptation would be of functional value where substrate concentration in situ is less than "saturated" relative to enzyme concentration (as for intracellular enzymes of intermediary metabolism). Since digestive enzymes ordinarily function under reaction conditions of zero-order kinetics, it might be anticipated that modifications with respect to molecular activity might be more important than modification with respect to substrate binding affinity. Examples of digestive enzymes which exhibit a temperature-dependent K_m' are shown in Figure 3.

The substrate binding affinities for pepsins isolated from cold-adapted fish differ from that of porcine pepsin in two respects. While the fish pepsins showed type 3 K_m'—temperature response, porcine pepsin exhibited type 2 response in the temperature range investigated (Fig. 3). Salmon pepsins have also been shown to have much higher K_m' values for the hydrolysis of acylated hemoglobin than mammalian pepsins (Owen, 1968). Two isozyme forms of Arctic cod pepsin separated by affinity chromatography had marked differences in K_m' (Table 2). One isozyme form had a K_m' similar to that of porcine pepsin and a second had a very high K_m' with a correspondingly high V_{max}. It is not yet known whether other pepsin sources from cold water fish have a similar distribution of pepsin isozyme forms. The data are of interest because the high V_{max} from of pepsin may present a mechanism for rapid digestion when the stomach contents are high in protein. Such forms of pepsin have not been reported previously and may have utility where a high turnover under conditions of zero-order kinetics is advantageous, such as in the production of protein hydrolysates.

The K_m' values for Greenland cod and bovine trypsins are also different. The Greenland cod trypsin showed type 3 K_m'—temperature response, while its bovine counterpart exhibited type 2 response, similar to the observation made with the pepsins (Simpson, 1984).

Thermodynamic Properties

When products form from reactants in biological reactions, they do so by overcoming an "energy barrier," the free energy of activation

Table 2. Kinetic Parameters for Arctic Cod (*B. saida*) Isozymes of Pepsin[a]

Source	K'_m (mM)	V_{max} (min^{-1})
Crude pepsin	0.40	133
Pepsin A (pure)	0.06	31
Pepsin B (pure)	1.33	556

[a]Substrate was 2% acid-denatured hemoglobin with sodium acetate-HCl buffer.
Source: Data from Arunchalam and Haard (1985).

(ΔG^*). The ΔG^* determines the velocity of a given reaction ($\Delta G^* = -RT \ln k$), and enzymes catalyze biological reactions by reducing the energy barrier. It follows, therefore, that for any given set of enzymes capable of driving a given reaction, that enzyme which is most capable of reducing the energy barrier will be the most efficient catalyst. The ΔG^* is related to the enthalpy of activation (ΔH^*) and the entropy of activation (ΔS^*) by the relation $\Delta G^* = \Delta H^* - T\,\Delta S^*$. It is to be implied from the relationship that both entropy and enthalpy factors contribute to the overall energy barrier. Generally, biologists have used the energy of activation (E_a) as a measure of the energy barrier, and hence the capacity of enzymes to catalyze reactions (Low et al., 1973). Since E_a is only directly related to ΔH^* ($E_a = \Delta H^* + RT$), only when the contributions from entropy factors are the same for all enzymes driving a given reaction will comparisons of E_a be valid estimates of these enzymes' abilities to reduce the energy barrier to facilitate overall reaction. However, E_a may be used together with substrate turnover numbers (V_{max}) to make reliable predictions of enzyme efficiencies, since V_{max} is related to the rate constant k, and hence to ΔS^* by the following relationships:

1. $k\ (sec^{-1}) = V_{max}/\text{mg enzyme} \times \text{mol. wt.} \times 1\ \text{min}/60\ \text{sec}$
2. $\Delta S^* = 4.576\ (\log k - 10.753 - \log T + E_a/4.576T)$

It has been demonstrated from thermodynamic parameters that cold-adapted poikilothermic enzymes are more efficient catalysts at cold assay temperatures than their homologs derived from homoiothermic species, as well as other warm-temperature-adapted poikilothermic organisms. For instance, Figure 4 summarizes thermodynamic parameters for an intracellular and an extracellular enzyme-catalyzed reaction and indicates that homologous enzymes from organisms adapted to different temperature regimes have ΔG^* values that are correlated with their respective habitat temperatures. However, the ΔH^* and ΔS^* values may differ considerably for homologous enzymes (Fig. 5). Similarly E_a values vary with the temperature preference of the organism from which the enzyme was derived (Fig. 6). Likewise, the E_a values for Greenland cod trypsin ranged from 5.8 to 8.5 kcal/mol and were considerably lower than values obtained for bovine trypsin, 11.2–13.4 kcal/mol (Simpson and Haard, 1984a).

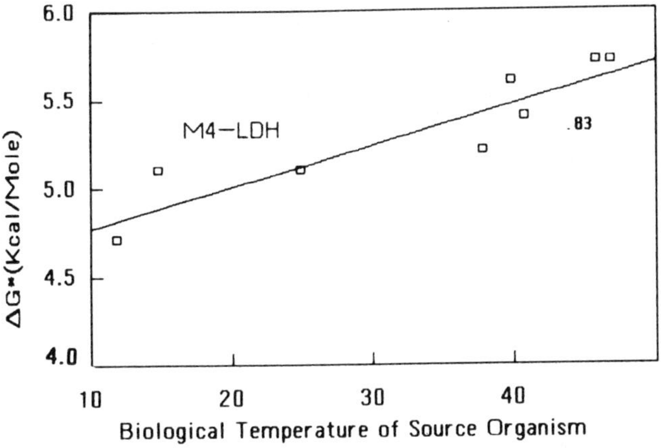

(a)

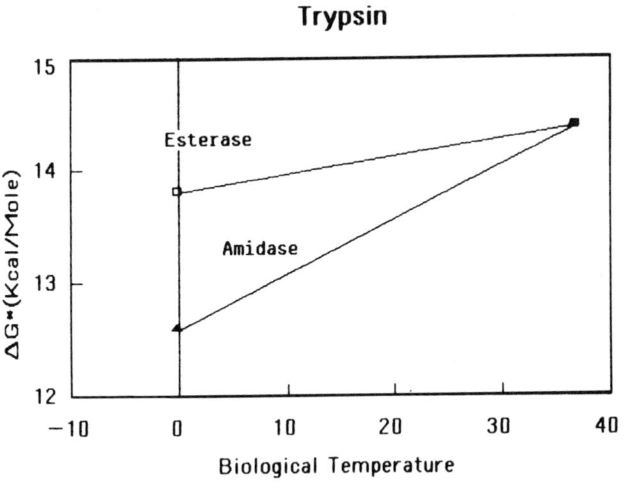

(b)

Fig. 4. Thermodynamic parameters for an intracellular and an extracellular enzyme-catalyzed reaction. (a) Data from Hochatchka et al. (1976); (b) data from Simpson and Haard (1984).

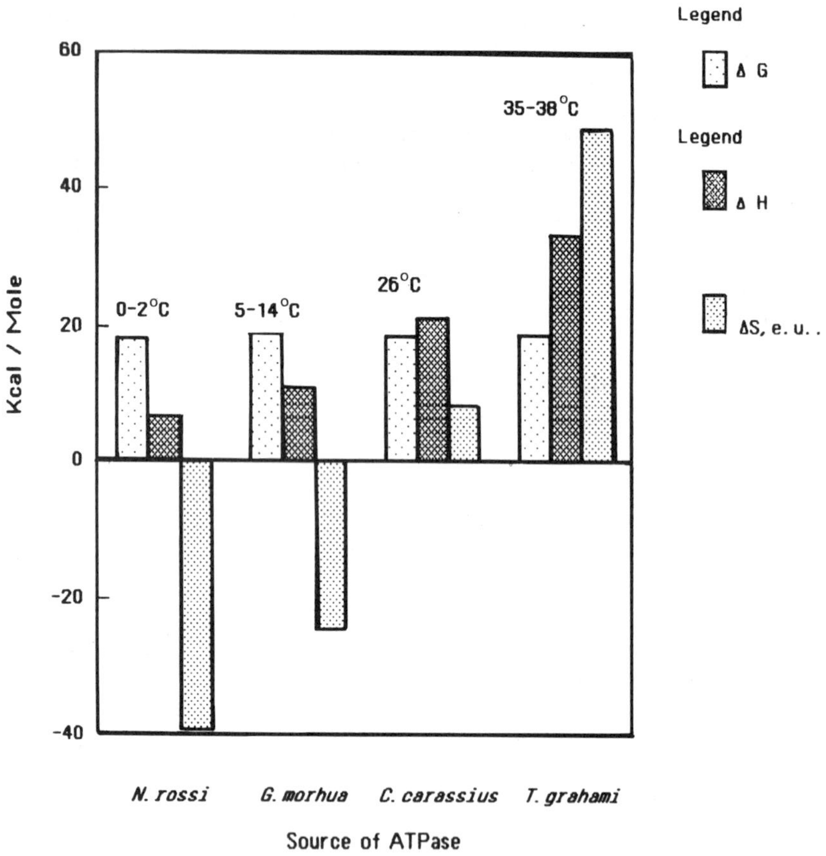

Fig. 5. Values of ΔH^* and ΔS^* for homologous enzymes. Fish from different environmental temperatures. Data from Hultin (1978).

Molecular Activity

For an enzyme to improve its performance at low temperatures, it has to either enhance its substrate binding capacity at low reaction temperatures or change its molecular activity, that is, its capacity to transform reactants to products. A large percentage of cold-adapted poikilothermic enzymes investigated generally have higher molecular activities than their homologs derived from warm-temperature-adapted organisms (Low and Somero, 1976; Simpson and Haard, 1984a; Somero and Low, 1976).

It also follows from the relationship $\Delta G^* = -RT \ln k$ that those enzymes that greatly reduce ΔG^* at lower reaction temperatures will have correspondingly higher reaction velocities at such temperatures.

The greater catalytic efficiency of enzymes from cold-adapted poikilotherms at low reaction temperatures has been attributed to the relatively more flexible structures of those enzymes which permit them to undergo conformational changes that favor higher reaction rates (Somero, 1975). The temperature coefficients Q_{10} for the hydrolysis of substrates by enzymes derived from cold-adapted organisms have also been demonstrated to be lower than those of their counterparts adapted to the warm environment (Cowey, 1967). It has also been amply demonstrated that there exists an inverse relationship between the catalytic efficiency of homologous enzymes derived from

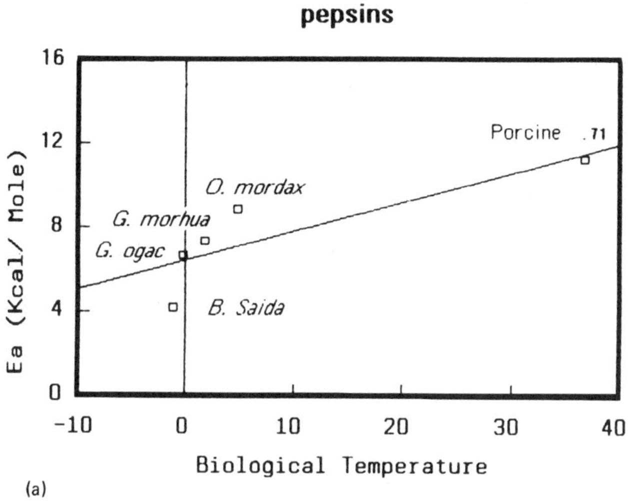

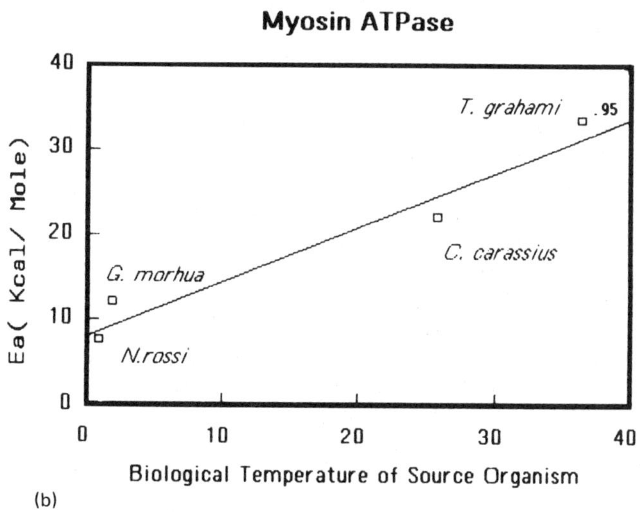

Fig. 6. Values of E_a versus temperature. (a) Data from Haard et al. (1982); (b) data from Hultin (1978).

Table 3. Molecular Efficiency of Bovine and Cod Trypsins

	$TN^a \times 10^2$ (at 25°C)			Physiological efficiency $\times 10^3$		
Enzyme source	Amidase	Esterase	Amidase/ esterase	Amidase	Esterase	Amidase/ esterase
Greenland cod	2.10	1.40	0.18	0.18	98.00	1.22
Bovine	0.30	0.29	0.03	0.03	182.60	0.13

[a] TN, turnover number.
Source: Data from Simpson and Haard (1984a).

organisms adapted to different temperature regimes and the habitat temperature of the organisms from which they are derived (Kaplan, 1965; Koffler et al., 1957; Light et al., 1969; Ushakov, 1967). Table 3 compares the molecular activities of trypsins derived from Greenland cod and ox at 25°C. The substrate turnover number for esterase and amidase reactions are greater for Greenland cod trypsin than bovine trypsin at all assay temperatures examined (Simpson and Haard, 1984a). Also, the cod enzyme is relatively more active as an amidase than as an esterase than is bovine trypsin. Hence the V_{max} data are consistent with the thermodynamic parameters, since both lines of study indicate that enzymes derived from cold-adapted poikilotherms are more efficient than their homologs derived from homoiothermic species.

Physiological Efficiency

The "physiological efficiency" of an enzyme has been defined as the ratio of its substrate turnover number to its substrate binding affinity, that is, V_{max}/K'_m (Fullbrook, 1983; Mihalyi, 1978; Pollock, 1965). This means that for a group of enzymes capable of catalyzing the transformation of a particular substrate to product(s), the enzyme with the highest V_{max}/K'_m ratio would be the most efficient to use to transform the substrate to product(s).

The relatively high K'_m and V_{max} values for Greenland cod trypsin appears to be compensatory, since the physiological efficiency (V_{max}/K'_m) of the two trypsins are similar at 5°C (Simpson and Haard, 1984a). However, at higher assay temperatures bovine trypsin exhibited greater physiological efficiency for the esterase reaction than the cod enzyme and lower efficiency for the amidase reaction (Table 3).

Temperature Optima and Thermostability

Findings from thermostability studies lend support to the theory of evolutionary adaptation to various thermal environments. With enzymes there generally is a direct relationship between the habitat temperature of the organism from which the enzyme is derived and the thermal stability of the enzyme. Investigation of the thermal stabilities of adolases, alkaline phosphatases, adenylate kinases, and cholinesterases derived from poikilotherms indicate that the enzymes derived from thermophiles tend to be more heat stable than their mesophilic counterparts (Ushakov, 1967). Additionally, the temperature optima for enzymes derived from various organisms are correlated with the habitat temperature of the organism (Abrahamson and Maher, 1967; Baslow and Nigrelli, 1964; Koffler et al., 1957).

Data supporting the hypothesis that there is a direct relationship between the thermal stability of an enzyme and the cell temperature of the organism it is derived from are also presented in Table 4. The temperature optima for pepsins from cold-adapted fish tend to be approximately 15°C lower than that reported for pepsins from mammalian organisms. The temperature stability of pepsins is also influenced by pH, so that there is greater instability observed at higher pH values. For example, Greenland cod pepsin loses 50% activity at pH 6.5 and 25°C in 60 min. On the other hand, the pepsinogen forms are stable at temperatures up to 45°C, even at neutral pH. Furthermore, Greenland cod trypsin is inactivated at temperatures greater than 40°C, whereas under the same conditions its bovine counterpart is stable up to 80°C. As cold-adapted enzymes are relatively easier to inactivate by heat, so are their zymogens relatively easy to activate. Figure 7 shows that fish pepsinogen activates several times faster at lower temperatures than its porcine counterpart (Squires et al., 1986a).

Structural Properties

Enzymic properties such as V_{max}, K'_m, temperature optimum, thermostability, and specificity are determined to a large extent by the primary structure of the particular enzyme. As the primary structures of proteins are genetically determined, they are subject to variation by the agency of mutation. The observation that the relative contributions of ΔH^* and ΔS^* to ΔG^* differs considerably for variants of the same enzymes derived from organisms adapted to different temperature regimes discussed earlier on has led to the inference that the probable basis for the observed differences must lie in the internal structures of the proteins (Somero, 1969). The greater V_{max} values of cold-adapted poikilothermic enzymes versus their warm-temperature-adapted homologs has been imputed to the relatively more flexible structures of the cold-adapted enzymes (Somero, 1975).

Table 4. Temperature Optima and Thermostability of Homologous Enzymes from Organisms Adapted to Different Temperatures

Enzyme	Source	Biological temperature (°C)	Temperature optimum (°C)	T_m (°C)
Pyruvate kinase[b]	Chicken	39	—	60
	Rabbit	37	—	62
	Mullet	18–30	—	58
	Toad	25–32	—	57
	Marine teleost	8–17	—	55
	Shark	8–17	—	52
	Rainbow trout	4–15	—	56
	Lobster	8–15	—	50
	Abalone	8–15	—	45
Pepsin[c]	Porcine	37	47	50
	Arctic cod	−2–2	32	32
	Atlantic cod	0–5	32	30
	Greenland cod	−2–2	30	30
	American smelt	5–10	30	35
Trypsin[d]	Bovine	37	45	80+
	Greenland cod	−2–2	30–35	40
Trypsin[e]	Bovine	37	50	—
	Greenland cod	−2–2	40	—
Ca^{2+}–ATPase[f]	Bluefin tuna	—	—	35
	Flatfish	—	—	32
	Mackerel	—	—	31.3
	Alaska pollack	—	—	26.4

[a] T_m values are taken as the temperatures at which heat inactivation of the enzyme began.
[b] Data from Low and Somero (1976).
[c] pH 1.9; data from Haard et al. (1982), Brewer et al., (1984), and Squires et al., (1986b).
[d] Benzoyl-DL-arginine p-nitroanilide (pH 8.2) as substrate; data from Simpson and Haard (1984a).
[e] With 2% casein as substrate; data from Simpson and Haard (1984b).
[f] For this enzyme T_m is defined as the temperature at which there is 50% inactivation of enzyme; data from Potter (1974).

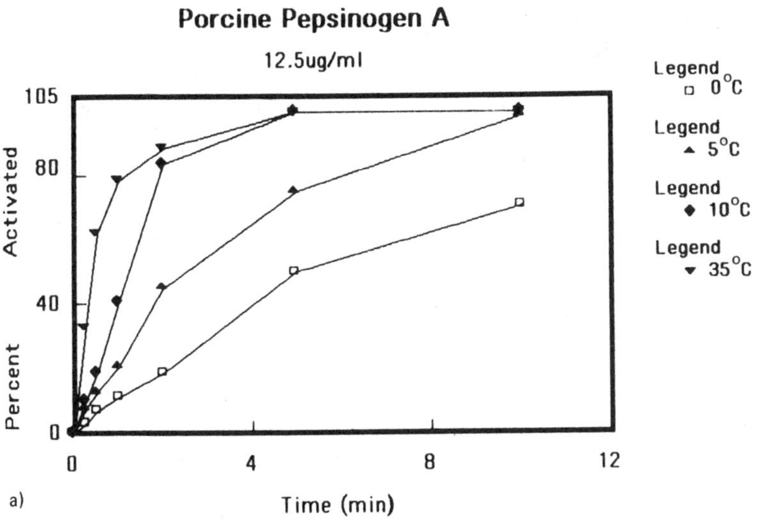

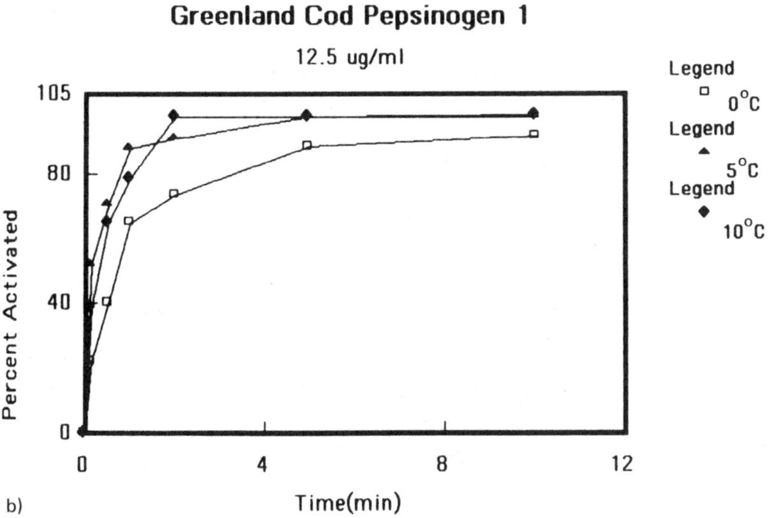

Fig. 7. Activation of fish and porcine pepsinogen. Data for (b) from Squires, Haard, and Feltham (1985).

Until recently the statements pertaining to the structures of the protein molecules from different temperature regimes were only highly plausible speculations deduced from indirect evidence such as amino acid composition and average hydrophobicity data. For example, it has been demonstrated that proteins from thermophilic organisms have distinctly higher hydrophobicities than their mesophilic counterparts (Bigelow, 1967; Hazel and Prosser, 1974). It has also been speculated that when organisms evolved from colder environments to inhabit relatively warmer habitats, they sacrificed some of the catalytic potential of their enzymes for increased thermal stability of their proteins to be able to survive. Such an adaptation would probably have been achieved through nonlethal mutations. The greater stability of proteins from thermophilic organisms has been attributed to greater hydrogen bonding (Koffler, 1957) more extensive hydrophobic interactions (Singleton and Amelunxen, 1973), and more pronounced disulfide linkages (Komatsu and Feeney, 1970).

However, a more recent study of the CD spectra of trypsins have borne out these speculations on the differences in the internal structure of proteins from different temperature regimes (Simpson and Haard, 1984b). At temperatures ranging from 0.2 to 35.3°C, Greenland cod trypsin contains 7.3–7.8% α-helix and 92.2–92.7% random coils, whereas bovine trypsin contains 11.5–12% α-helix and 88–89.5% random coils in this temperature range. Other lines of evidence supporting the fact that Greenland cod trypsin has a less-ordered structure than bovine trypsin have come from (1) their amino acid compositions, which indicates that Greenland cod trypsin has only 8 cysteine residues, as opposed to 12 in bovine trypsin. This means that, unlike bovine trypsin, which has six disulfide linkages, Greenland cod trypsin has only 4 potential disulfide pairs (Simpson and Haard, 1984b), (2) The average hydrophobicity ($H\Phi_{ave}$) of Greenland cod trypsin (0.86 kcal/residue) is lower than that of bovine trypsin (1.04 kcal/residue) (Simpson and Haard, 1984b). This observation also indicates that the contribution of hydrophobic interactions to the structural stability of trypsins is greater for bovine trypsin than Greenland cod trypsin, (3) The amidase and esterase activities of both trypsins are inhibited by the thiol reagents, 2-mercaptoethanol and dithioerythritol; however, the cod enzyme is more susceptible to inhibition by these reagents than bovine trypsin (Simpson and Haard, 1984b). This observation supports the amino acid composition data, which show that there are fewer potential disulfide pairs in the cod enzyme than in its bovine counterpart.

APPLICATIONS

Some of the properties of cold-temperature-adapted enzymes, such as thermal instability and higher molecular activity at low reaction temperatures, may be exploited in certain food processing operations. For example, cold-adapted gastric proteases and trypsins have been used to prepare cheese and prevent oxidized flavor development in raw milk, respectively, on a laboratory scale to exploit their lower thermal instability. Trypsin from a cold-adapted organism has also been used in fish fermentations to take advantage of its relatively higher molecular activity at low temperatures.

Preparation of Cheddar Cheese

Within the past 20 years there has been increasing concern over the short supply of chymosin needed in the production of various types of cheese. Traditionally the abomasum of suckling calves has been used as a source of chymosin. This enzyme is of special value in cheese making, because it converts the colloidal milk casein into a curd in such a way as to give high yields and desirable proteolysis in the aged cheese. Nearly all proteolytic enzymes will clot milk under appropriate conditions (Berridge, 1951). However, few enzymes are found to be adequate when the yield of curd, rheological properties of the cheese, off-flavor, and price are considered (de Koning, 1978). Most proteases are inferior to chymosin for cheese making because of their broader specificity for protein substrates. Excessive proteolysis during curding and subsequent steps in the cheese making operation lead to the above-mentioned deficiencies of the product. Given that gastric proteases from marine organisms are relatively unstable at temperatures above 30°C (see Table 4), it follows that it may be possible to rennet milk and subsequently heat-denature the coagulating enzyme during subsequent steps in the cheese making process. Recent studies have shown it is possible to prepare a satisfactory cheddar cheese with Atlantic cod pepsin as a rennet agent (Brewer et al., 1984). However, when the conventional cheddar cheese process is employed, there is somewhat more loss of fat and protein to the whey fraction (Table 5), indicating that additional protein degradation occurs during curd formation and the early stage of cheddaring.

The high molecular activity of fish pepsins at low reaction temperatures (Fig. 6) also occurs when milk is treated to initiate the clotting process (Fig. 8 and Table 6). The enzymic phase of milk clotting, involving hydrolysis of the phenylalanine—methionine bond of K-casein, can be separated from the nonenzymic phase, involving transformation from a sol to a gel, by carrying out the process at a temperature below 10°C (Fig. 9). Cold renneting of milk with a catalyst having a low temperature coefficient for the enzyme (see Table 6) can be accomplished with lower enzyme concentration, thereby conserving rennet and minimizing the presence of residual curd pepsin. An experiment where milk was treated with Atlantic cod pepsin showed that whereas nonprotein nitrogen (NPN) continued to increase after the enzymic phase of coagulation at 0°C, NPN did not increase when the milk temperature was increased to 39°C, thus causing clot formation and inactivation of the cod pepsin (Fig. 10).

Table 5. Analysis of Cheese and Whey Fractions

Clotting enzyme	Cheese wet weight[a] (g)	Cheese dry weight[a] (g)	Cheese (% fwb)		Whey (% fwb)	
			Fat	Protein	Fat	Protein
Chymosin	953.9	554.2	32.5	14.9	0.22	0.77
Porcine pepsin	914.0	503.6	29.9	13.9	0.25	0.79
Cod pepsin	956.1	569.8	26.6	14.2	0.36	0.86

[a] Yield of cheese from 8 liters of milk. All operations were the same, except for the clotting enzymes employed.
[b] Data normalized to 40% moisture content.
Source: Data from Brewer et al. (1984).

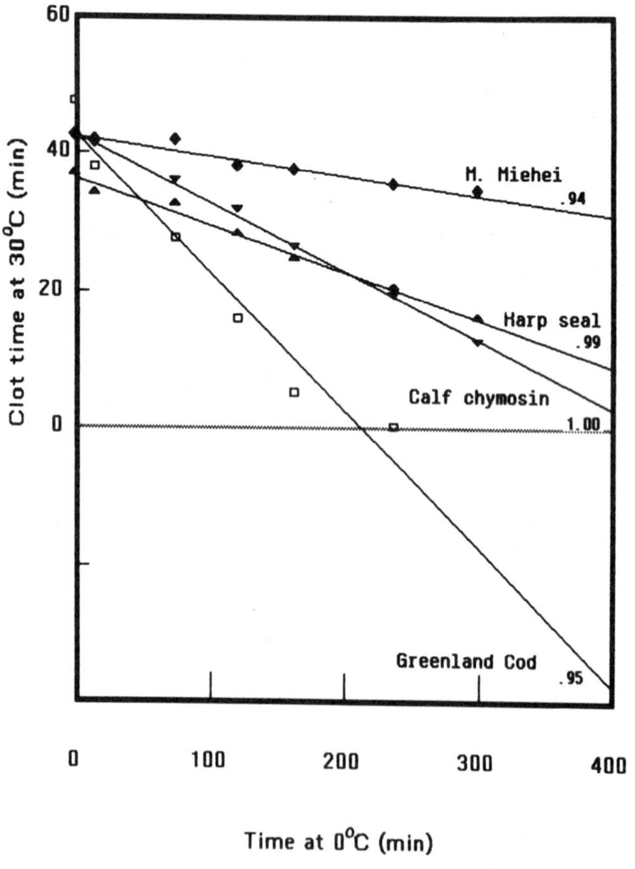

Fig. 8. Fish pepsin molecular activity.

Table 6. Temperature Coefficient for Milk Clotting

Enzyme source	Q_{10}
Mucor miehei	2.8
Calf chymosin	2.2
Calf rennet	2.0
Porcine pepsin	2.1
Harp seal protease	2.2
Greenland halibut	2.0
Redfish	1.9
Atlantic cod	1.7
Greenland cod	1.6
Thorny skate	1.6
Polar cod	1.4

Thus it appears that advantage can be taken of the catalytic activity at low temperature as well as the thermal instability of cod pepsin for the preparation of cheddar cheese. The cold rennet process has been employed successfully for the preparation of laboratory scale batches of cheddar cheese (Table 7).

Oxidized Flavor in Milk

Previous studies have indicated that the treatment of milk with bovine trypsin can prevent oxidized flavor in milk (Lim and Shipe, 1972). An experiment was designed to determine the efficiency of Greenland cod trypsin in preventing oxidized flavor with subsequent inactivation by pasteurization. That is, owing to the thermal instability of Greenland cod trypsin compared to bovine trypsin, the former enzyme can be inactivated by relatively mild heat treatments. The results of this experiment are summarized in Table 8. Both trypsins were similarly effective in preventing the oxidation of lipids at concentrations greater than 0.0013%; however, only the cod trypsin, and not bovine trypsin, was completely inactivated by the pasteurization process employed. Accordingly, there is an advantage in utilizing the trypsin from a cold-adapted fish, owing to its thermal instability, since residual enzyme would not be present to cause subsequent hydrolysis of milk proteins.

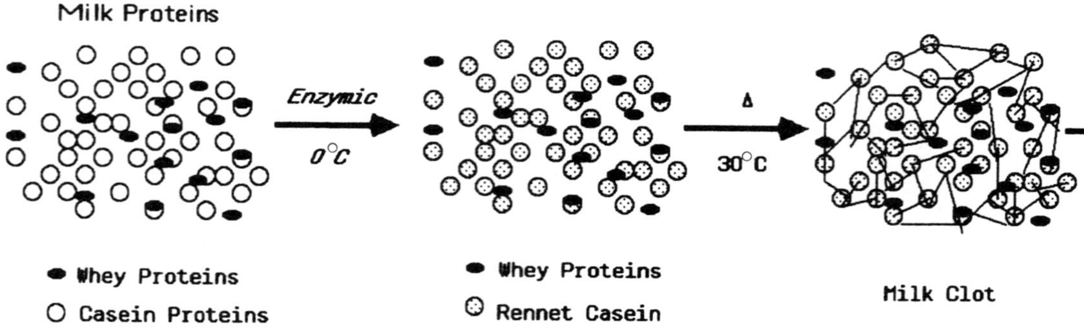

Fig. 9. Separation of the enzymic and nonenzymic phases of milk clotting.

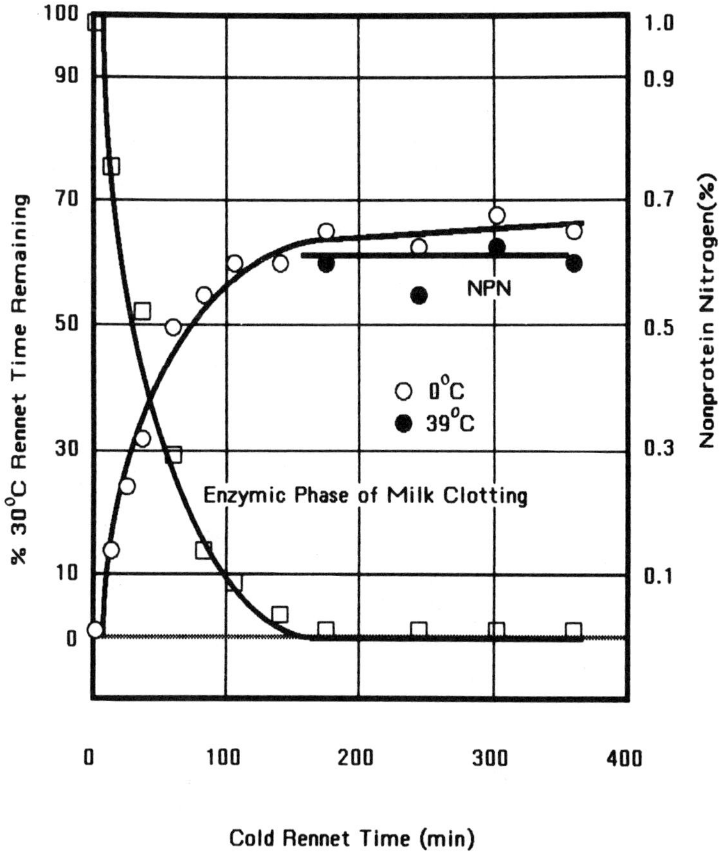

Fig. 10. Inactivation of cod pepsin in milk.

Fermentations

Attempts have also been made to exploit the relatively high molecular activity of cod trypsin at low temperatures by incorporating the enzyme into herring fermentations that proceed at 10°C. The preparation of brine-fermented round herring (matjes) is limited to certain seasons (usually spring) because of the balance of digestive enzymes in the fish at this time. Other studies have indicated that trypsin is an important component in matje fermentation (Orejana and Liston, 1982; Ritskes, 1971). Accordingly, an experiment was designed to compare the efficiency of bovine and Greenland cod trypsins in accelerating the fermentation of herring.

Table 7. Sensory Evaluation of Cheddar Cheese Prepared by Cold Rennet

Cheddar flavor intensity rank[a]	Sample	Process	Aging at (10°C (months)
1_a	Sobeys's (old)	Conventional	12–24
2_b	Sobeys's (medium)	Conventional	6–12
3_c	Sobeys's (mild)	Conventional	3–6
4_d	Cod pepsin	Cold rennet	3
5_e	Cod pepsin	Conventional	3
1_a	Kraft (old)	Conventional	12–24
$2_{a,b}$	Cod pepsin	Cold rennet	6
3_c	Kraft (medium)	Conventional	6–12
4_d	Cod pepsin	Conventional	6
5_e	Porcine pepsin	Conventional	6

[a] Numbers followed by the same letter are not significantly different ($p < 0.05$).

Table 8. Prevention of Oxidized Flavor in Milk by Trypsins

Sample	TBA no.[a]			Trypsin retained (%)
	24 hr	74 hr	288 hr	
Control	0.020	0.051	0.052	—
+ $CuCl_2$	0.033	0.064	0.067	—
+ $CuCl_2$; bovine trypsin[c]	0.012	0.018	0.002	47
+ $CuCl_2$; cod trypsin[c]	0.012	0.016	0.023	0

[a] The TBA no. is the thiobarbituric acid number, a measure of lipid oxidation; $CuCl_2$ (1 ppm) was added to milk samples to accelerate lipid oxidation.

[b] Milk was pasteurized at 70°C for 45 min after trypsin treatment.

[c] Trypsin (pure) was added at 0.005% of milk.

Source: Data from Simpson and Haard (1984c).

Table 9. Increase in Total and TCA-Soluble Proteins in Matjes

Herring	Trypsin added	Time[a] 6 days	12 days	18 days
Round	—	8.4	12.1 (66)	20.6 (49)
Gutted	—	3.1	6.9 (39)	11.1 (35)
Gutted	Bovine	3.3	9.0 (33)	13.0 (34)
Gutted	Cod	6.9	12.2 (30)	17.2 (37)

[a] Numbers in parentheses are the percentage of $A_{280\ nm}$ material soluble in 10% trichloroacetic acid (TCA). Fermentation was at 10°C in 10.6% salt, 2.22% sucrose, 0.03% sodium nitrate, and 0.29% benzoic acid.
Source: Data from Simpson (1984) and Simpson and Haard (1984c).

Removal of viscera from herring prior to fermentation reduced the formation of brine-soluble proteins and peptides (Table 9). Round herring had approximately twice the amount of protein in the brine as did gutted herring after 48 days. This demonstrates the need for viscera enzymes for normal matje fermentation. The characteristic flavor of matjes is due to soluble peptides and amino acids. Supplementing the fermentation of gutted herring with equivalent amounts of pure bovine and Greenland cod trypsins resulted in increased solubilization of protein. While the cod enzyme was effective in solubilizing protein, the percentage of solubilized protein which was soluble in 10% trichloroacetic acid (TCA) was substantially lower than the conventional matjes prepared with round herring. A summary of the major taste-active amino acids in matjes is shown in Table 10.

Similarly, the free amino acid concentration in conventional matjes (round) was twice that in the matjes prepared with eviscerated fish. Supplementation with trypsins resulted in increased free amino acid accumulation, notably in lysine and leucine. However, bovine trypsin appeared to be somewhat more effective than cod trypsin in promoting free amino acid accumulation. This was unexpected, since the data (Table 9) indicate that the cod enzyme is more active at the fermentation temperature employed. It would appear that the interplay between trypsin action and endogenous peptidase activity is complex.

Table 10. Major Taste-Active Amino Acids and Total Amino Acids in Matjes

Herring	Trypsin added	Tau	Ala	Gly	Leu	Ser	Arg	Lys	Total
Round	—	16.7	16.3	12.0	11.1	9.8	9.8	9.8	160
Gutted	—	12.8	0.4	8.5	5.9	4.7	3.1	6.8	78
Gutted	Bovine	10.0	10.7	10.4	13.0	7.1	9.2	13.9	135
Gutted	Cod	9.9	9.8	8.8	11.6	6.0	7.7	12.4	120

Source: Data from Simpson and Haard (1984c).

Sensory evaluation of the product by an unbiased panel was not supportive of the beneficial role of trypsin in supplementing matje fermentation with gutted herring (Table 11). While panelists preferred conventional matjes over herring which had been eviscerated prior to fermentation, they tended to rank trypsin-supplemented samples lower than the blander eviscerated control. The data indicate that other gut proteases and enzymes may be necessary to achieve a balanced flavor and texture. The data do, however, demonstrate the higher molecular activity of cold-adapted trypsin over bovine trypsin in solubilizing protein during low-temperature fermentation. It has also been shown that when squid was fermented with supplements of Greenland cod trypsin or bovine trypsin at 4°C, the cod enzyme is advantageous because of its higher molecular activity at the low fermentation temperature. In this case supplementation of the fermentation with trypsin improved the sensory score (Table 12).

Table 11. Sensory Evaluation of Matjes[a]

Herring	Trypsin added	Odor	Texture	Taste
Round	—	5.9	6.2	5.2
Gutted	—	6.0	5.5	4.7
Gutted	Bovine	4.6	4.8	3.5
Gutted	Cod	4.8	4.8	4.3

[a] Panelists were asked to rank coded samples on a 9 (excellent) to 1 (dislike) scale.

Table 12. Fermentation of Squid with Greenland Cod Trypsin Supplementation[a]

Treatment	Ala	Pro	Leu	Glu	Arg	Lys	Ser	Total	Sensory score[b] (overall taste)
No enzyme	16.2	12.9	11.6	11.5	9.0	8.1	6.3	75.6	5.9
Cod trypsin	20.9	16.2	16.5	16.4	13.0	13.4	7.9	104.3	6.7

[a] Fermentation was carried out as described in Table 9 at 4°C for 120 days.
[b] Sensory scores are on a 9 (excellent) to 1 (unacceptable) scale for taste preference.
Source: Data from Lee et al. (1982).

SUMMARY

The foregoing indicates that digestive proteolytic enzymes from cold-adapted fish possess unique properties when compared to mammalian proteases. It has been demonstrated that advantage may be taken of the thermal instability of these enzymes in certain food process operations where residual protease activity is undesirable. It has also been demonstrated that their high molecular activity at low temperatures may be used to advantage in low-temperature fermentations where proteolysis is desirable. This discussion demonstrates possible uses of fish processing wastes as industrial enzymes. In other areas of the world, such as in tropical waters, the digestive enzymes in fish offal may possess properties linked to high habitat temperature adaptation. The property may also be of use in different food and feed processing applications. Moreover, other classes of digestive enzymes from fish offal, such as lipases and carbohydrases, may also possess sufficiently unique properties to justify their use in certain situations. It is our belief that there exists an enormous potential for the recovery and use of enzymes from fish processing wastes.

REFERENCES

Abrahamson, Y. and Maher, M. (1967). The effect of temperature upon pancreatic amylase in selected reptiles and amphibians. *Can. J. Zool.* *45*:227–232.

Altschul, A. M. (1962). Seed proteins and world food problems. *Econ. Bot.* *16*:2–13.

Arunchalam, K. and Haard, N. F. (1985). Isolation and characterization of pepsin from polar cod (*Boreogadus saida*). *Comp. Biochem. Physiol.* *80*B:467–473.

Baldwin, J. (1971). Adaptation of enzymes to temperature: Acetylcholinesterase in the central nervous system of fishes. *Comp. Biochem. Physiol.* *40B*:181–187.

Baldwin, J. and Hochacka, P. W. (1970). Functional significance of isoenzymes in thermal acclimation: Acetylcholinesterase from trout brain. *Biochem. J.* *116*:883–887.

Baslow, M. H. and Nigrelli, R. F. (1964). The effect of thermal acclimation on brain acetylcholinesterase activity in killifish. *Fundalus heteroclitus*. *Zoologica* *49*:41–51.

Berridge, N. J. (1951). Rennin and the clotting of milk. *Adv. Enzymol.* *15*:423–448.

Bigelow, C. C. (1967). On the average hydrophobicity of proteins and the relation between it and protein structure. *J. Theor. Biol.* *16*:187–211.

Bobbitt, J. and Akenhead, S. (1982). Influence of controlled discharge from the Churchill river on the oceanography of Grosswater Bay. Labrador. *Can. Tech. Rep. Fish. Aquat. Sci.* *1097*:34–37.

Brewer, P., Helbig, N., and Haard, N. F. (1984). Atlantic cod pepsin—Characterization and use as a rennet substitute. *Can. Inst. Food Sci. Technol. J.* *17*:38–43.

Conrad, M. (1979). Mutation–absorption model of the enzyme. *Bull. Math. Biol.* *41*:387–405.

Conrad, M. (1983). In *Adaptability. The Significance of Variability from Molecule to Ecosystem*, Plenum, New York, p. 383.

Cowey, C. B. (1967). Comparative studies on the activity of D-glyceraldehyde-3-phosphate dehydrogenase from cold and warm-blooded animals with reference to temperature. *Comp. Biochem. Physiol.* *23*:969–976.

de Koning, P. J. (1978). Coagulating enzymes in cheese making. *Dairy Ind. Int.* *43*:7–12.

Demain, A. L. (1981). Industrial microbiology. *Science* *214*:987–995.

Fullbrook, P. D. (1983). Practical applied kinetics. In *Industrial Enzymology—The Application of Enzymes in Industry* (T. Godfrey and J. Reichelt, eds.), Nature Press, London, pp. 8–40.

Godfrey, T. and Reichelt, J. (1983). Introduction to industrial enzymology. In *Industrial Enzymology—The Application of Enzymes in Industry* (T. Godfrey and J. Reichelt, eds.), Nature Press, London, pp. 1–7.

Haard, N. F., Feltham, L. A. W., Helbig, N., and Squires, J. (1982). Modification of protein with proteolytic enzymes from the marine environment. *Adv. Chem. 198*:223–244.

Hazel, J. R. and Prosser, C. L. (1974). Molecular mechanisms of temperature compensation in poikilotherms. *Physiol. Rev. 54*:620–677.

Hebb, C., Stephens, T. C., and Smith, M. W. (1972). Effect of environmental temperature on the kinetic properties of goldfish brain choline acetyltransferase. *Biochem. J. 129*:1013–1021.

Hochacka, P. W. and Somero, G. N. (1971). Biochemical adaptation to the environment. In *Fish Physiology*, Vol. 6 (W. S. Hoar and J. D. Randall, eds.), Academic, New York, pp. 100–156.

Hochacka, P. W., Storey, K. B., and Baldwin, J. (1975). Design of acetylcholinesterase for its physical environment. *Comp. Biochem. Physiol. 52B*:13–18.

Hochacka, P. W., Norberg, C., Baldwin, J., and Fields, J. H. (1976). Enthalpy–entropy compensation of oxamate binding by homologous lactate dehydrogenases. *Nature 260*:640–650.

Hofer, R., Ladurner, H., Gattringer, A., and Wieser, W. (1975). Relationship between the temperature preferenda of fishes, amphibians and reptiles, and the substrate affinities of their trypsins. *J. Comp. Physiol. 99*:345–355.

Hoskins, M. A. H. and Aleksiuk, M. (1973). Effect of temperature on the kinetics of malate dehydrogenase from a cold climate reptile, *Thamnophis sirtalis parietalis*. *Comp. Biochem. Physiol. 45B*:343–354.

Hultin, H. O. (1978). Enzymes from organisms acclimated to low temperatures. In *Enzymes. The Interface Between Technology and Economics* (J. P. Danehy and B. Wolnak, eds.), Marcel Dekker, New York, pp. 161–178.

Kaplan, N. O. (1965). Evolution of Dehydrogenases. In *Evolving Genes and Proteins* (V. Bryson and H. J. Vogel, eds.), Academic, New York, pp. 243–277.

Koffler, H. (1957). Protoplasmic differences between mesophiles and thermophiles. *Bacteriol. Rev. 21*:227–240.

Koffler, H., Mallet, G. E., and Adye, J. (1957). Molecular basis of biological stability to high temperatures. *Proc. Nat. Acad. Sci. U.S.A. 43*:464–477.

Komatsu, S. K. and Feeney, R. E. (1970). A heat labile fructose-diphosphate aldolase from cold adapted Antarctic fishes. *Biochim. Biophys. Acta 206*:305–315.

Lee, Y. Z., Simpson, B. K., and Haard, N. F. (1982). Supplementation of squid fermentation with proteolytic enzymes. *J. Food Biochem. 6*:127–134.

Light, P., Dawson, W. R., and Shoemaker, V. A. (1969). Thermal adjustments in cardiac and skeletal muscles of lizards. *Z. Vgl. Physiol. 65*:1–14.

Lim, D. and Shipe, W. F. (1972). Proposed mechanism for the antioxygenic action of trypsin in milk. *J. Dairy Sci. 55*:753–758.

Linthicum, D. S. and Carey, F. G. (1972). Regulation of brain and eye temperatures by the blue fin tuna. *Comp. Biochem. Physiol. 43A*:425–433.

Litchfield, J. H. (1983). Single cell proteins. *Science 219*:740–746.

Low, P. S. and Somero, G. N. (1974). Temperature adaptation of enzymes: A proposed molecular basis for the different catalytic efficiencies of ectotherms and endotherms. *Comp. Biochem. Physiol. 49B*:307–312.

Low, P. S. and Somero, G. N. (1976). Adaptation of muscle pyruvate kinases to environmental temperatures and pressures. *J. Exp. Zool. 198*:1–11.

Low, P. S., Bada, J. L., and Somero, G. N. (1973). Temperature adaptation of enzymes: Roles of free energy, the enthalpy, and the entropy of activation. *Proc. Nat. Acad. Sci. U.S.A. 70*: 430–432.

Metz, F. E., Boyce, F. O., and Sigmiller, J. L. (1975). Process for making a barbecue sauce with a tenderizer. U.S. Patent No. 3,930,030.

Mihalyi, E. (1978). In *Applications of Proteolytic Enzymes to Protein Structure Studies*, 2nd ed., CRC Press, West Palm Beach, Fla. pp. 57–59.

Orejana, F. M. and Liston, J. (1982). Agents of proteolysis and its inhibition in patis (fish sauce) fermentation. *J. Food Sci. 47*:198–203.

Owen, T. G. (1968). Studies on peptic digestion in salmonid fish. M.Sc. thesis, University of New Brunswick.

Pollock, M. R. (1965). Purification and properties of penicillases from two strains of *Bacillus lichenformis*: A chemical, physiochemical and physiological comparison. *Biochem. J. 94*:666–675.

Potter, J. D. (1974). The content of troponin, tropomyosin, actin and myosin in rabbit skeletal muscle. *Arch. Biochem. Biophys. 162*:436–441.

Ritskes, T. M., (1971). Artificial ripening of maatjes-cured herring with the aid of proteolytic enzyme preparations. *J. Fish. Res. Board Can. 69*:647–654.

Simpson, B. K. (1984). Isolation, characterization, and some applications of trypsin from Greenland cod (*Gadus ogac*). Ph.D. thesis, Memorial University of Newfoundland, St. John's.

Simpson, B. K. and Haard, N. F. (1984a). Purification and characterization of Greenland cod (*Gadus ogac*) trypsin. 1. Kinetic and thermodynamic characteristics. *Can. J. Biochem. Cell Biol. 62*:894–900.

Simpson, B. K. and Haard, N. F. (1984b). Trypsin from Greenland cod, *Gadus ogac*. Isolation and comparative properties. *Comp. Biochem. Physiol. 79B*:613–622.

Simpson, B. K. and Haard, N. F. (1984c). Trypsin from Greenland cod as a food-processing aid. *J. Appl. Biochem. 6*:135–143.

Singleton, R. and Amelunxen, R. E. (1973). Proteins from thermophilic microorganisms. *Bacteriol. Rev. 37*:320–342.

Somero, G. N. (1969). Enzyme mechanisms of temperature compensations: Immediate and evolutionary aspects of temperature on enzymes of aquatic poikilotherms. *Am. Nat. 103*:517–530.

Somero, G. N. (1973). Thermal modulation of pyruvate metabolism in the fish *Gillichthys mirabilis*: The role of lactate dehydrogenases. *Comp. Biochem. Physiol. 44B*:205–209.

Somero, G. N. (1975). Temperature as a selective force in protein evolution: The adaptational strategy of "compromise." *J. Exp. Zool. 194*:175–188.

Somero, G. N. and Hochacka, P. W. (1971). Biochemical adaptation to the environment. *Am. Zool. 11*:159–167.

Somero, G. N. and Low, P. S. (1976). Temperature: A 'shaping force' in protein evolution. *Biochem. Soc. Symp. 41*:33–42.

Squires, J., Haard, N. F., and Feltham, L. A. W. (1986a). Pepsin isozymes from Greenland cod (*Gadus ogac*). 1. Purification and physical properties. *Can. J. Biochem. Cell Biol. 64*:205–214.

Squires, J., Haard, N. F., and Feltham, L. A. W. (1986b). Gastric proteases of the Greenland cod (*Gadus ogac*). II. Comparison of structural properties. *Can. J. Biochem. Cell Biol. 64*:215–222.

Ushakov, B. (1967). Coupled evolutionary changes in protein thermostability. In *Molecular Mechanisms of Temperature Adaptation* (C. L. Prosser, ed.), American Association for the Advancement of Science, Washington, D.C., pp. 107–129.

20

Bacterial Starter Cultures

PATRICIA M. WALSH and DALLAS G. HOOVER /
University of Delaware, Newark, Delaware

DAIRY STARTER CULTURES

The production of fermented dairy products, that is, cheese, yogurt, sour cream, butter, and buttermilk, depends greatly upon the activity of the lactic acid bacteria which are used as starter cultures (Table 1). These bacteria are responsible for the hydrolysis of milk proteins, lactose, and citrate and the production of acid and flavor compounds, as well as other characteristics of the end-product. The genetic instability of starter strains, bacteriophage infection, production of off-flavors, and insufficient development of acid during fermentation are costly problems for the dairy industry. Therefore there is a great deal of interest in the development of new and improved strains, in particular the construction of strains using the modern tools of molecular biology.

Since the early 1970s much research has focused on obtaining fundamental information on the genes, plasmids, bacteriophages, and gene transfer mechanisms of lactic acid bacteria, information that is essential to successful strain construction programs. This section of the chapter will review the plasmid biology and gene transfer mechanisms of the lactic acid bacteria, *Streptococcus*, *Lactobacillus*, and *Leuconostoc.*

Plasmids

Plasmids are important tools of biotechnology because of their roles in gene transfer as cloning vectors and conjugative plasmids. In the group N streptococci they have an added significance. Many

Table 1. Bacteria Used as Starter Cultures in Dairy Products

Product	Microorganisms added
Cheese	
Parmesan, Romano	Mixture of *Lactobacillus bulgaricus* and *Streptococcus thermophilus*
Cheddar, Colby	*Streptococcus lactis*, *Streptococcus cremoris*
Swiss, Emmenthaler	Mixture of *L. bulgaricus* (or *Lactobacillus lactis* or *Lactobacillus helveticus*), *S. thermophilus*, and *Propionibacterium shermanii*
Provolone	Mixture of heat-resistant *Lactobacillus* species and *S. thermophilus*
Blue, Gorgonzola, Roquefort, Stilton	*S. lactis*
Camembert	Lactic streptococci
Brick, Limburger	Mixture of *S. thermophilus* and *L. bulgaricus*
Brick, Limburger	Mixture of *S. lactis* and *S. thermophilus*
Muenster	Mixture of *S. thermophilus* and *Lactobacillus* species
Gouda, Edam	*S. lactis*
Mozzarella	Mixture of heat-resistant *Lactobacillus* species and *S. thermophilus*
Cottage cheese, cream cheese	*S. lactis* or *S. cremoris*; mixture of *S. lactis* or *S. cremoris* and *Streptococcus diacetylactis* (or *Leuconostoc* species)
Fermented milks	
Bulgarian buttermilk	*L. bulgaricus*

Source: Smith and Palumbo (1981).

important functional properties are linked to plasmid DNA in these bacteria (McKay, 1983).

With the development of techniques for plasmid analysis, McKay and co-workers became the first to isolate and physically characterize dairy streptococcal plasmids (Cords et al., 1974). It is now well established that most group N streptococci contain many diverse plasmids. The most thoroughly studied plasmid-related phenotype of group N streptococci is lactose metabolism. The ability to metabolize lactose is essential to successful dairy fermentations and its instability has been well documented (McKay, 1982). Conclusive evidence that lactose utilization is linked to plasmid DNA in *Streptococcus lactis* C2 was presented in 1976 (McKay et al., 1976). The transfer of lactose metabolism via a temperate phage induced from *S. lactis* C2 was correlated with the transfer of plasmid DNA. Since then, phenotypic, physical, and genetic evidence has linked plasmids to lactose utilization in many strains of group N streptococci (Kempler and McKay, 1979b; McKay et al., 1980; Snook et al., 1981; Davies and Gasson, 1981; Kondo and McKay, 1982b). A great deal of research effort has focused on the characterization of plasmids of group N streptococci. The development of efficient lysis procedures has greatly contributed to this effort (Klaenhammer et al., 1978; Yu et al., 1982; Anderson and McKay, 1983; Orberg and Sandine, 1984a).

Other metabolic traits have been correlated with plasmid DNA. Proteinase activity, the ability of the bacteria to degrade casein, providing the cells with needed nitrogenous compounds, has been conclusively linked to plasmid DNA in some strains (McKay et al., 1976; Gasson, 1983a). However, in other strains, like *Streptococcus cremoris* B1, the proteinase genes appear to be on the chromosome (Anderson and McKay, 1977). For still other strains the data are inconclusive, perhaps owing to the involvement of several plasmids or to chromosomal proteinase genes (McKay, 1983) and/or the frequent occurrence of plasmid deletions (Gasson, 1983a). *Streptococcus lactis* subsp. *diacetylactis* produces the flavor and aroma compound diacetyl from citrate. Phenotypic and physical evidence has linked citrate metabolism to a 5.5-Mdal plasmid (Kempler and McKay, 1979a; Davies and Gasson, 1981). Biochemical studies indicated that loss of the plasmid was correlated with loss of citrate permease activity. In some group N streptococci plasmids also appear to be involved in galactose metabolism (Park and McKay, 1982). and sucrose, mannose, glucose, and D-xylose metabolism (LeBlanc et al., 1980).

The ability to produce inhibitory substances such as nisin, diplococcin, and bacteriocin is linked to plasmids in many strains. LeBlanc et al. (1980) reported phenotypic and physical evidence for a 28-Mdal nisin plasmid in *S. lactis* 11454 (DR1251). Nisin production and resistance were conjugally transferred from strains of *S. lactis* to a nonproducing, plasmid-free strain of *S. lactis* and tentatively linked to a 30-Mdal plasmid (Gasson, 1984). Diplococcin production has been linked to a 54-Mdal conjugative plasmid in *S. cremoris* 346 (Davey, 1984). The production of bacteriocin-like substances was successfully linked to an 88-Mdal conjugative plasmid in *Streptococcus diacetylactis* WM4 (Scherwitz et al., 1983), to 39.6-Mdal plasmids in *S. cremoris* strains 9B4 and 4G6, and to a 75-Mdal plasmid in *S. diacetylactis* 6F7 (Neve et al., 1984).

Antibiotic-resistant plasmids do not appear to be as prevalent in group N streptococci as they are in other species of streptococci. McKay (1983) suggested that fresh isolates from raw milk might be a better source of resistance plasmids than are laboratory strains. Dobrzanski et al. (1982), however, successfully transformed *Bacillus subtilis* to kanamycin resistance using *S. lactis* 71 plasmid DNA, suggesting the existence of kanamycin-resistant plasmids.

The infection of starter cultures by bacteriophage is a major problem for the dairy industry. In some group N streptococci plasmids have been linked to phage resistance mechanisms. Sanders and Klaenhammer (1981) presented physical evidence that a restriction and modification system in *S. cremoris* KH is linked to a 10-Mdal plasmid. *Streptococcus lactis* IL594 has two plasmid-linked restriction modification systems, one of which has been genetically confirmed by conjugation (Chopin et al., 1984). Genetic evidence has linked a 40-Mdal conjugative plasmid of *S. diacetylactis* DRC3 to phage resistance due to restriction of phage growth (McKay and Baldwin, 1984). Resistance due to interference with phage adsorption has been linked to a 30-Mdal plasmid of *S. lactis* ME2 (Sanders and Klaenhammer, 1983) and to a 34-Mdal plasmid of *S. cremoris* SK11 (deVos et al., 1984).

Other traits which have been linked to plasmid DNA are resistance to arsenate, arsenite, and chromate and sensitivity to copper (Efstathiou and McKay, 1977). The instability of such starter culture traits as resistance to a lactoperoxidase—thiocyanate—hydrogen peroxide system (Auclair and Vassal, 1963), resistance to agglutinins (Auclair and Vassal, 1963), arginine hydrolysis in strains of *S. diacetylactis* (Truner et al., 1963), and slime production in *S. cremoris* strains (Forsin et al., 1973; Forsin and Pakkila, 1979) suggests that plasmid DNA may be involved (McKay, 1983).

The existence of plasmids in *Lactobacillus* species is also well established, although far less is known about them. The first evidence for plasmids in lactobacilli was reported in 1976 (Chassy et al., 1976). A 23-Mdal plasmid was isolated from *Lactobacillus casei* subsp. *casei* 69H and a 19-Mdal plasmid from *L. casei* subsp. *rhamnosus*. Plasmids have also been detected in strains of *Lactobacillus helveticus* (Smiley and Fryder, 1978; Klaenhammer, 1984), *Lactobacillus acidophilus* (Klaenhammer and Sutherland, 1980; Vescova et al., 1981), *Lactobacillus reuteri* (Vescova et al., 1981), *Lactobacillus fermentum* (Ishiwa and Iwata, 1980), *Lactobacillus plantarum* (Klaenhammer, 1984), and *Lactobacillus bulgaricus* (Klaenhammer, 1984). Plasmids have been linked to lactose fermentation in some strains of *L. casei* subsp. *casei* (Chassy et al., 1980).

Plasmid DNA in *Leuconostoc* species will be discussed later in this chapter.

Transduction

The first reports of bacteriophage-mediated gene transfer, transduction, in group N streptococci involved virulent phage which transferred tryptophan independence from *S. diacetylactis* (Sandine et al., 1962) and streptomycin resistance from *S. lactis* C2 (Allen et al., 1963). Subsequently research has generally concentrated on transduction involving temperate bacteriophage.

In 1973 McKay et al. reported the transfer of genes for lactose, maltose, and mannose utilization via a temperate phage induced from *S. lactis* C2. It was later shown that the genes for lactose metabolism (*lac*) and proteinase activity (*prt*) could be cotransduced (McKay and Baldwin, 1974). Further work with the C2 system resulted in the first confirmation of the linkage of *lac* genes to plasmid DNA (McKay et al., 1976). A plasmid-cured strain of *S. lactis* was transduced by phage induced from *S. lactis* C2. Lactose-positive (Lac^+) transductants contained a single plasmid of 20–23 Mdal, although the Lac plasmid of C2 is 30 Mdal. It was suggested that the bacteriophage head could not accommodate the entire plasmid and the plasmid was shortened during packaging (transductional shortening). Transductants have also been isolated in the C2 system in which the Lac plasmid or a portion of it is integrated into the bacterial chromosome (McKay and Baldwin, 1978). These transductants are stable for lactose metabolism and the 20- to 23-Mdal plasmid is not detectable.

The temperate phage of *S. lactis* 712 can transduce the 17-Mdal erythromycin resistance (Em^r) plasmid pAMB as well as *lac* genes (Gasson, 1982). Its lactose transduction system is very similar to that of *S. lactis* C2 (Davies and Gasson, 1981) and the phages of C2 and 712 have similar morphologies and identical DNA restriction patterns (Davies et al., 1981).

Transduction of *lac* genes also occurs via temperate phage induced from *S. lactis* C_2 (McKay et al., 1980) and from *S. cremoris* C3 (Snook et al., 1981). In the C3 system transductional shortening of the Lac plasmid occurred, and in some transductants no plasmids were detected.

Transduction may prove to be a useful technique for stabilizing plasmid genes, as well as for constructing families of smaller Lac plasmids.

Conjugation

Conjugation, the ability to transfer DNA via cell-to-cell contact, is widespread in the group N streptococci. The conjugal transfer of lactose metabolism was first reported in 1979 (Gasson and Davies, 1979; Kempler and McKay, 1979b). Gasson and Davies (1979, 1980b) described the transfer of lactose genes from *S. lactis* 712 to suitably marked 712 recipients, but they were initially unable to identify the lactose plasmid. Kempler and McKay (1979b) demonstrated the conjugal transfer of the 41-Mdal Lac plasmid of *S. diacetylactis* 18-16 to a plasmid-cured derivative of *S. lactis* C2. This provided the genetic evidence for the linkage of lactose metabolism to plasmid DNA in this strain. Subsequently McKay and co-workers studied the conjugal transfer of *lac* genes from *S. lactis* strains ML3 and C_2O, *S. diacetylactis* strains DRC3, 11007, and WM4 (McKay et al., 1980), and *S. cremoris* strains C3, R1, EB_7, and Z8 (Snook and McKay, 1981). The assignment of the *lac* genes to a particular plasmid was not always straightforward because the transconjugants often contained novel plasmids, more than one transferred plasmid, or no detectable plasmids. The transfer of chromosomal markers for streptomycin resistance and lactose has also been reported (McKay et al., 1980; Snook and McKay, 1981).

Some of the transconjugants from matings involving 712, ML3, and ML3 derivatives act as high-frequency donors and form cell aggregates in broth (Gasson and Davies, 1980b; Walsh and McKay, 1981; Snook and McKay, 1981). Novel 60-Mdal plasmids were isolated from some of these transconjugants (Walsh and McKay, 1981, 1982; Davies and Gasson, 1981). Detailed restriction enzyme analysis of the plasmids of ML3 and its transconjugants suggests that the 60-Mdal plasmid is a cointegrate of pSK08, the 33-Mdal Lac plasmid of ML3, and pRS01, a 27-Mdal plasmid of ML3 (Anderson and McKay, 1984). Anderson and McKay (1984) identified a restriction fragment associated with conjugal transfer ability and an inversion element involved in the cell aggregation phenotype located on pRS01 and presented evidence for an insertion sequence(s) on pSK08. It is likely that the same system exists in *S. lactis* 712 and may be prevalent among other strains of group N streptococci (Walsh and McKay, 1981; Anderson and McKay, 1984).

Conjugation has been used to study other plasmid-linked traits. McKay and Baldwin (1984) reported the conjugal transfer of a 40-Mdal plasmid, pNP40, in *S. diacetylactis* DRC3 associated with resistance to nisin and bacteriophage. This plasmid was transferred alone or cotransferred with the Lac plasmid. *Streptococcus lactis* IL594 also contains a conjugative plasmid linked to bacteriophage resistance (Chopin et al., 1984). The ability to produce inhibitory substances can be conjugally transferred from certain strains of group N streptococci. Conjugative bacteriocin plasmids were isolated from *S. diacetylactis* WM4 (Scherwitz et al., 1983), *S. cremoris* strains 9B4 and 4G6, and *S. diacetylactis* 6F7 (Neve et al., 1984), and a conjugative diplococcin plasmid was identified in *S. cremoris* 346 (Davey, 1984). Nisin resistance and production were cotransferred with sucrose-fermenting ability during conjugation with eight strains of *S. lactis* (Gasson, 1984). A 30-Mdal plasmid may be involved, but the results were inconclusive. The wide host range Em^r plasmid pAMB1, originally isolated from *Streptococcus faecalis*, has been conjugally transferred into strains of *S. lactis*, *S. cremoris*, and *S. diacetylactis* (Gasson and Davies, 1980a; Anderson and McKay, 1984), and strains of *L. casei* (Gibson et al., 1979) and *Lactobacillus salivarius* (Davies and Gasson, 1981). This plasmid has potential for use in in vivo and in vitro genetic studies and strain construction (Gasson, 1983b).

Conjugation has proved to be a useful tool in the genetic analysis of group N streptococci. It has been used to confirm plasmid-linked traits, in strain construction, and in basic genetic studies. It will likely continue to play an important role in the future.

Much less is known about conjugative plasmids in lactobacilli. Chassy and Rokaw (1981), however, have described the transfer of a Lac plasmid and small cyrptic plasmids between strains of *L. casei*. As more is learned about the plasmids of lactobacilli, more conjugation systems will likely be discovered.

Protoplasts and Cloning

Until recently, the use of recombinant DNA technology for strain improvement and the genetic analysis of lactic streptococci was prevented by the lack of a transformation system. Development of methodology for the production and regeneration of streptococcal protoplasts (Gasson, 1980; Kondo and McKay, 1982a; Okamoto et al., 1983; Yu et al., 1984) has helped to eliminate this roadblock. Both chromosomal markers and plasmids have been transferred through protoplast fusion in *S. lactis* 712 (Gasson, 1980). The long-awaited breakthrough, transformation, was reported in 1982 (Kondo and McKay, 1982b). Protoplasts of *S. lactis* ML3 derivatives were transformed with the 23-Mdal Lac plasmid pLM2103. Although the frequency of transformation was very low, about 8.5 transformants per microgram of DNA, in subsequent studies, Kondo and McKay (1984) increased the transformation frequency to $5 \times 10^3 – 4 \times 10^4$ transformants per microgram of DNA using pGB301, a 6.5-Mdal Em^r

Streptococcus sanguis cloning vector. Transfection of *S. diacetylactis* protoplasts with bacteriophage P008 has also been successful (Geis, 1982).

Now that a transformation system is available, work has begun on developing cloning systems for group N streptococci. The *S. sanguis* cloning vector pGB301 was used to clone the *lac* genes of *S. lactis* plasmid pLM001 into *S. lactis* LM0230 (Kondo and McKay, 1984). A *S. cremoris* cloning vector, constructed by inserting the genes for chloramphenicol resistance and Em^r from *Staphylococcus aureus* into an *S. cremoris* plasmid, pWV01, is now available (Kok et al., 1984). This vector, designated pGK12, can replicate in *Escherichia coli*, *B. subtilis*, and *S. lactis* and can transform *S. lactis* protoplasts. A system for cloning *S. lactis* genes into *S. sanguis* var. Challis has also been developed (Harlander and McKay, 1984; Harlander et al., 1984).

Transformation of lactobacilli has not yet been reported, but with the development of a method for preparing and regenerating *L. casei* protoplasts (Lee-Wickner and Chassy, 1984), successful transformation will likely soon follow. *Lactobacillus* genes have been studied by cloning them into *E. coli* (Lee et al., 1982; Davies and Gronenborn, 1982); however, this approach may not be successful for all genes. A transformation system for lactobacilli is definitely needed.

Conclusions

A great deal of progress has been made in the past 10 years or so. Plasmids have been identified in streptococci, lactobacilli and leuconostocs. In many strains important phenotypic traits such as lactose metabolism, proteinase activity, citrate utilization, and bacteriophage resistance have been linked to particular plasmids. In the group N streptococci genes can be transferred by conjugation, transduction, and transformation, and conjugation has been reported for strains of *L. casei*. It should soon be possible to construct starter culture strains that are genetically programmed to meet the needs of the dairy industry.

MEAT AND VEGETABLE STARTER CULTURES

The majority of advances in the genetics of starter cultures has been with those bacteria involved in the production of fermented milk products. As described earlier, the techniques for the genetic manipulation of dairy streptococci has developed to the point where practical improvement of these starter cultures is a reality. However, this cannot be said of those species involved in the commercial manufacture of fermented meat and vegetable products. Numerous reasons have been given for this technology gap:

1. Comminuted meat is of a particulate nature that makes experimental evaluation difficult. Meat has a natural microflora that cannot be effectively removed, and these meat microorganisms do contribute to the flavor, aroma, and texture of the finished products.
2. The entire dairy industry uses starter cultures, and this technology has had to develop and grow against the recurrent problem of bacteriophage, a problem not of great concern in meat and vegetable fermentations.
3. Many commercial meat fermentations still use natural fermentation or "back-slop" methods.
4. Use of starter cultures in the fermented produce area has just not been cost effective. Besides being cheaper, in some instances natural fermentations have been judged to produce a product superior to that made with starter cultures. This is because a number of microbial species are important in the fermentation.

However, in the fermented meat industry starter cultures are being used with increasing frequency. Over 50% of these foods now are produced with starter cultures (Smith and Palumbo, 1983). As the technology advances, controlled closed-vat fermentations will be adopted for the benefits of a greater yield of product with greater consistency, improved food safety, and shorter processing times. Eventually the technology will become cost effective. Presently in semidry and dry sausage manufacture, the U.S. Department of Agriculture does not require the use of starter cultures, but this has been recommended (American Meat Institute, 1982; U.S. Department of Agriculture, 1977; National Academy of Sciences, 1975). In the future, regulations will no doubt be written requiring their use.

Tables 2 and 3 summarize major meat, poultry, and vegetable products where bacterial starter cultures have been used. Table 2 also includes nonfermented meat and poultry products where lactic acid bacteria are added to extend shelf life.

Meat Starter Cultures

The final processing parameters necessary for a stable fermented meat product are (1) a pH less than or equal to 5.2 *and* a water activity less than or equal to 0.95 or (2) a pH less than 5.0 *or* water activity less than 0.91 (Leistner and Rodel, 1975). The first commercial meat starter culture used to achieve these specifications was a strain of *Pediococcus cerevisiae* that was selected for use in semidry sausages because of its high lactate production and the ability to survive lyophilization (Deibel and Niven, 1957).

Pediococci are similar to the dairy streptococci in that they are facultative, gram-positive cocci, are homofermentative, and produce no CO_2 in glucose utilization. Pediococci are microaerophilic and

Table 2. Bacteria Used as Starter Cultures in Meat and Poultry Products

Product	Bacteria
Semidry fermented meat sausages	
Lebanon bologna	Mixture of *Pediococcus cerevisiae* and *L. plantarum*
Summer sausage	*P. cerevisiae*
Summer sausage	*P. cerevisiae* and *L. plantarum* mixture
Cerevelat	*P. cerevisiae*
Cerevelat	Mixture of *P. cerevisiae* and *L. plantarum*
Thuringer	*P. cerevisiae*
Teewurst	*Lactobacillus* species
Pork roll	*P. cerevisiae*
Dry fermented meat sausages	
Pepperoni	Mixture of *P. cerevisiae* and *L. plantarum*
Dry sausage	*P. cerevisiae*
European dry sausage	*Micrococcus* species
European dry sausage	Mixture of *Micrococcus* and *Lactobacillus* species
Salami	Mixture of *Micrococcus* and *Lactobacillus* species
Salami	*L. plantarum*
Hard salami, Genoa	*Micrococcus* species; mixture of *Micrococcus* species and *P. cerevisiae*; mixture of *Micrococcus* species and *L. plantarum*
Fermented snack sausage	
Hot bar sausage	*P. cerevisiae*
Processed meat products	
Bacon	Lactic acid bacteria
Bacon	*L. plantarum*

Table 2. (Continued)

Product	Bacteria
Canned ham	Radiation-killed *P. cerevisiae*
Country-style ham	*P. cerevisiae*
Frankfurters	*Micrococcus* species; *Vibrio* species
Fresh meat	
Ground beef	Mixture of *S. lactis* and *Leuconostoc citrovorum*
Ground beef	*S. diacetylactis*
Ground beef	*L. bulgaricus; L. lactis; P. cerevisiae*
Ground beef	*L. brevis*
Beef longissimus dorsi steak	Mixture of *S. lactis* and *L. citrovorum*
Fermented poultry sausages	
Semidry turkey sausage	*P. cerevisiae*
Dry turkey sausage	*P. cerevisiae*
Dry turkey sausage	Mixture of *P. cerevisiae* and *L. plantarum*
Processed poultry products	
Smoked, vacuum-packed turkey	Radiation-killed *P. cerevisiae*
Cooked, mechanically deboned poultry meat	*P. cerevisiae* and/or *L. plantarum*
Fresh poultry meat	
Ground chicken	*P. cerevisiae* and/or *L. plantarum*
Mechanically deboned poultry meat	*P. cerevisiae* and/or *L. plantarum*
Eggs	
Pasteurized, liquid whole egg	*P. cerevisiae* and/or *L. plantarum*

Source: Smith and Palumbo (1981).

Table 3. Bacteria Used as Starter Cultures in Vegetable Products

Product (vegetable or fruit)	Bacteria
Pickles	
Carrots	Mixture of *L. plantarum*, *L. brevis*, *Leuconostoc mesenteroides*, and *Pediococcus cerevisiae*
Cucumbers	Mixture of *P. cerevisiae*, *L. plantarum*, and *L. brevis*; mixture of *P. cerevisiae* and *L. plantarum*; *L. plantarum*
Cucumbers, sliced	*L. plantarum*
Cucumbers, diced	*L. plantarum*
Mixed vegetables, green tomatoes, hot cherry peppers	Mixture of *P. cerevisiae* and *L. plantarum*; *L. plantarum*
Various vegetables, diced	*L. plantarum*
Olives	*L. plantarum*
Sauerkraut	*L. plantarum*

Source: Smith and Palumbo (1981).

nutritionally fastidious, and can grow at a pH of 3.5–3.8 in concentrations of sodium chloride of up to 8.0%. They are rarely found in dairy products; most pediococci cannot utilize lactose to a significant extent. Pediococci are classified as catalase variable, since some isolates possess non-heme catalase activity.

The nomenclature is somewhat confusing with regard to the genus *Pediococcus*. The eighth edition of *Bergey's Manual* (Buchanan and Gibbons, 1974) defined the species *P. cerevisiae*. *Pediococcus cerevisiae* generally has been the species name used for *Pediococcus* that are most active in food fermentations; however, in 1979 the Subcommittee of Lactobacilli and Related Microorganisms of the International Committee on Systematic Bacteriology declared the species *P. cerevisiae* invalid, and the species names *Pediococcus damnosus* and *Pediococcus pentosaceus* were defined, with rearrangement of the determinative characteristics for *Pediococcus* (Teuber and Geis, 1981). Presently the pediococcal species used as meat starter cultures are *Pediococcus acidilactici* and *P. pentosaceus* (Bacus, 1983). The name *P. cerevisiae* is still used by some people.

For practical purposes we will consider *P. cerevisiae* roughly equivalent to *P. acidilactici*, as has been suggested (Bacus, 1984), although some authors interchange *P. cerevisiae* with *P. damnosus* according to international nomenclature (Liepe, 1983).

The primary purpose of pediococcal starter cultures in meat is to produce lactic acid from the carbohydrate (usually glucose) added to the meat emulsion. The acid imparts a tangy flavor, alters the texture of the mixture (denatures protein, lowers water activity), and increases shelf life by inhibiting pathogenic and spoilage microorganisms. For semidry sausages (pH 5.3 or less, final moisture content of 40–50%, usually heated and smoked), *P. acidilactici* is the culture of choice. Its two best features are its high lactic acid production and tolerance to sodium chloride. *Pediococcus acidilactici* has a relatively high growth temperature (optimum growth temperature 40°C, maximum growth temperature 52°C), making it suitable for the traditional temperatures used in semidry sausage fermentation. Although the species does produce the important flavor compound, diacetyl, the major flavor attribute of significance contributed to most summer sausage-type products is the acid taste caused by the lactic acid. The other important flavors are derived from the salt, spices, sugar, and meat (Deibel et al., 1961).

For those dry sausages (pH 5.3 or less, final moisture content 25–45%, usually not smoked or heated) fermented at temperatures less than 32°C, *P. pentosaceus* is commonly used. This is because the species has a lower optimum growth temperature (35°C) and a lower maximum growth temperature (42–45°C) than *P. acidilactici*. Other contributing factors are the greater sensitivity of *P. acidilactici* to the antioxidants employed in dry sausage manufacture (i.e., BHA and BHT), and the ability of *P. pentosaceus* to rapidly ferment glucose at low temperatures when incubated in the presence of a manganese salt (Bacus, 1984).

When meats are fermented without addition of a starter culture, the predominant kind of microorganisms normally found are lactobacilli. Species of the genus *Lactobacillus* are facultative, gram-positive, asporogenous rods with complex nutritional requirements. Lactobacilli are able to break down hydrogen peroxide in the presence of myoglobin and thus are capable of retarding fat rancidity and the undesirable alteration of meat pigments. The lactobacilli have lower optimum growth temperatures than the pediococci. This characteristic makes them more suitable for dry sausage fermentations.

The species of *Lactobacillus* with the best fermentative performance in meats is *L. plantarum*. Other lactobacilli, such as *Lactobacillus brevis*, *L. casei*, and *Lactobacillus leichmanii*, have been isolated from fermented meats, but they do not predominate like *L. plantarum*. *Lactobacillus plantarum* grows well in the presence of more than 9% sodium chloride, is homofermentative, and tolerates acid pH (less than 3.8).

Other bacteria, yeasts, and molds indigenous to the meat contribute to taste, appearance, and texture. Those bacteria that play beneficial roles in flavor development include *Leuconostoc mesenteroides*, streptococci, salt-tolerant micrococci, and coagulase-negative staphylococci.

In Europe, where nitrate is used in the cure mix and fermentation times are extended, micrococci are incorporated into meat starter cultures. However, in the United States a straight nitrite cure is used which shortens the process time. The pan-curing fermentation step (reduction of nitrate to nitrite) is eliminated and makes the micrococci unnecessary as a starter culture. In Europe, whenever *Micrococcus* used as starter culture, a homofermentative lactic acid bacteria must be included to produce enough lactic acid to ensure a safe and organoleptically acceptable product with the proper shelf life.

Higher temperatures of fermentation are being used to increase starter culture proliferation and shorten incubation times. Unfortunately, these higher temperatures are also conducive to the growth of pathogens, such as *Staphylococcus aureus*. In dry sausage manufacture, where smoking is not common, *S. aureus* may be more of a problem if higher fermentation temperatures are used. The production of antimicrobial compounds other than lactic acid that are active against such pathogens as *S. aureus* would be a significant improvement in these starter cultures. These antimicrobial compounds would be important in nonfermented meat products that receive lactic acid bacteria for the purpose of preventing the growth of pathogens and spoilage microorganisms. Lactic acid bacteria are currently being used as nitrate reducers or preservatives in a number of nonfermented meat products (Smith and Palumbo, 1981).

Recent work from the University of Wisconsin has shown that the level of sodium nitrite can be reduced by 1/2 to 2/3 in bacon (from 120 ppm) without exposing consumers to the risk of botulism. This is accomplished by incorporating *P. acidilactici* and a fermentable sugar into the cure. When the bacon is temperature abused, *P. acidilactici* utilizes the sugar to produce lactic acid, lowering the pH, thus preventing the growth of *Clostridium botulinum* (Anonymous, 1984a,b).

There are many areas for improvement in meat starter cultures. Product failures caused by lack of process control still occur; stabilization problems remain. It would be suitable to develop or increase the production of lactic acid, flavor compounds, antioxidants, and antimicrobial compounds by starter cultures. To engineer bacteria for their improvement as starter cultures requires basic genetic techniques that allow incorporation and expression of the desired properties in the chosen strain. These techniques have not been developed for the key meat starter cultures.

At this time one of the few papers on pediococcal genetics is by Gonzalez and Kunka (1983), who conjugally transferred a broad host range resistance (R) plasmid (pIP501) from *S. faecalis* to *P. acidilactici* and *P. pentosaceus*, and from *P. pentosaceus* to *S. faecalis*, *S. sanguis*, and *S. lactis*. However, they were not able to do the same with another broad host range R plasmid from *S. faecalis*, pAMβ 1. The identification of plasmid-linked traits in pediococci would greatly aid the study of their gene transfer mechanisms. Thus far only bacteriocin activity has been associated with a pediococcal plasmid, a 13.6-Mdal plasmid in *P. pentosaceus* PC-39 (Daeschel and Klaenhammer, 1985).

The situation with *L. plantarum* is slightly more advanced, if only for the reason that significant work has been done with other species in the genus *Lactobacillus*. (These species are of dairy significance and have been described in the first section of this chapter.). Plasmids have been detected in *L. plantarum*. Nes (1984) examined six strains of *L. plantarum* used as starter cultures and found all of these to harbor one to six plasmids ranging from 1.35 to 15 Mdal. Klaenhammer (1984) has developed a low-temperature alkaline-detergent lysis method for rapid isolation of plasmid DNA in *Lactobacillus*. Using mutanolysin for cell lysis with two strains of *L. plantarum*, Klaenhammer detected plasmids that ranged in size from 1 to 10 Mdal.

The next step is to determine the phenotype of these plasmids. One would expect fermentation of lactose to be plasmid linked in *L. plantarum*, but this has not yet been confirmed.

Vegetable Starter Cultures

In North America use of bacterial starter cultures for vegetable fermentation is rare. Sauerkraut, pickles, and olives are the three major fermented plant products where starter cultures are most applicable; numerous articles have been written about their production (Pederson, 1960; Fleming, 1982; Vaughn, 1982; Fernandez-Diez, 1983; Stamer, 1983).

In comparing Tables 2 and 3, it is evident that the lactic acid bacteria involved in the fermentation of vegetables are also active in meat fermentations. An important distinction with vegetable fermentations is their multistage progression. Although not similar in all respects, the fermentation of sauerkraut, pickles, and olives can be described in three parts. For example, Stamer (1974) divided sauerkraut fermentation into three phases of microbial participation based on predominant microflora type:

Phase 1: undesirable flora which recede as a result of exposure to acid and anaerobiosis

Phase 2: a dominant heterofermentative lactic flora

Phase 3: an aciduric homofermentative population which stops fermentation.

Sauerkraut differs from pickles and olives in that it is not brined; the salt is directly added to the shredded cabbage. The finished sauerkraut is a result of both homofermentative and heterofermentative microorganisms. Because of this required balance of activities, sauerkraut has had less success for adaptation to starter culture technology than the brined produce (Stamer, 1974). Desirable properties of the sauerkraut can be altered by changes in the microbial population caused by shifts in salt concentration and temperature. Homofermentative and heterofermentative bacteria both produce lactic acid, but only the heterofermenters contribute such end-products as CO_2, ethanol, acetic acid, and acetaldehyde in amounts that contribute significantly to the flavor and aroma of good sauerkraut. Indeed, when the homofermenters dominate a fermentation, as happens when the fermentation temperature is too high, the sauerkraut will taste like acidified cabbage (Vaughn, 1982). No one strain has been found capable of producing a satisfactory sauerkraut (Stamer, 1968).

The predominant heterofermentative lactic acid bacteria during the middle stage of sauerkraut fermentation is *L. mesenteroides*. *Lactobacillus brevis* is often present but is not as active as *L. mesenteroides* (Pederson and Albury, 1969). *Leuconostoc mesenteroides* initiates the lactic fermentation of sauerkraut by producing acids and CO_2, thus lowering the pH and level of aerobiosis. This is the most important part of the fermentation, because if in 2 or 3 days the lactic acid bacteria have not established themselves, the fermentation will fail. The growth of *L. mesenteroides* prevents growth of undesirable aerobes, oxidation of vitamin C, and loss of the natural color of cabbage. It also stimulates the growth of other lactic acid bacteria by the production of lactic acid (Vaughn, 1982).

Leuconostoc mesenteroides functions as the primary heterofermentative bacteria in sauerkraut fermentation because it is active over wide temperature and salt concentration ranges with very short lag and generation times as compared to other lactic bacteria present (Stamer, 1975). However, increasing the salt concentration to above 2.5% will select for homolactic bacteria. Leuconostocs are fostered by low temperature (7–10°C) and low salt concentration (2.5%) (Pederson and Albury, 1950, 1954).

Like *Pediococcus*, the leuconostocs are facultative gram-positive cocci with complex growth factor and amino acid requirements. Leuconostocs usually occur in pairs and chains. The growth is dependent upon the presence of a fermentable carbohydrate; lactate, CO_2, and ethanol or acetate are formed from glucose. As with the taxonomy of *Pediococcus*, *Leuconostoc* is also in transition at the moment. The eighth edition of *Bergey's Manual* (Buchanan and

Gibbons, 1974) listed six species in the genus. More recent taxonomical studies (Garvie, 1983) suggest the inclusion of *L. mesenteroides*, *Leuconostoc cremoris*, and *Leuconostoc dextranicum* all under the species *L. mesenteroides*, with their phenotypic differences implied by subspecies designation (i.e., *L. mesenteroides* subsp. *cremoris*). This was concluded from DNA homology studies and dehydrogenase comparisons. The original species were based on important phenotypic differences, such as the functionality of *L. cremoris* as a dairy starter culture. Thus the original species definitions will probably continue to be used for working applications.

Cucumbers represent the largest crop grown in the United States for pickling (Vaughn, 1982). The sequence of events, active microflora, and process controls are very similar for the production of pickles and olives. The natural control points are salt concentration (5–8%), temperature (21–30°C), availability of fermentable material, and the relative numbers and types of microorganisms present at the onset of fermentation. Anaerobic conditions must be maintained.

A major difference in the microflora of pickles and olives as compared to the sauerkraut fermentation is that with a 5–8% brine *L. mesenteroides* never predominates the initial stages of the fermentation and may be absent throughout the incubation if the brine is at an 8% level (Vaughn, 1982). At the higher salt levels and with the pH approaching 3.7, *L. plantarum* will predominate, with *P. acidilactici*, *P. pentosaceus*, and *L. brevis* of limited occurrence.

Controlled fermentations are more prevalent in pickle manufacture than in olive fermentations. Etchells et al. (1973) developed a controlled fermentation method for pickles that has gained limited acceptance by the industry (Fleming, 1982). This procedure includes washing the cucumbers, acidifying brine with acetate, purging with nitrogen gas, and buffering the brine 18–24 hr after brining. *Lactobacillus plantarum* is either used alone or in combination with *P. acidilactici*. The fermentation at 25–30°C takes 7–12 days. This method results in increased yields and improved quality. A fermentation using starter cultures has been developed by Fleming et al. (1978) for cucumber slices as well.

The olive fermentation process is similar to pickle fermentation, with the exception of the longer incubation time. The minimum is usually 1 month for the fermentation of olives. As shown previously with the other fermentations of produce, three successive phases can be defined in olive fermentations (Vaughn et al., 1943). The first phase lasts 7 days and gram-negative bacteria such as *Aerobacter* and *Pseudomonas* are present with gram-positive bacteria, *Leuconostoc* and *Streptococcus*. There are also some yeasts present. The middle phase lasts until approximately day 21, with the gram-positive bacteria and *Aerobacter* persisting and the yeasts in decline. In the final phase the gram-negative bacteria have disappeared, with *L. plantarum* and *L. brevis* predominating.

Cruess (1930, 1937) first suggested the use of starter cultures for Spanish-style green olives. *Lactobacillus plantarum* was used extensively in California from 1937 to 1955, after which, for economic reasons, the use of starter cultures declined. When a fermentation needs an inoculation of lactic acid bacteria, brine from previous successful fermentation is used (Vaughn, 1975). However, studies have shown that controlled fermentations result in a profound improvement of texture, color, and other sensory qualities of the olive. For example, Balatsouras et al. (1983) found in work with Conservolia olives that addition of *L. plantarum* and fermentable sugars and a heat-shock treatment resulted in a complete fermentation with decreased incubation times. Acidification of the brine and the phenolic compounds of the olives had no effect on the lactic acid bacteria. One of the important variables that was found by Balatsouras and co-workers was the individuality of the starter culture strain used. Selection of the culture of *Lactobacillus* affected the outcome of the fermentation.

The benefits of controlled over natural fermentations has also been established with Manzanillo olives (Etchells et al., 1966; Fleming et al., 1973). Etchells et al. (1966) also discovered that strain selection was an important factor in the outcome of the fermentation.

The initial work in the genetics of *L. plantarum* and *Pediococcus* has already been discussed. Leuconostocs are bacteria which also have not received much attention in the development of techniques for their genetic modification. As a heterofermentative bacteria in a mixed culture fermentation, Leuconostoc is more complex with regard to its population dynamics, its nutrition, and how widely its fermentative performance will be affected by process controls and the buildup of metabolic products.

Plasmids in *Leuconostoc* were originally documented by O'Sullivan and Daly (1982). They examined 10 strains of *Leuconostoc* and found all of them to contain at least one plasmid, ranging from 2.5 to 40 Mdal. These authors correlated loss of lactose or citrate utilization with plasmid DNA loss, suggesting that these properties are plasmid linked.

Orberg and Sandine (1984b) examined plasmids from *Leuconostoc* species in conjunction with antibiotic resistance and antibacterial activity. They made two interesting suggestions: (1) Judging from the antibacterial substances produced by the *Leuconostoc* strains studied, one must be careful in the selection of a *Leuconostoc* for mixed-strain starter cultures, and (2) the similarity between *Leuconostoc* and dairy streptococci makes transfer of genetic elements between the two groups a strong possibility.

Summary

It is evident that there is a scarcity of information relevant to the genetics and physiology of starter cultures for meat and vegetable fermentations. Because of their commercial value, these bacteria are now starting to receive attention in these areas.

There is a trend for the use of higher fermentation temperatures for rapid acid production in shorter time periods for fermented sausages. This strategy reduces the production of flavor compounds by microflora, as well as the synthesis of antioxidants and antimicrobial compounds. Amplification of these desirable products by the appropriate microorganisms could allow for shorter fermentation times without loss of product quality. Shorter generation times for starter cultures at a lower temperature would lessen the opportunity for the growth of pathogens and undesirable chemical changes in meat products. These avenues should be investigated in both homofermentative and heterofermentative bacteria.

Lastly, with the world population continuing unabated, shortages of food are becoming more and more common. Food fermentations allow for a low-energy, natural method for food preservation, diversification, and waste utilization. Advances in the genetics of starter cultures and fermentation technology for indigenous foods in developing nations will assist in easing hunger.

REFERENCES

Allen, L. K., Sandine, W. E., and Elliker, P. R. (1963). Transduction in *Streptococcus lactis*. *J. Dairy Res.* *30*:351–357.

American Meat Institute (1982). *Good Manufacturing Practices, Fermented Dry and Semi-dry Sausage*, American Meat Institute, Washington, D. C.

Anderson, D. G. and McKay, L. L. (1977). Plasmids, loss of lactose metabolism, and appearance of partial and full lactose-fermenting revertants in *Streptococcus cremoris* B1. *J. Bacteriol.* *129*:367–377.

Anderson, D. G. and McKay, L. L. (1983). Simple and rapid method for isolating large plasmid DNA from lactic streptococci. *Appl. Environ. Microbiol.* *46*:549–552.

Anderson, D. G. and McKay, L. L. (1984). Genetic and physical characterization of recombinant plasmids associated with cell aggregation and high frequency conjugal transfer in *Streptococcus lactis* ML3. *J. Bacteriol.* *158*:954–962.

Anonymous (1984a). USDA proposal to permit 2/3 reduction in bacon nitrite levels. *Food Chem. News* *24*:50–51.

Anonymous (1984b). Bacon nitrite can be greatly reduced with no botulism risk, USDA says. *Food Chem. News* *22*:33–34.

Auclair, J. and Vassal, Y. (1963). Occurrence of variants sensitive to agglutinins and to lactoperoxidase in a lactenin-resistant strain of *Streptococcus lactis*. *J. Dairy Res. 30*:345–349.

Bacus, J. N. (1983). *Custom Cultures*™ *Technical Binder*, ABC Research, Gainesville, Fla.

Bacus, J. N. (1984). *Utilization of Microorganisms in Meat Processing*, Wiley, New York.

Balatsouras, G., Tisbri, A., Dalles, T., and Doutsias, G. (1983). Effects of fermentation and its control on the sensory characteristics of Conservolia variety green olives. *Appl. Environ. Microbiol. 46*:68–74.

Buchanan, R. E. and Gibbons, N. E. (1974). *Bergey's Manual of Determinative Bacteriology*, 8th ed., Williams & Williams, Baltimore.

Chassy, B. and Rokaw, E. (1981). Conjugal transfer of plasmid-associated lactose metabolism in *Lactobacillus casei* subsp. *casei*. In *Molecular Biology, Pathogenicity, and Ecology of Bacterial Plasmids* (S. B. Levy, R. C. Clowes, and E. L. Koenig, eds.), Plenum, New York, p. 590.

Chassy, B. M., Gibson, E. and Giuffrida, A. (1976). Evidence for extrachromosomal elements in *Lactobacillus*. *J. Bacteriol. 127*:1576–1578.

Chassy, B. M., Rokaw, E., and Giuffrida, A. S. (1980). Studies on the function and structure of lactose plasmids in *Lactobacillus casei* subsp. *casei*. *Plasmid 3*:235.

Chopin, A., Chopin, M. C., Moillo-Batt, A., and Langella, P. (1984). Two plasmid determined restriction and modification systems in *Streptococcus lactis*. *Plasmid 11*:260–263.

Cords, B. R., McKay, L. L., and Guerry, P. (1974). Extrachromosomal elements in group N streptococci. *J. Bacteriol. 117*:1149–1152.

Cruess, W. V. (1930). Pickling green olives. *Calif. State Agric. Exp. Sta. Bull. 498.*

Cruess, W. V. (1937). Use of starters for green olive fermentations. *Fruit Prod. J. 17*:1–12.

Daeschel, M. A. and Klaenhammer, T. R. (1985). Association of a 13.6 Mdal plasmid in *Pediococcus pentosaceus* with bacteriocin activity. In *Abstracts of the Annual Meeting of the American Society for Microbiology*, p. 31.

Davey, G. P. (1984). Plasmid associated with diplococcin production in *Streptococcus cremoris*. *Appl. Environ. Microbiol. 48*:895–896.

Davies, F. L. and Gasson, M. J. (1981). Reviews of the progress of dairy science: Genetics of lactic acid bacteria. *J. Dairy Res. 48*:363–376.

Davies, F. L., Underwood, H. M., and Gasson, M. J. (1981). The value of plasmid profiles for strain identification in lactic streptococci and the relationship between *Streptococcus lactis* 712, ML3 and C2. *J. Appl. Bacteriol.* *51*:325–337.

Davies, R. W. and Gronenborn, A. M. (1982). Molecular cloning of the gene for dihydrofolate reductase from *Lactobacillus casei*. *Gene* *17*:229–233.

Deibel, R. H. and Niven, Jr., C. F. (1957). *Pediococcus cerevisiae*: A starter culture for summer sausage. *Bacteriol. Proc.* 14–15.

Deibel, R. H., Niven, C. F., and WIlson, D. D. (1961). Microbiology of meat curing. III. Some microbiological and related technological aspects in the manufacture of fermented sausages. *Appl. Microbiol.* *9*:156–165.

DeVos, W. M., Underwood, H. M., and Davies, F. L. (1984). Plasmid encoded bacteriophage resistance in *Streptococcus cremoris* SK11. *FEMS Microbiol. Letts.* *23*:175–178.

Dobrzanski, W., Bardowski. J., Kozak, W., and Zajdel, J. (1982). Lactostrepcins: Bacteriocins of lactic streptococci. In *Microbiology—1982* (D. Schlessinger, ed.), American Society for Microbiology, Washington, D.C., pp. 225–229.

Efstathiou, J. D. and McKay, L. L. (1977). Inorganic salts resistance associated with a lactose fermenting plasmid in *Streptococcus lactis*. *J. Bacteriol.* *130*:257–265.

Etchells, J. L., Borg, A. F., Kittel, I. D., Bell, T. A., and Fleming, H. P. (1966). Pure culture fermentation of green olives. *Appl. Microbiol.* *14*:1027–1041.

Etchells, J. L., Bell, T. A., Fleming, H. P., Kelling, R. E., and Thompson, R. L., (1973). Suggested procedure for the controlled fermentation of commercially brined pickling cucumbers—The use of starter cultures and reduction of carbon dioxide accumulation. *Pickle Pak Sci.* *3*:4–14.

Fernandez-Diez, M. J. (1983). Olives. In *Biotechnology*, Vol. 5 (G. Reed, ed.), Verlag Chemie, Weinheim, pp. 379–399.

Fleming, H. P. (1982). Fermented vegetables. In *Economic Microbiology*, Vol. 7 (A. H. Rose, ed.), Academic, New York, pp. 228–258.

Fleming, H. P., Walter, Jr., W. M., and Etchells, J. L. (1973). Antimicrobial properties of oleuropein and products of its hydrolysis from green olives. *Appl. Microbiol.* *26*:777–782.

Fleming, H. P., Thompson, R. L., Bell, T. A., and Hontz, L. H. (1978). Controlled fermentation of sliced cucumbers. *J. Food Sci.* *43*:888–891.

Forsin, R. and Pakkila, M. (1979). Studies on slime forming group N *Streptococcus* strains V. Electrophoretic characterizaton of cell proteins associated with the particulate fraction. *Acta Univ. Oul. A78 Biochem.* *22*:1–13.

Forsin, R., Raunio, V., and Myllymaa, R. (1973). Studies on slime forming group N *Streptococcus* strains. I. Differentiation between some lactic *Streptococcus* strains by polyacrylamide gel electrophoresis of soluble cell proteins. *Acta Univ. Oul. A12, Biochem.* *3*:1–19.

Garvie, E. I. (1983). *Leuconostoc mesenteroides* subsp. *cremoris* (Knudson and Sorenson) comb. nov. and *Leuconostoc mesenterioides* subsp. *dextranicum* (Beijerinck) comb. nov. *Int. J. Sys. Bacteriol.* *33*:118–119.

Gasson, M. J. (1980). Production, regeneration and fusion of protoplasts in lactic streptococci. *FEMS Microbiol. Lett.* *9*:99–102.

Gasson, M. J. (1982). Identification of the lactose plasmid in *Streptococcus lactis* 712. In *Microbiology—1982* (D. Schlessinger, ed.), American Society for Microbiology, Washington, D.C., pp. 217–220.

Gasson, M. J. (1983a). Plasmid complements of *Streptococcus lactis* NCDO 712 and other lactic streptococci after protoplast-induced curing. *J. Bacteriol.* *154*:1–9.

Gasson, M. J. (1983b). Genetic transfer systems in lactic acid bacteria. *Antonie van Leeuwenhoek* *49*:275–282.

Gasson, M. J. (1984). Transfer of sucrose fermenting ability, nisin resistance and nisin production into *Streptococcus lactis* 712. *FEMS Microbiol. Lett.* *21*:7–10.

Gasson, M. J. and Davies, F. L. (1979). Conjugal transfer of lactose genes in group N streptococci. *Soc. Gen. Microbiol. Q.* *6*:87.

Gasson, M. J. and Davies, F. L. (1980a). Conjugal transfer of the drug resistance plasmid pAMβ in the lactic streptococci. *FEMS Microbiol. Lett.* *7*:51–53.

Gasson, M. J. and Davies, F. L. (1980b). High-frequency conjugation associated with *Streptococcus lactis* donor cell aggregation. *J. Bacteriol.* *143*:1260–1264.

Geis, A. (1982). Transfection of protoplasts of *Streptococcus lactis* subsp. *diacetylactis*. *FEMS Microbiol. Lett.* *15*:119–122.

Gibson, E. M., Chace, N. M., London, S. B., and London, J. (1979). Transfer of plasmid-mediated antibiotic resistance from streptococci to lactobacilli. *J. Bacteriol.* *137*:614–619.

Gonzalez, C. F. and Kunka, B. S. (1983). Plasmid transfer in *Pediococcus* spp.: Intergeneric and intrageneric transfer of pIP501. *Appl. Environ. Microbiol.* *46*:81–89.

Harlander, S. K. and McKay, L. L. (1984). Transformation of *Streptococcus sanguis* Challis with *Streptococcus lactis* plasmid DNA. *Appl. Environ. Microbiol.* *48*:342–346.

Harlander, S. K., McKay, L. L., and Schachtele, C. F. (1984). Molecular cloning of the lactose-metabolizing genes from *Streptococcus lactis*. *Appl. Environ. Microbiol. 48*:347–351.

Ishiwa, H. and Iwata, S. (1980). Drug resistance plasmids in *Lactobacillus fermentum*. *J. Gen. Appl. Microbiol. 26*:71–74.

Kempler, G. M. and McKay, L. L. (1979a). Charcterization of plasmid deoxyribonucleic acid in *Streptococcus lactis* subsp. *diacetylactis*: Evidence for plasmid-linked citrate utilization. *Appl. Environ. Microbiol. 37*:316–323.

Kempler, G. M. and McKay, L. L. (1979b). Genetic evidence for plasmid linked lactose metabolism in *Streptococcus lactis* subsp. *diacetylactis*. *Appl. Environ. Microbiol. 37*:1041–1043.

Klaenhammer, T. R. (1984). A general method for plasmid isolation in lactobacilli. *Curr. Microbiol. 10*:23–28.

Klaenhammer, T. R. and Sutherland, S. M. (1980). Detection of plasmid deoxyribonucleic acid in an isolate of *Lactobacillus acidophilus*. *Appl. Environ. Microbiol. 39*:671–674.

Klaenhammer, T. R., McKay, L. L., and Baldwin, K. A. (1978). Improved lysis of group N streptococci for isolation and rapid characterization of plasmid DNA. *Appl. Environ. Microbiol. 35*:592–600.

Kok, J., van der Vossen, J. M. B., and Venema, G. (1984). Construction of plasmid cloning vectors for lactic streptococci which also replicate in *Bacillus subtilis* and *Escherichia coli*. *Appl. Environ. Microbiol. 48*:726–731.

Kondo, J. K. and McKay, L. L. (1982a). Mutanolysin for improved lysis and rapid protoplast formation in dairy streptococci. *J. Dairy Sci. 65*:1428–1431.

Kondo, J. K. and McKay, L. L. (1982b). Transformation of *Streptococcus lactis* protoplasts by plasmid DNA. *Appl. Environ. Microbiol. 43*:1213–1215.

Kondo, J. K. and McKay, L. L. (1984). Plasmid transformation of *Streptococcus lactis* protoplasts: Optimization and use in molecular cloning. *Appl. Environ. Microbiol. 48*:252–259.

LeBlanc, D. J., Crow, V. L., and Lee, L. N. (1980). Plasmid mediated carbohydrate catabolic enzymes among strains of *Streptotoccus lactis*. In *Plasmids and Transposons: Environmental Effects and Maintenance Mechanisms* (C. Stuttard and K. Rozee, eds.), Academic, New York, pp. 31–41.

Lee, L. J., Hansen, J. B., Jagusztyn-Krynicka, K., and Chassy, B. M. (1982). Cloning and expression of the β-D-phosphogalactoside galactohydrolase gene of *Lactobacillus casei* in *Escherichia coli* K-12. *J. Bacteriol. 152*:1138–1146.

Lee-Wickner, L. J. and Chassy, B. M. (1984). Production and regeneration of *Lactobacillus casei* protoplasts. *Appl. Environ. Microbiol. 48*:994–1000.

Leistner, L. and Rodel, W. (1975). The significance of water activity for microorganisms in meats. In *Water Relations of Foods* (R. B. Duckworth, ed.), Academic, New York, p. 309.

Liepe, H. U. (1983). Starter cultures in meat production. In *Biotechnology*, Vol. 5 (G. Reed, ed.), Verlag Chemie, Weinheim, pp. 399–424.

McKay, L. L. (1982). Regulation of lactose metabolism in dairy streptococci. In *Developments in Food Microbiology*, Vol. 1 (R. Davies, ed.), Applied Science, London, pp. 153–182.

McKay, L. L. (1983). Functional properties of plasmids in lactic streptococci. *Antonie van Leeuwenhoek 49*:259–274.

McKay, L. L. and Baldwin, K. A. (1974). Simultaneous loss of proteinase- and lactose-utilizing enzyme activities in *Streptococcus lactis* and reversal of loss of transduction. *Appl. Microbiol. 28*:342–346.

McKay, L. L. and Baldwin, K. A. (1978). Stabilization of lactose metabolism in *Streptococcus lactis* C2. *Appl. Environ. Microbiol. 36*:360–367.

McKay, L. L. and Baldwin, K. A. (1984). Conjugative 40 megadalton plasmid in *Streptococcus lactis* subsp. *diacetylactis* DRC3 is associated with resistance to nisin and bacteriophage. *Appl. Environ. Microbiol. 47*:68–74.

McKay, L. L., Cords, B. R., and Baldwin, K. A. (1973). Transduction of lactose metabolism in *Streptococcus lactis* C2. *J. Bacteriol. 115*:810–815.

McKay, L. L., Baldwin, K. A., and Efstathiou, J. D. (1976). Transductional evidence for plasmid linkage of lactose metabolism in *Streptococcus lactis* C2. *Appl. Environ. Microbiol. 32*:45–52.

McKay, L. L., Baldwin, K. A., and Walsh, P. M. (1980). Conjugal transfer of genetic information in group N streptococci. *Appl. Environ. Microbiol. 40*:84–91.

National Academy of Sciences (1975). Prevention of microbial and parasitic hazards associated with processed foods. In *Fermented Foods, Fermented Sausages*, National Academy of Sciences, Washington, D.C.

Nes, I. F. (1984). Plasmid profiles of ten strains of *Lactobacillus platarum. FEMS Microbiol. Lett. 21*:359–361.

Neve, H., Geis, A., and Teuber, M. (1984). Conjugal transfer and characterization of bacteriocin plasmids in group N (lactic acid) streptococci. *J. Bacteriol. 157*:833–838.

Okamoto, T., Fujita, Y., and Irie, R. (1983). Protoplast formation and regeneration of *Streptococcus lactis* cells. *Agric. Biol. Chem. 47*:259–263.

Orberg, P. K. and Sandine, W. E. (1984a). Microscale method for rapid isolation of covalently closed circular plasmid DNA from group N streptococci. *Appl. Environ. Microbiol. 47*:677–680.

Orberg, P. K. and Sandine, W. E. (1984b). Common occurrence of plasmid DNA and vancomycin resistance in *Leuconostoc* spp. *Appl. Environ. Microbiol. 48*:1129–1133.

O'Sullivan, T. and Daly, C. (1982). Abstract. *Irish J. Food Sci. Technol. 6*:206.

Park, Y. and McKay, L. L. (1982). Distinct galactose phosphoenolpyruvate-dependent phosphotransferase system in *Streptococcus lactis*. *J. Bacteriol. 149*:420–425.

Pederson, C. S. (1960). Sauerkraut. In *Advances in Food Research,* Vol. 10 (C. O. Chichester, E. M. Mrak, and G. F. Steward, eds.), Academic, New York, pp. 233–291.

Pederson, C. S. and Albury, M. N. (1950). The effect of temperature upon bacteriological and chemical changes in fermenting cucumbers. *N.Y. State Agric. Exp. Stat. Bull.* 744.

Pederson, C. S. and Albury, M. N. (1954). The influence of salt and temperature on the microflora of sauerkraut fermentation. *Food Technol. 8*:1–5.

Pederson, C. S. and Albury, M. N. (1969). The sauerkraut fermentation. *N.Y. State Agric. Exp. Stat. Bull. 824.*

Sanders, M. E. and Klaenhammer, T. R. (1981). Evidence for plasmid linkage of restriction and modification in *Streptococcus cremoris* KH. *Appl. Environ. Microbiol. 42*:944–950.

Sanders, M. E. and Klaenhammer, T. R. (1983). Charcterization of phage-sensitive mutants from a phage-insensitive strain of *Streptococcus lactis*: Evidence for a plasmid determinant that prevents phage adsorption. *Appl. Environ. Microbiol. 46*:1125–1133.

Sandine, W. E., Elliker, P. R., Allen, L. K., and Brown, W. C. (1962). Genetic exchange and variability in lactic *Streptococcus* starter organisms. *J. Dairy Sci. 45*:1266–1271.

Scherwitz, K. M., Baldwin, K. A., and McKay, L. L. (1983). Plasmid linkage of a bacteriocin-like substance in *Streptococcus lactis* subsp. *diacetylactis* strain WM4: Transferability to *Streptococcus lactis*. *Appl. Environ. Microbiol. 45*:1506–1512.

Smiley, M. B. and Fryder, V. (1978). Plasmids, lactic acid production and N-acetyl-D-glucosamine fermentation in *Lactobacillus helveticus* subsp. *jugurti*. *Appl. Environ. Microbiol. 35*:777–781.

Smith, J. L. and Palumbo, S. A. (1981). Microorganisms as food additives. *J. Food Protect. 44*:936–955.

Smith, J. L. and Palumbo, S. A. (1983). Use of starter cultures in meats. *J. Food Protect. 46*:997–1006.

Snook, R. J. and McKay, L. L. (1981). Conjugal transfer of lactose-fermenting ability among *Streptococcus cremoris* and *Streptococcus lactis* strains. *Appl. Environ. Microbiol. 42*:904–911.

Snook, R. J., McKay, L. L., and Ahlstrand, G. G. (1981). Transduction of lactose metabolism by *Streptococcus cremoris* C3 temperate phage. *Appl. Environ. Microbiol. 42*:897–903.

Stamer, J. R. (1968). *Proc. Frontiers in Food Research*, N.Y. State Agric. Exp. Stn. June, p. 46.

Stamer, J. R. (1974). Fermented vegetables. In *Fermented Foods, Current Science and Technology*, N.Y. State Agric. Exp. Stn. Special Report No. 16.

Stamer, J. R. (1975). Recent developments in the fermentation of sauerkraut. In *Lactic Acid Bacteria in Beverages and Food* (J. G. Carr, C. V. Cutting, and G. S. Whiting, eds.), Academic, New York, pp. 267–281.

Stamer, J. R. (1983). Lactic acid fermentation of cabbage and cucumbers. In *Biotechnology*, Vol. 5 (G. Reed, ed.), Verlag Chemie, Weinheim, pp. 367–378.

Subcommittee on Lactobacilli and Related Microorganisms of the International Committee on Systematic Bacteriology (1979). Minutes of meeting. September, 1978. *Int. J. Bacteriol. 29*:435.

Teuber, M. and Geis, A. (1981). The family *Streptococcaceae* (nonmedical aspects). In *The Prokaryotes, A Handbook on Habits, Isolation, and Identification of Bacteria* (M. P. Starr, H. Stolp, H. G. Truper, A. Balows, and H. G. Schlegel, eds.), Springer-Verlag, New York, pp. 1614–1630.

Turner, N., Sandine, W. E., Elliker, P. R., and Day, E. A. (1963). Use of tetrazolium dyes in an agar medium for differentiation of *Streptococcus lactis and Streptococcus cremoris*. *J. Dairy Sci. 46*:380–385.

U.S. Dapartment of Agriculture (1977). The staphylococcal enterotoxin problem in fermented sausage. Task Force Report. F.S.Q.S., Washington, D.C.

Vaughn, R. H. (1975). Lactic acid fermentation of olives with special reference to California conditions. In *Lactic Acid Bacteria in Beverages and Food* (J. G. Carr, C. V. Cutting, and G. C. Whiting, eds.), Academic, New York, pp. 307–323.

Vaughn, R. H. (1982). Lactic acid fermentation of cabbage, cucumber, olives and other produce. In *Prescott and Dunn's Industrial Microbiology* (G. Reed, ed.), AVI, Westport, Conn., pp. 185–236.

Vaughn, R. H., Douglas, H. C., and Gililland, R. (1943). Production of Spanish type green olives. *Calif. Agric. Exp. Stat. Bull.* No. 678.

Vescova, M., Bottazzi. V., Sarra, P. G., and Dellaglio, F. (1981). Evidence of plasmid deoxyribonucleic acid in *Lactobacillus*. *Microbiologica 4*:413–419.

Walsh, P. M. and McKay, L. L. (1981). Recombinant plasmid associated with cell aggregation and high frequency conjugation of *Streptococcus lactis* ML3. *J. Bacteriol. 146*: 937–944.

Walsh, P. M. and McKay, L. L. (1982). Restriction endonuclease analysis of the plasmids in *Streptococcus lactis* ML3 and two recombinant lactose plasmids. *Appl. Environ. Microbiol. 43*: 1006–1010.

Yu, R. S.-T., Hung, T. V., and Azad, A. A. (1982). Rapid screening of highly purified plasmids in lactic streptococci. *Aust. J. Dairy Technol. 37*: 99–103.

Yu, R. S.-T., Kyle, W. S. A., Azad, A. A., and Hung, T. V. (1984). Conditions for the production and regeneration of protoplasts from lactic streptococci. *Milchwissenschaft 39*: 136–139.

FIVE

Regulatory and Social Aspects of Biotechnology

21

Regulatory Aspects of the Use of Modern Biotechnological Methods in the Food Industry

EDWARD L. KORWEK / Law Firm of Keller and Heckman, Washington, D.C.

INTRODUCTION

The commercial success of new technologies depends upon ease of entry into the marketplace of their derived products. Obtaining regulatory clearances to manufacture and market products of a new technology can involve millions of dollars and enormous expenditures of resources. Regulatory hurdles can also result in long delays in the delivery of useful products and drive up consumer costs. Products manufactured by the use of new technologies must also be assured as being as safe (and in some cases as effective) as their approved (1), conventionally made counterparts.

Use of new methods of manufacture, such as recombinant DNA (rDNA) and hybridoma techniques in place of conventional processes to prepare articles subject to the jurisdiction of the Food and Drug Administration (FDA) raises these general issues and, specifically, the question of "how" products made by such modern biotechnological methods will be regulated by the FDA under the Federal Food, Drug, and Cosmetic Act (2). This article discusses this question in the context of foods and food ingredients. Specifically, it discusses the FDA's premarket clearance authority, since not all food products require such clearances. Particular focus is on the FDA's authority over previously cleared food ingredients now manufactured

---

Portions of this article have been reprinted with permission from E. L. Korwek, FDA Regulation of Biotechnology as a New Method of Manufacture, *Food Drug Cosmet. Law J.* *37*:289 (1982).

by modern biotechnological methods and on whether changing the method of manufacture alters their approved status. Some discussion is also devoted to the authority of other agencies to regulate food products (3).

FDA POLICY

A few years ago the FDA established a Recombinant DNA Coordinating Committee composed of representatives of various offices. On January 7, 1983, the FDA became the first regulatory agency to announce how it would review applications for products prepared by modern biotechnological methods, particularly by use of the rDNA technique. A talk paper was issued, "Regulating Recombinant DNA Products," stating that rDNA-derived products would need new clearances from the FDA even if they were identical in structure to previously cleared or naturally occurring products. The amount of data required would vary, depending on a number of factors, such as the proposed use of the product, whether it is identical to a previously approved product, how long it is to be administered to patients, the previous clinical experience with conventionally produced products, and the applicant's clinical experience with rDNA-derived substances.

The exact scope of the talk paper is unclear, although its major thrust is obviously in the drug area, because of references to patients and clinical experiences. Nevertheless, because of the broad wording utilized, its ramifications seem more far reaching, perhaps even applying to rDNA-derived food ingredients. The ambiguity generated by the talk paper has not been resolved by more recent FDA statements. The agency has made it clear that it will evaluate rDNA-derived food additives on a case-by-case basis while generally viewing petitions along the lines of classic fermentation processes (4) and as requiring data similar to petitions for conventionally derived products (5). Other statements indicate, however, that the FDA needs to develop better ways to evaluate the safety of novel "foods" created through the use of biotechnology (6).

More recently, in December 1984, the FDA (and other regulatory agencies) issued in the *Federal Register* (7) some general statements and comments on its role in the regulation of products of modern biotechnological methods. It failed to mention the talk paper or otherwise speak of food ingredients intended for human use. The FDA's position in the talk paper regarding the submission of "new applications" for biotechnologically derived articles is only referred to indirectly and quite casually in the context of *animal* food additives and animal drugs. The agency states (8) that

> animal drugs and food additives produced by recombinant DNA technology must be the subject of an approval even if the active substance is shown to be identical or similar to the active substance in a food product produced by conventional methods.

This is a significant clarification of the general concept expressed in the talk paper insofar as biotechnologically derived food ingredients are concerned. As is discussed below, it is also a drastic departure from the law and the FDA's current practice.

THE FDA AND THE FEDERAL FOOD, DRUG, AND COSMETIC ACT

The FDA's authority over the use of differing methods of manufacture derives principally from the adulteration provisions of the Federal Food, Drug, and Cosmetic Act, which gives the agency regulatory authority over foods, drugs, medical devices, and cosmetics. The FDA's statutory mandate is to ensure that foods and ingredients thereof are safe, that drugs and medical devices, such as in vitro diagnostics, are both safe and effective, and that all are neither adulterated nor misbranded. Although the principal focus of the act is on products rather than methods of manufacture, this is an oversimplification of the extent of the agency's authority under the statute. Many regulations have been promulgated that are applicable to the manufacture of foods, drugs, and medical devices, called Good Manufacturing Practices Regulations (GMPs) (9), which pervasively govern nearly all aspects of manufacturing processes. Numerous other rules, discussed more fully below, also relate to methods of manufacture. Because the avowed purpose of all these regulations is to assure that foods are safe for human consumption and that drugs and medical devices are safe as well as effective, the FDA has significant authority to regulate methods of manufacture.

FOODS

The FDA's authority to regulate currently marketed foods and their ingredients now manufactured by biotechnology depends on both its statutory premarketing clearance authority and its general powers to protect the public from articles that are otherwise adulterated because of contamination with harmful or deleterious components. The availability of its premarket clearance authority is tied to the legal classification of the ingredient. Four classes of products exist in the food area over which the FDA has regulatory powers: food additives, generally recognized as safe (GRAS) substances, prior-sanctioned ingredients, and foods. The distinctions, which are based on the language of the act, have significance because the FDA's authority to require premarketing clearances is confined to only food additives.

Section 201(s) of the act defines the term *food additive* in relevant part to mean any substance that is not GRAS or prior sanctioned, the "intended use of which results or may reasonably be expected to result, directly or indirectly, in its becoming a component or otherwise affecting the characteristics of any food" (10). It includes not only those compounds added directly to foods (called direct additives), such as texturizers and flavoring agents, but also components of food packaging materials that migrate to food (called indirect additives). As discussed below, the term *food additive* is also broad enough to possibly encompass gene transfer in food plants and animals.

To understand the impact of changes in the method of manufacture on the regulatory status of food additives, it is important first to realize that the agency regulates additives on a generic basis. Once a food additive regulation is promulgated, all manufacturers of that additive may market it without obtaining premarket clearances, provided that the manufacturer's specific formulation satisfies the requirements of the applicable regulation and, further, that the additive is used in food manufacture in accordance with any conditions of use contained in the additive regulation. Marketing clearances are required, however, for new additives, that is, those not already the subject of food additive regulations, because such ingredients are presumed to be unsafe; hence they and foods containing them are adulterated unless regulations exist covering the intended uses for the additives (11).

Animal or human food additives meeting the criteria of the applicable FDA regulations but manufactured by the use of biotechnology should not require new premarketing clearances, although in light of recent FDA statements some question exists about the agency's position on this matter. Normally, because regulations for direct and indirect additives often contain criteria only for chemical structure (identity) and purity, as well as use limitations, the precise method of manufacture is usually immaterial to satisfying the requirements of the applicable regulations. For example, regulations applicable to white mineral oil and petrolatum specify only composition requirements and use limitations (12). Use of different methods of manufacture should therefore not affect the legal status of such approved food additives, unless the method changes the identity or creates impurities that make the additive adulterated. Food additives such as the amino acid L-alanine, which is used as a nutrient added to foods, if made by rDNA techniques, for example, should be able to be legally marketed once the requirements of the applicable regulation (13) have been met and if it is of otherwise suitable purity. In cases where food additive regulations specify manufacturing methods, such as in the regulations for glycerides (14), food additives in these and other such regulations that are now prepared by modern biotechnological methods would not be covered and hence would require new FDA clearances, unless they were GRAS or prior sanctioned.

The conclusion that biotechnologically produced additives meeting the requirements of the applicable regulations that specify no methods of manufacture can be marketed without premarketing clearances assumes that the additives are used in accordance with good manufacturing practice. The FDA's regulations defining the term *good manufacturing practice* require in relevant part that the quantity of the substance added to food not exceed the amount reasonably required to accomplish its effect in food and that the ingredient be of appropriate food grade and prepared and handled as a food ingredient (15). The requirement that an additive be of "appropriate food grade" basically means that it must be of a purity suitable for the intended use as a food ingredient (16).

Purity considerations are always important where a new method of manufacture is used to prepare an approved food additive. This is equally true in the case of biotechnologically produced additives, because use of the new method can produce a range of impurities different from those encountered with some traditional methods of manufacture. Biotechnologically produced additives must therefore not only meet the purity requirements specified in the applicable regulation but also otherwise be of suitable purity to avoid a charge of adulteration. In this regard, although FDA premarketing clearances must be obtained *only* for new "food additives," the FDA still has authority to protect the public from harmful products not having undergone premarket clearances under the adulteration and misbranding provisions of the act (17).

The statutory definition of a food additive specifically excludes substances that are GRAS or subject to a prior sanction. Although FDA premarketing authority over such ingredients is nonexistent, use of differing methods of manufacture can still affect the legal status of certain types of these ingredients. To understand whether and how use of biotechnology alters the GRAS or prior-sanctioned status of food ingredients made by conventional means, a review of the definitions for these terms and of the FDA's authority over these types of ingredients is necessary.

Prior-sanctioned substances are "grandfathered," that is, are those which had been specifically approved and marketed before enactment of the Food Additives Amendments in 1958. The GRAS substances are those generally recognized, among experts qualified by scientific training experience to evaluate the safety of food, as having been shown, through scientific procedures or, in the case of substances used in food prior to January 1, 1958, through either scientific procedures or experience based on common use in food, to be safe under the intended conditions of use.

The GRAS definition provides two ways to establish general recognition, depending on when the ingredient is used in food. To establish GRAS status for substances used in food after 1958, safety must be proven through scientific procedures, that is, scientific evidence of safety published in the literature or otherwise widely disseminated so as to become common knowledge among scientists knowledgeable about the safety of food ingredients. For food ingredients marketed before January 1, 1958, GRAS status can be established through scientific evidence published in the literature or common use in food, which means a substantial history of human consumption by a number of consumers.

Actually three ways exist to establish a GRAS position, which then can be used as a legal basis to market a substance. A manufacturer may seek the FDA's opinion through the filing of a GRAS affirmation petition or use an ingredient listed in the FDA's GRAS regulations, which contain two parts, Parts 182 and 184 (18), listing substances that are GRAS and those that have been affirmed as GRAS. Finally, a manufacturer may make an independent determination of GRAS status, which means establishing to his own satisfaction, without seeking FDA concurrence, that the statutory requisites for general recognition of safety have been met (19). Although the FDA has promulgated regulations in Parts 182 and 184 listing substances it recognizes as GRAS, these lists are admitted by the FDA not to be an all-inclusive compilation of GRAS substances (20); many GRAS food ingredients are not on the lists, such as fructose.

Marketing on the basis of a prior sanction is somewhat more difficult for two reasons. A letter or some type of documentary evidence is needed to establish that the FDA or the U.S. Department of Agriculture at one time considered the specific use of the substance as safe and had granted approval for that use prior to the effective date of the Food Additive Amendments to the act. In addition, according to the FDA, prior sanction status can be waived, so it must be shown that this has not inadvertently occurred. Waiver occurs when a GRAS affirmation or food additive regulation has been promulgated covering a substance alleged to be the subject of a prior sanction and the FDA has not been informed of the prior sanction during the rule making (21).

Because prior sanctions are considered to be generic, substances that are prior sanctioned should remain so even if manufactured by the use of biotechnology. The approval goes to the substance, and not its method of manufacture. The same considerations mentioned before of the necessity of identifying the chemical structure (identity) and establishing the purity of biotechnologically produced food additives therefore apply as well to prior-sanctioned ingredients.

In contrast, the use of biotechnology to prepare substances that have been affirmed as GRAS in Part 184 of the FDA's regulations affects their regulatory status. This is because the regulations in Part 184, which list substances that have been affirmed as GRAS, usually include general statements about the method of manufacture. Many ingredients that are the subject of the affirmed as GRAS regulations but which are now manufactured by modern biotechnological methods therefore would not meet the requirements of the regulation because conventional methods of manufacture are specified; they could not be marketed on the basis that they have been affirmed as GRAS. Although the GRAS status (or the safety) of any food ingredient is clearly related to its composition, the FDA has explicitly emphasized in promulgating these regulations in Part 184 that method of manufacture also can be a factor in determining the general recognition of safety. The agency might therefore view the use of biotechnology as also affecting the regulatory status of other GRAS ingredients as well, especially given its recent statements about animal food additives.

In the preamble to a *Federal Register* notice (22) defining criteria for the affirmation of GRAS status, the FDA noted that it is important to consider manufacturing processes in defining the substance that has been determined to be GRAS. The agency stated (23) that

> a determination of GRAS status is based on the composition of the ingredient. It may not be possible, however, to determine the precise composition by analysis. Especially in the case of contaminants present at very low levels, the complete composition of an ingredient will not be known unless it is tested for the presence of every conceivable contaminant. Such a process of complete testing would, of course, be prohibitively expensive. Instead of attempting to ascertain the composition of an ingredient . . . it may be more practical to define the substance in terms of its manufacturing process and to treat variations of the ingredient produced by new manufacturing processes as subject to independent review of their safety.

The agency continued its discussion of the relevance of method of manufacture to GRAS status stating (24):

> Processing information about a substance, as it serves to identify the substance and provide information on its safety, must be part of the generally available information for the substance to be affirmed as GRAS.

In light of the foregoing comments by the agency, use of different manufacturing processes may affect the regulatory status of all GRAS ingredients, whether or not they are the subject of the affirmed as GRAS regulations, because alternative methods of manufacture may alter the composition and hence toxicity of an ingredient (25). The FDA could view the use of different manufacturing processes as a factor in determining GRAS status *generally*, even though the language quoted above is in the specific context of the GRAS affirmation regulations of Part 184. Though the agency has acknowledged in some cases that a change in manufacturing process does not necessarily alter the GRAS status of an ingredient (26), it might view the use of modern biotechnological methods as presumptively affecting GRAS status because the techniques are not yet generally recognized methods of production. This means that the use of biotechnology to prepare GRAS ingredients listed in Part 182 could alter their regulatory status, even though regulations in this part are silent as to method of manufacture. The same consideration might also apply to ingredients previously marketed on the basis of independent GRAS determinations that are now manufactured by the use of biotechnology.

The view that a change in manufacturing process could affect the GRAS status of an ingredient *might* be overcome if a manufacturer could establish that the change has produced no alteration in the identity of the ingredient and that it is otherwise of suitable purity. In this case the substance might still be GRAS or eligible for affirmation as GRAS, although recent FDA statements alluded to previously suggesting that of new clearances are required for biotechnologically derived animal food additives may preclude the possibility of agency concurrence as to the GRAS status of biotechnologically derived food ingredients. Utilization of new processes may therefore require a food additive petition, or at least the adoption of additional specifications or limitations to assure that the new version of the ingredient is not significantly different from that which has been determined to be GRAS. As a practical matter, however, because biotechnology likely affects the purity of an ingredient, the FDA could also view the process as a food additive. Indeed, it has already regulated as food additives a number of microorganisms and enzymes used to prepare food ingredients (27).

Assuming that GRAS status can be preserved, ingredients listed in Part 182 that are made by biotechnology must be of food grade to be marketed, which means of a purity suitable for the intended use. This requires at least compliance with specifications for the ingredient listed in the *Food Chemicals Codex* (28). The *Codex* specifications generally represent acceptable levels of quality and purity for food-grade ingredients. The types and levels of impurities are based on those potentially present in the ingredients, taking into account the raw materials, processing chemicals, intermediates, and by-products associated with traditional manufacturing procedures. Since the *Codex* contains specifications only for ingredients prepared by conventional, recognized methods of manufacture, compliance with the requirements of the applicable monograph may not be enough (29). The manufacturer of biotechnologically produced ingredients listed in Part 182 must still ensure that, consistent with good manufacturing practice, the GRAS ingredient is of suitable purity. This means again, as with additives or other food ingredients, establishing that the use of biotechnology has not produced any harmful or deleterious components. Similar purity considerations would apply to ingredients that are marketed on the basis of an independent GRAS determination.

The last remaining important class of substances over which the FDA lacks premarketing clearance authority is food itself. Products that are foods, and not food additives, can be marketed without obtaining FDA clearances, although foods like food ingredients are still subject to the adulteration provisions of the act. Hence, the method of manufacture of a food, which is defined in the act in relevant part as articles used for drink or food for humans and other animals, or by a recent court case as items consumed for taste, aroma, or nutrition (30), is immaterial to its legal status, *provided* that the manufacturing method does not produce harmful components that may make the food adulterated. The regulatory distinction concerning foods versus food additives, however, is often academic. Because of the FDA's expansive interpretation of the term *food additive*, and because many foods marketed are used as components of other foods (e.g., beans in soup, tomatoes in sauce), a wide range of foods fall within the FDA's premarket clearance authority as food additives (31).

In summary, substances that are the subject of food additive regulations should not require premarketing clearances when manufactured by modern biotechnological methods, provided that they are of food grade and meet the requirements of the applicable regulations. This usually means demonstrating that they contain no significant levels of toxicologically important contaminants that are characteristic of the method of manufacture; that they meet the criteria specified in the regulations as to identity, purity, and use; and that they have the same chemical structure as the regulated materials, in the event the applicable regulations contain no or only general criteria as to identity. Similar identity and purity considerations apply to prior-sanctioned substances, so that the use of biotechnology instead of conventional methods should not necessarily change their regulatory classification.

The use of modern biotechnologies could alter the GRAS status of an ingredient, because the processes themselves have not achieved general recognition. The possibility exists, however, that if the identity and purity of biotechnologically produced ingredients can be firmly established, GRAS status may be preserved, although recent policy statements by the agency suggest otherwise. Substances that are the subject of GRAS affirmation regulations could not be marketed when made by nonconventional methods, unless a manufacturer asserts that they are otherwise GRAS on the basis of an independent determination.

ADDITIONAL REGULATORY CONSIDERATIONS

The use of modern biotechnological methods to alter the genetic makeup of food plants and food animals raises some additional, complex questions about the scope of the FDA's authority under the act, as well as that of the Environmental Protection Agency (EPA) under the Federal Insecticide, Fungicide, and Rodenticide Act (FIFRA) (32) and the U.S. Department of Agriculture (USDA) under such statutes as the Virus, Serum, and Toxin Act (VSTA) (33), which authorizes the USDA licensure of products such as vaccines used in the treatment of animal diseases (34).

The previously described definition of a food additive, which encompasses substances otherwise affecting the characteristics of food, raises the issue of whether genes inserted in plants to increase the yield, for example, are food additives that require premarketing clearances under the act. The same issue arises in the context of the genetic engineering of domestic food animals.

Alternatively, genes used to modify the characteristics of plants could be deemed pesticides. Pesticides, like food additives, require premarket clearances, but from the EPA instead of the FDA. A pesticide is defined in relevant part in the FIFRA to include not only conventional products such as insecticides and herbicides intended for preventing, destroying, repelling, or mitigating any pests, but also any substance or mixture of substances intended for use as a plant regulator (35). The term *plant regulator* is further defined in the FIFRA to mean any substance or mixture of substances intended, through physiological action, for accelerating or retarding the rate of growth or rate of maturation or for otherwise altering the behavior of plants or produce thereof; it does not include the substances intended for use as plant nutrients, trace elements, nutritional chemicals, plant innoculates, and soil amendments, such as vitamin–hormone horticultural products (36). Plant regulators registered as pesticides include daminozide, often used as a growth regulator for peanut plants that stimulates upright growth and reduces vegetative growth, promoting higher crop yields.

If the method of production of plants were regulatable under the act or the FIFRA, then either the FDA or the EPA, but not both, would be involved in oversight, since under the act a food additive cannot also be a pesticide, as the definition of a food additive excludes pesticides.

Genetic engineering of domestic food animals potentially creates even more complex regulatory issues. Similar to the considerations discussed above surrounding the use of genes to alter the characteristics of food plants, such genetic manipulation in animals could also be regulated as a food additive by the FDA. More importantly, however, depending upon the purpose for which the genes were introduced, genetic products could be regulated by the FDA as animal drugs under the act or by the USDA under the VSTA. The term *drug* is defined in relevant part under the act as articles intended for use in the diagnosis, cure, mitigation, treatment, or prevention of disease in humans or other animals; or articles (other than food) intended to affect the structure or any function of the body of humans or other animals. Since genetic manipulation would ordinarily affect the structure or function of animals, such as promote growth or milk production, inserted genes intended to accomplish such purposes could be considered drugs. Such genes might also be viewed as a special class of animal drugs, animal biologics, especially since DNA manipulation in animals might involve a vector, such as a virus.

The USDA regulations define an animal biologic as all viruses, serums, toxins, and analogous products of natural or synthetic origin, such as diagnostics, antitoxins, vaccines, live microorganisms, killed microorganisms, and the antigenic or immunizing components of microorganisms intended for use in the diagnosis, treatment, or prevention of diseases of animals (37). Under this definition, depending upon their intended uses, DNA or vectors containing manipulated DNA sequences could be viewed as biologics, which would need to be licensed by the USDA prior to marketing. Animal drugs, including biologics, are also exempt from the food additive definition under the act, so that genetic manipulation that was otherwise deemed to be encompassed by the definition of a drug would not also be considered a food additive. Dual regulation would thus be avoided.

Finally, the possibility of the use of such tests as DNA probes (38) or monoclonal antibodies (39) to detect microbial contamination of foods by *Salmonella* and other organisms raises the question of whether such detection methods are devices (40) under the act that require some type of clearance from the FDA prior to marketing.

CONCLUSIONS

One of the obvious conclusions from the foregoing discussion is that the use of modern biotechnological methods poses many old questions in a new context. Recognizing this is a step toward achieving rational regulation of articles now prepared by the new technologies. The FDA seems to be leaning toward classifying all articles now made by modern biotechnological methods as new, unapproved articles that require premarketing clearances and new, extensive safety (and efficacy) testing. A better approach to the regulation of biotechnologically produced articles, especially those in the food area, is to treat them like other articles where different, more conventional methods of manufacture are employed.

In the food area no compelling reasons exist for regulating currently marketed products now prepared by the new technology or the processes themselves in any special way, provided that biotechnologically produced food ingredients are demonstrably as safe as their conventionally manufactured counterparts. Gathering such evidence traditionally imposes significant responsibilities on manufacturers to establish the identity and ensure the purity of approved or otherwise legally marketed products made by different, conventional methods. Now in the context of biotechnologically produced food and food ingredients, having such data additionally encourages the agency not to develop excessive regulations or restrictive policies applicable to either the biotechnologies or to currently marketed articles now made by them. Such policies could impede commercial development and deprive the consumer of less expensive but equally safe products.

REFERENCES

1. The terms *FDA approved* and *approved products* and similar language are used broadly to mean federal agency clearances of articles such as food additives, drugs, and devices. Technically speaking, however, *approved* in the Food and Drug Administration (FDA) area implies licensing of a particular method of manufacture for a specific product. Thus the FDA does not approve food additives, because it promulgates regulations that permit their marketing by a variety of manufacturers. In contrast, the FDA "approves" drugs and class III devices in that it clears a specific product made by a particular method of manufacture. Each different manufacturer must obtain separate approval from the agency for his particular version of the approved product.

2. References which refer to the Federal Food, Drug, and Cosmetic Act cite first the section number of the act as enacted and, second, the corresponding section numbers as they appear in the *U.S. Code*. See generally Sects. 301, 401, 402, 403, 409, 501, 502, and 505; *U.S. Code 21*, Sects. 331, 341, 342, 343, 348, 351, 352, and 355 (1982).
3. For a review of other regulatory aspects of modern biotechnological methods, see E. L. Korwek and P. de la Cruz, *Rutgers Comput. Technol. Law J. 11*:301. E. L. Korwek, *Bio/Technology 2*:728 (1984); E. L. Korwek, *Bio/Technology 1*:757 (1983); E. L. Korwek, *Bio/Technology 1*:240 (1983); E. L. Korwek, *Food Technol. 37*:38 (1983); E. L. Korwek, *J. Parenteral Sci. Technol. 36*:251 (1982); E. L. Korwek, *Food Drug Cosmet. Law J. 37*:289 (1982); E. L. Korwek, *Gene 15*:1 (1981); E. L. Korwek, *U. Cincinnati Law Rev. 50*:284 (1981); E. L. Korwek, *Food Drug Cosmet. Law J. 35*:633 (1980) and reprinted with modifications in *Jurimetrics 21*:264 (1981).
4. *Food Chem. News 25*:2 (1983).
5. *Food Chem. News 26*:7 (1984).
6. *Food Chem. News 26*:18 (1984).
7. *Fed. Regist. 49*:50,856 (1984).
8. *Fed. Regist. 49*:50,879 (1984).
9. *Code Fed. Reg. 21*: Sects. 110 (umbrella food GMPs), 210 (drug GMPs), 820 (medical device GMPs), 211 (GMPs for finished pharmaceuticals), 225 (GMPs for medicated feeds), and 226 (GMPs for medicated premixes). The agency has even promulgated regulations, called Good Laboratory Practice for Nonclinical Laboratories, governing the conduct of laboratory studies that are performed to establish the safety of products submitted to the FDA for approval (*Code Fed. Reg. 21*:Sect. 58). The agency's authority to so thoroughly regulate all aspects of the manufacturing process has generally been upheld by the courts. The court in *National Association of Pharmaceutical Manufacturers v. FDA*, 637 Fed. Rep., 2nd ser. 877 (2d Cir., 1981), for example, has held that drug GMPs have the force of law.
10. Sect. 201(s), *U.S. Code 21*:Sect. 321(s) (1982).
11. Sect. 409(a) (2), *U.S. Code 21*:Sect. 348(a) (2) (food additive is unsafe and hence adulterated unless there is a regulation in effect describing the conditions under which it may be safely used). *Code Fed. Reg. 21*:Part 172 (1984), which contains food additive regulations, states that a specific food additive may be safely used in accordance with the conditions specified in the regulations, without regard to who manufactures them. A similar scheme of generic regulation is employed for over-the-counter drugs, which can be legally marketed by any

manufacturer once the requirements of the applicable monographs have been met (*Code Fed. Reg. 21*:Sect. 330.13, 1984).

12. *Code Fed. Reg. 21*:Sects. 172.878 and 172,880 (1984).
13. *Code Fed. Reg. 21*:Sect. 172.320 (1984).
14. *Code Fed. Reg. 21*:Sects. 172,828, 172.830, and 172.832 (1984).
15. *Code Fed. Reg. 21*:Sects. 172.5(a) (1) and 172.5(a) (2) (1984).
16. *Code Fed. Reg. 21*:Sect. 182.1(b) (3) (1984) states in reference to GRAS substances that GRAS ingredients shall be of appropriate "food grade," but the FDA Commissioner will offer an opinion upon request whether a substance is "of suitable purity for use in food." This apparently means that *food grade* refers to "of a purity suitable for the intended use." There is no reason to believe that the term *food grade* as applied to additives has any meaning different from that used to describe GRAS ingredients, even though the term is not currently defined for additives. In this regard the *Food Chemicals Codex*, National Academy of Sciences–National Research Council (NAS-NRC), 1st ed., 1966, p. v., contains a letter from James Goddard, then Commissioner of the FDA, stating that the agency will regard specifications in the *Codex* as defining *appropriate food grade* for *both* GRAS substances and food additives, implying that *food grade* means the same for both ingredients.
17. For an extensive discussion of the adulteration provisions of the act and their potential applicability to biotechnologically derived foods, see M. J. Brace, *Am. Univ. Law Rev. 33*:899 (1984).
18. *Code Fed. Reg. 21*:Parts 182 (list of GRAS substances) and 184 (list of substances affirmed as GRAS). Between 1958 and 1962 ingredients were listed in the FDA's regulations as GRAS in Part 182 without a detailed scientific review of all available data. Beginning in 1969, however, the FDA began a systematic review of the status of ingredients listed in Part 182, and all determinations of GRAS status pursuant to this review are then announced in Part 184 [*Code Fed. Reg. 21*:Sect. 170.30(e)].
19. *Fed. Regist. 39*:34,188 (1974). Here, in the promulgation of a food additive regulation for citric acid, the agency states in the preamble to the regulation that "[the Act] does not require that a food manufacturer consult with, or obtain the approval of, the [FDA] before using a food ingredient on the ground that it is GRAS for the use involved." When GRAS status is based on scientific procedures, the burden is on the manufacturer to prove that experts would agree that a substance is safe, and not that it actually is safe [*United States v. 41 cases, More or Less*, 420 Fed. Rep., 2nd ser. 1126 (5th Cir. 1970), p. 1131].

20. *Code Fed. Reg. 21*:Sects. 170.30(d) and 182.1(a) (1984).
21. *Code Fed. Reg. 21*:Sect. 181.5(d) (1984).
22. *Fed. Regist. 41*:53,600 (1976). Preambles constitute advisory opinions unless otherwise repudiated by the agency or overruled by a court [*Code Fed. Reg. 21*:Sect. 10.85(d) (1), (1984)].
23. *Fed. Regist. 41*:53,603 (1976).
24. *Fed. Regist. 41*:53,604 (1976).
25. *Fed. Regist. 39*:34,194 (1974). (The preamble to proposed regulations governing GRAS status states that method of manufacture is relevant to affirming a substance as GRAS because "other processes . . . may significantly alter the composition, and perhaps the toxicity, of the ingredient.")
26. *Fed. Regist. 41*:53,603 (1976). Here the agency states that "[a] determination that an ingredient produced by one manufacturing process is GRAS does not exclude the possibility that the ingredient produced by a different manufacturing process is not also GRAS."
27. *Code Fed. Reg. 21*:Sects. 173.145 (enzyme used in the production of sugar), 173.160 and 173.165 (organisms used to make citric acid).
28. The *Food Chemicals Codex* specifications are regarded by the FDA as defining "appropriate food grade" for GRAS substances listed in Parts 182 and 184. In *Code Fed. Reg. 21*:Sect. 170.30(h)(1) (1984) it is stated, for example, that GRAS substances must comply with applicable food grade specifications of *Codex*.
29. The latest edition of the *Codex* states the following:

> [I]t is obviously impossible to provide limits and tests in each monograph for the detection of all possible unusual or unexpected impurities. . . . The limits and tests provided are those considered to be necessary according to currently recognized methods of manufacture and are based on information available to or provided to the Committee on Codex Specifications. If other methods of manufacture or other than the usual raw materials are used, or if other possible impurities may be present, additional tests may be required and should be applied, as necessary, by the vendor or user to demonstrate that the substance is suitable for its intended application in foods or in food processing. [NAS–NRC, *Food Chem. Codex* 3rd ed., p. 3 (1981)].

30. *Nutrilab, Inc. v. Schweiker*, 713 Fed. Rep., 2nd ser., 335 (7th Cir., 1983), p. 338.

31. In 1972 FDA Commissioner Edwards testified that the term *food additive*

> is not limited to the artificial or synthetic chemicals that the public most often associates with it. It includes . . . fabricated food. This means that, for example, the components of beef stew—the carrots and meat as well as emulsifiers or stabilizers—must either be GRAS or [the] subject of a food additive regulation. . . . [U]nder modern methods of processing and packaging, virtually the entire food supply must be classified either as GRAS or as regulated food additives, or they may not lawfully be permitted to be used as part of the daily diet.

In *Monsanto v. Kennedy*, 613 Fed. Rep., 2nd ser., 947 (D.C. Cir. 1979), manufacturers of acrylonitrile bottles challenged the FDA's expansive interpretation of the definition of a food additive. In this case involving the use of acrylonitrile to fabricate beverage containers, the FDA sought to ban the use of acrylonitrile copolymers, since they were unapproved food additives. Because containers invariably retained a residual level of acrylonitrile monomer that failed to react completely during the manufacturing process, the FDA argued that the second law of thermodynamics leads to a scientifically indisputable prediction that there would be some migration of acrylonitrile into food sufficient to make it a "food additive." The Circuit Court rejected this argument, noting that the Commissioner has the discretion to disregard *de minimis* levels of migration (*Nutrition and Human Needs: Hearings before the Select Committee and Nutrition and Human Needs, U.S. Senate*, 92nd Congress, 2nd Session, Part 4B, 1972, p. 954).

32. *U.S. Code 7*:Sects. 136–136y (1982).
33. *U.S. Code 21*:Sects. 151–158 (1982).
34. For an extensive discussion of FDA and USDA jurisdiction over genetic manipulation utilized in the food area, see M. J. Brace and D. Jones, *Food Drug Cosmet. Law J. 38*:273 (1983).
35. *U.S. Code 7*:Sect. 136(u) (1982).
36. *U.S. Code 7*:Sect. 136(v) (1982).
37. *Code Fed. Reg. 9*:Sect. 101.2(w) (1984).
38. R. Fitts, *Food Technol. 39*:95 (1985).
39. J. A. Mattingly et al., *Food Technol. 39*:90 (1985).
40. For a discussion of FDA regulation of biotechnologically derived devices, see E. L. Korwek, *Food Drug Cosmet. Law J. 37*:289, 302–305 (1982).

22

Biotechnology and Food: A Social Appraisal

JEFFREY BURKHARDT,* LAWRENCE BUSCH, WILLIAM B. LACY, and MICHAEL HANSEN† / University of Kentucky, Lexington, Kentucky

There can be little doubt that the new biotechnologies are having and will continue to have significant impact on the practice of food processing, agriculture, and related research and development. From plant and animal improvement to any number of food processing techniques, biotechnology holds the promise of contributing to the provision of more efficient production techniques and superior food products. Moreover, the new biotechnologies have the present and future potential not only for changing food production and processing, but also for altering the institutional structure of agriculture. Though it is not yet clear what the ultimate impacts of biotechnology on those institutional arrangements might be, we can begin to assess the likelihood of certain transformations.

In this paper, we focus on the institutional changes likely to occur as a result of the introduction of the new biotechnologies into food production and processing. Our assessments of the current and projected impacts of biotechnologies are based upon over 100 interviews with scientists and research administrators in public and private sector research institutions concerning their views of the scientific, institutional, and societal importance of biotechnology in food and agricultural research and agriculture. First we examine the changing institutional context within which biotechnological research and development is taking place. Then we examine the social and economic impacts that biotechnology is likely to have. In the third section, we discuss the decisions that must be made by actors

Current affiliations:
*University of Florida, Gainesville, Florida
†Institute for Consumer Policy Research, Mt. Vernon, New York

in the food and agricultural research system: bench scientists, administrators, and the larger public. Finally, we argue that an imperative of responsibility to future generations must govern our decisions over biotechnology and food.

INSTITUTIONAL CONTEXT

A major determinant of the extent to which the new biotechnologies will have a significant impact on food, agriculture, and agricultural research is the institutional structure and climate wherein biotechnological R&D is undertaken. A major feature of this institutional context is the division of labor between the public sector institutions and private industry. Traditionally, the public sector research institution has been responsible for longer-term, higher-risk R&D. Private sector institutions have focused upon shorter-term, profit-oriented projects. Furthermore, the mission-oriented nature of public research institutions has tended to emphasize research and service to a number of publics or client groups: farmers, processors, inputs suppliers, consumers. Alternatively, the R&D enterprise in the private sector has been geared specifically toward the interests of the firm. The upshot of this is that the criteria for the choice of research problems and the development of technologies, management strategies, and so forth, have differed between the public and private sectors. Scientists and administrators in both the public and private sectors repeatedly stated in our interviews that these different research agendas will both affect, and be affected by, the increasing move toward biotechnological research.

Public Research Agenda

Public sector research has had a broad agenda, which included the quality of farm life, sustainability of farm production, yield, environmental safety, as well as broader consumer interests. Various programs, departments, and disciplines addressed these concerns. For example, traditional plant breeding programs tended to emphasize primarily research on variety development or improvement, while other disciplines focused on the impacts that new varieties might have on farm structure and markets. While most R&D was geared toward considerations of efficiency and productivity, the fundamental criterion of service to the public implied a broader orientation for the public institution as a whole.

Historically, the funding structure for agricultural research facilitated broad-based and/or long-term developmental projects of the land grant system. Hatch funds or federal "formula funding" and related state funds accounted for the major source of an institution's support, and U.S. Department of Agriculture (USDA) or state grants and contracts were the major sources of supplemental support for individual scientists (Busch and Lacy, 1983). This situation is changing. Hatch or federal formula funding is now a relatively small portion of total funds; USDA and other competitive grants, grants from commodity associations, state grants and contracts, and more recently, large corporate grants, are replacing the traditional "institutional" funding for the experiment stations.

The shift from institutional funding is partly the result of the eclipsing of public agricultural research at the federal level by basic science, medical, and military research. While agricultural research was the most visible of all federal research in 1940, today it is just a small portion of the total research budget. In addition, there is increased pressure on public institutions for accountability in research, teaching, and extension. Since colleges of agriculture report directly to and are directly funded by the respective state legislatures, program justifications are a fundamental component of the annual budgetary request. In many states population shifts toward urban areas have redistributed the rural–urban balance in the legislatures, making traditional programs more difficult to defend. And colleges of agriculture have become submerged in large state universities.

The population shift toward urban areas has also contributed to a major shift in the purpose and function of the Land Grant Universities (LGU). The LGU system was established in 1862 to counter the growing elitism of private universities. The LGU had a mission orientation to serve the needs of rural people. Its purpose was to educate the rural masses and to improve the quality of rural life, by doing research on the pressing social and agricultural problems of the day. Scientists were rewarded for being good teachers and, later, for doing applied research that addressed social problems. Over time, however, the LGU seems to have lost this component of its mission orientation (Schuh, 1984) as the rural population steadily declined in numbers and power. This decline, coupled with the pervasive views that rural areas are more backward than urban areas and that basic science is more interesting and better than applied science, encouraged the LGU system to shift its focus more toward high technology and basic science. Furthermore, criticism of the agricultural research establishment—voiced in the Pound (National Academy of Sciences, 1972) and Winrock (Rockefeller Foundation, 1982) reports—as being pedestrian has also spurred the shift toward more glamorous basic science. Indeed, colleges of agriculture increasingly emphasize the academic criteria of basic science—for example, number of publications in peer-reviewed journals (Busch and Lacy, 1983)—and deemphasize teaching and applied work, such as variety development, when evaluating agricultural researchers for promotions. Rethinking of the traditional goals of the experiment station, and of public institutions in general, is well underway.

Accountability, demands for scientific productivity, funding shortages (or at least great competition for funding), and the decline in the rate of growth of agricultural productivity appear to have encouraged experiment station directors to view favorably the new biotechnologies. Given the economic and structural aspects, as well as the inherent importance of scientific knowledge in this area, it is likely that public universities will seek to hire more young faculty to do predominantly biotechnological research. And biotechnology is a prime candidate for receiving a high priority among the various goals that an experiment station can pursue. Various science policy groups (Joint Council for Food and Agricultural Sciences, 1984; National Association of State Universities and Land Grant Colleges, 1983; USDA, 1983; Experiment Station Committee on Organization and Policy, 1984) have targeted biotechnology as the first priority in goals for scientific research. These factors only reinforce what we have heard in our interviews—that biotechnology is perceived as the key to the future of public agricultural research and development.

Private Sector Agenda

Private sector R&D has tended to focus upon efforts to (1) truncate the time and space within which production or processing take place and (2) increase the precision of techniques or technologies for production or processing. These factors affect profitability of production and processing and hence are not unexpected primary considerations of private firms. Indeed, in private sector plant improvement programs—mostly performed by seed companies that are increasingly controlled by large agrichemical firms—the emphasis has been on rapid development of varieties for potential marketability. It is for this reason that private firms are extremely interested in the new biotechnologies. For example, rather than requiring acres of land for field plots and 8–10 generations for the development of a new variety, cell and tissue culture techniques allow one to grow thousands of plants, to screen them for useful variants in Petri dishes, and to reduce dramatically generation times via the use of double haploids. In this respect, increased use of biotechnology in the private sector is eminently reasonable: It contributes toward the further "rationalization" and control of an important and profitable sector of the food industry.

Adoption of this technology by the private sector is a manifestation of the trend, begun in handicrafts in the eighteenth century and now apparent throughout agriculture, toward industrialization, that is, systematizing a number of related technologies, either in one place or under control of a single agent, in order to increase the efficiency of a production process. Moreover, history has shown that there are clear market advantages for firms which are early adopters of techniques or technologies which increase efficiency in this way. In a competitive market system there is an incentive to engage in R&D which is geared toward further control and systematization of a production process. There are not only clear advantages in terms of immediate profits to be gained from early adoption of the new technology; the potential to increase significantly a firm's market share exists as well, guaranteeing a profit stream over the long term (Busch et al., 1984). These factors have joined together to induce the production and processing sectors of market economies to pursue technologies which might provide the competitive edge (Cochrane, 1979). The overall result is that the economy as a whole tends toward complete industrialization, and, to the extent that a few firms manage to lead the way in control over technological progress, there will be increased monopolization or concentration of markets as well.

In agriculture this trend was first apparent in the food processing sector of the industry. As early as 1785, Oliver Evans had designed a fully automated, continuous process flour mill (Bathe and Bathe, 1935). By 1789 bread-kneading machines were in operation in Genoa. Hog slaughtering was a partially automated process as early as the 1830s (Giedion, 1975). Later in the nineteenth century pasteurization brought regularity and mass production to milk and cheese processing. More recently poultry production has been fully industrialized by a massive increase in flock size and assembly line processing techniques.

Close behind the processing arena has been the farm equipment industry. As early as the 1830s stationary steam engines were in use on American farms. By 1880 four-fifths of all wheat was reaped by machine (Giedion, 1975). The advent of the tractor at the turn of the century further increased the area that could be cultivated by a single man.

Clearly, then, some segments of the agricultural production and processing system industrialized early, and some later. Similarly, in some segments of the system the concentration of production or processing in the hands of a very few firms occurred earlier, while in others later. Farm machinery became concentrated relatively early (Blair, 1972), while concentration in vegetable processing and farming is still underway (Busch et al., 1984; USDA–Economic Research Service, 1978–1985).

The important point in this regard is that R&D geared toward industrialization will contribute toward concentration—but only if the industry is not already concentrated. That is, where a firm's market share can be increased dramatically by the introduction of a new technology, there is even greater incentive to develop or adopt a new technology. Indeed, it is not surprising that great attention is being paid by chemical and pharmaceutical firms to new technological developments in plant and animal improvement, since market shares can be significantly increased in these areas.

Until recently the very biological character of agricultural products acted as a barrier to complete control over their production and processing. The new biotechnologies, however, hold the potential for providing that control. For example, bovine growth hormone (BGH) appears capable of increasing per cow milk production by 10–40%. Only one or two manufacturing plants would be able to supply all the BGH needed by the nation's dairy farmers. Widespread adoption of BGH is likely to lead to increased herd size (Kalter, 1984) and perhaps a geographical redistribution of the dairy industry as well. Similarly, the development of flavor enhancers, new fermentation techniques, and even the production of certain types of processed foods in vitro is now within the horizon of possibility. It has even been suggested that agriculture might be replaced by genetically engineered foodstuffs.

Legislation and court decisions have provided further impetus for industry's move in this direction. Before the Second World War private firms involved in agriculture were confined largely to the manufacture of farm machinery and the processing of farm products. In part as a result of the war, private sector interest in chemical R&D increased considerably, including the development of the agrichemical industry. More recently, the passage of the Plant Variety Protection Act (PVPA) in 1970 allowed the patenting of most sexually reproducing plant varieties and made variety development more profitable. This in turn led to major changes in the seed industry. Large multinationals, primarily agrichemical and pharmaceutical companies, rapidly began buying seed companies. Acquisitions were so extensive in 1971 that half of the annual meeting of the American Seed Trade Association (ASTA) was devoted to a special symposium entitled "How to Sell Your Seed Company" (Mooney, 1980). By 1980 five companies, all with less than 10 years of experience in plant breeding, owned 30% of all U.S. plant variety patents. In fact, 72% of all the patents issued went to six crops, where a handful of multinational firms clearly dominate the industry (Mooney, 1983). The net effect of the PVPA was to stimulate capital investment and economic concentration in the seed industry. A similar effect, of particular importance for food processing, has been brought about by the 1980 Supreme Court decision permitting the patenting of novel life forms (see *Diamond v. Chakrabarty*, U.S. Patent No. 447,303,313, 1980). After the Chakrabarty decision patent activity in the field of genetic engineering jumped dramatically. A number of patent applications had been suspended pending resolution of the case. Since 1980 patent activity in genetic engineering has increased at over twice the rate of other technologies compared to 1974-1980 rates (NAS, 1984).

In the private sector R&D has been and is still motivated by the fact that returns to research may be captured by those doing (or paying for) the research. Patent laws further ensure that new processing techniques and machinery might yield a satisfactory rate of return. In contrast, returns to most research in the public sector could not be captured in a similar fashion, and there has been little motivation for so doing. Besides its mission, public agricultural research has had the luxury of pursuing R&D which is not necessarily commercially oriented. As we suggest below, however, biotechnology may contribute toward a change in this situation.

IMPACTS

The social and scientific impacts of the new biotechnologies are occurring, and will continue to occur, within this complex institutional milieu. Part of our assessment of these technologies is that they are in large measure being used by the experiment stations, USDA Agricultural Research Service (ARS) and the universities as both scientific tools and a means to secure funding. Indeed, biotechnology is viewed as essential to the continued existence of the public institutions. Private corporations are using the new biotechnologies as means for securing profits and increasing market shares but, most immediately, for redirecting public research. The most noticeable and important changes will thus occur in the public research institutions. These changes and their implications for the products and information emerging from public institutions will affect the structure of agriculture and hence the larger society.

New Agenda for Public Research

The most significant impact of biotechnology on public sector agricultural research is the increasing importance of the private sector's research agenda for public research. The scientific and commercial potential of biotechnology, and decreasing federal monies for research, have led to increasing university-industry ties. The private sector provides 13% of all funds expended for biotechnological research in the state agricultural experiment stations (SAES), while the national average of private funds for university research in general is 3-4% (NASULGC, 1983). In addition to higher funding levels, the nature of private sector grants has changed. Previously, most grants were fairly small, went to individual scientists, and came with few overt strings attached. For example, a pesticide company might give $10,000 to an SAES for testing a particular pesticide. Now much larger grants are often given to a department or institution, with specific conditions. The research, even though often of a basic nature, is viewed as proprietary. Any patents for products or procedures developed from such research are, at the least, shared with the granting company. The potential profits to be made from such patents are enormous. Many SAES are spending much time and money determining how to establish guidelines for a university/industry research contract. In addition, SAES view royalties and licensing fees from patents in general and the legal protection of new plant varieties as potential sources of income to support research (NASULGC, 1983).

The investment of capital in the SAES, almost always tied to exclusive release of technology via patent rights, is viewed as a disturbing development by many scientists. In interviews both public and private sector scientists stressed the detrimental effects of granting private patents for work done in the public sector. They wondered whether it represented a conflict of interest and stressed that work done in the public sector should be available to the public. In addition, many thought it might unduly influence public sector research toward narrower private sector goals. As one scientist said, "This establishes a dangerous precedent; it diverts researchers from unbiased basic research of benefit to the general public to biased research oriented to specific money making objectives. It also uses tax funded money and facilities for the benefit of the exclusive grantors."

Such strong sentiments were not restricted to the scientists themselves. A number of research directors for seed companies stressed that private sector grants should come with "no strings attached." In addition, an American Seed Trade Association (ASTA) survey of its membership revealed that a large majority of the seed companies responding were strongly against the use of venture capital for SAES research when it is tied to exclusive release (ASTA, 1984). Nevertheless, the trend has been and probably will continue to be toward more capital investment in biotechnological R&D in the public sector.

Despite the efforts of SAES directors and concerned scientists to slow this trend, the specter of the money to be made will probably decrease the flow of information among scientists. This is perhaps inevitable with private sector grants. Scientists often must delay public discussion of such work, or its results, until it has been reviewed by the sponsoring company. Even some scientists with public funding feel inhibited about discussing their work for fear that some private company with the money, equipment, and time will utilize their ideas and perform the experimental work before they can. The harm done by restricted scientific communication is not clear, but many scientists, in both the public and private sectors, view such secrecy as detrimental to science. Indeed, most maintain that the free flow of new information is fundamental to the practice of good science.

Concern regarding conflicts of interest will probably continue. Several lawsuits challenging use of public research facilities for private gain have already been brought, for example, the case of *California Rural Legal Assistance v. The Regents of The University of California* (1980). Perhaps National Association of State Universities and Land Grant Colleges (NASULGC) guidelines will determine how conflicts of interest might be avoided. However, the proprietary interests of companies in the products of sponsored research will never totally prevent such situations from arising.

Public Resource Allocation

An additional impact we can project is that there is likely to be a significant increase in the concentration of scientific talent at a small number of public institutions. For example, every state could afford and has had a conventional plant breeding program. Every state cannot afford and will not be able to have a comprehensive plant biotechnology program. Instrumentation costs are particularly expensive ($125,000–$150,000 just for initial lab setup). Minimum funding levels of $100,000 per year per grant are necessary, according to SAES directors, for adequate funding of biotechnology research. Such funding levels are 1.7 times higher than current funding levels for National Science Foundation grants and 2.8 times higher than those for USDA competitive grants (NASULGC, 1983). Starting salaries are much higher for scientists trained in the new biotechnology, owing to their relative scarcity and the higher demand for them in the private sector. These factors should lead to concentration of scientific talent in a few states and in the private sector.

In the long run this situation may reverse itself. The demand for new biotechnologists may decline somewhat as some venture capital firms go bankrupt. The supply may increase as some universities are able to mount needed training programs. Since there are no restrictions on entry into biotechnology, as there are on physicians and plumbers, new entrants' salaries may decline. As the techniques and procedures become more established and routinized and instrumentation costs decline, perhaps even faster than scientists' salaries, lower-paid technicians may even replace some scientists. In the meantime, however, the costly programs will have significantly reduced the number of less costly "traditional" programs, particularly in the plant and animal sciences.

Changing Disciplinary Focus

The third impact of biotechnology may be the deemphasis and even phasing out of certain traditional research and instructional programs. This is clearest in plant improvement. From the point of view of chemical companies and their seed company subsidiaries, experiment stations should do basic research and produce "enhanced germplasm" that can be developed into new varieties by the seed companies. The new biotechnologies are viewed as the tools for doing such basic research. Pressure on public sector institutions from industry to abandon varietal breeding, from administrators for greater productivity, as well as the lure of large amounts of private money for biotechnology research, has led to a change in disciplines in the SAES. An additional 108 full-time equivalent (FTE) scientists will be added in the biotechnology disciplines (plant and animal sciences, as well as food science) in the next 2 years (NASULGC, 1983). Interviews of SAES directors by the authors make clear that many of these positions will be obtained by reducing the scope of conventional breeding programs. As plant breeders retire, many have been and will continue to be replaced by molecular biologists. A similar process appears to be occurring within the Agricultural Research Service (ARS). The 6-year plant for 1984–1990 calls for ARS scientists to emphasize basic science (i.e., molecular biology) and germplasm enhancement and to deemphasize varietal breeding and some small commodity programs (USDA–ARS, 1983). In fact, the plan calls for a reduction of $2 million for breeding of horticultural crops.

A survey of public breeding programs (in the SAES) of horticultural and sugar crops reveals a projected 22–55% reduction in the number of programs and a 13–39% reduction in FTE Scientists by 1990 (Kalton, 1984). Much of this reduction will be due to the termination of smaller programs, especially in the minor crops. This survey raises a number of disturbing questions.

Who will do the breeding for the minor crops? The problem of minor crops is very similar to that of orphan drugs. The market is either limited or insufficiently profitable. As a result, the private sector invests most heavily in major crops and also pressures the public sector to focus on these crops (through grants, contracts, consulting, and even legislative pressure). The public sector also focuses on major crops as a result of state and national funding practices. Furthermore, with public funds available for biotechnology programs involving only a few crops, research is likely to follow the interests of the most powerful commodity associations which tend to represent the major crops. A consequence of this is likely to be a decrease in the breeding of minor crops, and therefore in the number of food crops available for human use.

Some private sector breeders are aware of the problem and want the public sector to continue minor crop breeding (Kalton, 1984).

Furthermore, who will train the next generations of plant breeders? There is a growing demand for breeders in the private sector (Kalton, 1984), in seed companies, biotechnology firms, and biotechnology departments in large corporations. Even varieties and hybrids developed in tissue culture laboratories need to be grown out in the field. The problem is that as LGU's move toward the emphasis on biotechnology or basic research in general, and breeding programs become deemphasized, there may be no one to train future breeders. Plant breeding cannot be learned solely from books: One must have practical experience. The only way to obtain this experience is in the process of breeding, supervised by an experienced breeder. If public breeding stops, both the public and private industry are likely to suffer.

The Bioproduct Market: Farmers

A more immediate impact of the use of biotechnology in both public and private sector R&D will be felt in the bioproduct market, especially seed. Public sector commitment to more basic research has contributed toward and accelerated a shift of varietal breeding from the public to the private sector. Until 1923 the USDA regularly distributed free seed, collected from around the world, to farmers who wanted to test them on U.S. soils. As the techniques and effectiveness of plant breeding improved, the distribution of free seeds stopped; instead, state agricultural experiment stations (SAES) began to disseminate new varieties developed by public sector breeders to the seed companies who multiplied and sold them to farmers. The development of hybrid corn shifted the division of labor again. Experiment stations gradually shifted to the development of parent material and significantly reduced the production of finished products for hybrid crops. The growth of the seed development (as opposed to multiplication) industry put increased pressure on the public sector to cease producing finished varieties. The American Seed Trade Association (ASTA) began to encourage this as early as 1923 (ASTA, 1984). As was noted, many station directors stated that they support this move, given the current economic situation of public R&D.

It is important to note that the continuation of this trend is likely to affect farmers dramatically. For example, as the production of finished seed is moved more and more to the private seed industry, product differentiation of the type found with other consumer goods is likely to invade the farm sector. Farmers may be faced with a bewildering array of seed varieties. Given this, advertising is likely to play a much greater role in seed sales than it has in the past. It may be difficult for farmers to distinguish between product differentiation and significant varietal differences.

Most important, however, are the kinds of varieties which may be available to farmers. Given the technical requirements of genetic engineering, the first traits to be introduced into plants will have to be genetically simple ones. At present, herbicide tolerance has received the most interest, since it is usually a single gene trait (Barton and Brill, 1983). Just as importantly, there is a large and expanding market for herbicides. Between 1971 and 1982 herbicide use in the United States rose from 44 million to 100 million kg/year, while the acreage on which herbicides are used nearly doubled (Mathiessen and Kohn, 1984). The annual U.S. market was \$2.2 billion in 1980 and is predicted to grow to \$3.6 billion by 1990 (Chandler, 1985). Consequently, most major chemical firms have already staked a claim in herbicide resistance. The implication of this is that farmers may find themselves increasingly tied to the use of chemicals, despite recent calls by the American Farm Bureau Federation (AFBF) for reductions in chemical inputs on economic grounds (AFBF, 1984).

Other developments in biotechnology will also affect farmers' decisions about which varieties to grow. For example, most biotechnology companies working with tomatoes are trying to increase total solids. Increasing total solids decreases water content, thereby greatly increasing case yields (the amount of canned product per unit weight of harvested tomatoes), but not necessarily crop yields. An increase in total solids of 1% is worth an estimated \$75 million annually (Davenport, 1981). Since processors either pay no bonus, or a very small one, to growers for increased solids tomatoes, the processors gain the vast majority of benefits from higher solids tomato. Furthermore, canners will only buy those tomato varieties which appear on their processing industry's acceptable list, thereby heavily influencing which varieties the farmers grow.

Similar points can be made in regard to genetically engineered bioproducts available for animal production. In the field of animal production technical breakthroughs will significantly affect the structure of the market. At present experiments are underway to insert genes into beef cattle, sheep, and pigs to increase the production of the growth hormone throughout the body, thereby increasing size. Indeed, some have speculated that they will be able to produce cattle the size of elephants (U.S. Office of Technology Assessment, 1984) and "super-sheep" (Miller, 1985). The initial objective of these experiments, though, is to increase the efficiency of converting feed into protein, either through faster growth rates or greater size with the same quantity of feed. Increased efficiency and faster growth rates would mean lower feed costs and a shortening of the time the animal would need to spend in a feedlot, resulting in higher turnover and greater profit for the farmer. Undoubtedly, early adopters of this animal technology will have an important market advantage. It is likely, in fact, that a large number of cattle, sheep, and dairy farms will simply disappear, while those remaining will increase in herd size.

Important market impacts will also occur as a result of in vitro production of plant-based flavors and scents. For example, the Swiss firm Firmenich recently signed an agreement with DNA Plant Technology (DNAP) to use biotechnology to manufacture chemical flavors and scents (Orr, 1985). The basic idea is to isolate the plant cells responsible for synthesizing flavors and scents (e.g., mint, vanilla, sage) and then genetically engineer them to increase the production of these chemicals in a cell culture system. The commercial potential of these technologies would be enormous. The logical extension of this work would be the in vitro production of many processed foods such as juices, pastes, and sauces. The tremendous market restructuring resulting from the adoption of these production processes would significantly affect the production of many foods.

The Public: Consumers

The agricultural production system is a complex interweaving of many kinds of enterprises, from R&D organizations to grocery stores, and the ultimate product of this system is food and fiber to be purchased and consumed. Therefore, whatever changes biotechnology produces in the R&D agenda, in resource allocation, and in the restructuring of production and processing will affect consumers. Clearly, changes in the nutritional value of genetically engineered foodstuffs would have direct effects, as would increased chemical additives. Less direct, however, are changes in the overall agricultural market. As we have noted, new technologies tend to affect markets, and the trend in agriculture has been toward increasing concentration of markets in the hands of a few producers and processors. Whether or not the monopoly power—the power to affect price levels and the allocation of resources—will have negative impacts, we cannot know now. Economists argue that increased concentration inevitably creates disutilities in terms of allocative efficiency (Blair, 1972). This kind of impact would, however, be felt only over the long term.

The private sector is eager to renegotiate with public sector institutions the division of labor over R&D and products and services coming out of the public sector. Though certainly less immediately noticeable than health, environmental, or economic impacts, changes such as these would undoubtedly affect the broader public as well.

The specific impacts of the redirected mission of public sector research efforts on the public—as both consumers and citizens—will probably depend upon the extent to which the general public accepts this realignment of university–industry relations. Perhaps the most important point in this regard is that public officials may themselves be affected by any significant public concern over the social, scientific, and institutional impacts of the use of the new biotechnologies in agricultural R&D, food production, and processing.

ACTORS

This appraisal of the impacts of biotechnology in the institutional structure of agricultural R&D and agricultural production and processing is not exhaustive. However, there are questions that arise from our review concerning decisions which have been and remain to be made in regard to the use of biotechnology as both a scientific and institutional tool. As our assessment of the institutional context and projected impacts suggests, some of the most important decisions regarding the shape of the food and agricultural sciences, and the research institutions in which they are practiced, have already been made. There remain, however, decisions about the future of the public and private sector R&D efforts and the shape and direction of science. Whose decisions are they? Whose responsibility is it to make them? Finally, on what basis should they be made?

To begin with, the actors must be identified. Clearly, decisions are made by bench scientists, actively engaged in research and development, whether "traditional" or biotechnological. These include researchers in the public sector (SAES, ARS), as well as scientists employed by major corporations, seed companies, or venture capital firms. Research administrators are significant decision makers as well: experiment station directors, agricultural college deans, and research administrators in private corporations. For the public sector we must include legislators at the state and federal level and USDA officials at any number of levels as well. The bottom line is, however, the public: consumers of the end result of the food production and processing system also have decisions to make. Scientific and institutional implications of the use or adoption of any technology ultimately affect us. As such, these decisions and the imperatives that govern them are of vital concern to all of us.

Scientists

The first and most immediate decision makers are practicing bench scientists. The major decision they must make is this: Will they, should they, opt to use the various biotechnologies as another "tool in the toolbox" for the pursuit of knowledge, and for improved production and processing techniques? Certainly the promise of biotechnologically improved food production, of greater control over processing techniques, and, fundamentally, of the further truncation of the time and space so long a crucial limiting factor in agricultural production and processing are strong inducements to move in the direction of biotechnological R&D. There is also the promise of forefront research and publications. And the increasing availability of large sums of research support, particularly from private industry, make movement into, or reinforced commitment within, biotechnology even more attractive.

Public Sector Scientists

To be consistent with the tradition of scientific objectivity, professionalism, and mission orientation, public sector scientists must appraise the legitimate appeals of this kind of research, as opposed to its "hype" and "glitter." In the course of our interviews scientists have stated repeatedly that the growing institutional commitment to biotechnology may be nothing more than publicity or marketing but that there are good and bad points to this. On the one hand, scientists assert that it is desirable for science to receive additional financial support; that private and public funding sources are increasing for biotechnology in plant, animal, and food science, can only benefit the pursuit of these sciences. On the other hand, they also see the danger of a backlash for false or unfulfilled promises. At the very least, the kinds of commitments in resources necessary for biotechnological research raise the question of the social value of those commitments. Thus, even in the work of the individual scientist, accountability is a fundamental issue. Accountability to society in the context of publicly sponsored mission oriented research has always been of prime importance. The issue is even more pronounced now. Biotechnological research may be the best new scientific "tool in the toolbox"; it is also, as we have noted, a tool for institutional change.

Private Sector Scientists

Decisions such as these are not confined to scientists in the public sector. Interviews with scientists in private industry indicate that there are questions private scientists have, and decisions they must make, as well. Private sector scientists also voice concern about the hype and glitter of biotechnology; for them, however, more than the mission of their institution is at stake. Either they produce results from the use of biotechnology or they are fired or their firm is defunct. Pressure such as this forces inevitable questions about inadequate and unsafe testing and experimentation.

While agricultural of food-related biotechnological research may hold the same health or safety risks as research in pharmaceuticals, it has not been generally regarded as such. Consequently, there have been fewer regulatory efforts aimed at private agricultural R&D than at pharmaceuticals.

Common Concerns

There are issues and decisions common to both public and private sector scientists as well. Conflicts of interest and limitations on scientific communication were constantly raised in our interviews as matters of serious concern to scientists in both private industry and the public sector. If there is, however, one overarching concern, it is the notion of accountability, not just to society or the company, but to science. It is accountability to the practice of sound, well-conceived, cautious, candid, and responsible science with which they must contend. Certainly no one can or has the right to expect that each practicing scientist *fully* explore the social, environmental, or institutional consequences of the practice of his or her craft. Yet the issues and impacts that we have raised here are relevant to even the everyday scientific decisions made at the bench level.

Administrators

Directors of SAES and R&D administrators in the private sector have the greatest singular influence on the extent to which the new biotechnologies have their projected impacts. Their decisions are key ones. Yet they also act under important constraints.

Public Sector

Experiment station directors are accountable to higher-level university administrators, the USDA, and legislators for broader concerns such as productivity, nutrition, and service to constituencies and clients. The shape and direction of a particular institution, program, or department are fundamentally affected by the director's own commitments. As such, the station director's appraisal of the social and scientific importance of biotechnology is crucial: The implementation of a biotechnology institute or program is the director's responsibility. With this, perhaps, no station director would disagree. The nature of the key decision maker's role, however, involves not only fiscal, administrative, or personnel responsibilities; it necessarily involves *ethical* ones as well, insofar as people are directly affected by actions both by the director and through his or her office. Internally, hiring, promotion, requests for research support, leaves, assistants, and so forth, involve ethical choices, since the allocation of scarce resources is fundamentally an allocation away from somebody toward someone else. Even when based on efficiency, productivity, legislative mandate, or some other such "objective" value criterion, these decisions have ethical overtones. There is perhaps no better characterization of what ethics involves than that one's actions affect the lives of others. Clearly, through the station director's actions, some people are benefited and some may be harmed.

This is not to suggest that decisions station directors have made regarding the increased use of biotechnological research in the public sector are unethical ones. Indeed, administrators repeatedly stated that their concern is to benefit as many people through this move as is possible, that is, to serve the greatest good of the greatest number. The decision they must face is whether *in fact* the increased commitment to basic or biotechnological research does benefit the greatest number. We have already noted that the increasing linkage between the university and private industry will change client groups and redirect research and development toward the further industrialization and concentration of food production and processing. Although institutional survival must be considered, decisions about how far the mission orientation of the public institution can be pushed in response to these internal and external pressures cannot be made lightly.

However, the constraints under which public administrators make their decisions may seem to diminish the force of any ethical responsibility we wish to attribute to them. Inside the institution there are pressures from below. Scientists make demands, require support, and voice displeasure or indignation at institutional moves. Often the administrator has come from their ranks. What impacts institutional actions have are often, then, a collective responsibility, with the administrator as the nominal "agent" of the whole. At the same time there are pressures from above. Legislators who pay the bills demand results. This pressure from above or outside of the research institution is the real constraint on administrators' decision-making criteria. Simply, biotechnological research holds the promise of generating financial support. As such, administrators in the public sector have looked to it as the key to continued institutional prosperity. The ethical dimensions of their decisions are ultimately affected by these overarching economic considerations.

Private Sector

Similar decisions have been made, and remain to be made, by private industry's research administrators. Unless they are chief executives or very high-ranking officers of the corporations engaged in biotechnological research, they are perhaps no freer to dictate the course of their institution's R&D effort than are station directors free to ignore legislative mandates. As in the public sector, private R&D administrators do have the power to decide specifics, for example, hiring and firing, what projects to be undertaken, what levels of productivity should be achieved, and, ultimately, decisions affecting the profitability of the firm's R&D effort. Responsibilities such as these imply an ethical dimension as well. Decisions affect not only scientists working for the firm but also stockholders, officers, and, eventually, the public. Particularly, safety considerations, the reasonableness of risk, and the long-term viability of projects are fundamental components of the decisions private administrators have to make.

Even with this decision-making power, the private administrator is constrained by the market. Biotechnological R&D has to produce marketable products or feasible changes in processing techniques. That the number of biotechnology firms is rapidly decreasing because of unfulfilled expectations exacerbates the external pressure to bring products or processes out as quickly as is possible. This, however, is where hard decisions and basic responsibilities lie, since an honest appraisal of the prospects of biotechnological research must be made. To commit resources here, with only a remote chance of return on the investment, violates the most basic canon of business: profitability. Thus the ethical responsibilities here are affected by economics.

Institutional Actors

Overtures by large agribusinesses, particularly petrochemical subsidiaries in agriculture, toward universities and experiment stations are more than accidental: They are required by the logic of increased agricultural R&D aimed at private gain. In a word, it is economically necessary for firms to seek out the best scientific talent which might aid in the quick, scientifically sound development of agricultural products. As such, many of the impacts of biotechnology on science and society are the direct result of agribusiness actions. If we judge such impacts to be unacceptable, concomitant responsibilities on the part of private industry to cease such actions immediately come to exist.

Whatever the real technical or scientific possibilities of the employment of biotechnologies in agriculture research and whatever the potential profitability of the products of such research, major corporations are acting on the belief that biotechnology will yield some benefit. They are willing to invest huge sums of money in private contracts with universities and to establish institutes. The responsibility for the massive move into biotechnology rests in large degree with these corporations. The question is, however, what it is that biotechnology will do and is doing for these firms. These corporations certainly hold the key to the future of biotechnology in agriculture.

The financial exigencies of public sector, especially experiment station research, have forced the increased alliance with industry. External and internal research agendas have moved public research toward biotechnology. Public benefit and some private benefit from such research may take a long time to materialize. There are, however, more immediate benefits which biotechnology research and development by public researchers for private industry can yield. Certainly there are tax breaks for such endowments to the university. More significant is the power that private industry now has over the research agendas in the public sector. Perhaps this power should not be overestimated. Still those corporations are in large measure responsible for this shift in mission and ultimately the public accountability of public research institutions.

Leaders in the public sector are, however, responsible as well. Congress, the USDA, and state legislatures have made and will continue to have to make difficult decisions affecting the nature and direction of public sector research. The resources entrusted to legislative bodies and government agencies carry with them the responsibility that these bodies thoroughly inform themselves—and the public they serve—of all the social and scientific implications of the move to increased biotechnological research. This implies that an understanding of the impacts of the new collaborative public–private efforts on the broader public is a fundamental responsibility. Clearly some investigation and analysis has already been done. However, continued "social impact assessment" (Friedland and Kappel, 1979) and, more importantly, public promulgation of the results of those assessments, must be a first priority for these governmental institutions. On such important issues as the nature of public institutions, the direction of science, and ultimately the structure of the food production–processing–delivery system, our commitment to democratic decision making entails public knowledge of the range of alternatives available.

The Public

In the final analysis, the major responsibility for any and all of the impacts of biotechnology is ours. We, as citizens, decide. We need to decide for what ends science is to be funded and used, the goals of public sector research institutions, and, most importantly, the proper division of labor between public research institutions and private corporations. To make these decisions we must inform ourselves of the possible impacts of science on society. Only then can we address these impacts.

Whatever scientific prospects the new technologies may hold, they also have economic and ethical dimensions. They are capable of being used for good or ill. Judgments about the goodness or badness of the various impacts we have posited here will no doubt vary among citizens. Have we as citizens considered that our present decisions affect future generations, people whose choices and opportunities are either expanded or constrained by ours? Judgments about the goodness or badness of the new technologies, and their social and scientific effects, must be made in light of the interests of even far-off future human beings. Fairness, justice, and, indeed, the pursuit of science present us with the following imperatives.

IMPERATIVES

In a recent book philosopher Hans Jonas (1984) argues that the decisions we have to make as individuals and members of institutions must be responsible to future humanity. What this implies is that a full awareness of the consequences of our actions, stretching as far into the future as our present vision and imagination can project, is fundamental. In this chapter we have employed what Friedland (Friedland and Kappel, 1979) has called a "projective analysis"—using every conceptual device at hand in an attempt to understand as clearly as possible where present actions, trends, and possibilities might lead. There are undoubtedly lacunae in our projections. What remains is for us to suggest that Jonas' prescriptions can help guide present decisions about the use of biotechnology in food production and processing and R&D designed to better the food system. In particular, the imperatives of responsibility for each of us are the following:

1. The imperative to assess adequately the future health risks associated with the use of biotechnology in agricultural research and agricultural practice.
2. The imperative to assess adequately the future environmental consequences of the use of biotechnology in agriculture and agricultural research.
3. The imperative to assess adequately the future benefits and burdens associated with the transformation of institutions.
4. The imperative to assess adequately the benefits and costs to the quality of human life associated with a profound change in the nature and focus of science resulting from increased biotechnological research and development.

This last responsibility is the overarching one, in our judgment: What kind of science will we leave future generations? Will it be, as those concerned would hope, ameliorative, humane?

Health Risks

Already, the National Institutes of Health have guidelines for grading health risks associated with the use of biotechnology for those institutions receiving funding from them. There are requirements for various levels of containment for biomaterials and safety standards for procedures, testing, development, and so on. Recently the U.S. Office of Science and Technology Policy (OSTP) has proposed a "coordinated framework for the Regulation of Biotechnology," to augment the National Institutes of Health guidelines by coordinating them with guidelines in agriculture and other areas so that "everyone will reap the benefits of this exciting biological revolution" (OSTP, 1984). Licensing for the use of biotechnology in each of these fields would be required. Obviously these guidelines are socially responsible, although an internally generated and enforced set of similar guidelines and procedures would be desirable for all institutions and individuals working in the biotechnological area. In particular, private industry should generate such guidelines; without them, more governmental regulation might come into being, since many risks are already judged to be inconsistent with the public interest.

There are questions which might arise concerning any guidelines, internal or external. While some biomaterials resulting from biotechnology do currently pose health risks, it might be argued that agricultural biomaterials do not and cannot exhibit these risks in the way that pharmaceuticals might. Or, if they do, it is only in a very indirect way, through environmental or even economic effects on health. How, for instance, can improved varieties adversely affect health? Or, for that matter, how might a bioengineered tomato having higher solids affect health? The issue in the "Ice Minus" case is that an agricultural bioproduct could cause enough environmental harm to affect peoples' health. However, this is over the very long term.

More immediate health hazards may emerge with respect to nutrition and processing. Some scientists claim that biotechnology has the potential to replace agriculture, as foodstuffs become totally genetically engineered. How will this affect the nutritional quality of the foods we produce and consume?

Therefore assessment of future health risks is fundamental. Perhaps no demonstrable risks will come to exist through the use of biotechnology, but perhaps some will. It is necessary that approaches be developed for assessing future, projectible risks associated with the use of biotechnology in food production and processing and with the associated R&D. Better risk assessment models can be employed (Thompson, 1983–1984). Speculation is even justifiable. If harm might result, the fundamental maxim of responsibility to future humanity would demand a reconsideration of safety measures. The imperative to consider health-related consequences is encumbent upon both private and public research institutions and individuals therein.

Environment

There are many environmental issues associated with food production and processing: for example, reduced genetic diversity, chemical abuse, erosion, and lowered water quality. Some of these have connections to the health risks we referred to above, and similar points concerning responsibility can be made. There are, however, other considerations regarding responsibilities to the future over environmental issues.

Much current agricultural practice is a direct assault on the environment, on land, water, plant, and animal materials. A maxim of Do No Harm to the environment implies that we must be concerned about how agriculture is practiced. As we have argued in this chapter, agriculture in the Western World is becoming increasingly industrialized; this implies that it is becoming increasingly uniform and increasingly dependent upon external inputs in the form of machinery and chemicals. The environmental consequences of agricultural practice in these terms are presently just becoming evident. What, however, will the future environment be like if we continue such practices? And, more to the point, how will the use of biotechnology be linked to environmental consequences of future agricultural production? These questions cannot be answered in the abstract. They require careful attention to what biotechnological R&D can do to the environment, either directly or through its impact on production and processing. There exists an imperative to consider possible future environmental effects in all present decisions about the use of biotechnology. Furthermore, what kinds of biotechnological research should we engage in? Given alternative agricultural techniques, alternative specifications of desirable characteristics in plants and animals, alternative harvesting processes, and so on, and the relative impacts the alternatives might have on the environment, biotechnological research should perhaps be geared to these ends. This may be either in addition to or instead of the current trend toward research supportive of increased industrialization and concentration. At the very least, these other techniques and products should be considered. When judged to be of more substantial environmental, health, institutional, and human benefit, they should be pursued.

Institutions

We have noted the rapidity of private entry into the biotechnology arena and the not so gradual realignment of the division of labor between private industry and public sector research institutions. Inevitable questions remain about the long-term results of these new alliances: What do we want our future society to look like? What missions do we want our public institutions to pursue? What goals, values, interests, and needs do we want addressed? How are benefits and burdens of agricultural research, and agriculture in general to be distributed?

It is not our place to answer these questions here. Rather, let us suggest that, as important as they are, we, as a society, must not simply let historical trends happen. Individuals and institutions, through their actions, shape the present, and as a result of those actions the stage is set for future acts. The decisions of the present set the terms and conditions for markets, negotiations, directions, and agreements, for the very long term. And thus the imperative arises that we address, in the most explicit terms, the issue of what we want the future of our agriculturally oriented institutions to be. This includes the market. We have noted that there are projectable consequences of private industry pursuing profits. We have also noted the apparent necessity of private funding of some public research. Yet questions about the reasonableness or legitimacy of some private sector activities and industry–university relationships cannot be simply taken as answered. There is a fundamental imperative that we ask ourselves: Is this the direction in which we want food production and processing and related R&D to proceed?

Science

As important as the practice of science and technology is to our knowledge of ourselves, our environment, and our institutional arrangements, we often presume that science, like the nature it studies, should simply take its course. But our view of the use of biotechnology and the implications it has for food, agriculture, and society suggests a different perspective. However strongly or weakly we choose to make the claim that there are values in science, it is nonetheless true that science affects us. We are responsible for the science we practice, for the knowledge, products, and processes which result from that practice. Therefore science cannot simply take its course; it must be addressed in terms of its likely effects.

Biotechnological research in food production and processing, as in other arenas, presents us with a dilemma in this regard. Clearly biotechnological research holds promise for an improved human condition. Yet it has also been shown to be potentially a tool for the further industrialization of agriculture, for securing profits and market shares of private interests and funding for public sector research and education. It is therefore a tool for redistributing the benefits and burdens of agricultural production, processing, and R&D. The responsibility for each of these institutional mores is not, however, biotechnology. It is not to be praised or blamed in and of itself. Rather, responsibility lies with those who do, move, manipulate, use, or abuse biotechnology and the processes and products which result. In the final analysis the impacts of the new biotechnologies in the present and in the far distant future are our present responsibilities. Responsibilities to future generations of human beings—and perhaps to plant and animal species as well—demand present consideration of those impacts.

There is thus one further imperative. Biotechnological research is only one aspect of an increasing trend in contemporary Western society toward a reductionist view, seeing "wholes" as only sums of increasing smaller parts. Is this the kind of philosophical orientation we wish to maintain and continue through our future research? Although obviously more speculative than much of the above, this question still needs to be addressed. How shall we view the world? And what shall our science of that world be? Narrow, submolecular, instrument dependent? Broad, global, open? Perhaps these are false dichotomies. Perhaps they can be integrated into a science that magnifies human possibilities and the human spirit in the same moment it investigates the meaning of life in the most microbiological fashion. Our responsibility to the future, as well as to the present, is to consider such a science.

REFERENCES

American Farm Bureau Federation (1984). Statement to the Subcommittee on Agricultural Research and General Legislation of the Senate Nutrition and Forestry Committee, Washington, D.C.

American Seed Trade Association (1984). Report of the Public Research Advisory Committee, Washington, D.C.

Barton, K. A. and Brill, W. J. (1983). Prospects in plant genetic engineering, *Science 219*: 689–693.

Bathe, G. and Bathe, D. (1935). *Oliver Evans: A Chronicle of Early American Engineering*, Historical Society of Pennsylvania, Philadelphia.

Blair, J. M. (1972). *Economic Concentration*, Harcourt Brace Jovanovich, New York.

Busch, L. and Lacy, W. B. (1983). *Science, Agriculture, and the Politics of Research*, Westview Press, Boulder.

Busch, L., Silver, J. L., Lacy, W. B., Perry, C. S., Lancelle, M., and Deo, S. (1984). The relationship of public agricultural R&D to selected changes in the farm sector. Report to the National Science Foundation, Lexington, Ky.

Chandler, J. M. (1985). Economies of weed control in crops. In *The Chemistry of Alleopathy* (A. C. Thompson, ed.), American Chemical Society, Washington, D.C.

Cochrane, W. W. (1979). *The Development of American Agriculture: A Historical Analysis*, University of Minnesota Press, Minneapolis.

Davenport, C. (1981). Sowing the seeds—Research, development flourish at DeKalb, Pioneer HiBred. *Barrons 61*:9–10, 33.

Experiment Station Committee on Organization and Policy (1984). *Research 1984*. ESCOP, Washington, D.C.

Friedland, W. and Kappel, T. (1979). *Production or Perish: Changing the Inequities of Agricultural Research Priorities*, Project on Social Impact Assessment and Values, University of California, Santa Cruz.

Giedion, S. (1975). *Mechanization Takes Command*, Norton, New York.

Joint Council for Food and Agricultural Sciences (1984). *Biotechnology in Agriculture*, U.S. Department of Agriculture, Washington, D.C.

Jonas, H. (1984). *The Imperative of Responsibility*, University of Chicago Press, Chicago.

Kalter, R. J. (1984). *Biotechnology and the Dairy Industry: Production Costs and Commercial Potential of the Bovine Growth Hormone*, Cornell University Department of Agricultural Economics, Ithaca, N.Y.

Kalton, R. (1984). Who is going to breed the minor crops and train the next generation of plant breeders? *Seed World 122*:16–17.

Mathiessen, C. and Kohn, H. (1984). In search of the perfect tomato. *Nation 239*, July 7–14:14.

Miller, C. (1985). Australian "super-sheep": Genetic studies prompt environmental concern. *Genet. Eng. News 5*:116.

Mooney, P. R. (1980). *Seeds of the Earth*, Inter Pares, Ottawa.

Mooney, P. R. (1983). The law of the seed: Another development and plant genetic resources. *Dev. Dialogue 1–2*:104.

National Academy of Sciences (1972). Report of the Committee on Research Advisory to the Department of Agriculture, Washington, D.C.

National Academy of Sciences (1984). *Genetic Engineering in Plants*, NAS, Washington, D.C.

National Association of State Universities and Land Grant Colleges (1983). *Emerging Technologies in Agriculture: Issues and Policies*, Progress Report II.

Orr, T. (1985). DNA plant technology plots trajectory from lab to marketplace. *Genet. Eng. News 5*:107.

Rockefeller Foundation (1982). *Science For Agriculture*, Rockefeller Foundation, New York.

Schuh, G. E. (1984). Revitalizing the land grant university, miscellaneous publication, Strategic Management and Research Center, University of Minnesota.

Thompson, P. (1983–1984). Risk, ethics, and agriculture. *J. Environ. Syst. 13*:135–153.

U.S. Department of Agriculture, Agricultural Research Service (1983). *Agricultural Research Service Program Plan, 6 Year Implementation Plan, 1984—1990*, Department of Agriculture, Washington, D.C.

U.S. Department of Agriculture—Economic Research Service (1978–1985). *Vegetable Situation Report*, USDA, Washington, D.C.

U.S. Office of Science and Technology Policy (1984). Proposal for a coordinated framework for regulation of biotechnology. *Fed. Reg. 49*:50856–50877.

U.S. Office of Technology Assessment (1984). *Commercial Biotechnology*, Government Printing Office, Washington, D.C.

ACKNOWLEDGMENTS

The material in this chapter is based upon work supported by the National Science Foundation and the National Endowment for the Humanities under grant No. RII-8217306. Any opinions, findings, conclusions, or recommendations expressed in this publication are those of the authors and do not necessarily reflect the views of these organizations.

Index

Acidic compounds, 174
  analysis of, 174
Acidophilus milk, 106
Acids, edible, 68
Activity, biological, 152, 154
Additives, 101
Administrators, 592
  private sector, 592
  public sector, 593
Adsorbent culture, 308
Aerobacter, 546
Affinity sensors, 234
Aflatoxin, 114
Agar, 293, 300, 301
Agarose, 300
Agarose gel electrophoresis, 146
Agitator, 207, 208
Agrobacterium tumefaciens, 13, 333
L-Alanine, 61
Algae, 46
Alginate, 30, 65, 67, 290, 291, 295, 305
Amaranthus tricolor, 121
American Seed Trade Association (ASTA), 582, 584
Amines, analysis of, 170
α-Amylase, 394, 395, 396, 397, 398, 495
β-Amylase, 394, 395, 398, 419
Analysis, 163, 167, 170, 174, 177, 179
Animal feed, 433
Anther culture, 321, 329
Antibiotic, resistance to, 532
Anticodon, 142
Antimicrobial systems, 33
Amino acids, 42, 63, 70, 71, 100, 103, 115, 156, 199, 373
  analysis of, 167
  essential, 42, 199
  production of, 72
  requirements, 71
Aminoacylase, 72
Aminoacyl-t RNA, 142
Animal cell
  culture methods, 253
  growth of, 254
  technology of, 267
Aroma, 74, 82
  concentrates, 74
  evaluation, 84
  formation, 75
  production, 74, 75, 84

Arginine, 71
Ascorbic acid, 100, 101, 107, 112, 116, 120, 121
Ascomycetes, 437
Asepsis, 215
Aseptic condition, 201
Aspartame, 61, 157
  synthesis of, 427
Aspartic acid, 61, 71
Aspergillus awamori, 398, 399
Aspergillus niger, 398, 399, 404
Autoradiograms, 154
Auxin, 271

Bacillus amyloliquefaciens, 396, 397
Bacillus coagulans, 396
Bacillus licheniformis, 396, 397
Bacillus stearothermophilus, 396, 397
Bacillus subtilis, 396 397
Bacteria, 40
Bacteriocin, 531, 535, 536
Bacteriophage, 140, 532, 533, 534, 536
Baking, 428
Barley, 397, 419
Beer, 295
Beets, fermented, 111
6-Benzylaminopurine (BAP), 275
Biobased processes, 22
  annual turnover in, 22
  classification of, 23
Biocatalyst, 288, 295, 306, 308
Bioconversion, 413
Biology, molecular, 333
Biomass, 289
  economics of, 364
Bioprocess
  complexity of, 223
  control, 223, 224
  modelling of, 245
  reproducibility of, 223
Bioproducts, 588
  market, 587
Bioprotein, 43
Bioreactors, 214, 295, 305
  fluidized bed, 218, 219
  hollow fiber, 218, 220
  immobilized, 217, 218
  membrane, 218
Biotechnology
  definition of, 4
  impact of, 22, 37
  limiting factors in, 33
  regulatory aspects of, 559
  social appraisal of, 577
Biotransformation, 61, 72
Blood processing, 193
Bread aroma, 82
Breeding programs, 586
Brewing, 193
Butter aroma, 74, 80
  application of, 81
  concentrates, 80
Buttermilk, 106
By-products, 39

Cacao bean, 461
  tissue culture, 464
Calf milk replacers, 417
Callus, 271, 324
Calorimetry, 236
Candida utilis, 200
Capsaicin, 301
Carbohydrase, 393
Carbohydrate, 29, 193
  analysis of, 170
  processing of, 29
Carotenoids, 157
Carrageenan, 30, 290, 292, 304

Cell
animal, 253
division of, 272, 302
growth of, 302
habituated, 280
heterotrophic, 278
immobilization of 60, 61
287
line, 257, 259
lysis of, 197
microbial, 288
plant, 86, 116, 271, 287
reactors, 295, 308
recycle systems, 220
separation, 220
tumor-derived, 261
undifferentiated, 278
viability, 278, 308
Cell culture
animal, 253
imitation of, 255
plant, 86, 116, 118, 120,
122, 271, 287, 295, 461,
473, 483
Cellobiohydrolase, 394, 395,
403, 404
Cellular genetics, 337
Cellular growth, 193
genetic, 325
Cellulomonas fimi, 401, 403
Cellulase, 49, 201, 275, 350,
352, 437
Cellulose, 49, 201, 350
crystalline, 51
degradation, 50, 51
Centrifugation, 198
Caotropica anions, 376
Chemical modification, 378
Chemostat, 215
Cheese, 106, 108, 112, 413,
429, 514
cheddar, 109, 515
cottage, 108
flavor, 432, 80
ripening, 432
Chitosan, 292, 301, 304
Chlorogenic acid, 96, 99, 114
Chloroplast, 332
Cholesterol, 115
Chromatography, 198
Chromosome, 329
number, 325
aberrations, 280
Chymosin, 429, 495
Citraconylation, 382
Citrate, 531, 536
Citric acid, 68
production of, 247
Cleavage, 145
Clonal propagation, 323
Cloned genes
isolation, 9
transfer, 9
Clones, 139, 331
screening of, 151, 154
selection of, 140, 154
Cloning, 322, 336, 536
molecular, 153
vector, 144
vehicles, 139
Chlostridium thermocellum, 400,
401
Coagulation, 198
Cod, 519, 523
Code, genetic, 140, 143
Codon
nonsense, 143
start, 142
stop, 142
triplet, 142
Coentrapment, 294
Cofermentation, 294
Coimmobilization, 62, 294
Cold adaptation
molecular, 501
enzymic, 499
Collagen, 293
Colony hybridization, 153
Computer
software, 244

[Computer]
tasks, 242
Conjugation, 534
Consumer product, 589
synthesis of, 23, 27
Contamination, 203, 209
Control
direct digital, 243
set point, 243
Control
computer, 210
feedback, 210
process, 210
Cooling panel, 209
Copolymerization, 308
Corn sweetener, 443
development of, 444
economics of, 458
marketing, 458
properties, 447
types, 446
Corn syrup
composition, 446
functional properties of, 445
Cottonseed meal, 113
Coumarin, 181
Crop improvement, 119, 120
Crosslinking, covalent, 289, 290
Culture
medium, 195, 198, 205, 264, 274
seed, 195
stock, 195
Curdlan, 67
Cyanogenic glycosides, 96, 114
Cyclone, 205
Cysteine, 71
Cytokinin, 271
Cytoplasm, 332
Cytoplasmic
genes, 332
traits, 332

Dahi, 106, 108
Dairy starter cultures, 529
Dairy products
cultured, 106, 112
fermented, 529
fermentation of, 115
Density determination, 230
Dextran, 66
Dextrose, 451
feed stock, 453
saccharification, 452, 453
Diacetyl, 531
Diagnostic kits, 253
2,4-Dichlorphenoxyacetic acid (2,4-D), 275
Differentiation, 276, 463
Digestibility, 98, 100, 103
Dimethallylaminopurine, 275
Dimethylsulfoxide (DMSO), 305
Diplococcin, 531
Disciplinary focus, 586
Distillation, 199
DNA
cloning, 139
cytoplasmic, 327
fragmentation, 140, 143, 145
fragments, 139, 147, 150
isolation, 140, 143
mitochondrial, 332
nuclease, 144
polymerase, 141
probes, 569
purification, 140, 143, 145
recombination, 140, 559
synthetic, 152
Dough, fermentation of, 106

Electroelution, 145
Electrostatic interaction, 372
Embryo culture, 271
Embryogenesis, 275
Enantiomer separation, 168, 169, 178, 179

ncapsulation, 289
ndoglucanase, 394, 395, 400, 401, 402, 403
nergy of activation, 506
ntrapment, 289
  microbial cells, 289
  plant cells, 300
Environment, 598
Environmental Protection Agency (EPA), 568
Enzymatic treatment, 102
Enzyme, 31, 63, 74, 156, 200
  aroma-forming, 75, 81
  cold-adapted, 495
  degradation, 227
  digestive, 504
  engineering, 12
  extracellular, 200
  homologous, 508
  hydrolytic, 425
  immobilized, 56
  intracellular, 200
  macerating, 47
  modification, 227
  pectin-splitting, 47
  processing, 32
  production of, 193
  sales of, 31
  soluble, 46
  technology, 413
  thermistors, 234
  use of, 31
Epigenetic, 280
Escherichia adecarboxylata, 405
Escherichia coli, 7, 429
Ethanol, 62, 194, 291, 297
Eukariotes, 139
Eukaryotic
  cells, 139
  genes, 139
Evaporation, 200
Expression, 141
Extraction, 198
Farmers, 587
Fat splitting, 74
Fatty acids, 41, 79, 436
  composition of, 469, 474
Federal Food, Drug and Cosmetic Act, 561
Federal Insecticide, Fungicide and Rodenticide Act (FIFRA), 568
Feedback inhibition, 226
Feedstocks, 38
Fermentation, 102
  aerobic, 194, 200, 206
  anaerobic, 194, 207
  bacterial, 211, 215
  batch, 195
  computer-aided, 239
  continuous, 195, 215
  design, 201, 203
  effects of, 102, 112, 114
  fed batch, 197, 199
  immobilized cell, 220
  operation, 201
  pilot plant, 214
  processes, 193, 199
  systems, 193
  yeast, 211, 215
Fermentation processes, 193, 199
  substrates for, 39
Fermenter
  air lift, 200, 216, 217
  configuration, 214
  fed batch, 215
  harvest, 197
  parameters, 211
  scale up, 212
  stirred batch, 214
  tower, 216, 218
Filter
  absolute, 194
  sterile, 194
Fish
  enzymes, 495, 496
  offal, 498

Flavonoids, 181, 279
Flavorants, 157
Flavors, 28, 514
  enhancers, 75
  mushroomlike, 82
  oxidized, 517, 520
Flocculation, 199
Fluorescence, 232
  quenching, 233
Food
  fermented, 85
  functionality, 298
  industry, 21, 580
  modification of, 23
  natural, 308
  nutritional quality, 95, 298
Food additives, 23, 561
  modification of, 23
  synthesis of, 23
Food and Drug Administration (FDA), 261, 559
  authority of, 261, 561
  policy of, 560
Food Chemical Codex, 566
Food processing, 21, 33
  biobased, 21
  effects of, 98
Food production, trends in, 14
Fossil resources, 38
Fragrances, 28
Fructose, 291
  products, 457
Fruits
  aroma, 81
  enzymes, 75
  liquefication, 47
  products, 48
Functional properties, 65
Fungi, 40

Gametoclonal variations, 321, 326
Gametoclones, 327
Gari, 113
Gas chromatography (GC), 164, 166, 170, 176, 178, 179, 181
GC-MS technique, 166, 169, 173
Gel
  entrapment, 287
  porosity, 287
  stability, 287, 308
Gellan, 15
Gene
  amplification, 151
  cloned, 9
  cloning, 144
  eukaryotic, 154
  expression, 6
  functional, 139
  insertion, 140, 147
  isolation, 9
  regulation, 6, 280
  selection, 140
  structural, 150
  transfer, 9
Generally recognized as safe (GRAS) substances, 562, 565
Genetic, 3
  cellular, 329, 337
  code, 140, 143
  cytoplasmic, 333
  engineering, 272
  manipulation, 8
  marker, 330
  molecular, 329, 334
  pediococcal, 543
  principles of, 4
Genomic banks, 11
Germination, 116
Glucan structure, 357
Glucoamylase, 353, 395, 396, 398, 399, 400, 419
Gluconic acid, 10
δ-Gluconolactone, 70
Glucose, 291
Glucose isomerase, 58, 419 456
α-Glucosidase, 394, 395, 400
β-Glucosidase, 394, 395, 404, 405
Glutamate, 292, 297
Glutamic acid, 71

lutamine synthetase, 52
luten decomposition, 52
lycosides, 181
ossipol, 95, 99
rains, 104, 110, 113
reen revolution, 13
rowth
  anchorage-dependent, 263
  animal cells of, 254
  exponentional, 196
  nutrient-limited, 196
5'-Guanosine monophosphate, 76
Guanylic acid, 157
Gums, 15

Ham, cured, 109
Harvest valve, 202
Haploid, 326, 329
  doubled, 326, 328
  plants, 327, 328
Heat
  exchange, 209
  metabolic, 196, 209
  source, 209
  transfer, 201, 208, 214, 216
  treatment, 98, 100
Heavy metals, 41
Hemicellulase, 275
Hemicellulose, 275
Heredity, analysis of, 5
High-fructose corn syrup (HFCS), 58, 62, 448
  composition, 448
  process technology, 449, 450
  producer, 449
High-performance liquid chromatography (HPLC), 164, 167, 168, 170, 172, 174, 177, 179, 181
Hold-up time, 207
Homogenization, 198
Homopolymeric tailing, 151
Host cell, 139
HPLC-MS technique, 165
Hybrid, 329
  seed, 323
  design, 217
  somatic, 329, 330, 331, 332
Hybridoma, 559
Hydrocolloid, 63
  natural, 64
Hydrogen bonding, 372
Hydrophobic interaction, 374

Idli, 103
Immobilization, 61
  of microbial cells, 288, 295
  of plant cells, 300, 295, 306, 307, 335
  of whole cells, 287
Immunological detection, 153
Impeller, tip speed of, 213
Inactivation, insertional, 152
Indoleacetic acid (IAA), 275
Inosinic acid, 157
Isomerate sugar, 58, 62
Isomerization, 453
  process, 454
Institutional,
  changes, 577, 591
  context, 578
Instrumentation, 210
Interfaces, 241
Introns, 151
Invert sugar, 62
Irradiation, 100, 266

Kefir, 106
Kinetin, 275, 484
Klyveromyces fragilis, 404, 405
Klyveromyces lactis, 352
Koumiss, 106

Laboratory requirements, 262
Lactase, 59, 531, 532, 534, 535, 536
Lactic acid, 70, 291, 293

[Lactic acid]
bacteria, 529
Lactobacillus, 529, 532, 533, 535, 536
Lactobacillus acidophilus, 108
Lactobacillus brevis, 541, 544
Lactobacillus casei, 541
Lactobacillus leichnamii, 541
Lactobacillus plantarum, 541 543, 545
Lactoferrin-lactoperoxidase, 417
Lactoperoxidase, 416
Lactose, 352
intolerance, 60, 102, 106
Lag period, 195
Leuconostoc, 529, 533, 536, 546
Leuconostoc mesenteroides, 542, 544
Linkers, 151
Lipases, 74, 426, 436
Lipids, 181
biosynthesis of, 473
classes, 465, 470
content, 466
production of, 461, 483
synthesis of, 461
total, 465, 474
Lipolyzed
butterfat, 74
products, 75
Lipopolysaccharides, 41
Liquefaction-dextrinization reaction, 451
Lysine, 71
Lysozyme, 413, 415

Macerase, 275
Macerates, 48
Macronutrients, 103, 274
Male sterility, 323, 332
Malic acid, 61, 69
Mass spectra, 169, 173, 176, 178, 180
Mass transfer, 289, 308
Mass transfer rate, 212
Matjes, 519, 521, 522
Meat, 74, 100
aroma, 74
fermented, 109, 112
products, 106
starter cultures, 536, 537
Medium
inlet, 205
sterile, 194
Membrane
hollow fiber, 218, 296, 305
microfiltration, 218
microporous, 218
reactor, 287, 305
ultrafiltration, 218
Meristem culture, 324
Meristematic areas, 277
Messenger RNA, 141, 150
Metabolic studies, 271
Metabolites, 287, 289, 306
Methanol, 41, 200, 353
Methionine, 71
Methyl ketones, 79
Michaelis-Menten kinetics, 501
Microbial biomass, 40
Microbial cells
entrapment, 289
stability, 294
Microbial protein, 41
Microcarrier, 263
Micronutrients, 103, 274
Microorganism, 40
phototrophic, 40, 41
composition of, 364
Milk
clotting, 432
flavor, 517, 520
products, 76
Mineral oil, 41
Miso, 103
Mitochondria, 332, 334
Molecular activity, 508
activity, 508
adaptation, 501
biology, 333

[Molecular activity]
  cloning, 139, 153, 393
  genetics, 334
Monellin, 157
Monochlonal antibodies, 24, 569
Monosodium glutamate (MSG),
    75, 200
Morphogenesis, 275
Mutagenesis, cellular, 329
Mutation, 280
Mutant, 8
  isolation, 329
  lines, 330
  production, 271

Napthyleneacetic acid (NNA),
    275
Natto, 105
Natural food, 308
Nisin, 531, 534, 535
Nitrates, 107, 120, 121
Nitrosamines, 101, 115
Nonaqueous, 428
Nucleic acid, 40, 371
Nucleobases, analysis of, 177
Nucleoprotein, 363, 371, 372
  amino acids of, 380
  dissociating, 376
  composition, 379
Nucleosides, analysis of, 177
Nucleotides, 79
  analysis of, 177
Nutrients, 289
  availability of, 197
Nutrition, 37
Nutritional quality, 95, 97,
    118
Nutritional stress factor, 5, 97,
    112, 116, 119

Oilseeds, 104, 110, 113
Olives, 43, 546
Oncogenesis, 260
Oncom, 105, 113
Organic acids, 63
Organism washout, 215, 219
Oxalate, 95, 120, 121, 301
Oxygen
  consumption, 209
  dissolved, 196, 205, 321
  transfer, 201, 205, 206, 210,
    212, 216
  transfer coefficient, 205, 207
  transfer rate, 205
  uptake, 210
  uptake rate, 206, 212

Packaging of food, 193
Papain, 495
Passenger DNA, 139, 148
Peas, fermented, 111
Pectinase, 275
Pediococcal genetics, 543
Pediococcus acidilactici, 540, 545
Pediococcus cerevisiae, 537, 540
Pediococcus damnosus, 540
Pediococcus pentosaceus, 540
Pepsins, 505
Peptides, 54
  distribution of, 56
Permeabilization of plant cells,
    306, 307
Phage resistance, 532, 535
Phenolics, 181
Phenylalanine, 61, 71
Phospholipids, 181, 428
Phosphorylation, 383
Photosynthesis, 275
Physiological efficiency, 510
Physiological state of cells, 224
Phytic acid, 95, 99, 102, 112,
    114, 120
Pickles, 111, 543
Pigments, 157, 301
Plant biotechnology program,
    585
Plant cell
  immobilization, 300, 307, 335

[Plant cell]
reactor, 305
systems, 302
Plant food, 116
Plant tissue, degradation of, 48
Plant tissue culture, 86, 116, 118, 271, 287, 295, 461, 473, 483, 486
food application of, 120, 122
history, 462
lipid production for, 461
methods in, 271, 462, 483
Plant varieties, new, 321
Plant Variety Protection Act (PVPA), 582
Plasmid, 151, 529, 543, 546
bacterial, 140
DNA, 141, 144
vector, 149
Plastein reaction, 74
Poikilothermic organism, 499
Pollen, 328
Polyacrylamide, 290, 293
Polysaccharides, 29, 41, 60, 157
application of, 30
functional properties of, 65
market volume of, 30
microbial, 53, 64, 66
natural, 64
production of, 29
sources, 30
Polyurethane foam, 305
Pontryagin's maximum principle, 246
Potato virus, 436
Poultry feed, 434, 436
starter cultures of, 538
Precipitation, 198, 200
Premarketing clearance, 562
Preservation
chemical, 100
food, 98, 102
system, 413, 416
Private sector R & D, 580
Process
optimization, 246
simulation, 245
Process control, 223, 243
computer-aided, 238
developments in, 238
Processing, effect of, 98
Processing aid, 23, 31
production of, 23
Product
growth-associated, 197, 200
non-growth-associated, 197, 200
purification, 197, 198, 212
recovery, 197, 198, 212
Productivity
microbial, 363
of plant cells, 288
Prokaryotes, 139, 154
Propagation, 271
Protein, 52
amino acids of, 373
availability, 99
bitterness of, 55
functional properties of, 363, 368
functional requirements of, 369
hydrolysis, 55, 106
nonconventional, 52
quality, 98, 101, 116
recovery, 368
separation, 385
succinylated, 382
Proteinase, 52, 301, 496, 531, 533, 536
Protein efficiency ratio, 103
Protoplast, 9, 272, 325, 331, 333, 535, 536
formation, 9
fusion, 330, 332, 535
Public research agenda, 578
Public resource allocation, 585
Pullulan, 76

Racemates, 72
Racemic mixtures, 72
Raffinose, 102
Raw material, 28
Reactor, 296
  air lift, 295, 305
  continuous, 305
  fluidized bed, 305
  immobilized cell, 95, 298, 299, 305, 308
  packed bed, 305
  stirred tank, 295
Recombinant DNA, 8, 140, 147, 253, 559
  techniques, 154
Recombinant DNA technology
  application of, 155
  future of, 158
Recombinant organism, 200, 215
Reduction of RNA, 386
Regulation, metabolic, 226
Regulatory
  aspects, 559
  authority, 261
  consideration, 568
Rennet, 431, 432
Rennin, 15, 201
Replication, 141
Research and development
  private sector, 580
  public sector, 578
Respiration, 235, 302
  endonuclease, 145, 147
  enzyme, 151
  fragment, 144
  map, 148
  site, 145
  system, 532
Retention
  data, 178
  indices, 166, 176, 180
Reverse reaction, 425
Reverse transcriptase, 151
Ribonuclease, 371
5'-Ribonucleotide, 75
Ribosome, 141, 372
RNA polymerase, 141
Roquefort aroma, 78
Rushon turbine, 207

Saccharification, 157, 452, 453
Saccharomyces carlsbergensis, 400
Saccharomyces cerevisiae, 211, 294, 349, 356
Saccharomyces diastaticus, 399, 400
Salting, 100
Sample port, 204
Sanitary, 201
  design, 202
Sauerkraut, 111, 113, 543
Sausages
  dry, 541
  fermented, 109
  raw smoked, 80, 82
  semi-dry, 541
Scale up, 212, 306, 308
Schwanniomyces castellii, 400
Scientific communication, restricted, 584
Scientist, 590
  private sector, 591
  public sector, 591
Secondary metabolites, 288, 298, 306, 308, 322, 335, 336, 337
Seed, hybrid, 323
Seed oil
  plant, 486
  production of, 486
Segregation, 332
Selective media, 153
Sensor, 234, 237
Separation
  of food, 98, 102
  mechanical, 98
  physical, 98
Serum, 259, 265
Silage, 433, 434
Simplex method, 246

Single-cell protein, 13, 40, 42, 44, 156, 217, 347
  cellular lysis, 356
  flavor of, 355
  functional properties of, 357
  genetic engineering of, 348
  modification of, 347
  nutritional quality of, 354
  prospects of, 358
  production of, 44, 200, 347
  substrate, 350
  toxic components of, 356
  utilization of, 347
Smoking, 100, 101
Social appraisal of biotechnology, 577
Solanine, 96
Somaclonal variation, 321, 325, 326, 337
Somatic
  embryo, 322
  embryogenesis, 464
  hybrid, 329, 330, 331, 332
Sour cream, 106
Soy protein, 200
Sparger, 202
Stachyose, 102
Staphylococci, 542
Staphylococcus aureus, 542
Starch, 353, 419, 451
Starter culture, 80, 82, 106, 157
  bacterial, 529
  dairy, 529
  meat, 537
  poultry, 538
  vegetable, 540, 543
State Agricultural Experiment Stations (SAES), 583
Static head, 213
Steam seal, 204
Strand
  coding, 142
  template, 142
Sterile filtration, 266
Sterility, 201, 323, 332
Sterilization, 201
Streptococcus, 529, 530
Streptococcus cremoris, 531, 532
Streptococcus lactis, 531, 532, 534
Streptococcus sanquis, 536
Stress factor, 117
  nutritional, 95, 97, 112, 116, 119
Stress tolerance of plants, 116, 118
Structure-function relationship, 358
Subcultivation, 257
Succinylation, 379
Sunflower meal, 113
Suspension, growth in, 263
Sweetener, 25, 157, 443
  consumption of, 26
  market of, 25
Symba process, 353
Synthetic DNA, 152
Synthesis termination of, 142

Tannin, 95, 120
Target gene, 144
Tartaric acid, 69
Tempeh, 103, 110, 113, 140
Temperature coefficient, 509
Templates, 141
Thaumatin, 157
Thermomonospora YX, 401
Thiaminases, 96, 101
Thioglycerides, 96
Threonine, 71
Ti-plasmid, 13, 333, 334
Tissue culture
  animal, 253
  medium, 272
  plant, 86, 116, 118, 120, 122, 271
Technology, 271
Toluene, 305

Trait, expression of, 140
Transcription, 141
Transduction, 533, 536
Transesterification, 426
Transformants, 140
Transformation, 151, 260, 333, 535, 536
  in vitro, 257, 259
Translation, 142
Transposon, 9
Trichoderma reesei, 437, 438
Trichoderma reeset, 402, 403
Triglyceride synthesis, 428
Trypsin, 519
  inhibitor, 96, 114, 116, 120
Tryptophan, 62, 71, 278, 292, 293
Tumorigenic state, 260
Turnips, 111
Two-phase system, 308
Tyramine, 115
L-tyrosine, 62

Unit operation
  biological, 101
  effect of, 101
  organization of, 99
Ultrafiltration, 198
United States Department of Agriculture (USDA), 568

Vaccine, 253
Variability, genetic, 338
Variants, 325, 330
Vector, 139, 140
  choice of, 147
  DNA, 139
Vegetable, fermented, 111, 113
  liquefication of, 47
  product, 48
  of starter culture, 536, 543
Viability of plant cell, 302
Virus, 331, 334
  animal, 140
  eradicated plant, 323
  free plant, 324
  infection, 324
  potato, 436
Virus, Serum and Toxin Act (VSTA), 568
Vitamin C, 100, 101, 107, 112, 116, 120, 121
Vitamins, 63, 99, 100, 106, 112, 116
Volatiles, analysis of, 9

Waste
  product, 39
  treatment, 24, 33
Wheat, 397, 398
Wheat flour, 113
Whey, 59, 60, 291, 352
  fermented, 77
  lactose-hydrolyzed, 59
Whole cell immobilization, 287
Whole wheat flour, 113

Xanthan, 15, 65, 66

Yeast, 10, 40, 62
  alcohol-producing, 62
  amino acid of, 380
  composition, 365, 379
  functional properties of, 368
  fusion, 10
  hybridization, 10
  mineral content of, 366
  nutritional value of, 366
  proteins of, 365, 367, 379
  torula, 200
  vitamin content of, 366
Yogurt, 106, 108

Zeatin, 275
Zymomonas mobilis, 294